Geotechnical Slope Analysis

Geotechnical Slope Analysis

Robin Chowdhury
Faculty of Engineering, University of Wollongong, Wollongong, Australia

With contributions by:

Phil Flentje
Faculty of Engineering, University of Wollongong, Wollongong, Australia

Gautam Bhattacharya
Department of Civil Engineering, Bengal Engineering and Science University, Shibpur, Howrah, West Bengal, India

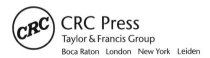

CRC Press
Taylor & Francis Group
Boca Raton   London   New York   Leiden

CRC Press is an imprint of the
Taylor & Francis Group, an **informa** business

A BALKEMA BOOK

CRC Press/Balkema is an imprint of the Taylor & Francis Group, an informa business

© 2010 Taylor & Francis Group, London, UK

Typeset by Vikatan Publishing Solutions (P) Ltd, Chennai, India.
Printed and bound in Great Britain by TJ International Ltd, Padstow, Cornwall

Published by: CRC Press/Balkema
           P.O. Box 447, 2300 AK Leiden, The Netherlands
           e-mail: Pub.NL@taylorandfrancis.com
           www.crcpress.com – www.taylorandfrancis.co.uk – www.balkema.nl

Library of Congress Cataloging-in-Publication Data

Chowdhury, Robin.
    Geotechnical slope analysis / Robin Chowdhury ; other contributors, Phil Flentje,
    Gautam Bhattacharya.
    p. cm.
    Includes bibliographical references and index.
    ISBN 978-0-415-46974-6 (hardcover : alk. paper) 1. Slopes (Soil mechanics) I.
    Flentje, Phil. II. Bhattacharya, Gautam. III. Title.

    TA710.C5466 2010
    624.1'51363–dc22

                                                    2009026758

ISBN: 978-0-415-46974-6 (Hbk)
ISBN: 978-0-203-86420-3 (eBook)

To those progressive readers
who gently asked about
a second edition of "Slope Analysis"
and also to earnest new readers

Contents

About the Author

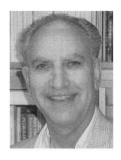

Dr Robin Chowdhury

Dr Robin Chowdhury, well known internationally as a geotechnical engineer and scholar, is an Emeritus Professor at the University of Wollongong, Australia. He completed his PhD from the University of Liverpool, England in 1970 and has devoted more than three decades to teaching, research and scholarship. His early work was concerned with factors influencing slope stability, landslide occurrence and mechanisms and with the concepts and methods of deterministic geotechnical analysis. Subsequently he devoted considerable attention to the development and application of probabilistic approaches and reliability analysis. He also made a sustained contribution to the understanding and simulation of progressive failure. In recent years Robin has emphasized the linking and integration of regional slope studies with site-specific slope engineering assessments. He has also advocated the adoption of an interdisciplinary approach for geotechnical engineering projects and, in particular, for landslide management. His recent work has been concerned with the assessment of geotechnical hazard and risk as well as with observational approaches which include modern methods of field monitoring.

Other contributors

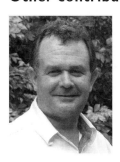

Dr Phil Flentje

Dr Phil Flentje, a recognised expert in Slope Engineering and Landslide Management, is a Senior Research Fellow at the University of Wollongong, Australia. His education and training is in Engineering Geology and Geotechnical Engineering. He completed his PhD at the University of Wollongong (NSW, Australia) in 1998. He developed a comprehensive GIS-based approach for regional studies concerning the occurrence, frequency and impact of landslides. In his subsequent work he has developed models for the use of landslide inventories, the assessment of landslide susceptibility, hazard and risk. His current activities include web-based real-time monitoring of slope deformations, pore pressures and associated structural displacements as part of a regional assessment of landslide activity and frequency. His research also embraces analysis of rainfall with its spatial and temporal variability and landslide-triggering rainfall thresholds/alerts.

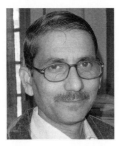

Dr. Gautam Bhattacharya

Dr. Gautam Bhattacharya, an experienced academic and researcher, is currently the Head of the Department of Civil Engineering, BESU, Shibpur, and also the Vice-Chairman, Calcutta Chapter of the Indian Geotechnical Society. His interest in the subject of slope stability developed during his doctoral research at IIT Kanpur (1985–1990). His thesis was concerned with the application of numerical methods in slope analysis. He has since been engaged in teaching this subject and in pursuing research on both deterministic and probabilistic approaches of analysis of unreinforced and reinforced slopes under static and seismic conditions. He has teaching, research and consultancy experience in the field of geotechnical engineering for about three decades.

Preface

Significant advances have been made in the knowledge and practice concerning slope analysis during the three decades that have passed since the publication of the first edition of this book. In this second edition, an effort has been made to highlight the most important developments and the attention of readers is drawn to current and future challenges. For a number of reasons, including the increasing frequency and impact of natural hazards such as landslides triggered by rainstorms and earthquakes, the importance of slope analysis has increased significantly.

This book is still primarily about geotechnical aspects of slope analysis for individual sites. However, regional studies of hilly and coastal areas are now increasingly being undertaken all over the world, with outcomes such as maps of landslide susceptibility and hazard. Thus site-specific slope analyses can be placed, assessed and validated in their appropriate contexts. New and versatile tools such as Geographical Information Systems (GIS) enable the assembly, organization, display, updating, analysis and synthesis of spatial and temporal data on a wide range of factors that influence slope stability and reliability. It is necessary for the slope engineer to be aware of these developments even when concerned primarily with investigations and analyses at individual sites.

Recognition of the importance of uncertainties in geotechnical engineering has ensured an increasing role for probabilistic approaches. For both site-specific and regional studies concerning slope stability, probabilistic perspectives are almost essential. Knowledge, skill and judgment are, however, required to decide the proper role and application of methods within a probabilistic framework. Because the subject is so important, basic probability concepts are introduced at an early stage of this book (Chapter 3). A complete chapter is devoted to comprehensive coverage of probabilistic methods relevant to slope analysis (Chapter 10).

Two major triggering factors for slope instability and landsliding are rainfall of high magnitude and strong ground motion due to earthquakes. References are made in Chapters 1 and 2 to pore water pressure changes associated with rainfall (decrease of suction in unsaturated slopes or increase of pore water pressure in saturated slopes) leading, in turn, to decrease of shear strength and factor of safety of slopes. The subject is followed up in chapters 4 and 5 which deal primarily with limit equilibrium methods of analysis although some attention is given to the post-failure behavior and landslide dynamics including exceptional landslides. Seismic analyses of slopes are covered in Chapter 9 with particular emphasis on the application of limit equilibrium and sliding block models. An up-to-date though brief review of regional studies of earthquake effects on slopes is included in this chapter.

Stress-deformation methods are considered in Chapter 6 and the significance of recent research is highlighted. Chapter 7 concerns the role of initial stresses and the simulation of change in a stress field associated with progressive failure. This chapter includes a discussion of two alternative explanations for the catastrophic Vaiont slide. Chapter 8, concerning plasticity solutions has been suitably updated. There are frequent references to mechanisms of progressive failure throughout the book. In particular, it is shown in Chapter 5 that the influence of strain-softening and stress redistribution on the factor of safety of a slope can be studied within the framework of limit equilibrium methods.

The role of observation and monitoring and, in particular continuous (real-time) monitoring is highlighted in a chapter on urban slope stability within a specific study area (Chapter 11). Case studies of back-analysis are followed up by a discussion of rainfall analysis and the assessment of rainfall thresholds for landsliding. This chapter also highlights the importance of a comprehensive landslide inventory for the modeling of landslide susceptibility and hazard on a regional basis.

While references are made to the adverse impacts (economic, human safety, environmental) of slope instability and landsliding, a detailed coverage of the subject of landslide risk assessment and management is outside the scope of this book. Brief references are also made to the implications of climate change (e.g., sea level rise, increased variability of rainfall) on the frequency and impact of landslides. However, detailed coverage of these topics is outside the scope of this book.

There has been a tremendous increase in the power of computers and considerable progress has been made in the development of specialized software based on both traditional and sophisticated methods of analysis relevant to slope stability under static or dynamic conditions. Discussion of the merits and limitations of different types of slope stability software is outside the scope of this book. Nevertheless, one must acknowledge that the use of such software will grow. Hopefully, geotechnical engineering of slopes will be enhanced in the process. However, if there is excessive dependence on computer software, basic concepts and principles may tend to be forgotten. Moreover, the assessment of the reliability of such software must be taken up seriously by the geotechnical engineering profession. Otherwise, inconsistencies and contradictions may be overlooked and the right balance between available knowledge, accurate analysis and engineering judgment may not be attained.

While I have decided to retain, as far as possible, the format and flavour of the original book, significant improvements have been made by including examples and case studies wherever possible. While trying to make the book more reader-friendly and helpful to students, the unique personality of the original book has been retained. In particular, there is continued emphasis on basic principles and frequent discussion of issues which are critical to conceptual clarity, genuine scholarship and progressive practice.

I appreciate the help and collaboration of Phil Flentje and Gautam Bhattacharya. Chapter 11 is essentially Phil's contribution in which I played only a subsidiary role. Phil has also been helpful on a number of issues throughout the period of writing despite many other demands on his time. Gautam played a significant role as a patient reviewer of successive drafts of this book. He has been prompt in his responses and persistent in getting his points across but always with great courtesy. He also worked out the numerical solutions for most of the example problems. Several months after he agreed to work on this project, he was appointed to the Headship of his Department at BESU in Shibpur. He did not falter in his commitment in the face of his increased workload and responsibility. It has been a pleasure to work closely with Phil and Gautam. To the extent that this book has achieved its aims, they both deserve credit for their contributions. However, the responsibility for any faults or errors is entirely mine.

Robin Chowdhury
May 9, 2009
Wollongong, New South Wales, Australia

Acknowledgements

The writing of a book such as this is a major undertaking. In this instance, I learnt that updating a book can be as hard a task as it is to write a completely new one. For sustained effort required for a challenging project, one is grateful for the goodwill and support of family, friends and colleagues. One must, however, express special appreciation for those who have directly facilitated the implementation of the project.

It is a pleasure to acknowledge the cooperation of support staff at the Faculty of Engineering, UOW. In particular, I wish to acknowledge Roma Hamlet for the assistance in word processing of some early sections of the book and Peter Turner and Leonie Mcintyre of our IT-section for assistance.

In updating drafts of the manuscript, Miss Mitali Mondal provided considerable secretarial support to Gautam Bhattacharya at BESU. Her role is greatly appreciated.

I acknowledge Paul Bryden of GEO-SLOPE International for access to "Geostudio Professional" software used by Phil Flentje for slope stability analyses described in Chapter 11.

I am thankful to Randall W. Jibson of U.S. Geological Survey for providing a link to the website containing his software for seismic analysis of slopes based on the sliding-block concept.

I wish to thank Alex M. Dunstan of RTA (Roads and Traffic Authority, New South Wales) for providing the photo used on the book cover.

Every effort has been made, throughout this book, to refer to the correct sources of tables, figures and other information.

Finally, it must be said that a continuous process of learning is a pre-requisite for attempting to write a book concerned with the fundamentals of the subject as well as with the most recent developments in the field. I owe a debt of gratitude to researchers and scholars from whose work I have gained understanding and insight into various aspects of the subject of slope analysis.

Robin Chowdhury

Preface to the first edition

The subject of slope analysis is a fascinating one both from theoretical and practical points of view and has attracted the attention of researchers and scholars in diverse fields such as soil mechanics, rock mechanics, engineering geology and geomorphology. Over the last few decades excellent books have been written in each of these disciplines with important sections devoted to aspects of slope stability analysis. An integrated treatment covering the analysis of both soil and rock slopes has seldom been presented in sufficient detail. It has sometimes been stated that many slope problems defy a theoretical or analytical treatment. While such statements emphasise the complexity of factors which influence the performance of slopes, they also indicate the need for refinements in available methods of analysis and for the development of new concepts and approaches.

The main aims of this book may be summarised as follows:

1   To outline the fundamental principles of slope analysis and to explore both similarities and differences in soil and rock slopes.
2   To discuss the assumptions underlying both simple and so-called 'rigorous' methods of analysis.
3   To highlight the importance of factors which influence slope performance and especially to consider the role of progressive failure.
4   To discuss the use of alternative methods of analysis and to present information on new concepts and new approaches to analysis.

This book is meant for the senior undergraduate and graduate student, the researcher as well as the practitioner. The material has been arranged in a form convenient for the undergraduate student who may have only an introductory background in one of the disciplines mentioned above. New concepts and approaches are introduced gradually and as a consequence of discussion of conventional ideas and practices. The graduate student and researcher will find many references to the most recent developments. Issues of real significance in research such as progressive failure and probabilistic concepts are dealt with throughout the book and there is a consistent emphasis on the need to distinguish between assumed models and practical realities.

For the practitioner comprehensive information on the choice, use and limitations of conventional methods of analysis is provided in chapters 3 and 4. In Appendix II slope stability charts are included for 'total stress' as well as 'effective stress' types of analysis and information is also provided to enable location of critical slip circles. The practitioner must never lose sight of the assumption of a circular failure surface on which these and similar charts are based. One is tempted to quote from the Terzaghi lecture of Wilson (1970):

"... As my first illustration I had intended to use an example of ground movements during a classical circular arc failure. After a diligent search of literally hundreds of case histories in my files, not one such example could be documented. Undaunted I turned to colleagues for help. When their efforts were likewise unproductive, I decided to limit the topic to non-circular failure surfaces, but with particular emphasis on progressive failure...". It is hoped that this book will stimulate renewed awareness of important issues in slope analysis. Such an awareness is necessary if significant progress is to be achieved in the near future.

Dr. James V. Hamel of Pennsylvania read the first draft of this book with keen interest and conveyed his detailed comments with exemplary promptness. His comments, often supported by references to published and unpublished material, were very useful during the preparation of the final manuscript and resulted in significant revisions of parts of chapters 2, 3 and 4. It is with pleasure and gratitude that I acknowledge his assistance and the contribution he made to a lively correspondence on slopes which started in 1973. I look forward to our first meeting in the second half of 1978. Mr. Brian Cousins very kindly arranged for the use of tracings of his charts and provided information concerning their use. Mrs. Adell Smith typed the manuscript with care and patience and I express my sincere appreciation for her efforts and for those of Roger McAlister who assisted with the line drawings. At the University of Wollongong I have received encouragement from everyone and must mention, in particular, Professor L. Michael Birt, Vice Chancellor, Professor C.A.M. Gray and Associate Professor R.W. Upfold. Finally I record with pleasure the affection and support of my wife Nancy, daughter Rita and especially little son Vivek.

R.N. Chowdhury
April 14, 1978
Wollongong, New South Wales, Australia

Chapter 1

Aims and overview – slopes, geology and materials

1.1 INTRODUCTION

The construction, design, remediation and maintenance of slopes have always formed an important area of geotechnical engineering which is often termed as 'slope engineering'. The wide variety of applications of slope engineering include excavations, hill roads, railway lines, embankments, earth dams, reservoirs, open-cut mines, urban development of hilly areas, protection of river banks and coastal slope stability. The study and analysis of slopes is essential for understanding their performance and, in particular, their stability, reliability and deformations. Thus geotechnical engineers often seek to calculate values of quantitative indicators of performance such as the factor of safety (safety factor), lateral deformation, and probability of failure and reliability index. Important concepts of geomechanics and, in particular, of soil mechanics have been vitally important for developing the basic mechanistic models of slopes and the associated methods of analysis, both simple and sophisticated. However, it is widely recognized that interdisciplinary approaches are required for a complete understanding of slope performance and for the choice of realistic models and methods of analysis for specific sites. Geoscientists have made significant contributions to the understanding of natural slopes, their evolution and performance over the long-term. To that end, they are concerned with modeling natural and other processes much more than considering specifics of stability analysis, slope design and remediation which are understood to be the main concerns of geotechnical engineers. However, the input of geoscientists is often valuable for slope engineering including the development, choice and use of mechanistic models. In fact, a geotechnical engineer would start detailed modeling after studying the geological report of a site and often after considering the specific observations made by an engineering geologist.

1.2 OVERVIEW OF RECENT DEVELOPMENTS AND TRENDS

1.2.1 Increasing frequency and impact of disasters from slope failures and landslides

Over the last few decades, the frequency and consequences of disasters associated with natural events and human activities, around the world, has increased significantly and this trend continues. In addition to enormous economic losses resulting from slope failures and landslides, considerable loss of life and injury also occur especially as a result of catastrophic events. The number of people killed, injured or displaced globally due to natural hazards during the 20th century has been presented by Bryant et al. (2005) based on data published in 1992 by the World Health Organization (WHO) and supplemented by other information. This is reproduced as Table C1.1 in the Appendix to this chapter. The fatalities and other numbers are considerable for most categories and it is significant that many of the highest consequence events have occurred in relatively less developed countries. As a separate category, landslides are responsible for more than 60,000 reported deaths and more than 3 million homeless. It should be noted, however, that additional losses caused by landslides would be included in the data for other categories in this table such as earthquakes and tropical cyclones. Another investigation, specifically for landslides, has been summarized by Petley et al. (2005) and some of the information is reproduced in Table C1.2 in the Appendix to this Chapter. Again it is important to note that the total number of deaths as well as the number per million of the population are both significantly higher for most of the underdeveloped parts of the world. The main reasons include the increase in the frequency of hazards as well as the increase in elements at risk and their vulnerability. Major contributing factors include the growth of urbanization, lack of adequate planning for development of hilly areas and marginal lands and inadequate management of hazards. There is an increasing recognition of the need for assessment of landslide susceptibility and hazard and for landslide risk management.

The occurrence of disasters cannot be attributed to natural processes alone. While natural factors are dominant features of hazards, disasters often occur due to increased vulnerability of communities and infrastructure resulting from excessive urban development, inadequate infrastructure, poor quality control, incomplete understanding of hazards and of vulnerability and lack of action to mitigate risk.

1.2.2   Climate change, global warming and sea level rise

Global warming and climate change are now widely accepted as phenomena that have been in progress for more than a century and expected to worsen over the next 50 years even if the global community takes concerted action to reverse the human-induced causes. Focused research is urgently required to model the effects of climate change on hilly regions, coastal areas as well as infrastructure and other assets involving slopes (see, for instance, McInnes et al., 2007). It is expected that climate change will lead to even more unfavorable conditions for slope stability and thus to increasing susceptibility and hazard of landsliding. This is primarily because of the expected increase in the variability of rainfall and the expected increase in sea levels. Responding to the effects of climate change will thus require more flexible and robust strategies for assessment of landslide susceptibility, innovative engineering solutions in some situations, pro-active risk management in most cases as well as mitigation of the effects of landslide disasters which cannot be prevented. Slope analysis will continue to be one of the important tools for most such strategies, other tools being modern observational approaches, early warning systems, reduction of vulnerability of people, systems and infrastructure, and other preventive measures.

1.2.3 Built slopes – lessons from the catastrophic impacts of Hurricane Katrina

Catastrophic losses occurred in New Orleans (USA) following the landfall of Hurricane Katrina on August 29, 2005 due to the failure of the Hurricane Protection System (HPS) of which the constructed earth structures (levees) were the most important part. In the Greater New Orleans area, there were 1503 deaths (without including several hundred during the evacuation process), direct economic losses in the range of 75–150 billion US dollars, indirect losses of similar magnitude and 400,000 people were initially displaced. Among the broad lessons to be learnt from the catastrophic disaster, contributors to Katrina (2008) refer to the need for sensible land use policies and management. Cities should be developed in locations where a high level of protection can be provided for a large number of people and to their homes and businesses. The exposed location of New Orleans meant that it was not economically feasible to provide such a level of protection. The following comment in one of the contributions to Katrina (2008) is especially pertinent:

> "With both projected sea level rise and continuing warming of the Gulf waters, the hurricane risk for the area is likely to increase in the decades ahead".

Yet, the important lessons are not being learnt at the national, state and local administration levels. For example, redevelopment is being carried out on the pre-. Katrina footprint despite the overall decrease in the population.

Other broad lessons from the investigation of the disaster include the following (Katrina, 2008):

- Enough resources were not devoted to the defense of critical parts of the HPS. Levees were constructed with locally available materials dredged from the excavation of shipping channels. Large portions of the levees thus comprised uncompacted soils with poor resistance to erosion. Initial cost savings achieved by using such materials were vastly exceeded by the losses arising from the catastrophic failures including loss of life and economic losses.
- Resources were not devoted in a timely manner to complete the final stages of some sections of the levee system. Consequently those sections of the levee system were vulnerable to overtopping during the storm surge. Thus overtopping occurred after the landfall of Hurricane Katrina, leading to flooding and associated losses.
- However, overtopping alone (without the failures or breaches of the levee system) would have caused only one third of the flooding that occurred and recovery efforts would have been more efficient and capable of being executed faster.
- Overtopping scour protection was not incorporated in the HPS. Breaches were caused by erosion after overtopping. Thus the lack of erosion protection proved enormously costly.
- Roller compacted levees performed well while hydraulic fill levees performed poorly.
- In some instances, adequate allowance was not made in the geotechnical design for uncertainties in shear strength of levee materials and foundations. In one case, shear strength was significantly overestimated in one part of the foundation due to limited site investigation. Variability in shear strength was not provided for.

- Uncertainties due to imperfect knowledge should be provided for in adopting the minimum factors of safety for design. For example, investigations revealed that there was a change in failure mechanism as a gap or crack developed on the flood side of a levee-I wall system due to the deflection of the I-wall.

  In one case the factor of safety was found to be 1.28 without the gap but only 0.98 with the gap. In another case, the factor of safety was 1.52 without the gap but only 0.99 with the gap. The minimum factor of safety of about 1.3 adopted for design was based on analysis without the gap. Consequently the formation of the gap was responsible for the occurrence of failures.

- Based on the above, there is need for a system with resilience in the HPS to consider conditions and forces beyond its design and to provide for variability. Moreover, there should be conservatism to allow for knowledge deficiency.

- Risk-based planning and design approach is important so that a system performance can be evaluated and not just the performance of its individual components. The performance of each component and the consequences of that performance should thus be evaluated in relation to the impact on the system as a whole.

1.2.4   New developments related to slope analysis

With increasing frequency and adverse impact of landslides and failures of earth structures, slope engineering and, therefore, slope analysis have assumed increasing relevance and importance. Moreover, new developments of great value to geoscientists and geo-engineers have occurred over the past few decades, as outlined in the following sub-sections. Recent decades have also been characterized by the growth of computing power and increasingly efficient hardware and software. Some of these developments have had the effect of shifting the focus inevitably from site-specific to regional studies within hilly areas.

Landslide susceptibility and hazard may not correspond directly to geotechnical performance indicators such as 'factor of safety' and 'probability of failure' used for site-specific studies.

Definitions of performance indicators will be considered in the following chapters including aspects relating to time (temporal context). For example, one must consider return periods of triggering factors such as landslide-triggering rainfall. A simple example is the need to consider an average annual probability of failure in a region or within a particular zone rather than just the site-specific probability of failure corresponding to the calculated mean safety factor at an individual site.

1.2.5   Importance of probabilistic analysis

Geotechnical engineers have increasingly recognized the importance of probabilistic approaches for analysis and decision-making. In particular, slope analysis can benefit greatly from the adoption of methods and techniques within probabilistic framework. Basic concepts of probability are introduced in Chapter 3 of this book and applications to slope analysis are detailed in Chapter 10.

Probability concepts are important for both site-specific and regional studies concerning slopes. Both qualitative and quantitative assessments of landslide susceptibility and hazard require a good grasp of probability concepts. Important aspects of a regional case study concerning urban slope stability and landsliding are discussed is in chapter 11 of this book.

The benefits of adopting a formal probabilistic approach go well beyond complementing traditional, deterministic analyses or simply replacing the factor of safety by the reliability index or probability of failure as performance indicators. A number of examples are given in chapter 10 to illustrate the significant advantages in developing new perspectives for slope analysis within a probabilistic framework.

Similarly, the potential benefits of using a formal probabilistic approach go well beyond the judicious use of empirical relationships that may be developed between factors of safety on the one hand and probability of failure on the other, as proposed by Silva et al. (2008). This important subject is discussed further in chapter 12, the concluding chapter.

1.2.6 GIS-based methods and analyses

With a shift in focus to regional assessments, the concepts and principles of slope analysis may receive inadequate attention from students, scholars and professional engineers. It is, therefore, important to place the subject of slope analysis, once again, in its proper perspective while recognizing the power and value of the new developments. Consider, for example, the development of Geographical Information Systems (GIS) which has revolutionized the way in which a variety of spatial data can be handled, checked, analyzed, manipulated, synthesized and updated (Carrara and Guzzetti, 1995). GIS has proved to be a powerful tool for working with large bodies of data, deriving suitable spatial and temporal parameters and performance indicators and for displaying information in a suitable form such as maps. Moreover, GIS-based maps can be updated, altered and enhanced with the availability of additional data or better quality data or as a consequence of improved knowledge about any aspect of a project. Most books concerning landslides, published in the last decade, have devoted considerable attention to regional studies but while some have covered GIS-based methods and techniques (for example, Turner and Schuster, 1996), others have not (for example, Lee and Jones, 2004). Of course, books devoted to detailed geotechnical investigation and remediation of landslides concentrate primarily on site-specific studies (for example, Cornforth, 2005, 2007).

1.2.7 Assessments concerning very large landslides

Throughout this book, there are references to some major landslides such as the 1963 Vaiont slide (refer sections 1.10.6, 2.3.4, 5.6.5, 7.15–7.18). Major landslides provide evidence of unusual phenomena and raise important questions concerning causes, mechanisms of failure and about post-failure landslide dynamics. Consequently, research studies associated with such landslides facilitate progress in the understanding and analysis of slope failures and landslides.

Initial assessments concerning landslides of relatively large magnitude (often millions of cubic meters in volume, travelling at high velocities and attaining large run-out distances) and of relatively low frequency are generally carried out by geoscientists. An outstanding compilation of such assessments is contained in a volume on catastrophic landslides edited by Evans and DeGraff (2002) which is part of the Geological Society of America Series entitled 'Reviews in Engineering Geology'. The adverse impact of many such landslides on urban areas including housing, roads, railways and other engineering infrastructure can be enormous. Thus the involvement of geotechnical engineers in studying the occurrence and impact of such landslides should increase. It is important to note that understanding the causes, mechanisms and dynamics of such landslides requires the application of engineering principles and, in particular, the basic and advanced concepts of geomechanics. As in the case of much smaller and less destructive landslides, the triggering factors of catastrophic landslides are varied although heavy rainfall and earthquakes are the dominant triggers. For example, an overview of catastrophic landslides of South America in the twentieth century, carried out by Schuster et al. (2002) included 23 landslides in the period 1941–1994. Amongst these, 10 were triggered by heavy or prolonged rainfall, 5 by earthquake shaking, 3 by valley down-cutting due to long-term erosion, 2 by failure of natural dam, 1 by volcanic activity and 1 by leakage from man-made pond.

1.2.8 Landslide frequency related to magnitude

In general, the temporal frequency of occurrence of any natural event like a catastrophic landslide is inversely proportional to its magnitude. The larger the magnitude, the lower is the expected annual frequency of occurrence or greater is the return period. However, the actual frequency of occurrence of an event of given magnitude is highly variable, being dependent on a number of factors such as location, geology, geomorphology and size of the region under consideration. For example, McSaveney (2002) described four high velocity rock avalanches/ falls which occurred in the Mount Cook National Park, New Zealand between Dec. 1991 and February 1996. Their locations and volumes in million cubic meters are: Mount Cook (9.4–14.2), Mount Fletcher I (>7.8), Mount Fletcher II (>about 5) and Mount Thomson (0.1). The frequency of a collapse greater than one million cubic meters in the Park was estimated as 1 per 20–30 yr. However, the smallest magnitude event (Mount Thomson) was regarded as an annual event in the Park but as a 1 per 10 yr event at the location itself, near Mueller Glacier. In contrast, many other mountainous regions in the world are far less prone to landsides; thus, in a region of the same size as the Mount Cook National Park, a high velocity landslide in the size range (0.1–1) million cubic meters would be a much less frequent event. In some regions such a catastrophic landslide would be regarded as a rare event within an engineering time-scale.

1.2.9 Assessing regional landslide susceptibility and hazard

Considering the spatial and temporal variability of factors which influence slope stability (e.g., variability in slope inclination, slope length, local geology, groundwater conditions, vegetation etc.) the availability of a GIS framework is, of course, more valuable for regional assessments than it may be for site-specific studies. Thus it is important to distinguish between the role of site-specific and regional studies on the one hand and between qualitative and quantitative studies on the other. A range of GIS – based methods have been developed for assessment of the landslide susceptibility and hazard of hilly areas. Some of these methods are considered qualitative and others quantitative; some make greater use of statistical techniques of analysis than others. Most of these methods are based on the synthesis or overlap of several factor maps, each detailing the distribution of one influencing factor. (Refer to chapter 11 for a regional case study.)

Recent developments include the use of computer intelligence and knowledge-based methods which take into consideration the location and distribution of existing landslides in a region, in addition to the relevant influencing factors.

The tools and techniques for regional studies are thus improving significantly. However, the value and significance of results depends on the range and quality of data as well as the adequacy of the modeling method used. What may be regarded as a good quantitative approach for a regional study may not be good enough or sufficiently quantitative for a site-specific study. While qualitative methods do have a role even for site-specific assessments, detailed quantitative analyses are required for high priority sites. Therefore, geotechnical slope analysis methods must be strengthened to be of value for such detailed site-specific studies. Extension of geotechnical quantitative methods to regional studies is also desirable. Relatively simple methods, such as 'infinite slope analysis' (see chapter 4), have been used successfully for regional studies within a GIS framework.

1.2.10 Development and use of slope stability software

Another recent trend has been the development and use of versatile and user-friendly slope stability software as a logical and inevitable follow-up to computer-based methods which had already been in use for several decades. The use of manual analyses and slope stability charts is indeed rare now. Most of the popular software is that based on the limit equilibrium concept utilizing either a deterministic framework or a probabilistic one or both. Such a software product may offer a choice among individual methods of limit equilibrium analysis, 'simplified' and 'rigorous' (chapters 4 and 5 of this book). Software products for stress-deformation analyses based on finite-difference, finite-element and other methods have also been developed. More sophisticated software have also been developed which can handle, three-dimensional effects, non-linear behaviour, simulation of earthquake shaking, liquefaction and other phenomena. Software with capabilities for linked seepage and limit equilibrium analyses have been developed as also for coupled stress-deformation analyses. The use of any software assumes prior knowledge of the concepts and methods of slope analysis. Moreover, intelligent choice of software would require the user to have broad knowledge of the subject, and in sufficient depth. Ironically, however, the availability of such a variety of software has tended to discourage a detailed or deep study of the basics and may thus inhibit an informed selection and use of these analytical tools.

1.2.11 Need to strengthen the fundamentals of geomechanics and slope analysis

Thus the fundamentals of slope analysis require renewed and continuing emphasis. However, the development of new perspectives, methods and tools is very important. Consequently, much greater flexibility is required in the application of the fundamentals of geomechanics in general and slope analysis, in particular. The importance of the basic concepts and methods must again be presented, the advantages of each method and its limitations highlighted and the correct assessment and use of software products encouraged. Moreover, students and scholars must be encouraged to look at the wider picture rather than be limited by what available software offers. It is interesting to note that the principles of geomechanics, developed more than 70 years back, and which are the basis of geotechnical slope analysis, continue to be accepted and affirmed (for example, see Terzaghi et al., 1996).

It is also important to highlight areas that have received relatively little attention. For example, the adverse effects of erosion processes on natural slopes and man-made soil structures, such as embankments, are well known. Following intense rainstorms, it may be difficult to separate the effects of erosion from landsliding at certain sites. While the hydraulic aspects of erosion processes are well developed as a result of research, geotechnical aspects have been neglected. Facilitating the progress of slope engineering requires that assessments of slope failures and landsliding take into consideration erosion processes as well. The tragedy of hurricane Katrina, for example, includes the failures of levees by overtopping. A strategic systems approach would need to combine conventional geotechnical analysis with a consideration of erosion processes as well. Recently a beginning has been made to focus attention on the need to develop the geotechnical aspects of knowledge concerning erosion of soil and rock. Four case histories of soil and rock erosion were considered by Briaud (2008) and two of these are relevant to slopes. One provides an explanation of the process of rock cliff erosion while the other (New Orleans levees case history) concerns erosion by overtopping of levees.

1.3 MAIN AIM AND SCOPE OF THIS BOOK

As stated above, the aims of slope analysis range from regional to site-specific studies and from qualitative to quantitative methods. The whole spectrum of analysis methods is, of course, important. However, the concepts and techniques of geotechnical engineering are essential for site-specific, quantitative studies. Therefore, except for chapter 11, the main emphasis in this book is on geotechnical analysis involving quantitative methods which have generally been applied to individual slopes. New tools and techniques, such as GIS, facilitate application of such quantitative analyses within a regional context. So far, however, only the simplest method, the one-dimensional 'infinite slope analysis' has been used in this way.

This book deals with the concepts and methods of geotechnical analysis, deterministic and probabilistic. While concentrating on individual slopes (site-specific analyses) several references are made to regional studies. The detailed presentation of the latter is outside the scope of this book. Many of the methods used for regional studies have been developed by geoscientists and primarily involve manipulation and interpretation of observational and historical data. These methods cannot be described as engineering approaches.

It must be stated that observational data concerning a specific site are often useful for calibration and improvement of site-specific, geotechnical studies which focus on the mechanics of soil and rock behavior. On the other hand, most regional studies analyze and interpret observational data in an empirical manner or using statistical techniques. Of course, field checking helps to validate the results of such regional studies which may not place due emphasis on the mechanics of slope behavior.

Although this book is primarily concerned with quantitative, site-specific geotechnical studies, the importance of regional perspectives is highlighted wherever necessary. With the development of versatile tools and techniques of analysis and synthesis such as GIS, one can have access to fairly reliable regional perspectives and scenarios. Therefore, wherever possible, geotechnical slope analyses should be considered in relation to the overall regional picture rather than in isolation. Conversely, regional studies implemented with methods outside the geotechnical engineering framework must be tested and calibrated with detailed geotechnical slope analyses at selected locations.

With that clear understanding of the complementary role of regional and site-specific studies, let us deal with the aims of geotechnical analysis in more detail.

1.4 AIMS OF GEOTECHNICAL SLOPE ANALYSIS

Geotechnical slope analysis should consider the basic concepts of geomechanics such as effective stress, shear strength, stability, and deformation and failure mechanisms. Modern slope analysis must also consider probability concepts in relation to safety and failure. Both deterministic and probabilistic perspectives are important. Terms such as probability, likelihood, and hazard have increasingly become accepted by the geotechnical engineering profession and this has brought their perspectives closer to those of geoscientists. Consequently, infrastructure managers, other stake holders and the public are also attuned to accepting outcomes in probabilistic terms where it is difficult to talk in terms of certainties.

The primary purpose of geotechnical slope analysis in most engineering applications is to contribute to the safe and economic design of excavations, embankments, earth dams and spoil heaps. Preliminary analyses assist in the identification of critical geological, material, environmental and economic parameters. Therefore, the results are of value in planning the detailed investigations of major projects. Subsequent analyses enable an understanding of the nature, magnitude and frequency of slope problems that may require to be solved. Previous geotechnical and engineering geological experience of an area is always valuable in dealing with slopes in general and slope analyses in particular. Evaluation of slope stability is often an inter-disciplinary effort requiring contributions from engineering geology, soil mechanics and rock mechanics. The main recognized aims of slope analysis may be summarized as follows.

- To assess the stability of different types of slopes under given conditions.
  Often it is necessary to assess the stability separately for short-term (end-of-construction) and long-term conditions. Analytical studies are essential in many cases before suitable cut or fill slopes can be designed with confidence. Such studies enable economical use to be made of materials, labor and resources.
- To assess the possibility of landslides involving natural or existing man-made slopes.
  The influence of proposed modifications to an existing slope can be studied in an organised manner. Similarly, comparative studies can be made to assess the

value of proposed preventive or remedial measures. Sensitivity analyses can be made to study how variations in material and field parameters of uncertain magnitude might affect stability.

- To analyze slips and landslides that have already occurred and to assist in the understanding of failure mechanisms and the influence of environmental factors.

    Such analyses, often called 'back-analyses', can provide reliable information about the average shearing resistance of natural slope materials. Actual failures can be considered as large-scale shear tests and enable comparison with strength parameters obtained from laboratory tests and field investigations.

- To enable the redesign of failed slopes, and the planning and design of preventive and remedial measures where necessary.

    Data from instrumented slopes, embankments and earth dams can be evaluated with confidence if a suitable method of slope analysis is used.

- To enable a study of the effect of exceptional loadings such as earthquakes on slopes and embankments.

- To understand the development and form of natural slopes and the processes that have been responsible for different natural features.

The manner in which contemporary processes and changes can influence slope form is of general interest in applied geomorphology. At the same time there is increasing recognition of the practical value of such studies with regard to proposed and existing developments in hilly areas.

The analysis of real slopes involves consideration of a variety of factors including topography, geology and material properties.

Often some idealization of problems is required for clarity and for the effective application of basic concepts. In the following sections, attention is given to some of these factors after a brief discussion of individual types of slope problems.

1.5 NATURAL SLOPES – REGIONAL AND SITE-SPECIFIC ANALYSES

Consideration of the stability of natural slopes is often a very important part of planning and development of hilly regions. Some regions may still be forested and almost undisturbed; some may have been deforested but with little urbanization while others may be already urbanized to a certain extent and, in some cases, with pressures for growth in extent or intensity of development or both. The extension of urbanization to sensitive parts of such regions often increases the susceptibility to landsliding. Both regional and site-specific analyses are appropriate for dealing with geotechnical assessments in hilly regions. For long-term planning, a regional perspective is of particular importance. Since only a limited amount of data and resources are available in the initial stages of development, only qualitative studies are feasible. As more and more data and resources become available, quantitative studies and analyses should be carried out.

It is appropriate to consider here, very briefly, the question: 'How is a qualitative analysis carried out and how are the findings presented?'

Qualitative appraisal of individual sites is based on site inspection, consideration of all available information on geology, geotechnical aspects, topography and other regional characteristics followed by careful exercise of professional judgment. Relative stability of individual sites is then described by choosing from a limited range of indicators of landslide susceptibility such as: very high, high, medium, low and very low susceptibility. These terms are considered again in chapter 3 after defining the most commonly used performance indicators.

Once the resources become available for detailed site-specific studies at individual sites, detailed geotechnical data can be acquired and analytical approaches based on fundamentals of geomechanics can be utilized. The stability and reliability of a slope are then described quantitatively in terms which are quite different from the qualitative description mentioned above. These quantitative indicators, deterministic and probabilistic, such as factor of safety, failure probability and reliability are first considered properly in chapter 3 and then discussed or used in the following chapters.

It is equally appropriate to consider here, very briefly, the related question: 'How are regional studies, qualitative and quantitative, carried out and how are the results presented?'

Using a modern GIS framework and utilizing all the topographical information, a digital elevation model (DEM) is developed for the whole study area. Such a model is useful for deriving important parameters at individual points such as slope angle, slope direction, curvature etc. GIS-based maps of geology, existing landslides, and vegetation are also developed. Based on a synthesis of these maps and other relevant information, it is then possible to demarcate zones with landslide susceptibility indicators within a limited range such as: very high, high, medium, low and very low susceptibility. Thus a regional map of landslide susceptibility is obtained for the study area. Different susceptibility maps may be prepared for different types of landslides such as slides, falls and debris-flows. To go further and assess hazard, additional information is required such as landslide magnitude (volume) and frequency. Thus additional data, research information and appropriate analyses would be required to develop hazard maps from susceptibility maps.

As the quality and range of data improve to a significant extent, such a regional study can be greatly improved over time with the use of more refined analyses while adopting sophisticated methods of synthesis and interpretation. Efforts must be made for validation of the outcomes in order to establish the reliability of the modeling procedure.

The results are presented in the same form as for a qualitative regional study, i.e., in terms of zones of landslide susceptibility ranging from very high to very low susceptibility. As stated above, significant additional information, research results and analyses are required to develop hazard maps from susceptibility maps. For a comprehensive discussion of concepts and methods of regional slope and landslide analysis, qualitative and quantitative, the reader may refer to Aleotti and Chowdhury (1999).

1.6 NATURAL SLOPES – FACTORS AFFECTING STABILITY

Natural slopes in soil and rock are of interest to civil and mining engineers, engineering geologists, applied geomorphologists, soil scientists, and environmental managers.

The material composing any slope has a natural tendency to slide under the influence of gravitational and other forces (such as those due to tectonic stresses, seismic activity etc.) which are resisted by the shearing resistance of the material. Instability occurs when the shearing resistance is not enough to counterbalance the forces tending to cause movement along any surface within a slope. Natural slopes which have been stable for many years may suddenly fail due to one or more of the following main causes (which are also discussed in other appropriate sections of the book).

- External disturbance in the form of cutting or filling of parts of a slope or of ground adjacent to it resulting in an alteration of the balance between forces tending to cause instability and forces tending to resist it.
- External disturbance in the form of seismic activity (earth tremors or earthquakes).
- Infiltration of precipitation (rainfall, snow-melt) into the ground leads to decrease in shear strength in two ways depending on whether the soil mass is saturated or unsaturated (see chapter 2):

  - Increase of pore water pressures within a saturated soil slope (e.g., rise in water table).
  - Elimination of suction or negative pore water pressure in an unsaturated soil slope.

  The role of rainfall as a triggering factor for slope instability and landsliding is discussed further in section 1.9.5. Attention is given to flow of groundwater and seepage analyses in section 1.9.6.

  The proportion of precipitation (rainfall, snow-melt) which infiltrates into the ground can be vastly different in undisturbed areas with vegetation cover in comparison to deforested and disturbed areas. Thus, decrease in shear strength due to rainfall infiltration is highly influenced by significant changes in the surrounding areas such as deforestation, filling of valleys, disturbance of natural drainage characteristics, urbanization and construction of reservoirs.

  Of course, for a region with given characteristics, the greater the precipitation, the greater the infiltration and hence, greater the effect on soil strength and slope stability. Consequently exceptional rainstorms often lead to widespread landsliding, especially in deforested and disturbed regions.

- Excavation or cutting in a saturated, cohesive soil (soils with low permeability) causes negative excess (transient) pore water pressures as a consequence of this unloading process (see chapter 2 for the relevant concepts). Consequently, the shear strength and hence slope stability are increased in the short-term. As time passes, these transient negative pore water pressures dissipate. After years or decades (depending on the permeability), pore water pressures increase to equilibrium values. Consequently, shear strength and slope stability decrease and the slope may fail.

- Progressive decrease in shear strength of slope materials:
  This may be due to significant deformations which do not appear to constitute instability but lead to it. Such deformations may occur due to sustained gravitational forces and slope disturbances of intensity not high enough to cause

complete failure. Deformations often occur along major natural discontinuities, ancient slip surfaces and tectonic shear zones within a slope.

- Progressive change in the stress field within a slope:
Every natural geological formation has an 'initial' stress field which may be significantly different from the one considered in terms of the weight of the material alone. Initial lateral stress at any location may not have a simple or direct relationship with the vertical stress computed from gravitational considerations. The unique 'initial' stress field of any slope depends on its geological background and other natural factors. The stress history of slope materials is a very important factor. Attempts have been made in recent years to develop methods for the prediction of initial stresses in soils on the basis of laboratory tests. However, it is recognized that reliable information is best obtained from in-situ measurement in soil and rock. In some cases these measurements present considerable difficulties (Wroth, 1975).

A change in the initial stress field may also occur due to causes similar to those which produce a progressive decrease of shear strength. Release of stresses may accompany or follow most forms of slope disturbance. Often this leads to changes in both the magnitude and orientation of the stresses.

- Weathering:
It is now widely recognized that weathering may occur at a rate rapid enough to be of concern in the design of engineering works. Therefore, it is important to consider not only the existence of weathering which has occurred in the past but also the possibility of continued and even accelerated weathering. Weathering of soils and rocks destroys bonds and reduces shear strength. Bjerrum (1967) suggested that the weathering of shales and over-consolidated clays (clays which have experienced a higher overburden pressure in their past than their present overburden pressure) increases their recoverable strain energy and consequently their capacity for progressive failure. This occurs due to the destruction by weathering of diagenetic bonding in these materials. Weathering may be accelerated by slope disturbance and by exposure to atmospheric and other agencies such as stream action.

Differential weathering of interbedded weak and strong rocks often leads to instability. Rockfalls from vertical or sub-vertical cliffs occur without any warning as a consequence of such a long-term process of differential weathering.

Many failures of natural slopes are imperfectly understood and there may be other critical factors which influence the long-term stability of natural slopes. In rocks a slow and cumulative process of deterioration and destruction depending on climatic factors is always at work and thousands of years may elapse before a slope fails. According to Bjerrum and Jorstad (1968) the following factors are of primary importance in the time-dependent process leading to rock slides:

- The presence of a system of joints known as valley joints along which rock masses are often detached during slides.

The occurrence of large residual stresses in natural formations is well known and it is believed that valley joints are often formed by further stress changes and uneven deformations which occur during the formation of valleys. The release of strain energy stored due to large overburden in previous geological periods has thus an important role to play in the development of such joint systems. Each system at a particular depth is associated with a different stage of erosion in a rock mass.

The phenomena of valley stress relief and valley rebound and their geotechnical and geological implication have also been emphasized by Ferguson (1967, 1974), Matheson and Thomson (1973) and Matheson (1972).

- The presence of residual ground stresses which have still not been relieved during the formation of valley joint systems.
- The presence of water in open joints of rock masses which influences stability by exerting a direct outward force as well as by decreasing the effective stress and hence the shear strength on failure surfaces (refer to chapter 2 for discussion of the principle of effective stress in soil and rock).
- The fluctuation of water pressure in a joint system, causing cumulative opening of joints during periods of high water pressure following precipitation.

The wedging of crushed rock in joints often prevents them from returning to their original position after opening under high water pressures. Fatigue failure may also result due to fluctuations of pressure leading to further extension of open joints through intact rock. Thus gradually the proportion of a potential failure plane passing through jointed rock is increased to a critical value. At such a stage further decrease of the area of intact rock is no longer consistent with slope stability.

The foregoing remarks were made in the context of hard rock slopes. However, there are similar processes at work in soil slopes. The cumulative influence of natural processes on long-term stability can rarely be quantified. In many instances concerning both soil and rock slopes a significant level of uncertainty exists with regard to stability and this has been emphasized by Peck (1967, 1977).

- Existing slip surfaces or shear zones
  It is most important to draw a clear distinction between natural slopes with or without existing slip surfaces or shear zones. Knowledge of the existence of old slip surfaces makes it easier to understand or predict the behaviour of a slope. Such surfaces are often a result of previous landslide or tectonic activity. Morgenstern (1977) has emphasized that shearing surfaces may also be caused by other processes including valley rebound, glacial shove, periglacial phenomena such as solifluction and non-uniform swelling of clays and clay-shales. The shearing strength along surfaces produced by these phenomena is reduced to residual values (see chapter 2 for discussion of the concept of residual strength). It is not always easy to recognize landslide areas (while postglacial slides are readily identified, pre-glacial surfaces may lie buried beneath glacial sediments) or locate existing shear surfaces on which previous movements have occurred. However, once pre-sheared strata have been located, evaluation of stability can be made with confidence.

  There are two main reasons for this: (1) renewed movements in these slopes are likely to occur along existing slip surfaces and (2) residual strengths operative on such surfaces can be determined or inferred with greater certainty than shear strengths of unsheared, in-situ soils and rocks. On the other hand, evaluation of stability of slopes with no previous landslide activity and no existing shear surfaces is a far more difficult task.

1.7 BUILT SLOPES, UNREINFORCED AND REINFORCED

1.7.1 Unreinforced slopes

Built slopes may be considered in three main categories: (a) Excavations or cuts (b) Embankments, levees, earth dams and (c) Spoil or waste heaps.

1.7.1.1 Excavations or cuts

Shallow and deep cuts are of major interest in many civil and mining engineering operations. The aim is to design a slope with such a height and inclination as to be stable within a reasonable life span and with as much economy as possible. Such design is influenced by geological conditions, material properties, seepage pressures, the possibility of flooding and erosion, the method of construction as well as the purpose of a particular cutting. In open-cut or surface mining operations, excavations may be carried out in several steps or benches and the stability of individual benches must be ensured as well as that of the entire cut. Steep cuts may sometimes be necessary in many engineering applications so that preventive and protective measures are part of the initial design. In some situations the stability at the end of construction of a cutting may be critical. On the other hand many cut slopes are stable in the short-term but may fail without much warning many years later. The reasons for such failure have been given in the previous section concerning natural slopes. The most well known example is that of failures of cut slopes in London clay (Skempton 1964, 1970). (For a discussion of relevant concepts and case histories refer to chapters 2 and 5). Making cut slopes so flat that they are stable for an indefinite period of time would often be uneconomical and sometimes impractical. On the other hand, slopes which are too steep may remain stable for only a short time and pose real danger to life and property. Frequent failures would also involve tremendous inconvenience and the expense of repairs, maintenance and stabilisation measures.

1.7.1.2 Embankments, levees and earth dams

Fill slopes involving compacted soils include railway and highway embankments, earth dams and levees. The engineering properties of materials used in these structures are controlled by the method of construction and the degree of compaction. The analysis of an embankment, properly designed and constructed, does not generally involve the same difficulties and uncertainties as does the stability of a natural slope or an excavation. However, it is vitally important for earth structures to perform adequately during extreme natural events.

1.7.1.2.1 Example of levee failures in New Orleans

The catastrophic disaster in New Orleans, USA, following the landfall of Hurricane Katrina on August 29, 2005, was largely the consequence of inadequate design and performance of the levee system or the Hurricane Protection System (HPS). Reference has already been made to the scale of the disaster and to some of the important lessons to be learnt from it, based on comprehensive post-failure investigations. (Katrina, 2008).

Some failures of the New Orleans levees occurred as a result of erosion following overtopping. Thus the design height was inadequate for the storm surge and also there was no provision of an erosion protection system in the design of the HPS. Moreover, if there had been an erosion protection system, overtopping would have caused only one third of the flooding that occurred and the recovery efforts would have been executed more efficiently and completed much faster.

Other levee failures in New Orleans occurred even before overtopping because of poor construction materials, inadequate investigation, overestimation of shear strength, and failure mechanisms which had not been considered in the design. Six breaches of the flood protection system which occurred under the thrust due to water pressure from the storm surge, were investigated by Duncan et al. (2008). Four of these were not caused by overtopping but by one of the following factors:

Shear failure in weak foundation clay,
Internal or subsurface erosion, and
High pore water pressures combined with low friction angle of loose sand.

The flood protection system often consisted of the levee and an I-wall. As a result of the deflection of the I-wall during storm surge, a gap formed along the full length of the I-wall right to its base on the flood side. This gap had an important influence on the failure mechanism and also increased the lateral force on the wall significantly. It was found that the factor of safety decreased by a significant proportion when the gap was included in the limit equilibrium analyses (Brandon et al., 2008). In one case, the gap reduced the calculated factor of safety from 1.28 to 0.98 and in another case from 1.52 to 0.99. Both calculations were based on assumed slip surfaces of circular shape. Noncircular slip surface assumption gave similar location of critical slip surface to that of circular slip surface but the factor of safety was about 6% smaller.

1.7.1.2.2 *Analyses for different stages and observational approach*

For a built-up earth structure, independent analyses are required for the following critical conditions:

(i) end-of-construction (ii) long-term condition (iii) rapid draw-down (for water-retaining structures such as earth dams) and, (iv) seismic disturbance.

In recent years the advantages of an observational approach have been demonstrated and it is usual to monitor the performance of embankments and earth dams during and after construction (Peck, 1969; Casagrande, 1950). The construction of test sections of embankments is particularly useful for large projects.

It is often necessary to consider the stability of an embankment-foundation system rather than that of an embankment alone. In major projects it is often economically feasible to conduct comprehensive and detailed investigations of foundation conditions. However, in many cases embankments have to be built on weak foundations so that failures by sinking, spreading and piping (a phenomenon associated with internal soil erosion and its progression) can occur irrespective of the stability of embankment slopes. Terzaghi and Peck (1967) have given guidelines for assessing and ensuring stability against such failures.

1.7.1.2.3   Failure of Teton Dam

A well known example of a major slope failure due to piping and internal erosion is that of the Teton Dam, Idaho, USA on June 5, 1976 (US Dept. of Interior, 1977). Internal erosion and piping occurred in the core of the dam deep in the right foundation key trench, where a grout curtain had been installed to a certain depth. Soil particles moved through channels along the interface of the dam with the highly pervious abutment rock and talus. The volcanic rocks at the site were intensely fissured and water was able to move rapidly during reservoir filling. The wind-deposited clayey silts of very low permeability used for the core and key trench were found to be highly erodible. An independent review panel concluded that the use of this material adjacent to intensely jointed rock was a major factor in the failure. They also felt that the geometry of the key trenches favored arching which, in turn, resulted in the reduction of normal stresses and consequent development of cracks in the erodible fill. Cracking by hydraulic fracturing was considered to be another possibility since calculations showed that water pressure at the base of the key trench could have exceeded the sum of lateral stresses in the impervious fill and its tensile strength. Whatever the initial cause of cracking, it led to the opening of channels through the erodible fill. Once piping began it progressed rapidly through the main body of the dam leading to complete failure.

R.B. Peck, one of the experts on the review panel, commented as follows: "It is perhaps paradoxical that if, on the one hand, the grout curtain were not effective, failure would result directly from the under seepage, whereas, on the other hand, if the grout curtain were fully effective, failure would tend to develop as a result of hydraulic fracturing."

He concluded that the design lacked adequate defenses against several combinations of unfavorable circumstances, combinations of which were unfortunately not visualized or foreseen.

1.7.1.3   Spoil or waste heaps

The stability of spoil heaps consisting of mining and industrial waste is being recognized as a problem of major importance in view of (i) many disasters which have been a consequence of failures of spoil heaps, (ii) the growing magnitude of wastes requiring to be disposed in this manner, and (iii) the scarcity of adequate sites for waste dumps. Until 50 to 60 years ago spoil heaps had little or no compaction control and in many cases compaction was not even considered. Similarly there was little control on the composition of material of dumps. During the early 1970s, compaction was emphasized as part of the operations and considerable government regulatory control began to be exercised on refuse and mine waste piles, tailings dams and industrial waste disposal areas in USA, Canada, the U.K and some other developed countries. In many cases, there is now increasingly effective control on material composition and compaction. There are some instances in which particulate wastes may be uniform in composition and engineering properties. However, in general, the problems are somewhat different from those concerning embankments due to differences in methods of construction, uncertainties in geotechnical characteristics and foundation conditions which are often unfavorable. The solution of these problems is greatly complicated where there is inadequate control on composition, location and compaction of the refuse materials (see Blight, 1977).

Despite the progress in knowledge about the need for compaction of a built-up earth mass, poor construction practice may occur. As stated in section 1.2, significant lengths of the levees in New Orleans were constructed with locally available materials dredged from the excavation of shipping channels and comprised largely uncompacted soils of variable quality with poor resistance to erosion. Post-failure investigations led to the expected conclusion that levees made with roller compacted soils performed far better than hydraulic fill levees. There may be initial cost savings in adopting locally available materials but the cost penalties are huge when lack of adequate performance leads to failures with catastrophic losses (Katrina, 2008).

Where refuse materials are placed in a loose state, shear failure is often followed by 'static liquefaction' (complete loss of strength) with catastrophic consequences. Fortunately such occurrences are now rare because of increasing awareness leading to regulation and control. Initiation of instability is often a result of inadequate drainage in wet, saturated dumps. Failure may also occur due to overtopping caused by inadequate spillway capacity in tailings dams.

Bishop (1973) discussed the stability of tips and spoil heaps with special reference to his wide experience in the U.K. He pointed out that the failure of tips is controlled not only by the character of the tipped material but also by the mechanical properties of the natural strata on which tips are located. The brittleness of both natural and artificial material has a significant influence on whether failure is likely to be catastrophic or not (brittleness index and its significance are discussed in chapter 2). Unfavorable geological conditions (such as those in which high excess pore water pressures can develop within the natural strata due to loading by tips and spoil heaps) are significant in the development of extreme forms of movement e.g., flow slides. Materials of high brittleness index are especially liable to progressive failure (see chapter 2). An appreciation of the possibility of progressive failure is necessary for the safe design of spoil heaps. Particular care is required when waste dumps are located on sloping ground (such locations are sometimes unavoidable). In seismically active areas the stability of spoil heaps must be carefully evaluated for dynamic loading conditions.

1.7.2   Reinforced slopes

The stability of a slope can be improved by incorporating one or more layers of reinforcing elements at different elevations within the body of the slope. These elements may include materials such as steel strips, steel grids, geotextile fabrics, geogrids and high strength steel tendons. Applications include reinforced fill slopes, reinforced embankments on weak foundations, reinforced earth walls, use of soil nails and the use of anchors in soil and rock cuttings or natural slopes. Natural slopes may also be strengthened by incorporating reinforcing elements. The term 'reinforced soil' or 'reinforced earth' is often used to describe the composite structure made of a soil mass with reinforcing elements within it.

Basic concepts of geomechanics and probability presented in the following chapters (chapters 2 and 3) are applicable to reinforced soil as well as to unreinforced slopes. However, in order to use stability models such as limit equilibrium methods presented in chapters 4 and 5, additional terms representing reinforcing forces must be included in the equilibrium equations. By incorporating reinforcement, a slope with a desired level of stability can be built with a steeper inclination than is possible to achieve without reinforcement. Similarly an embankment on weak foundation can be built to a desired level of safety with a greater height with reinforcement at the base than is possible to achieve without such reinforcement. Detailed discussion of reinforced slopes including the mechanical properties of reinforcement materials and design guidelines can be found in specialist publications such as Koerner (1998) and FHWA (2000). Essential considerations in analysis include the tensile strength of reinforcing elements, their stiffness and their pull-out resistance. An important consideration in design is the durability of reinforcing elements over the design life of the structure. Thus, factors affecting corrosion of steel reinforcement must be identified and the rate of deterioration estimated. For geotextiles and geogrids, the effects of creep, long-term deterioration and installation damage have to be considered. Another application of geotextiles and geomembranes is the construction of liners for hazardous-waste landfills. For example, it is of interest to consider the components of the liner at the Kettleman Hills waste landfill, which failed by sliding on interfaces within the composite liner (Mitchell et al., 1990; Seed et al., 1990).The liner included three geomembranes, six geotextiles, three layers of granular fill and two layers of compacted clay.

1.8 GEOMORPHOLOGY AND SLOPES

Geomorphology is concerned with the nature and origin of landforms, with the study of processes of landform development and with material composition. The shape of the earth's surface is subject to significant change over time due to dynamic processes. These processes are a consequence of the interaction between the physical settings on the one hand and the forces and energy provided by external agents on the other. The rate of change can be highly variable in both its spatial and temporal aspects because of the variability of factors such as location, topography, geology, climate and the frequency and magnitude of the external events. Understanding of geomorphologic processes helps a geotechnical engineer to place site-specific geotechnical data in its proper context, to carry out better engineering analyses and to better evaluate hazard and risk. Different aspects of the role and benefits of geomorphology for engineers have been presented in a volume edited by Fookes et al. (2005) which has 27 chapters including those on landslides, soil erosion, coastal environments and urban geomorphology. A stage may not yet have been reached for engineering geomorphology to be considered as a discipline in itself. However; a book has recently been devoted to the subject (Fookes et al., 2007).

It has been estimated that over half of the world's population lives in urban areas and thus the adverse consequences of urbanisation are enormous in scope and global in their reach and spread. The process of urbanisation often alters geomorphologic processes and thus it is important to understand the nature of such changes.

Geomorphologists are concerned not only with types of processes but also with the rate and frequency of each process. For instance, in relation to slopes they are concerned with (i) transport-limited processes in which weathering rates are potentially more rapid than transport processes, resulting in development of thick soil cover and (ii) weathering-limited processes in which transport processes are potentially more rapid than weathering so that only a thin soil cover can develop. Traditionally, geomorphology has been theoretical in its aims. However, there is growing evidence of interest in 'applied' aspects of the subject among geomorphologists, engineering geologists and geotechnical experts. Applied geomorphology is concerned with contemporary processes and their influence on landforms and, as such, it also embraces the role of man in changing or altering the physical environment. An appreciation of geomorphology is useful in understanding the complex phenomena with many interacting factors which control landforms. It is also very useful in establishing a geological framework of sites for many aspects of geotechnical work.

A geomorphologist is concerned with the relationship of slope form to stability. Therefore, the parameters of significant interest include the inclination, length, curvature and aspect of natural slopes. Slopes similar in inclination, materials and geology may behave differently depending on their aspect which may control moisture, seepage and pore water pressures, Surface drainage patterns often directly reflect the nature of underlying soil or rock (Eckel, 1958).

Some workers have suggested a morphometric approach to the study of landslides (Crozier, 1973). This consists of defining a number of unique indices based on the form of a landslide. For example, the depth to length ratio may be a key factor in indicating the process responsible for a slide. Identification of landslide-prone situations and sites on the basis of (i) aerial photographs, (ii) land-systems mapping and (iii) geomorphological mapping is one of the most useful contributions geomorphology can make in practical problems involving slopes (Brunsden et al., 1975). Geomorphological mapping attempts to identify and classify slopes, recognise past and present processes and the relationship between form and processes occurring within the slope materials (i.e. soil and rock). The role of geomorphology in environmental management has been discussed with practical examples by Cooke and Doornkamp (1974). Carson and Kirkby (1972) have produced a work on slopes from a geomorphological view point.

While geomorphology is often important for understanding regional landslide susceptibility especially in urban areas, it may also be useful for site-specific assessments of slope stability and understanding of individual landslides. This is as true of ordinary failures of natural and man-made slopes as of exceptional failures such as the very large and catastrophic 1963 Vaiont (or Vajont) slide which has been the subject of many studies and is discussed in some detail in chapter 7. For example, Hendron and Patton (1985) carried out a reassessment of the geological, hydro-geological and geotechnical factors relevant to the 1963 Vaiont) slide. They came to the conclusion that the 1963 slide was the reactivation of an old slide which occurred probably in postglacial times. The evidence cited in support of this conclusion included many aspects of the surface morphology such as enclosed depressions, bulging slopes, altered drainage, and related patterns seen on air photos. In combination with geological features mapped by other geotechnical investigators before and after the 1963 landslide, surface morphology was also cited as evidence for the conclusion that most of this huge slide moved as a single unit.

1.9 TYPES OF SLOPE MOVEMENT AND LANDSLIDES

1.9.1 Processes and types of slope movement

1.9.1.1 Introduction

Many classifications of landslides have been given e.g., Eckel (1958), Varnes (1958), Zaruba and Mencl (1969), Varnes (1978) and Cruden and Varnes (1996). There are several basic types of slope movement. In general, it is important to distinguish among three basic types: 'slides', 'falls' and 'flows' (see Figure 1.1). There are other types of movement such as 'spreads' and also combined and complex landslides which include more than one of the basic types mentioned above.

Within each category or type of landslide, movement can be and often is extremely rapid, although some slides occur very slowly. Rates of movement range from extremely slow to extremely rapid. Varnes (1978) suggested 60 mm/year as the demarcation between extremely slow and very slow movements and 3 m/second as the demarcation between very rapid and extremely rapid movement. Cruden and Varnes (1996) proposed 5 mm/sec as the demarcation between very rapid and extremely rapid movement and 16 mm per year as the demarcation between very slow and extremely slow movement. The probable destructive significance of landslides was proposed by considering 7 classes of velocity. At one extreme, extremely rapid movement (velocity class 7) is likely to cause catastrophic damage and many deaths and, at the other extreme, extremely slow movement (velocity class 1) would be imperceptible without instruments and construction on such a landslide site might be permissible with precautions. Even for landslides with velocity class 2 (very slow movement), some permanent structures might remain undamaged by movement.

In their Table 3.6, Cruden and Varnes (1996) summarise the estimated landslide velocities of 16 historical landslides from 1932 to 1970. At one extreme, are the Elm and Goldau landslides which caused 115 and 457 deaths respectively (estimated velocity 70 mm/sec for both, velocity class 7) At the other extreme is the Fort Peck Spillway slide which caused no deaths but required flattening of slopes (estimated velocity 0.02 m/year, velocity class 2).

The effects, occurrence and mechanisms of catastrophic landslides over the last century have been discussed in Evans and Degraff (2002).

1.9.1.2 Landslide mechanisms and activity

Slides involve shear failure and may be translational or rotational in character (or a combination of rotation and translation). Translational slides often involve movement along marked discontinuities or planes of weakness. Rotational slips have a failure surface which is concave upwards and occur in both soil and rock formations. The reactivation of existing slides must be distinguished from new or first-time slides. Existing landslide sites may be dormant or active and the frequency of reactivation may vary greatly from one slide to another in the same region. Cruden and Varnes (1996) refer to the following states of activity: active, suspended, reactivated, dormant, stabilized and relict. They also refer to different distributions of activity and different styles of activity.

Falls are confined to surface zones in soil (soil falls) or rock (rock falls) and are preceded by the formation and enlargement of cracks and removal of base support of individual blocks or masses. Rockfalls may be caused by frost shattering, chemical decomposition, temperature variations, the wedging effect of roots and water pressure. Toppling failures of rock are common in situations where the vertical line through the centre of gravity of individual blocks (which have lost lateral support) falls outside of their respective bases (Figure 1.1).

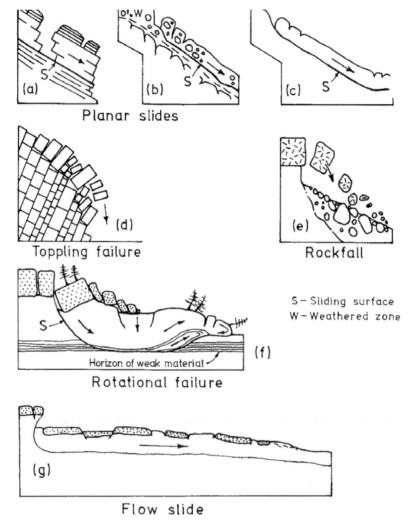

Figure 1.1   Types of slope movement (after Blyth and de Freitas, 1974). Permission requested, see page 714, No 45.

Depending on the relative orientation of a slope and its discontinuities, failures may involve detachment of small or large wedges in rock, so that failure is essentially three-dimensional in character. On the other hand, movement along only one main discontinuity gives a two-dimensional, slab-type failure. Flows range from slow to extremely rapid and occur mostly in unconsolidated materials. Varnes (1958) mentions the following types of flow:

(i) rock fragment flows (ii) sand run (iii) loess flow (iv) sand or silt flow (v) slow earth flow (vi) rapid earth flow (vii) debris avalanche and (viii) debris flow.

1.9.1.3   Very slow movements including creep

Slopes also undergo creep movements which are often so slow as to be imperceptible (e.g., 0.1 cm to few cms per year). Distinction must be drawn between surface creep of a seasonal nature and continuous or depth creep. Continuous creep occurs under the action of low shear stresses and may continue for long periods without resulting in failure. Many slides occur as a result of the acceleration of creep movements which have been going on for a long time (sometimes many years). Thus continuous or depth-creep may be part of a process of progressive failure. Continuous creep is more common in argillaceous (clayey) soils and rocks than in granular soils and harder rocks.

Solifluction movements occur in periglacial areas due to annual freeze-thaw processes. Such movements are a form of seasonal creep and their influence generally extends only to shallow depths. In certain areas there may be no present-day periglacial activity but such processes may have occurred in the past. Previous periglacial activity is often evidenced by zones and surfaces of weakness in a soil mass which are re-activated by any form of development or disturbance. These surfaces may be located at significant depths below the present-day ground surface. Geotechnical aspects of periglacial features in Britain have been discussed by Weeks (1969), and Higginbottom and Fookes (1970).

1.9.1.4   Progressive and retrogressive slides

Finally it is important to point out again that slope, movement and landsliding is a continued process and often multiple as well as complex landslides occur. For example, the development of a slide into a slide-flow is quite common. Similarly, some rockfalls may develop into flows or avalanches. Depending on the geological setting, the nature of materials involved and the triggering factors, there can be many types and mechanisms of failure and thus many complex landslide types.

For example, considering just clay slopes, Skempton and Hutchinson (1969) have suggested a classification of (a) basic types of mass movement shown here in Figure 1.2 and (b) multiple and complex landslides shown here in Figure 1.3.

The diagrams in Figure 1.3 indicate that landslide occurrence in clays often includes processes of progression and retrogression of the landslide mass. Such processes may also occur when landslides occur in other types of soil or in rock. Many examples of rock falls, slides and avalanches have been provided by different contributors to the volume on catastrophic landslides edited by Evans and Degraff (2002).

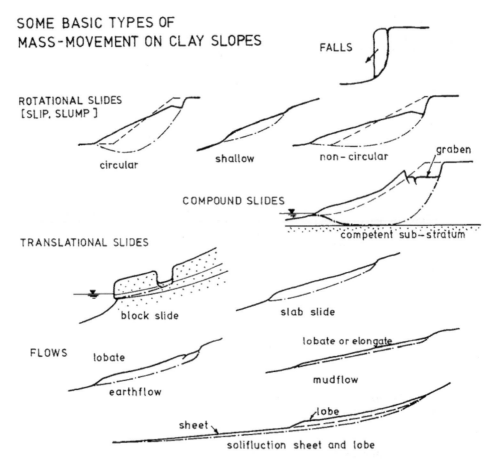

SOME BASIC TYPES OF MASS-MOVEMENT ON CLAY SLOPES

FALLS

ROTATIONAL SLIDES
[SLIP, SLUMP]

circular   shallow   non-circular   graben

COMPOUND SLIDES

TRANSLATIONAL SLIDES

competent sub-stratum

block slide   slab slide

FLOWS   lobate

lobate or elongate

mudflow

earthflow

lobe

sheet

solifluction sheet and lobe

Figure 1.2 Types of movement in clay slopes (after Skempton and Hutchinson, 1969). With permission, see page 713, No 1.

1.9.1.5   *Examples of landsliding in the study area of chapter 11*

Seven photos are included in the Appendix to this chapter in order to illustrate the main landslide types triggered by rainfall in the Illawarra region of the state of New South Wales, Australia. Urban landsliding in this region is discussed in chapter 11 of this book. In that chapter, the reader will find brief descriptions of regional setting, topography and geology. The contents of chapter 11 also include landslide occurrence, analysis and the monitoring of rainfall, subsurface movement and pore water pressure. Modeling of landslide susceptibility and hazard are also outlined briefly.

Referring to the photos in the Appendix to this chapter, brief information follows. The approximate landslide volumes are sourced from the landslide inventory for this study area (see chapter11).

Figure C1.1 is an example of a slide in fill and colluvium along a suburban road (approx. volume 7900 cubic meters). The occurrence of this type of landslide after significant magnitude of rainfall may be considered relatively frequent* in this region.

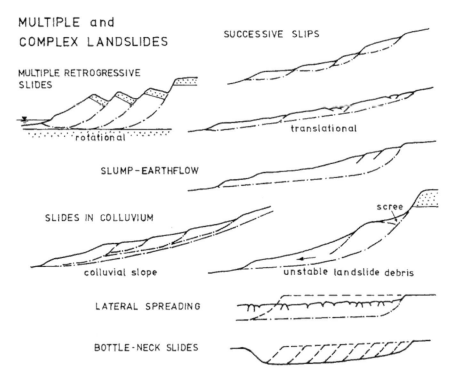

MULTIPLE and
COMPLEX LANDSLIDES

SUCCESSIVE SLIPS

MULTIPLE RETROGRESSIVE
SLIDES

rotational

translational

SLUMP-EARTHFLOW

SLIDES IN COLLUVIUM

scree

colluvial slope

unstable landslide debris

LATERAL SPREADING

BOTTLE-NECK SLIDES

Figure 1.3 Types of movement in clay slopes (after Skempton and Hutchinson, 1969). With permission, see page 713, No 1.

Figure C1.2 is an example of a complex slide-flow which occurred after very high rainfall, over a 4-day period, in August 1998 (approx. volume 14,300 cubic meters). The occurrence of this type of landslide is relatively infrequent* in this region.

Significant details concerning the August 1998 rainfall event are presented in chapter 11. The reader will find references to magnitude of rainfall, its variation over the four day period and to spatial distribution of rainfall over a particular duration.

Figure C1.3 is an aerial photograph of a railway embankment failure in 1988 at Coledale which developed into a slide and then transformed into a flow, demolishing a house and killing two persons. (approx. volume 25,200 cubic meters). This event was also triggered by very high rainfall and may be considered as relatively infrequent* in this region.

There has been reference to several contributing factors to this tragedy such as deficiencies in construction, maintenance and management of the railway embankment (Davies and Christie, 1996).

---

* Accurate estimates of the frequency of different landslide types are difficult to make. The qualitative terms used here such as "relatively frequent", "relatively infrequent" and "relatively rare" in the context of this region are based on limited experience and data.

Figure C1.4 is an aerial photograph of the rock fall at Dombarton (approx. volume 80,000 cubic meters). This site had a history of rock fall occurrence preceding this large event. Moreover; underground coal mining had been carried out for many decades, at relatively shallow depths, in the vicinity of the site. Thus mining activity could have been one of the contributing factors to the development of the rock fall or as a final trigger for its occurrence. Such a large rock fall is a relatively rare* event in the region and is the culmination of loss of cliff stability over a period of decades.

Figure C1.5 is an example of a rock fall triggered by heavy rainfall (approx. volume 6,000 cubic meters). This type of rock fall is more frequent than the major rock fall at Dombarton.

Figure C1.6 shows a hazardous section of the coast road (Lawrence Hargrave Drive) subject to rockfalls, slides and flows, all types triggered generally by rainfall. After a number of geotechnical risk studies, this hazardous section of road was considered to represent unacceptably high risk to road users (persons travelling by car or other vehicles).

Thus the road was closed for a couple of years and a number of alternatives were considered for reducing the magnitude of risk to human safety to an acceptable level. Continuation of a number of remedial measures, some already carried out over many years, were estimated to reduce the risk significantly but not to acceptable levels. Thus, a decision was made to construct a by-pass bridge which can be seen under construction in this photo.

Figure C1.7 shows the same site after the bridge was completed. The bridge was named "Sea Cliff Bridge".

The photo on the cover of this book shows a view of this section of road before the construction of Sea Cliff Bridge.

1.9.2   Pre-failure and post-failure movements

Pre-failure movements are of considerable interest and may give a warning of impending danger. Consequently, observations of such movements are often very valuable as indicated by Wilson (1970). Magnitude of movements depends on the thickness of soil or rock involved. Movements may be hardly noticeable for thin soil layers but quite large for deep masses. Saito (1965) has suggested that pre-failure movements may be used to estimate the time to failure on an empirical basis. Broadbent and Ko (1972) studied rheological aspects of rock slope behaviour and found that (i) movements are usually initiated by a temporary excess in external forces (ii) velocity of movement decays if this excess is eliminated (iii) repeated applications of an impulse cause successive increases in velocity and displacement (iv) displacement is a function of the failure surface characteristics (v) empirical rules can be devised to formulate action concerning control and prevention of active slope failure. Rock slope performance has also been discussed by others in Cording (1972).

---

* Accurate estimates of the frequency of different landslide types are difficult to make. The qualitative terms used here such as "relatively frequent", "relatively infrequent" and "relatively rare" in the context of this region are based on limited experience and data.

Movements during failure depend not only on the nature and extent of slope materials involved but also on the shape of the slip surface. The manner in which the shear strength varies with strain and displacement is extremely important in this regard. For brittle materials, in which there is a sudden drop of strength after the peak value has been reached, considerable acceleration of movements can occur. In some materials such as extra-sensitive or 'quick' clays, remolding results in almost complete loss of strength and consequently speeds of movement are very large. There are other factors which may control the speed of landslides. For instance, the transformation of a slope from a high initial stress field to a state of limit equilibrium may have a strong influence on whether the movement is accelerated or stabilised. This subject is discussed in considerable detail in chapter 7 and the concepts developed are successfully used to explain the well known Vaiont slide of 1963 in the same chapter.

Post-failure movements often occur on existing slip surfaces at rates which may be regarded as low to moderate. These movements may be caused by changes in pore water pressure or due to any external disturbance. In some soils the movement during initial failure is such as to bring the slipped mass into a position of relative stability and there may be no post-failure movements. Mudflow movements may occur where the initial slide has remolded the soil or rock into a broken and softened mass. These movements are therefore faster than post-failure movements of landslides in general.

1.9.3   Failures of slopes in poorly compacted fill

The occurrence of failures in slopes comprising loosely deposited fill is neither surprising nor uncommon. Sometimes the consequences of poorly compacted fills can be catastrophic. As a relatively recent example, one may consider the levee failures in New Orleans after the landfall of Hurricane Katrina in August 2005. As pointed out in sections 1.2 and 1.7, an important contributing factor to some of these failures of the levee system was the use of hydraulic fill in their construction. Levees built in this manner were largely uncompacted (Katrina, 2008).

Uncompacted soil structures perform poorly because their shear strength is low and its value decreases further as pore pressures rise after rainfall. A relatively low degree of compaction of saturated fill has another important consequence once shear failure starts. The loose, saturated fill then tends to contract. However, drainage cannot occur in the short-term. Thus the tendency to contract results in further increase of pore water pressures. Consequently, the combination of low degree of compaction, saturation and deformation associated with initiation of shear failure has a considerable influence on the speed of movement of such slope failures which can reach high magnitudes with catastrophic consequences. The term 'static liquefaction' is often used to describe the complete loss of soil shear strength under these circumstances.

An example of high speed of fill slope movements is the failure of fill slopes at Sau Mau Ping, Hong Kong in 1976, which resulted in the loss of many lives (Govt. of Hong Kong, 1977). Failures in natural and artificial slopes in Hong Kong often occur during periods of heavy rainfall when a seepage condition develops in these slopes to varying depths. At Sau Mau Ping, investigations by an expert panel revealed that the wetted surface layers of the fill were in a loose condition and had not been properly compacted. Tests showed that the material had low shear strength with a tendency to decrease in volume during shear. This tendency for volume decrease under undrained conditions led to increased pore water pressures after initial failure, thus reducing strength to such an extent that the material was liquefied. The resulting mud avalanche occurred with considerable speed. The subject of pore water pressure, its influence on shear strength, its variation during loading and unloading, i.e., the generation of 'excess pore water pressures', is discussed in chapter 2.

The causative mechanism of rainfall-induced failures in slopes of loosely compacted fill, derived from completely decomposed granite in Hong Kong, have been further explored by Chen et al. (2004). They do acknowledge that, as far back as 1977, 'static liquefaction' was considered to be the process involved in such slope failures where the soil mass moves rapidly as a flow. However, their recent research suggests that these fill slopes are largely unsaturated and that suction contributes to their shear strength (see chapter 2). Rainfall infiltration reduces soil suction and thus the shear strength. If this reduction in shear strength is sufficiently large, it can become the triggering factor in initiating slope instability. Yet the consequent stages of excess pore pressure development, occurrence of static liquefaction and the acceleration of the speed of movement can only be explained on the basis of a fully saturated soil mass. Only in a saturated soil mass would excess pore pressures be generated during the early stages of shear failure under undrained conditions. Further research must establish precisely how, during rainfall infiltration, an unsaturated soil mass is converted into a fully saturated one. The authors have not elaborated on this process. However, they have discussed the practical implications of the mechanism of failure for the upgrading and repair of fill slopes in Hong Kong.

Slope stability issues including mechanism of rainfall-induced failure of soil slopes have also been explored by Collins and Znidarcic (2004). The effects of both negative and positive pore water pressures on the stability of initially unsaturated slopes were considered and a method developed for predicting the change in the factor of safety. The results included the time and depth of failure in relation to soil slope and rainfall data. A case study from Santa Cruz (California, USA) was studied as part of the research.

1.9.4   Some observed data concerning magnitude of movements in soil and rock slopes

Skempton and Hutchinson (1969) have compiled available data on pre-failure movements in clay slopes observed over periods of up to 7 years. Reported movements vary in magnitude from 35 cms to 250 cms and in rate from 2 cm/year to 30 cm/day. Examples of post-failure movements with average velocities up to 600 cm/year and maximum velocities up to 6 cm/day were given for slopes of inclination varying from 7.5° to 13°. Mudflow movements with average velocities from 5 m/year to 25 m/year and maximum velocities from 25 cm/day to 50 cm/day were noted for slopes of inclination 7.5°–9°, the period of observation being 1 to 20 years. Hamel (1972) reported very slow movements before a rock slide occurred due to increased water pressure resulting from freezing and blocking of natural drainage channels in a slope. The crack at the rear of the rock slide took several years to develop but failure, when triggered by water pressure, occurred suddenly. Post-failure movements along existing shear surfaces may not occur in the same directions as the original movements.

This is important because there is likely to be potential for faster movement oblique to previous direction of movement. (The sliding mass may have reached a position of comparative stability in the previous direction of movement so that potential for further movement is not high in that direction). Hamel (1976) reported movements which occurred oblique to the direction of previous shearing.

Hamel (1973a) reported different magnitudes of movement in the Bearpaw clay shale slopes adjacent to Fort Peck Dam Powerhouse in Montana, USA. Rates of movement varying from 6 to 60 cms/year are characteristic of creep-type movements of old slide masses. Short term movements of old slide masses, which have been slightly disturbed, range from 60 to 300 cms/year. High movement rates of up to 30 cms/day are characteristic of initial failures or re-activated slides following a major disturbance such as rise in pore water pressures or excavation. When the factor of safety along an existing slip surface is even slightly higher than one, movement rates are small. As the magnitude factor of safety falls below one, even small changes in its value can lead to large movements.

1.9.5   Rainfall as a triggering factor for slope failures or for the occurrence of landslides

A soil or rock mass often contains water within its pores spaces between solid particles or within the discontinuities such as joints and faults. This water may be flowing or static. The magnitude of pore water pressure may be determined by the static or seepage conditions unless it is held under artesian conditions when the magnitude may be higher than that based on either of the other two conditions. In many parts of the world, rainfall is an important source of groundwater and of the water that flows through slopes and especially natural slopes. (Other forms of precipitation such as snowmelt also contribute to groundwater flow and to seepage through slopes in some areas of the world). Consequently, pore water pressure within a slope may increase when rainfall magnitudes are relatively high and decrease when rainfall magnitudes are relatively low. The rate of increase or decrease of rainfall-induced pore pressures is controlled by the permeability of a soil or rock mass. The coefficient of permeability of different soils and rocks can vary vastly by several orders of magnitude. Moreover, a slope and adjacent soil mass may be comprised of layers with very different coefficients of permeability.

For water-retaining earth structures or earth dams, the seepage of water in relation to the reservoir level is often a more important consideration than the seepage of water from rainfall. However, 'mounding' of the top seepage line in an earth dam may occur after heavy rainfall as briefly discussed in the next sub-section.

According to the principle of effective stress, discussed in chapter 2, high pore water pressure within a slope means lower shear strength. Moreover, as will be clear from chapters 4 and 5, decreased shear strength means decreased stability. Consequently, if rainfall magnitudes affecting a slope are high enough, the slope may fail. The extent of slope movement at a particular site, the extent and volume of material involved and the speed of failure depend on many factors. It is important to note that many slope failures or landslides can occur in a given region after very high magnitude rainfall (an exceptional rainfall event). One such event, the August 1998 event (Flentje and Chowdhury, 1999), occurred in the Illawarra region of the State of

New South Wales, Australia and some details are given in Chapter 11 of this book. In order to analyse a rainfall event and assess its significance it is important to consider antecedent rainfall magnitudes for different periods before any particular date. For example, an antecedent period of one week may be significant for one region while an antecedent period of one month or more may be significant for another region. Moreover, shallow debris-flows are often triggered by intense rainstorms of short duration whereas deep-seated landslides are triggered by antecedent rainfall (high cumulative rainfall) over days or weeks often combined with intense rainfall over a much shorter period.

It is important to determine the return periods associated with different rainfall magnitudes in order to assess the hazard of landsliding. The estimation of rainfall magnitude which will lead to landsliding is often called 'rainfall threshold'. In order to investigate the rainfall thresholds for landsliding, it is useful to plot rainfall intensity against rainfall duration. Combinations of these two parameters associated with landslide occurrence or recurrence can be used to establish a threshold envelope. An example has been discussed by Flentje and Chowdhury (2001) and comparison made to published correlations as well. The spatial variation of rainfall during a rainstorm is also of significant interest in understanding landslide distribution within a region. One such exercise, carried out in detail for an exceptional rainfall event, has been reported by Murray (2001) and Flentje and Chowdhury (2001).

Rainfall thresholds may be used for developing landslide alert or warning systems based on weather information in general and rainfall magnitudes in particular. Uncertainties associated with such thresholds must be recognized even for the specific regions for which they were developed. Such uncertainties are unavoidable because it is seldom possible to have reliable data for all the landslide occurrences in a region and for all the landslide-triggering rainfall events. Then there are uncertainties associated with a particular method of analysis. Different methods of analyzing rainfall, assessing landslide triggering thresholds, real-time monitoring or alert or warning systems have been discussed in a number of papers over the last two decades and these include Aleotti and Chowdhury (1999), Ko Ko et al. (2003), Dai and Lee (2003), Aleotti (2004), Chien-Yuan et al. (2005), Flentje and Chowdhury (2002; 2005a,b), Walker (2007), Guzzeti et al. (2007) and Bunce (2008).

A review of several approaches and methods used worldwide to study the analysis of rainfall in relation to landsliding has been made by Bunce (2008). His focus was on the estimation of landslide risk to railways. For one of his case studies, the Maple Ridge site, he concluded that a precipitation induced landslide warning system and a hazard detection system would reduce the probability of a fatality by 39% and 80% respectively. In the Wollongong area of New South Wales Australia, an alert during a major rainstorm in August 1998 proved successful and useful in mitigating risk. The alert was based on a careful assessment of rainfall magnitudes over the first few days of the rainstorm event.

For geotechnical slope analysis of individual slopes and landslide sites, it is necessary to assess the pore water pressures within the slope and this can only be done by seepage analysis or subsurface measurement and monitoring or both. Consequently, seepage analysis is a very important aspect of geotechnical engineering in general and slope engineering in particular. While modeling and analysis based on assumption of steady seepage (time-independent seepage) through a saturated medium may suffice in most cases, more advanced modeling and solutions are required for assessing the conditions within unsaturated soils during rainfall infiltration. The main differences in the mechanical behavior of saturated and unsaturated soils are explored briefly in Chapter 2. However, detailed coverage of unsaturated soil mechanics is outside the scope of this book. Details of subsurface instrumentation and monitoring are outside the scope of this book. However, the use of data from such monitoring and the advantages of both periodic and continuous (real-time) monitoring are briefly outlined in respect of one region in Chapter 11 of this book.

Availability of simple and advanced seepage solutions is discussed below. The coverage of the vast subject of seepage modeling and the development of seepage solutions is outside the scope of this book. However, the simplest seepage solutions and their use in stability analysis of slopes are presented in Chapter 4. Moreover, a detailed new solution is proposed for the draw-down condition which is so important for water-retaining structures such as earth dams.

1.9.6 Available methods for seepage analysis

The determination of pore water pressures is facilitated by the theory of seepage based on Darcy's law of flow which proposes a linear relationship between velocity of flow and hydraulic gradient. Closed-form, numerical and graphical solutions have been developed for seepage problems and reference may be made to books such as Harr (1962), Cedergren (1967), Lambe and Whitman (1969) for solutions of practical use. The graphical flow-net approach is often very valuable in practical applications concerning slopes. Harr (1977) has demonstrated the solution of seepage problems on the basis of theory of probability. Anisotropy and non-homogeneity of a medium with respect to permeability can be tackled by both numerical and graphical methods based on seepage theory. Some closed-form solutions to such problems are also available. Such solutions are often valuable in providing a means of checking approximate solutions.

Sophisticated numerical methods such as the finite-element method (FEM) have been developed over the last 40 years to solve a variety of engineering problems including those concerned with stress-deformation and seepage in soil and rock masses. Even complex problems of groundwater flow under two-dimensional and three-dimensional conditions can be analyzed by such versatile methods. Applications include both confined and unconfined flow such as seepage through and beneath earth and rock fill dams. Both steady seepage and unsteady or transient seepage through slopes can be analyzed by these methods.

The assumption of a saturated soil or rock medium is common in most analytical and numerical solutions for seepage. However, unsaturated soils are found in many parts of the world. For example, many rainfall-triggered landslides occur in the unsaturated tropical soils of Hong Kong. For unsaturated soils, it is incorrect to analyze seepage on the basis of a steady state model or to make the assumption of a fully saturated soil or rock medium. However, advanced numerical methods like FEM facilitate the solution of different types of problems involving unsteady seepage. The infiltration of rainfall through unsaturated soil is just one type of unsteady seepage.

While seepage through natural slopes reduces the stability of natural slopes and such reductions are routinely considered in geotechnical analyses, rainfall effects on built-up slopes like earth dams may receive much less attention. This is because prominence is rightly given to pore water pressures associated with (i) seepage of reservoir water from the upstream face of a dam to its downstream face, and (ii) rapid drawdown of water below the reservoir-full condition to lower levels.

However, rainwater infiltration may cause the top seepage line (phreatic surface) to rise or 'mound' provided the rainfall intensity, frequency and duration are sufficient. This mounding will then reduce the safety of the dam .The problem of 'mounding' is one of transient seepage and an approximate solution has been proposed by Schmertmann (2006) who has concluded from his investigations that significant reductions in slope stability can occur as a result of mounding. He claims that in exceptional circumstances, mounding can reduce the stability of an earth dam slope by as much as 50%.

Seepage forces at different points are directly proportional to respective pressure gradients which may also be determined from seepage solutions. The direction and magnitude of seepage forces is of obvious importance in problems of slope stability. Further, their role in possible failures of embankments and dams due to internal erosion and piping cannot be over-emphasised. Pore water pressures and adversely directed seepage pressures, in natural slopes, excavations, embankments and fills, can be relieved by adequate drainage measures. In the foundations of dams, undesirable seepage can be reduced by key trenches, grout curtains etc.

1.10   GEOLOGY AND SLOPES

Understanding of the geology of a region is of paramount importance in tackling problems concerning slopes and slope development. Local geological details often have a considerable influence on the performance of individual slopes. The reader would have encountered several references to such factors in the previous sections of this chapter. Thus slope stability evaluation is often an inter-disciplinary endeavour requiring concepts and expertise from engineering geology, soil mechanics and rock mechanics. In order to be successful any method of analysis must give due consideration to significant geological features. Awareness of geology is necessary for appropriate idealisation of ground conditions and the development of realistic geotechnical models. Adequate engineering-geological information facilitates the choice of a suitable method of analysis. For instance, geological complexities of a site may dictate that sophisticated methods of analysis are used only after a thorough and detailed site investigation. If it is not economically feasible to conduct such investigations, simple methods of analysis only should suffice. The results of analysis may be evaluated in the light of geotechnical as well as engineering-geological experience and precedent in the area. On the other hand, if geological conditions are uniform, refined analytical methods may be justified after a routine though reliable investigation and testing programme. Indeed if (in the latter case) resources are limited, simple methods of analyses may be used with confidence with only occasional checks on the basis of more accurate methods. Geologic awareness is also of great value in planning site investigation and testing programmes. The role of geology in relation to slope stability has been emphasised, among many others, by Terzaghi (1950), Terzaghi and Peck (1967), Zaruba and Mencl (1969), Eckel (1958), Deere and Patton (1971) Terzaghi et al. (1996), Turner and Scuster (1996), Evans and Degraff (2002), Fookes et al. (2005, 2007).

Basic concepts concerning geological materials (i.e. soil and rock) are discussed subsequently. In this section attention is restricted to aspects like fabric, geological structure, ground water, in-situ stresses etc.

1.10.1   Fabric

Discontinuities in geological materials may range in size from microscopic mineral fabric to major joints and bedding planes. Mineral fabric many be well developed in some rocks to be influential in their engineering characteristics. For example the fabric of schists, slates and laminated clays results in marked anisotropy in their strength and deformation behaviour. In some cases, the delicacy of mineral fabric may result in almost complete loss of strength on disturbance. Such behaviour has been observed in Scandinavian and Canadian extra-sensitive or 'quick' clays. Both micro and macro fabric are often important and it is useful to have details of mineral orientation, stratification, fracture, shear zones, joints and faults. It is usually for the expert engineering-geologist to determine which features are of primary or secondary importance in a given situation. To some extent the importance of different features also depends on the size of the area being studied.

1.10.2   Geological structure

Structure plays a dominant role in the behaviour of slopes and is, therefore, of primary importance to engineering geologists and geotechnical engineers. In sedimentary rocks, the succession, thickness and attitude of beds are of direct relevance to considerations of potential instability. These features also help in understanding slope development processes, formation of valleys, ridges, escarpments and the development of residual and colluvial soils. Other major and minor structural features such as folds, faults and joints must always be carefully studied and mapped. For general discussions of geological structure and its engineering significance the reader may consult books on engineering geology e.g., Blyth and de Freitas (1974), Attewell and Farmer (1976). For slope studies, recognition of the following is of paramount interest:

1   Sequences of weak and strong beds (interbedded weak and strong layers):
    Weak rocks like clay-shales and clay-stones are often critical in the development of slope instability.
2   Thin marker beds such as coal and clay seams and carbonaceous shale:
    These beds are often missed in routine investigations. Their presence is useful in establishing stratigraphic correlations and in determining the extent of previous tectonic and landslide activity.
3   Old failure surfaces or shear zones:
    The critical importance of these zones and the processes which are responsible for their formation have been discussed in section 1.6. The fact that shear strength along such surfaces is reduced to a low residual value due to large deformations must always be borne in mind.

Folds are a consequence of the bending of earth's crust and may vary in size from microscopic to very large extending over miles. The strata are called competent if they behave in a brittle manner during folding and incompetent if they deform by ductile flow. Faults frequently occur in rocks as fractures are developed due to a relief of accumulated stresses. Stress relief results in relative displacement of the two sides of a fracture. Joints are formed due to similar causes but do not involve relative displacement. There is a wide variation in the size, spacing and extent of joints in rock. Reference to typical spacings is made in section 1.12 (see Table 1.5). The formation of valleys often results in compression faults in valley bottoms and tension fractures in valley walls. These effects are marked in sedimentary rocks of variable hardness as discussed by Ferguson (1967, 1974) who noted that in the Allegheney Plateau the fractures in valley walls were near vertical and parallel to the strike. Horizontal movement of valley walls produced compression forces within the valley bottoms causing failure in the form of arching, thrust faulting and formation of bedding plane faults and mylonite zones. The phenomenon has also been studied by Deere and Patton (1971).

1.10.3 Geological structure and tendency of slope movement

It is easy to show with a simple calculation that a steep hard rock slope can be stable with a height of thousands of feet if it is free of discontinuities, even if the lowest realistic value is chosen for rock strength. This was done by Terzaghi (1962) who emphasised the importance of discontinuities, water pressure in discontinuities and water seepage forces within a rock mass. Assuming that there are no seepage forces, the orientation of a slope with respect to significant discontinuities influences the possibility of relative movement and the manner in which it may occur. Figure. 1.4 shows possible relationships between joint planes in bedrock and slope stability as discussed by Terzaghi (1962). The figure shows relationship of the critical slope angle to the angle of dip of the main joint plane and the angle of friction along the joints. The relationship is shown when there is one set of joints as well as when there are two sets of joints. The angle of friction along discontinuities (such as joints) depends on a number of factors such as roughness, waviness and continuity of joints, weathering products filling the discontinuities and their mechanical properties. Gouge material may separate two rock surfaces and the strength of a gouge-rock interface may sometimes be lower than that of the gouge material itself. The degree to which gouge or infilling material controls stability depends on its thickness and extent and on the proportion of the slip surface which passes through it. The strength of gouge-filled discontinuities has been discussed by many workers in recent years as summarised in several papers by Barton (1973, 1974 and 1976).

The effect of structure on the slope stability of an excavation in uniformly dipping strata as discussed by Blyth and de Freitas (1974) is shown in Figure 1.5. The excavation is parallel to the strike of the strata with tendency of movement along their dip and along one set of joint surfaces (the other set is vertical).

The two slopes of the cutting have different stability. If the axis of the slope were located differently, failure by detachment of wedges would be likely as shown for section across CD. In the latter case a different overall stability angle would result.

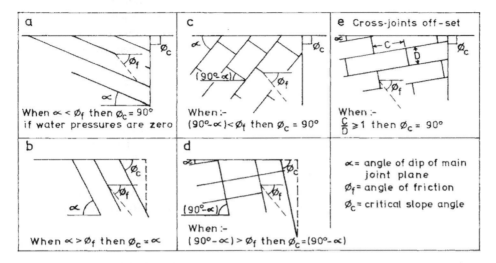

Figure 1.4 Effect of structure on rock slope stability. Relationship between joint planes and critical slope angle (after Cooke and Doornkamp, 1974) (based on Terzaghi, 1962). With permission, see page 713, No 2.

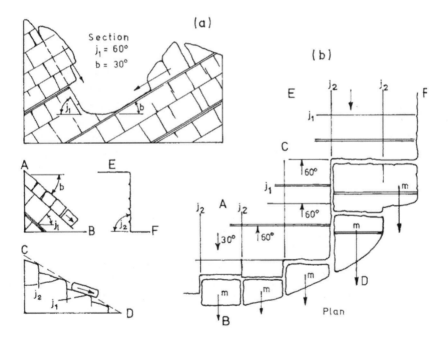

Figure 1.5 Effect of structure on stability showing j_1, j_2 – joint sets, b – bedding, m – blocks sliding into cutting (after Blyth and de Freites, 1974). Permission requested, see page 714, No 45.

Structure has also a direct influence on the possibility of the occurrence of rock-falls and toppling failures (Figure 1.1) which are often of considerable magnitude and significance in natural slopes and excavations.

1.10.4 Ground water

Geology influences the flow of groundwater, its direction, pressure and gradient at any point within a slope. Water can influence the strength of the materials by (1) chemical alteration and solution, (2) reduction of apparent cohesion due to capillary forces which disappear on submergence or saturation, (3) increasing pore water pressures with consequent reduction of shear strength as discussed in detail in chapter 2, (4) the mechanism of softening particularly applicable to strength reductions in stiff-fissured clays as discussed by Terzaghi (1936, 1950) and Terzaghi and Peck (1967). References to the mechanism of softening are made in chapters 2 and 5.

Rainfall infiltration into the ground and its effects have been outlined briefly in sub section 1.9.5 while available methods of seepage analysis have been outlined briefly in sub section 1.9.6. As stated earlier increase of pore water pressures due to the flow of ground water is an important factor in the development of slope failures and the occurrence of landslides. In particular the presence of groundwater under pressure, often facilitates severe slides of the flow type. However, such slope failures have also been triggered by seismic events, in materials thought to be dry at the time of failure.

Terzaghi and Peck (1967) have given an interesting example of failure of a slope in weathered rock (Figure 1.6). Seepage occurred into the weathered rock due to the filling of an adjacent reservoir. Whereas steep, near-vertical slopes of an excavation remained stable, much flatter slopes at lower levels failed. This was obviously because the pore water pressure was high at these levels in relation to the overburden pressure of the weathered material. Examples were also given by Terzaghi and Peck to illustrate the influence of geological details and pore water pressure on slope stability. Figure 1.7(a) shows a plain slide in varved clay when the pore water pressures are negligible. Figure 1.7(b) shows a sudden spreading failure which occurs when the pore water pressure in the silt layers is equal to the overburden pressure. Geological conditions favourable to spreading failure are illustrated in Figure 1.7(c).

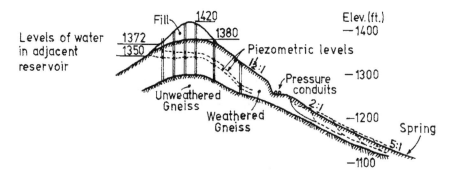

Figure 1.6 Slope failure in weathered rock. Steep slopes near conduits unaffected while gentler slopes show instability (after Terzaghi and Peck, 1967). Permission requested, see page 714, No 44.

1.10.5   Seismic effects

Many major and minor landslides have resulted from seismic activity and it is often important to consider the likely effect of earthquakes on slopes. While the main geological features of a slope are always important for stability evaluation, it has been established, over decades of observation and analysis, that minor geological details can have a significant influence on the behaviour of slopes under static loads. These details also have a significant influence on slope stability during earthquakes. Earthquakes result in increased shear stresses under dynamic conditions (cyclic loading). Moreover, for saturated, cohesionless soils, excess or transient pore water pressures are generated during such dynamic loading. Consequently, the shear strength decreases and even a complete loss of shear strength can occur. Such a loss of shear strength in cohesionless soil under dynamic loading is called earthquake-induced liquefaction and should be distinguished from 'static liquefaction' to which reference has been made in earlier sections of this chapter.

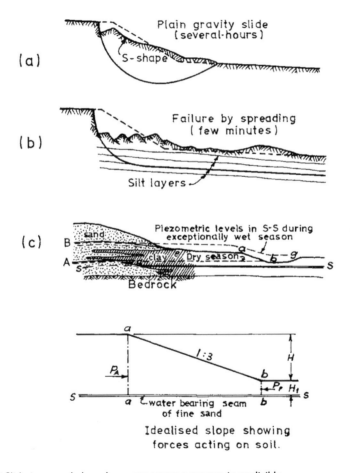

Figure 1.7 (a) Slide in varved clay when pore water pressure in negligible.
(b) Slide in varved clay if pore water pressure in silt layers is equal to overburden pressure.
(c) Geotechnical conditions favourable to spreading failure. (after Terzaghi and Peck, 1967). Permission requested, see page 714, No 44.

Liquefaction of small sand and silt lenses within a slope can result in progressive failure of materials which are relatively insensitive to seismic disturbance. Seed (1968) has discussed many examples to show how minor geological details have been extremely important in the development of landslides caused by earthquakes. A full chapter of this book is devoted to earthquake effects on slopes and to seismic slope analysis (see chapter 9).

1.10.6   Ground stresses or 'initial' stresses

The importance of initial stresses has already been mentioned earlier and methods of analyses which take such stresses into consideration are discussed in chapters 6, 7 and 8.

The geology of an area is of immense importance in considering the presence and nature of these 'initial' stresses. These stresses are a result of gravitational loading, tectonic activity, weathering, erosion and other processes. Many structural features are produced by stress relief. Considerable stress release activity is thought to be an important feature at the site of the famous Vaiont rock slide in Italy discussed by Muller (1964) and by others to some of whom reference has been made elsewhere in this book (see chapter 7, in particular) The importance of high lateral stresses in overconsolidated clays and clay-shales has been discussed by Bjerrum (1967) and in hard rocks by Bjerrum and Jorstad (1968).

1.10.7   Weathering

The importance of weathering has already been mentioned in section 1.6(g) According to Blyth and de Freitas (1974) chemical changes due to weathering can occur very quickly (e.g., a matter of a few days). The rate of such decrease will depend not only on the slope materials but other factors such as climate, drainage characteristics and geological details. Terzaghi and Peck (1967) consider the degree of bonding of shales to be far more important than chemical weathering. This is because weakening of bonds by a network of joints (due to removal of overburden or load by geological processes) may extend to a depth considerably greater than the depth of chemical weathering. Destruction of diagenetic bonding by weathering in overconsolidated clays and clay-shales has been discussed by Bjerrum (1967). Studies of the influence of weathering on the engineering properties of soils have also been made by Chandler (1969, 1972).

The weathering profile of a slope has an important influence on its permeability characteristics. Relict geological structures such as joints, bedding planes and faults influence the nature of the weathering profile. Deere and Patton (1971) have discussed the importance of the weathering profile in slope stability problems concerning residual soils. They show how a critical sequence of weathering zones (as regards strength and permeability) can develop in igneous and metamorphic rocks. For example a sequence of low strength, low permeability zone overlying a high penneability zone often leads to instability. Table 1.1 gives the description of a generalised weathering profile for igneous and metamorphic rocks.

1.10.8   Previous landslide activity

The geology of an area is very valuable in understanding both recent and ancient landslide activity. Many features may he explained only in terms of difficult climates and

Table 1.1 Description of a weathering profile for igneous and metamorphic rocks (after Deere and Patton, 1971). With permission, see page 713, No 3.

Zone and description	Relative permeability	Relative strength
Residual soil		
IA – top soil, roots, organic material, zone of leaching and eluviation, may be porous	medium to high	low to medium
IB – clay-enriched, also accumulation of Fe, Al and Si	low	commonly low high if cemented
IC – relict rock structures retained, silty grading to sandy material, less than 10% core stones, often micaceous	medium	low to medium relict structures very significant
Weathered rock		
IIA – Transition zone, highly variable soil-like to rock-like, fines common, coarse sand to fine sand spherodial weathering common	high	medium to low where weak structures and relict structures are present
IIB – partly weathered rock, rock like soft to hard rock, joints stained to altered, some alteration to feldspars and micas	medium to high	medium to high
Unweathered rock		
No iron stains to trace along joints – no alteration of feldspars and micas	low to medium	very high

rainfall patterns in the past. The recognition of areas in which there may be ancient slip surface is facilitated by geological studies and considerations.

1.11   THE NATURE OF SOILS

Soils are particulate materials in which the void spaces between particles may be filled with liquid or gas or both. There is a tremendous range and variety in the particle sizes and shapes of natural soils. Powerful electron microscopes are required to observe the finer clay-size soil particles. Water is the most common liquid and air the most common gas in the soils. Water may contain different types and quantities of dissolved electrolyte. The mechanical properties of soils are related to the interactions among the solid, liquid and gas phases. Fundamental understanding of soil behaviour requires knowledge of mineralogy. Physico-chemical aspects of soil behaviour have been discussed by Mitchell (1976). Gravels, sands and most silts are composed of non-clay minerals such as quartz, feldspar and mica. Quartz, which occurs in abundance, has a very stable crystal structure. Feldspars are weak and less stable and occur less abundantly in soils than in igneous rocks. Mica occurs in stacks of layers bonded weakly together and its presence increases compressibility under loading as well as swelling due to unloading. Elongated and plate-shaped particles of different minerals may be associated with preferred orientations which have a marked influence on mechanical behaviour. The latter also depends on the composition, porosity and surface texture of coarse-grained soils.

Most of the fine particles in soils are composed of clay minerals which usually exhibit plasticity when mixed with certain quantities of water. Clay minerals are silicates of calcium and aluminum with basic structures such as the silica tetrahedron and the aluminum or magnesium octahedron. Water is strongly adsorbed by the clay-minerals. The structure and properties of adsorbed water are different from those of normal water and it plays an important role in soil behaviour. Differences in clay minerals arise from the manner in which sheets of the basic structural elements are arranged and held together in layers. The most common clay minerals are kaolinite, illite and montmorillonite. Interstratification of layer types can lead to mixed-layer clays. Due to weathering, hydrothermal alteration or both, clay minerals are often found in the joints, shears and faults even in non-argillaceous rocks. Therefore clay minerals often have a significant influence on the behaviour of rock masses. Mineralogy influences the mechanical properties of soil directly as well as through its control on shapes, sizes and surface characteristics of particles and through its role in the interactions between the solid and liquid phases of soil. These relationships have been discussed in depth by Mitchell (1976). Mineralogy has a strong influence on Atterberg Limits which are determined in most problems of soil mechanics to identify and classify soils. However, it is not possible to determine the type and proportion of different clay minerals from these limits of consistency.

It is important to remember that in soils interatomic bonds are stronger than interparticle bonds. Consequently deformations are predominantly due to movements between particles and groups of particles. Deformation of individual particles is usually unimportant at stress levels of interest in slope stability problems. The crushing of particles of coarse-grained soils at high normal stresses may sometimes be of significance e.g., in high earth dams.

Mechanical properties of some soils may also be influenced considerably by cementation among particles. Loss of cementation bonds can drastically reduce the strength and stability of cemented soils. In some situations, there is a gradual transition from rock-like behavior to soil-like behavior and it may be difficult to distinguish between soft rock and hard soil.

The origin and history of soil deposits are extremely important because they largely determine soil characteristics including composition, structure and mechanical behaviour. This has been discussed and emphasised by Terzaghi and Peck (1967), Peck, Hanson and Thornburn (1974), Lambe and Whitman (1969) and Mitchell (1976) among others. The depositional history and stress history of soils is often extremely important and it is useful to distinguish between

(a) normally consolidated or normally loaded soils which have never in their history experienced an effective overburden pressure greater than their present overburden pressure and (b) overconsolidated or preconsolidated soils which have been subjected in the past to an effective overburden pressure greater than their present pressure. The highest previous pressure is important and known as the preconsolidation pressure. There are significant differences between the mechanical behaviour of these two types of soils as discussed in chapter 2. The degree of overconsolidation is given by the ratio of the maximum past pressure and the present overburden pressure.

In overconsolidated soils lateral stresses higher than gravitational stresses exist, the magnitude depending on the degree of overconsolidation.

It is also useful to distinguish between residual soils and transported soils and to learn about the processes of transportation and the depositional environment. The latter influences interparticle forces and structure. For a discussion of the properties of residual soils and the behaviour of slopes in such soils the reader should also refer to Deere and Patton (1971) and Blight (1977).

Many soils and particularly clays are weakened by joints and fissures which may have an important influence on the engineering properties of the soils. There are many soils with special characteristics such as quick clays which exhibit a dramatic loss of strength on remolding and collapsing soils which undergo large volume decrease when saturated. Bjerrum (1973) discussed the engineering behaviour of special and structurally unstable soils. Knowledge of soil formation, deposition and subsequent history is also useful in understanding deviations from homogeneity and isotropy in many soils. Fabric or the arrangement of particles and particle groups and pore spaces in a soil is also important and can help in understanding the soil behavior (see Rowe, 1972.) Many features in the macrofabric such as stratification, fissuring and voids may have a dominant influence on problems relating to the mechanics and hydraulics of both cohesive and cohesionless soils. The development of micro-fabric in fine-grained soils like clays is often related to the interactions in the clay-water-electrolyte system.

For typical soils in a natural state Table 1.2 shows the void ratio e (the ratio of volume of voids to volume of solids, the water content w (the ratio of weight of water to weight of solids), the dry unit weight γ_d (the ratio of weight of solids to volume of soil including the voids) and the saturated unit weight γ_{sat} (the ratio of total weight to total volume). The water content shown here is for soil when it is saturated (all the voids filled with water).

Approximate values of unconfined compressive strength q_u of clay soils are given in Table 1.3 which also shows common descriptions of consistency. It must be emphasised that the values given in this table are only approximate and are based on the experience of Terzaghi and Peck in USA, especially in the Great Lakes region of the midwest.

Table 1.2 Void ratio, water content and unit weight of typical soils (after Terzaghi and Peck, 1967). Permission requested, see page 714, No 44.

Description	Void ratio e	Water content w%	Unit weight (Kg/m³)	
			Dry (γ_d)	Saturated (γ_{sat})
Uniform loose sand	0.85	32	1430	1890
Uniform dense sand	0.51	19	1750	2090
Mixed grained sand loose	0.67	25	1590	1990
Mixed grained sand dense	0.43	16	1860	2160
Glacial till, very mixed grained	0.25	9	2120	2320
Soft glacial clay	1.2	45	–	1770
Stiff glacial clay	0.6	22	–	2070
Soft slightly organic clay	1.9	70	–	1580
Soft very organic clay	3.0	110	–	1430
Soft bentonite	5.2	194	–	1270

In the case of cohesionless soils, density is directly related to shear strength. The range of angles of shearing resistance ϕ in the loose, medium and dense conditions is shown by Table 1.4. The minimum values shown (i.e., for loose state) are often called the ultimate values of ϕ. (The angles of repose of cohesionless soils correspond to these values). The values at other densities are the corresponding peak values of the angles of shearing resistance. The concept of an angle of shearing resistance for any soil is discussed in chapter 2 in connection with the Mohr-Coulomb theory of strength.

The properties of natural soils depend on the proportion of different sizes of fine grained and coarse grained materials and on their mineralogy. The properties also depend on the process of formation, density and stress history. Thus the angle of shearing resistance ϕ of talus and taluvial material may range from $18°$ to $53°$ depending on the gravel fraction and the values of ϕ for residual soils may range from $20°$ to $50°$ depending on the clay fraction. (The percentage less than 2 micron or 0.002 mm is often called the clay-size fraction.) As clay fraction increases ϕ value decreases. The mineralogy of the clay fraction is of course important. Montmorillonite gives lowest ϕ values; Illite and Kaolinite give higher values respectively. Reference to residual friction angles (or residual angles of shearing resistance, often much lower than the peak values) is made in the next chapter.

The properties of compacted soils used in the construction of embankments and earth dams depend to a significant extent on the method of compaction, the

Table 1.3 Approximate unconfined compressive strength q_u of clay in terms of consistency-values from Terzaghi and Peck, 1967. Permission requested, see page 714, No 44.

Consistency	q_u Kg/cm^2	Remarks on field identification
Very soft	0.25	Exudes from between fingers when squeezed in hand
Soft	0.25–0.5	Moulded by light finger pressure
Medium	0.5–1.0	Moulded by strong finger pressure
Stiff	1.0–2.0	Indented by thumb
Very stiff	2.0–4.0	Indented by thumb nail
Hard	over 4.0	Difficult to indent by thumb nail

Table 1.4 Range of values of angle of shearing resistance ϕ for cohesionless soils (after Hough, 1957, and Lambe & Whitman, 1969). With permission, see page 713, No 4.

Description	ϕ Values in degrees when soil compaction is		
	Loose	Medium	Dense
Non-plastic silt	26–30	28–32	30–34
Uniform fine to medium sand	26–30	30–34	32–36
Well graded sand	30–40	34–40	38–46
Sand and gravel	32–36	36–42	40–48

Note: Within each range, assign lower values if particles are well-rounded or if there is significant soft shale or mica content, higher values for hard, angular particles. Use lower values for high normal pressures than for moderate normal pressures.

compaction effort and the moisture content at which they are compacted. The proportion of different soil sizes and the moisture content have a great influence on the efficiency with which the soils can be compacted and on the resulting mechanical properties. Similarly, permeability is determined by the composition and compaction and whether soil is compacted wet or dry of optimum moisture content (that moisture content which corresponds to maximum dry unit weight for given compaction effort). For a discussion of the properties of compacted soils and of their use in embankments and earth dams the reader should refer to Sherrard et al. (1963), Terzaghi and Peck (1967), Hirschfeld and Poulos (1973) and Resendiz (1977).

1.12   THE NATURE OF ROCKS

Rocks are aggregates of crystals and amorphus particles which may be cemented together to varying degrees. Individual crystals may vary in size from fraction of a centimeter to several centimeters. Igneous rocks consist of minerals such as quartz, plagioclase, pyroxene, mica etc. Sedimentary rocks consist of clay minerals, calcite quartz etc. together with detrital particles and pebbles from other rocks. Metamorphic rocks are produced by the action of temperature and stress or both on sedimentary or igneous rocks. The mechanical properties of rocks may be influenced by particle size, the properties of crystals and their preferred orientation. In sedimentary rocks porosity plays an important part. Fabric and texture often give important indications of mechanical behaviour. Most igneous rocks have a dense interlocking fabric while many sedimentary rocks such as shales and sandstones are laminated. Therefore the latter often exhibit directional differences (anisotropy) in their mechanical properties (e.g., strength, shear modulus etc.) while the former do not. Many metamorphic rocks such as slate, talc and mica-schist have well developed foliation planes and also exhibit anisotropy.

The behaviour of rock masses is controlled not only by lithology or rock type but also by structural features and discontinuities as discussed in earlier sections. Discontinuities such as bedding planes, cracks, joints, fissures and faults may have a predominant influence on the behaviour of slopes and are, therefore, significant in any analysis. Firstly, structural features may control the mobilisation of shear strength and hence stability directly. Secondly, they may drastically increase the magnitude of the permeability (the rate at which water can flow through a rock mass). The permeability of intact rock is often insignificant as compared to that of a rock mass. The latter is often called the secondary permeability. Thirdly, pore water pressures and directions of flow of water (and hence seepage forces) are often related to the size, spacing, orientation and distribution of discontinuities. Table 1.5 shows a suggested descriptive terminology for joint spacings. The importance of weathered material (gouge) in the discontinuities has already been mentioned (section 1.10.3). The shear strength of gouge and gouge-rock interface and the thickness of gouge determine the extent to which it may influence stability.

Geological data collection and its graphical presentation with particular reference to rock slopes have been discussed by Hoek and Bray (1974, 1977). In three-dimensional rock slope problems graphical techniques such as equal area projection or stereographic projection may be of great value to the engineer.

Table 1.6 shows typical unit weights and range of shear strength parameters of different types of rock mass. Typical ϕ values for rock discontinuities and gouge are shown in Table 1.7. Table 1.8 shows typical permeability coefficients of rock and soil.

Deere and Patton (1971) compiled separate tables for shear strength parameters of igneous, sedimentary and metamorphic rocks. These tables should prove to be of immense value in practice (see Appendix I).

Table 1.5 Terminology for joint spacings (after Deere, 1963). With permission, see page 713, No 5.

Descriptive term	Spacing
Very close	less than 5 cm
Close	5 cm–30 cm
Moderately close	30 cm–1 m
Wide	1 m–3 m
Very wide	greater than 3 m

Table 1.6 Typical rock properties (after Hoek and Bray, 1974). With permission, see page 713, No 6.

Rock mass	Unit weight Kg/m³	Friction angle ϕ degrees	Unit cohesion c Kg/m²
Granite	2614	30–50	9800–30,000
Quartzite	2614	30–45	–
Sandstone	1950	30–45	4900–14,600
Limestone	3169	30–50	4900–14,600
Porphyry	2580	30–40	9800–30,000
Shale	2400	27–45	2400–9800
Chalk	1760	30–40	2400–9800

Table 1.7 Typical ϕ values of joints and materials filling joints and faults (after Hoek, 1970). With permission, see page 713, No 7.

Description	ϕ values in degrees
Andesite joints	31–45
Chalk	35–41
Porphyry joints	40
Sandstone joints	27–38
Shale joints	37
Clay gouge (remolded)	10–20
Calcitic shear zone material	20–27
Shear fault material	14–22

Table 1.8 Permeability of soils and rocks (after Hoek and Bray, 1974). With permission, see page 713, No 6.

	k-cm/sec	Intact rock	Fractured rock	Soil
Practically Impermeable / Low discharge Poor drainage	10^{-10} 10^{-9} 10^{-8} 10^{-7} 10^{-6} 10^{-5} 10^{-4} 10^{-3} 10^{-2}	Slate Dolomite Granite	Clay-filled joints Joint rock	Homogeneous clay below zone of weathering Very fine sands, organic and inorganic silts, mixture of sand and clay, glacial till, stratified clay deposits
High discharge Free drainage	10^{-1} 1.0 10^{1} 10^{2}	Limestone Sandstone	Open- jointed rock Heavily fractured rock	Clean sand, clean sand and gravel mixtures Clean gravel

Deere and Patton (1971) compiled separate tables for shear strength parameters of igneous, sedimentary and metamorphic rocks. These tables should prove to be of immense value in practice (see Appendix I).

Table C1.1 Number of people killed, injured or displaced globally due to natural hazards during the 20th century (based upon WHO, 2002). Tsunami statistics updated to 26th of December, 2004. Before then, tsunami ranked eighth in terms of death in the 20th century. [Modified from Bryant et al. (2005)].

Type of hazard	Global deaths	Golbal deaths (%)	Global injuries	Global homeless	Largest death toll event and date	Death toll of largest event
Floods	6851740	66.01	1033572	123009662	China, July 1931	3700000
Earthquakes	1816119	17.50	1147676	8953296	Tangshan, China, July 1976	242000
Tropical cyclones	1147877	11.06	906311	34272470	Bangladesh, Nov 1970	300000
Tsunami[1]	337693	3.25	125789	1500000	Indian Ocean, Dec 26 2004	228432
Volcano	96770	0.93	11154	197790	Martinique, May 1902	12000
Landslides, avalanches, mud flows	60501	0.53	8071	3759329	Mount Huascaran, Peru, 1970	18000
Extra-tropical storms	36681	0.35	117925	12606891	Northern Europe, Feb 1953	2541
Heat wave	14732	0.14	1364	0.00		3000
Tornado	7917	0.08	27887	575511	India, May 1998	400.00
Cold wave	6807	0.07	1307	17340	Bangladesh, Apr 1989	800.00
Fires	2503	0.02	1658	140776	India, Dec 1982	800.00
Total	10379340	100.00	3382714	185033065	USA, Oct 1918	1000

[1] Data from national geophysical data centre tsunami database (2005) and Intergovernmental oceanographic commission (2003).

Table C1.2 Landslide fatality data for the period 1980 to 2000 for the main continental areas [after Petley et al. (2005)].

Continent	Deaths	Population density	Total population in million	Deaths per million per year
N. America	62	16	307	0.01
Europe	535	30	795	0.03
Africa	612	26	860	0.03
S. Asia	2596	305	1300	0.1
E. & SE. Asia	5125	193	2205	0.11
Australaisia	119	4	33	0.17
C. Asia	1958	9	80	1.17
S. America	57365	19.5	351	7.78
C. America	38250	64	174	10.47

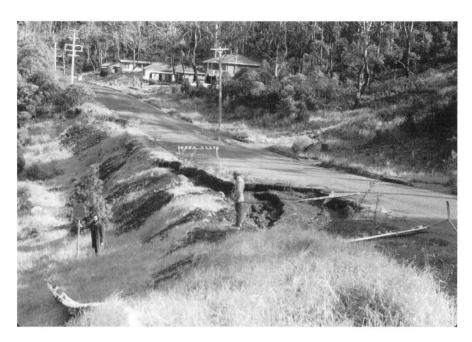

Figure C1.1 Slide in coalwash fill and colluvium along Alanson Avenue (Photo by Ann Young 1974 (Young, 1976)). (See colour plate section).

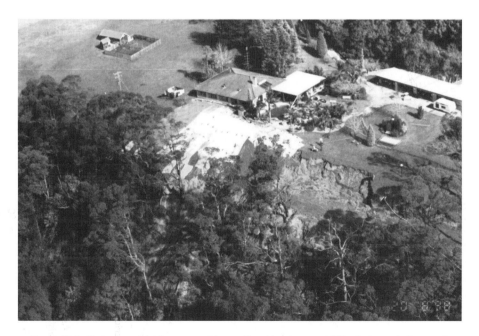

Figure C1.2 Complex slide-flow near Mount Kembla, August 1998. Coloured sheets of plastic cover parts of the slide close to the house (Photo, courtesy of NSW Police and Wollongong Geotechnical Team). (See colour plate section).

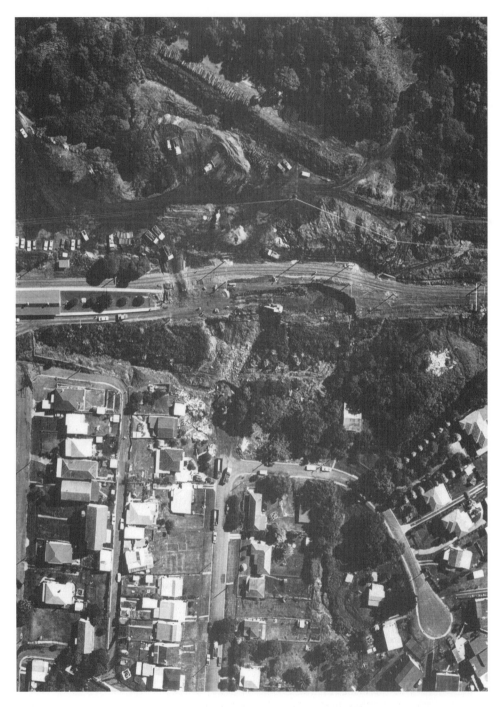

Figure C1.3 Vertical aerial photograph of the Coledale Landslide (slide-flow) which occurred on the 30th April, 1988. This landslide destroyed a house and caused two fatalities. (Photo, courtesy of the New South Wales Railway Services Authority). (See colour plate section).

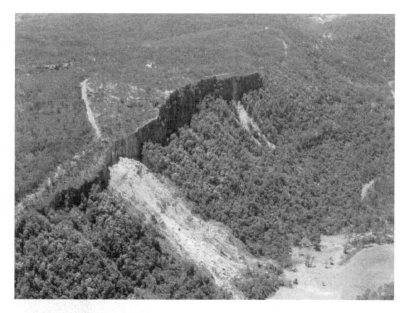

Figure C1.4 Oblique aerial photograph of a rockfall at Dombarton (Photo by Ann Young 1974). (See colour plate section).

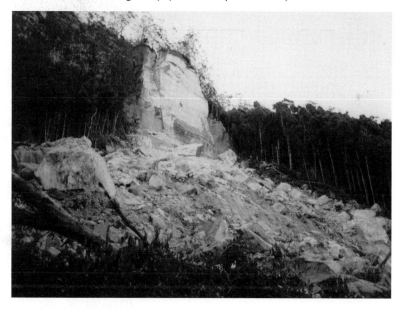

Figure C1.5 The Mount Barrengarry rockfall occurred in the early morning of the 29th of June, 1997, during heavy rainfall in the Kangaroo Valley southwest of Wollongong. The rock fall involved approximately 6000 m^3 of Hawkesbury Sandstone bedrock. The ensuing debris flow also involved approximately 15000 m^3 of additional colluvium on the slopes below (underlain by Kangaloon Sandstone). The debris flow completely destroyed up to 2Ha of dense forest. The toe of the flow stopped several metres upslope of the Fitzroy Falls to Kangaroo Valley Road. (See colour plate section).

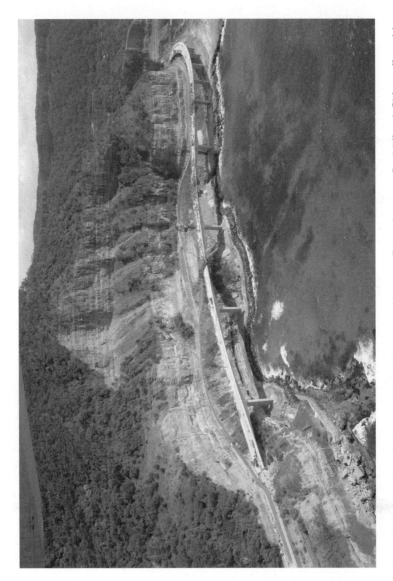

Figure C1.6 A section of the coastal road, Lawrence Hargrave Drive, between Coalcliff and Clifton affected by falls, slides and flows. Over a 1km section the road was bypassed by a bridge (later named the Sea Cliff Bridge), shown here under construction during 2005. (See colour plate section).

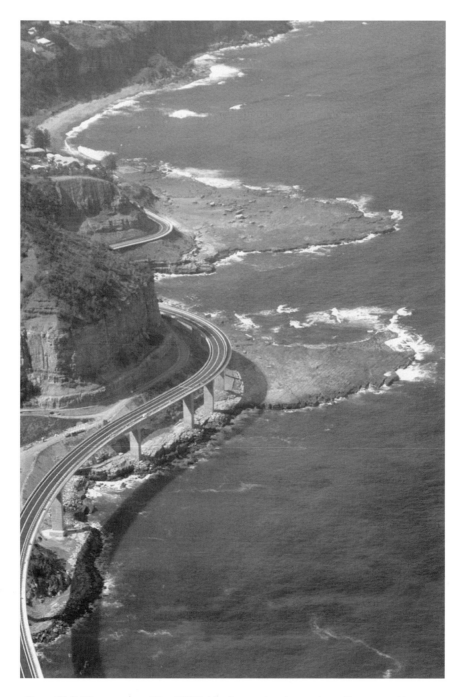

Figure C1.7 The completed Sea Cliff Bridge by-passing the section of Lawrence Hargrave Drive affected by landslides. The cover of this book shows a view of the area taken prior to the bridge construction. (See colour plate section).

Chapter 2

Basic geotechnical concepts

2.1 INTRODUCTION

Any method of analysis is based on concepts which are either universally accepted within the appropriate discipline or well advanced on the way to such acceptance. An understanding of concepts is not only necessary for the study and development of existing methods of analysis but also for initiating new approaches and ideas with regard to analyses and analytical techniques. The early development of both soil mechanics and rock mechanics was based in part on a broad acceptance of existing concepts relating to mechanics as such. Many of these concepts and, in particular those relating to continuum mechanics, are still accepted, although not without question. However, there has been an increasing recognition of fundamental differences between particulate (or jointed), multiphase materials on the one hand and solids on the other. By about the middle of the twentieth century, a great deal of progress had been made towards an understanding of the behaviour of real soil and rock masses. For example, it is now known that apparent and real differences in strength and deformation characteristics of clays and sands are due to real differences in their particle shapes and sizes, structure, mineralogy and permeability. Before the advent of modern soil mechanics, sand was considered to be a frictional material while clay was considered to be different from sand because it was 'cohesive' with zero angle of internal friction. It is now known that both cohesive and cohesionless soils are frictional in character and that no clay has a real value of $\phi = 0$. It is true that, in some situations, a saturated clay behaves apparently like a "$\phi = 0$" material. This is a consequence of the undrained response of such a material of very low permeability. Such behaviour can be adequately understood in terms of the principle of effective stress discussed in subsequent sections.

Every method of analysis requires some assumptions to be made before it can be applied to real problems. The importance of these assumptions can only be appreciated fully when the concepts underlying a particular method have been understood. Unfortunately, many of the assumptions tend to be forgotten after continued use of a popular method of analysis. In such situations, there is a likelihood of growing divergence between the objectives of analysis and the real significance of the results actually obtained. In order to ensure that a method of analysis enables progress towards realistic solutions, it is of paramount importance to keep firmly in mind the underlying basic concepts as well as the assumptions, implicit or otherwise.

2.2   STRESS AND STRAIN

The complexity of soils and rocks is such that many simplifying assumptions are necessary before the principles of mechanics can be applied to geotechnical problems. The most important and common assumption, often unstated, is that a mass of soil or rock can be regarded as a continuum with specified properties. Frequently situations arise in which some departure from the concept of a continuum is implied. References to some such situations are made throughout this book.

2.2.1   Elastic (recoverable) stresses and strains in soil and rock

The concept of stress and strain is fundamental in mechanics. The distinctive feature of soil and rock mechanics is that stress increment must be distinguished from stress level and that stress-paths (discussed in section 2.5) may be important particularly for soils. (Stress analysis is discussed in chapter 6 in which the importance of incremental analysis is explained). Before loads are applied to a soil or rock material, a significant state of stress may already exist in it. The application of loads results in stress increments. These in turn cause strains or increments of strain. Strains may also be influenced by the existing initial stresses since the new stresses (the sum of the initial stresses and the stress increments) must be considered in relation to any criterion of yield or failure. In the development of stress-strain theories, it is often necessary to adopt an elaborate notation which distinguishes between stress level and stress increment and between strain and strain increment. Such a notation, though useful, would be cumbersome for the purposes of this book. Relationships between stress and strain must in general be regarded as relationships between increments in these quantities. The reader will be alerted where both increments and levels of stress or strain are being discussed together in any section of this book. Comprehensive notation will be used where necessary.

Three components of normal stress σ_x, σ_y, σ_z and three components of shear stress τ_{xy}, τ_{yz}, τ_{zx} are required to represent the general state of stress at a point. This set of 6 stress components is also called the stress tensor. These may also be represented by σ_{ij} where subscript i refers to the direction normal to the plane on which the component acts and j to the direction of the component itself. The stress state at a point is completely defined by three principal (normal) stresses σ_1, σ_2, σ_3 in the three mutually perpendicular directions 1, 2, 3, which are inclined to the co-ordinate system x, y, z. If the three principal stresses are equal in magnitude and direction, the stress state is called spherical or hydrostatic. Unequal principal stresses may be resolved into one spherical or octahedral normal component σ_{oct} (also called the mean normal stress) and three deviatoric components t_1, t_2, t_3 whose resultant is called the octahedral shear stress τ_{oct} where:

$$\sigma_{oct} = \frac{1}{3}(\sigma_1 + \sigma_2 + \sigma_3), \quad \tau_{oct} = \sqrt{t_1^2 + t_2^2 + t_3^2}$$

$$t_1 = \frac{1}{3}(\sigma_2 - \sigma_3), \quad t_2 = \frac{1}{3}(\sigma_3 - \sigma_1), \quad t_3 = \frac{1}{3}(\sigma_1 - \sigma_2)$$

$$(2.1)$$

The strain tensor also consists of three normal components ε_x, ε_y, ε_z and three shear components γ_{xy}, γ_{yz}, γ_{zx} and together they may be denoted by ε_{ij}. If material behaviour in any loading increment can be regarded as linearly elastic and isotropic, two elastic constants are required to represent the relationship between the components of stress and the components of strain. These are the modulus of elasticity E and the Poisson's ratio v. Alternatively, the bulk modulus K and the shear modulus G are sometimes used and these are easily obtained in terms of E and v as follows:

$$K = \frac{E}{3(1-2v)} \quad G = \frac{E}{2(1+v)} \tag{2.2}$$

The directions of principal stresses are collinear with the corresponding directions of principal strains in isotropic materials. Theories of anisotropic elasticity are sometimes applied to geotechnical problems. Even with the assumption of a plane of isotropy (e.g., a plane parallel to the direction of bedding or strata, implying a transversely isotropic material), five independent elastic parameters are required to describe the relationship between components of stress and the components of strain. Moreover the principal axes of stress are no longer collinear with the principal axes of strain.

Often laboratory or field experiments are conducted to obtain mechanical properties of soils and rocks. These experiments involve particular conditions of symmetry or restraint and it is useful to compare the stress situation in the experiment to that in a given field problem. Consider the well known cylindrical compression test with axial stress σ_a and radial stress σ_r. The octahedral normal and shear (deviatoric) components of stress are:

$$\sigma_{oct} = \frac{1}{3}(\sigma_a + 2\sigma_r), \quad \tau_{oct} = \frac{\sqrt{2}}{3}(\sigma_a - \sigma_r) \tag{2.3}$$

On the other hand, a plane-strain compression test involves deformation in one plane, e.g., a plane defined by two directions a and r; the strain and deformation being zero in the direction perpendicular to this plane. The normal and shear stresses in that direction may be obtained by equating the expressions for corresponding strains to zero. Assuming elastic behaviour during a load increment, the octahedral normal and shear components of stress are:

$$\sigma_{oct} = \frac{1}{3}(\sigma_a + \sigma_r)(1+v), \quad \tau_{oct} = \frac{1}{3}(\sigma_a - \sigma_r) \tag{2.4}$$

Note the dependence of σ_{oct} on Poisson's ratio, v which is different from Equation 2.3. Similarly, expressions may be developed for a cross-anisotropic (or transversely isotropic) material with five independent elastic parameters referred to earlier. In the latter case, the orientation of principal stresses with respect to the orientation of the plane of isotropy assumes major importance, and particular care must be taken when the plane of isotropy is oblique to the principal axes or to the plane of deformation.

2.2.2   *Irrecoverable strains in soil and rock*

Geomechanics deals with multiphase materials like soil and rock which include, in general, solids, air and liquid (usually water). The pore fluids, air and water, play a significant role in the stress-strain behaviour of a soil. For saturated soils (voids completely filled with water), only the solid and liquid phase need to be considered and, for dry soils, only the solid and air phases. However for unsaturated soils, also called partially-saturated soils, all three phases (solid, liquid, and air) must be considered. Both recoverable (elastic) and irrecoverable strains are associated with applied normal and shear stresses and thus both will contribute to deformations. Moreover, stress-strain behaviour is often non-linear. Under certain conditions, the assumption of linear-elastic behaviour may be a good approximation but this should be justified on the basis of evidence from testing or field performance.

Irrecoverable volumetric and shear strains are particularly important in soils and are associated with volume changes which occur due to the water and air phases. Air is compressible but water and solid phases are relatively incompressible. Therefore, irrecoverable volume changes in a saturated soil can only occur if boundary conditions allow the drainage of water in and out of the soil mass. A soil mass is dilatant if volume increases under applied stresses and this occurs in relatively dense soils and, for a fully saturated soil under (i) drained conditions, would be associated with intake of pore water, and, (ii) under undrained conditions, would be associated with decrease in the pore water pressure. Further references to these effects are made in the following sections and elsewhere in the book, where appropriate. In contrast to dilatant behaviour, compressive behaviour of a soil mass occurs in relatively loose soils and, for a saturated soil under (i) drained conditions, would be associated with drainage of water out of the mass, and, under (ii) undrained conditions, would be associated with increase in the pore water pressure. Either dilatant or compressive behaviour can also occur in a dry or a partially saturated (unsaturated) soil, depending on the relative density and other conditions.

The relative importance of elastic and irrecoverable strains to geotechnical performance depends on the type of project. For example, only elastic foundation deformations are important for a building located on rock or dense soil and the magnitude of these deformations must be within permissible limits for the building as a whole. On the other hand, slope stability is often adversely affected by irrecoverable or permanent deformations and, therefore, understanding why and how such deformations occur is vitally important. Apart from deformations within a homogeneous soil or rock mass, relative movement along existing discontinuities (joints, faults, bedding planes, slip surfaces etc.) can occur under applied stresses. Generally these are irrecoverable deformations and highly significant for adverse change in stability conditions.

2.3   THE PRINCIPLE OF EFFECTIVE STRESS IN SOIL AND ROCK

2.3.1   *Saturated soil*

The discovery of the principle of effective stress by Terzaghi around 1920 marks the beginning of modern soil mechanics. The appreciation of this principle is also essential in many problems of rock mechanics. Consider three principal stresses σ_1, σ_2, σ_3 at any point in a saturated soil mass and let u be the pore water pressure at that point.

Effective principal stresses σ_1', σ_2', σ_3' are defined as follows:

$$\sigma_1' = \sigma_1 - u, \quad \sigma_2' = \sigma_2 - u, \quad \sigma_3' = \sigma_3 - u \tag{2.5}$$

Compression, distortion and a change of shearing resistance are exclusively due to changes in the effective stresses. Therefore changes in u are significant when these changes lead to changes in the effective stresses. For example a change Δu may occur due to drainage and volume change in a saturated soil mass without alteration in the total stresses. Such a change would increase the effective stresses. On the other hand, simultaneous identical changes in total stress and pore water pressure have no effect on effective stress.

In general there is an effective normal stress σ' corresponding to a total normal stress σ ($= \sigma' + u$). The distinction between total and effective does not apply to shear stress. Since water carries no shear stress, the principle of effective stress implies that there is no distinction between a 'total' and 'effective' shear stress in a soil mass. The principle of effective stress is discussed with historical background in Terzaghi (1960).

For fine-grained soils, Mitchell (1976) drew attention to the influence of physicochemical forces which might influence Terzaghi's effective stress equation but concluded that the simple equation was quite accurate for most soils.

2.3.2   Unsaturated soil

The pore water pressure can be negative in fine-grained, unsaturated soils. In order to define effective stress in such partially saturated soils, Bishop (1960) proposed the following equation:

$$\sigma' = \sigma - u_a + \chi(u_a - u_w) \tag{2.6}$$

in which u_a is the pressure in the air, u_w the pressure in the water and χ is a parameter which depends on the degree of saturation. (χ has values equal to 0 and 1 for dry and saturated soils respectively but determination of χ values for intermediate conditions is difficult). For saturated soils Equation (2.6) reduces to the simple Terzaghi equation for effective stress.

Skempton (1960) suggested that the principle of effective stress in the original simple form given by Terzaghi may not be sufficiently accurate for homogeneous rock or concrete even when these materials are fully saturated. The effective area of interparticle contact and the relative compressibilities of the solids, on the one hand, and of the rock or concrete materials, on the other hand, are important in this regard. Skempton proposed the following equations for shear strength and volume change respectively and then examined them in relation to available data concerning saturated rock and concrete.

For shear strength,

$$\sigma' = \sigma - \left\{1 - \frac{a_c \tan \psi}{\tan \phi'}\right\} u$$

(2.7)

and, for volume change,

$$\sigma' = \sigma - \left\{1 - \frac{C_s}{C}\right\} u$$

in which a_c is the effective area of inter-particle contact, C_s is the compressibility of the solid phase, ψ its intrinsic friction angle, ϕ' the effective angle of internal friction in terms of Coulomb's equation of shear strength (see section 2.4) and C the compressibility of the mass of rock or concrete or soil. For soils the terms in brackets approximate to unity with the result that Terzaghi's simple equation is obtained. This explains its continued success in soil mechanics. However, for concrete and rock, the terms C_s/C and $(a_c \tan \psi/\tan \phi')$ are not negligible. Consequently, Terzaghi's simple equation is not always applicable.

A rock mass often contains discontinuities and it is pertinent to consider whether Skempton's objection to the Terzaghi equation applies for points within or along such a discontinuity. The answer to this question is extremely important since such a situation is quite different from that of homogeneous rock or concrete on the one hand and soil on the other; and yet discontinuities may be critical with regard to the behaviour and stability of a rock mass. It must be recognised that the properties of a discontinuity are important in determining the answer. For instance the value of a_c in an open joint may be small. Again if a joint is filled with soil-like materials such as gouge, the Terzaghi effective stress equation would be applicable within it. Therefore it is not surprising that most slope stability problems in rock masses have been tackled with success on the basis of the simple equation. However, this is an area worthy of further study and research. There are many discussions of effective stress in rocks which show that Skempton's (1960) contribution is not widely known. Brace and Byerlee (1966) presented evidence to show that the principle of effective stress in its original form was valid for many rocks and they did not mention the importance of factors appearing in Skempton's equations. On the other hand Heard (1960) found the strength of Solenhofen limestone to be practically independent of pore pressure. According to one point of view this could be attributed to the low porosity of these rocks. It may be recalled that Terzaghi (1945) proposed the following equation:

$$\sigma' = \sigma - \eta u$$

(2.8)

in which η is a value normally less than unity for rock materials and equal to unity when the surfaces of joints are considered. This parameter represents the relationship between the projected area of voids and the total projected area of the surface of rupture.

2.3.3   Different types and sources of pore water pressure

Pore water pressures due to submergence or seepage must be distinguished from excess pore water pressures generated in most cohesive soils by loading or unloading. The tremendous importance of excess pore water pressures in slope stability problems is discussed separately in section 2.8. Pore water pressures due to seepage may be estimated by using closed-form, graphical or numerical solutions for any given problem with known boundary conditions. As stated in chapter 1, a solution is often obtained in the form of a flow net consisting of a family of flow lines and a family of equipotential lines. For a medium with isotropic permeability the members of one family of curves always intersect the members of the other family at right angles. At any point, the direction of a flow line represents the direction of seepage and seepage force. An equipotential line joins points with equal total head (sum of position head, pressure head and velocity head; of these the velocity head is negligible in most problems of flow through porous media). Procedures for drawing flow nets are well established even for anisotropic and layered media (e.g., Taylor, 1948; Harr, 1962; Cedergren, 1967). For other closed-form, numerical or probabilistic solutions to seepage problems the reader may also refer to Harr (1962, 1977) and Zienkiewicz (1971).

While seepage solutions in general, and flow nets in particular, are often useful, there may be considerable uncertainty with regard to details of subsurface conditions. Soil exploration may not identify important geological details which have a considerable influence on pore water pressures. Artesian conditions and perched water tables may also exist. In view of these factors, field measurements of pore water pressure by piezometers installed at different points are always valuable and sometimes essential. Several types of piezometers have been developed and there is increasing recognition of the need for field measurements of pore water pressure in soils and rocks. For urban slope stability assessments, the importance of monitoring pore water pressures is highlighted in chapter 11 of this book.

2.3.4 Reservoir filling and artesian pressures – an example, the 1963 Vaiont slide

Analyses of the huge and catastrophic 1963 Vaiont slide have been carried out by many investigators and references to some of them are made in chapter 7. In most of these analyses the importance of changing pore water pressures along the chair-shaped slip surface has been recognised. This slide occurred at the site of the Vaiont dam-reservoir system during a period of reservoir filling. It is the most famous example of the catastrophic failure of a reservoir slope. In fact, there were several periods of observed movement of the landslide mass, separated by periods of stability. The reservoir level was lowered after significant movement was observed and then raised again. Unfortunately, the final slide movements were so sudden and rapid that lowering the reservoir level, in that instance, was out of the question.

There have been many studies of the Vaiont slide and most investigators agree that pore water pressure distribution along the slip surface changed in two ways. One important cause of change was the raising or lowering of reservoir level and the other cause was the pore pressure increase over a part of the slip surface due to infiltration of rainfall over an extended period of time.

Some investigators have gone further and suggested that cumulative rainfall over the surrounding area led to the development of very high artesian pore water pressures over the upper part of the slip surface. However, this is, by no means, the only hypothesis concerning the reasons for the Vaiont catastrophe (refer also to chapter 7 and, in particular section 7.17). Unfortunately, detailed data on subsurface movements and pore water pressures are either completely lacking or very scarce because of lack of systematic instrumentation as part of a subsurface observational programme. However, there are some isolated data although their reliability has not been established. At one stage of reservoir filling, during a period of low to moderate rainfall, water levels 90 m above the reservoir level are reported to have been recorded by a piezometer "probably located not far from the slip surface".

Hendron and Patton (1985) suggest that this site (the site of the Vaiont slide) is "... a near classic case of an inclined multiple-layer artesian aquifer system at and below the surface of sliding." Thus they tried to explain the occurrence of the slide on the basis of very high artesian pore pressures having developed over the upper part of the slip surface. They also made some time plots of reservoir levels against cumulative precipitation, highlighting the pore water pressure conditions during observed periods of landslide movement. By extrapolation they assessed that a cumulative 30-day rainfall of 700 mm would cause sliding without a reservoir. In fact only 500 mm per month was realised during the four year period of the record. Thus the 1963 slide could not have been caused by rainfall alone. However, if an old landslide occurred on this site, as has been claimed with some justification, the 700 mm monthly rainfall must have been exceeded at the time of that old landslide. The reservoir level for landsliding to occur without any rainfall was estimated to be in the range 710–720 m. The design full supply level was 722.5 m. Had this level been reached, it was argued, the Vaiont landslide might have occurred even if antecedent rainfall had been very low (refer to more details in sections 5.6.5, 5.12.7 and 7.17).

2.4   SHEAR STRENGTH OF SOILS

2.4.1   Dry or saturated soils

The most widely used theory of soil strength is the Mohr-Coulomb theory which may be expressed by the following equation:

$$s = c + \sigma \tan \phi \qquad (2.9)$$

in which s is the shear strength or the shear stress along the failure plane, σ is the normal stress at failure on the failure plane, c is the unit cohesion and ϕ is the angle of internal friction. This equation is often written in a modified form, to take account of the principle of effective stress, thus:

$$s = c' + \sigma' \tan \phi' \qquad (2.10)$$

in which σ' $(=\sigma - u)$ is the effective normal stress on the failure plane at failure when the pore water pressure is u. Note that the parameters c and ϕ in Equation (2.9) have in general different values from the parameters c' and ϕ' in Equation (2.10). The former are referred to as 'total stress' parameters and the latter as 'effective stress' parameters. The latter are often used with a prime suffix e.g., c' and ϕ' as in Equation (2.10).

2.4.2   Unsaturated soils

In general, throughout this chapter, effective stresses and effective stress parameters are implied unless otherwise stated. However, the prime suffix will be used to denote effective stress parameters when there is likelihood of confusion between the two sets of parameters. Equation (2.10) is also referred to as the Terzaghi-Coulomb equation since it is based on the principle of effective stress discovered by Terzaghi.

At this stage it is important to consider the special case of unsaturated soils. The drained shear strength of unsaturated or partially saturated soils may be expressed by including an additional linear term which is the product of the suction (the difference between the negative pore water pressure and the pore air pressure) and a related parameter that can be expressed as the tangent of a friction angle ϕ^b different from the internal friction angle ϕ'.

$$s = c' + (\sigma - u_a)\tan\phi' + (u_a - u_w)\tan\phi^b \tag{2.11}$$

in which $(u_a - u_w) = u_s$ is the matric suction, and $\tan\phi^b$ represents the rate of increase of shear strength with increase in matric suction. Fredlund and Barbour (1992) discussed the application of this equation to slope stability problems in unsaturated soils. They summarised data from various authors indicating values of ϕ^b in degrees ranging from 13.8° to 21.7° for soils with internal friction angles in the range 22.5° to 35.3°. The mechanics of unsaturated soils and its application has also been considered in detail by Fredlund and Rohardjo (1993).

Based on experimental evidence, a somewhat different approach has been proposed in which the third term, again a function of suction, may be regarded as another cohesion intercept. The relationship is presented below and was proposed by Abramento and Carvalho (1989). The third term is the product of parameter b and suction raised to the power parameter a:

$$s = c' + \sigma'\tan\phi' + b(u_s)^a \tag{2.12}$$

Terzaghi et al. (1996) quote the following results of tests carried out in the suction range of 4 MPa: $a = 0.5$ and b is in the range 2 to 10, being dependent on the internal friction angle and effective normal stress.

This last term may be considered as a suction-related cohesion intercept which can provide a significant contribution to shear strength of partially saturated soils such as residual soils and fills above the water table. For example, for a soil with $b = 6$ and $a = 0.5$ and a modest suction of 100 kPa, the suction-related cohesion intercept is 60 kPa which is significant for stability. A perfectly stable slope in such a partially saturated soil might fail after submergence or flooding or after rainfall infiltration which results in elimination of the negative pore pressure or suction.

2.4.3   Slope failures involving unsaturated soil slopes

Slope failures after significant rainfall are generally associated with saturated soils in which positive pore water pressures increases to a critical value. On the other hand, the mechanism of rainfall-induced failure in unsaturated soil slopes is associated with the elimination of suction or negative pore water pressure. Appreciating this important distinction is critical to an understanding of issues concerned with slope stability in unsaturated soils. Thus it is useful to refer here to typical examples of failures in natural slopes, fill slopes and mining spoil under unsaturated conditions.

In many parts of the world, shallow failures of unsaturated soil slopes above the water table occur after significant rainfall. The occurrence of such failures in natural slopes within Hong Kong has frequently been noted in the literature. However failures of unsaturated fill slopes are not uncommon and reference was made in chapter1 to a catastrophic slide involving such a slope in Hong Kong.

The mechanism of strength loss after submergence of an unsaturated hill slope has also been associated with the disastrous 1997 Thredbo landslide which occurred near a ski resort in the snowy mountainous region of New South Wales, Australia, causing a dozen deaths and huge economic loss (Hand, 2000).

Another important application of unsaturated shear strength concerns the building-up of mining spoil piles associated with open-cut (open-pit) mining operations. The deformation and potential failure of these massive earth structures formed by dumping of mining spoil must be considered very carefully. Failure of the spoil pile has significant economic consequences (apart from safety aspects including human safety). Any such failure causes a huge disruption in the mining operations with associated economic loss.

These spoil piles may be as high as 100 metres as reported by Richards (1982) for the open-pit coal mines at Goonyella in Queensland, Australia. The shear strength of unsaturated spoil in the upper parts of the spoil pile (the dry areas) is high. In the lower parts near the pit floor, where the spoil has been remoulded by the massive shear strains occurring during the spoiling operations, the shear strength is relatively low. Richards (1982) presented results showing the increase of shear strength with increasing suction. Following rainfall there is consolidation of the spoil and also saturation occurs in the lower areas. Thus suction is eliminated and shear strength decreases.

More importantly, the residual shear strengths are significantly lower than the peak strengths [read the following sub-sections for concept of residual shear strength; typical values of these shear strength parameters for the spoil at Goonyella are quoted from Richards (1982) at the end of sub-section 2.4.7].

2.4.4   Factors influencing shear strength parameters

Figure 2.1(a) shows a straight line Mohr-Coulomb envelope, which represents Equations (2.9) and (2.10). It is so called because it represents a common tangent or envelope to different Mohr-circles at failure. Any stress state may be represented by a Mohr circle drawn from the major and minor principal stresses. However these circles lie below the Coulomb envelope unless they represent stress states at failure.

The shearing resistance (and hence the values of c and ϕ) of a soil is influenced by its void ratio, mineralogy, pore fluid composition, structure, stress level, stress history, strain and rate of strain. Uncemented sands and normally-consolidated clays (clays which have never been subjected to an overburden pressure greater than their present overburden pressure) show a zero or near zero cohesion intercept in terms of effective stresses for the stress range of interest in most stability problems. Values of

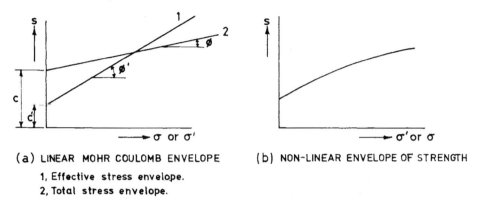

(a) LINEAR MOHR COULOMB ENVELOPE   (b) NON-LINEAR ENVELOPE OF STRENGTH

1, Effective stress envelope.
2, Total stress envelope.

Figure 2.1 Types of shear strength envelope.

shear strength parameters for different soils are determined using different types of experiments, different drainage conditions, stress paths and rates of loading. Total stress parameters would usually be obtained from undrained tests in which the pore water pressure may or may not be measured. Effective stress parameters may be obtained from drained tests or those undrained tests in which pore water pressure is measured. For most soils the magnitude of c is greater than that of c' and the magnitude of ϕ is less than or equal to that of ϕ'. These basic relationships ($c > c'$ and $\phi < \phi'$) are useful for a quick check on the reliability of test data.

The Mohr-Coulomb theory proposes a linear strength envelope. However, the strength envelope for some soils may be curved (Figure 2.1b). It is, therefore, important to use a range of normal stresses for testing which corresponds to the stress levels of interest in a given problem. Decrease of friction angle with increasing normal stress has been reported for granular soils by Vesic and Clough (1968) and Banks and MacIver (1969) who noted a linear relationship between zero cohesion peak friction angle and the logarithm of mean effective normal stress. Hamel (1973b) noted a similar relationship for desert alluvium.

2.4.5 Measurement of shear strength under different drainage conditions

Laboratory tests for shear strength parameters should always be conducted by competent personnel under the close personal supervision of a geotechnical expert. Some reputable geotechnical experts personally check all test results before using values in analysis or design. The importance of sampling, sample selection and test procedures on the interpretation of test results and selection of design values etc. cannot be over-emphasised. It is necessary to distinguish clearly between strength obtained from remoulded specimens and that from undisturbed specimens. Remoulding of soil destroys its original structure and alters its mechanical behaviour. While it is difficult to obtain truly undisturbed specimens, it is possible to minimise the extent of disturbance by the adoption of proper sampling procedures. Sensitive soils lose a large proportion of their strength due to disturbance or remoulding and exceptional care is required in sampling and testing such soils (sensitivity is the ratio of undisturbed strength to remoulded strength at unaltered water content. This value may be as high as 50 for some extra-sensitive or 'quick' clays found in different locations in the world, notably within Canada and Scandinavia).

Three types of shear tests, depending on drainage conditions are commonly employed for testing of soils: (1) In undrained tests, no drainage is permitted during the application of either normal or shear stresses. These tests are also called quick tests (notation: Q tests or UU tests). (2) In fully drained tests, also called consolidated-drained tests, drainage is permitted during the application of the normal load. Only when consolidation of a specimen is complete under a normal load, is the specimen sheared. Drainage is again permitted during shear. To achieve complete drainage of cohesive soils many days may be required for each test. Therefore they are referred to as slow tests (notation: S tests or CD tests). (3) In consolidated undrained tests, drainage is permitted during the application of normal load but such consolidation is followed by shear under undrained conditions. These tests are also called consolidated-quick tests (notation: R tests, CQ tests or CU tests). The consolidation phase may be carried out under (a) isotropic or equal principal stresses (CIU tests), (b) anisotropic or unequal principal stresses (CAU tests) or (c) conditions of no lateral strain (CK$_0$U tests).

Most of these types of test can be performed in direct shear and simple shear apparatus as well as in triaxial or cylindrical compression apparatus. However, in practice triaxial compression test is used for UU, CU and CD tests while direct shear is commonly used only for CD tests (although it can be used for other types of test as well). An excellent discussion of procedures for triaxial testing to suit different types of soil stability problems is given by Bishop and Henkel (1962). They discuss standard as well as special tests. The relevance of the triaxial test in soil stability problems has also been discussed by Bishop and Bjerrum (1960), Lowe (1967) and Johnson (1975). The last two references are especially useful in respect of earth dams.

Before laboratory tests can be performed it is necessary to extract samples from the ground. Sampling involves disturbance and it is particularly difficult to obtain reliable samples of cohesionless or sensitive cohesive soils. Further, a consequence of sampling is that the state of stress in the sample is altered from its original condition in the ground.

In view of these recognised difficulties, in-situ tests or field tests have often been used in geotechnical engineering practice. The most common test for cohesionless soils is the standard penetration test. The number of blows required for a foot of penetration of a standard sampler have been correlated empirically with the relative density and hence the angle of shearing resistance. For determining the in-situ undrained cohesion of soft clays, the shear vane test is very popular. This parameter is useful for analysing the end-of-construction stability of slopes in soft clays (see chapter 5). If a soft clay is anisotropic (e.g., undrained cohesion different in horizontal and vertical directions), strength variation with direction can be found by using vanes of different sizes. Among other in-situ methods are those involving the use of pressuremeters including self-boring devices designed to cause minimum soil disturbance (Windle and Wroth, 1977).

2.4.6 Peak, ultimate and residual shear strength

The shear strength of soils decreases from a peak to ultimate value at large strains. However, the decrease is marked only in the case of dense sands and heavily over-consolidated clays and is not significant for loose sands and normally-consolidated (or normally-loaded) clays. The shear strength along a well defined failure surface reduces at large displacements to a value referred to as the residual shear strength. This strength is considered to be independent of stress history and original structure.

In recent literature the terms 'ultimate shear strength' and 'residual shear strength' have sometimes been used synonymously. This can be misleading and must be avoided particularly when discussing the mechanical behaviour of cohesive (or clayey) soils. Dense sands and heavily overconsolidated clays exhibit dilatancy or a tendency to increase in volume during shear. Therefore undrained shear of such soils results in reduction of pore water pressure and consequent increase of effective stress whereas drained shear results in increase of water content (assuming saturated conditions). Drained stress-strain behaviour of such dense soils is brittle compared to that of nor-mally consolidated clays and loose sands. The latter soils tend to decrease in volume during shear so that their water content decreases during drained shear and effective stresses decrease during undrained shear (due to increase in pore water pressure). Typical stress-strain curves are shown in Figure 2.2.

Figure 2.2(b) may be considered typical for clays deforming under drained shear. Shear deformation curves under undrained conditions would differ from correspond-ing curves under fully drained conditions. A complete set of curves for drained shear deformation of saturated soil would include a plot of volumetric strain as a function of shear strain or deformation. In contrast, for undrained shear of saturated soil, a plot of pore water pressure as a function of shear strain or deformation would be included. Undrained peak and residual shear strengths would, in general, differ from the corresponding drained shear strengths.

It is also important to note that clays from different regions of the world can vary significantly in their behaviour depending on the composition, clay mineralogy envi-ronment, and depositional history and several other factors.

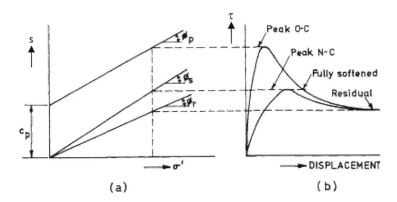

Figure 2.2 (a) Peak, residual and fully-softened shear strength envelopes for an overconsoli-dated clay (b) comparison of shear stress-displacement curves of normally consoli-dated (N-C) and overconsolidated (O-C) clays at a given effective normal stress.

Both dense and loose soils change in volume with increasing strain only till the ultimate condition is reached. In drained shear, the water content decreases for normally consolidated (N-C) clay and increases for overconsolidated (O-C) clay. At this stage (ultimate condition) water content does not change with further shear distortion. In undrained shear of saturated clay, the pore water pressure increases for N-C clay but decreases for O-C clay due to dilatant behaviour. Roscoe et al. (1958) referred to 'ultimate state' as the 'critical state'. Fissured overconsolidated clays lose their strength with time due to a process of softening discussed originally by Terzaghi (1936) and also subsequently by Skempton (1948, 1970). Softening occurs as a result of water infiltration in the fissures and joints leading to swelling and associated weakening of the clay. In the fully softened condition a stiff-fissured clay has a near zero cohesion intercept in terms of effective stresses and according to Skempton (1970) the shear strength is close to the critical state strength or the ultimate strength. Skempton recognised the difficulty of defining and determining the true critical state of real clays exhibiting bonding, sensitivity and preferred particle orientation. Critical state concepts were developed for saturated remoulded clays assuming somewhat idealised conditions as discussed in Schofield and Wroth (1968). However, on the basis of available evidence it appears that the shear strength parameters of a fully softened, stiff fissured clay are very close to that of the same clay if remoulded and tested after normal consolidation in the laboratory.

Further reduction in the shear strength of a clay beyond the ultimate or critical state value (or beyond the fully softened value in the case of a stiff fissured clay) may occur along continuous shear surfaces or slip surfaces and is always associated with large deformations. The limiting strength under such conditions is the residual shear strength which may be considerably lower than the ultimate, critical state or fully softened strength (Figure 2.2).

2.4.7   *Factors influencing residual shear strength*

Residual shear strength decreases in a general way with increasing plasticity index and clay fraction of any soil. However, empirical correlations, e.g., Voight (1973), cannot be relied upon because of numerous exceptions from such correlations. Typical values of residual ϕ for clays range from 8° to 18° although values lower than 8° have also been reported in different parts of the world. Residual shear strength is independent of the initial moisture content or stress history of a soil specimen and depends mainly on the percentage and mineralogy of the clay fraction. To a lesser extent residual shear strength is influenced by the pore fluid composition and particle sizes, shapes etc. of the non-clay fraction.

Residual shear strength envelopes are often curved and care should be exercised in interpreting and comparing values of residual ϕ quoted in different papers. Sometimes confusion may also arise between values of residual ϕ measured in the laboratory and values inferred from back-analyses of slope failures. The post-peak shearing displacement required to cause a reduction in the angle of shearing resistance to a residual value varies with soil type, normal stress on the shearing plane, test conditions and sample size. In this connection it is extremely important to note that much larger displacements are required for progress to residual conditions in the field than in the laboratory (Skempton, 1964, 1970; James, 1971a and b). Moisture content in the shear zone at the residual state appears to decrease linearly with increase in the residual shear strength (Chowdhury and Bertoldi, 1977).

Residual strengths measured in the laboratory using multiple-reversal shear box tests have sometimes given results different from those obtained using ring shear tests (Bishop et al., 1971). It is, therefore, probable that residual values operative in the field may differ from values measured in the laboratory. The ring shear apparatus has been developed and improved over the decades since 1971 and one version is the Bromhead apparatus. Field residual shear strengths continue to be compared with laboratory measurements (Bromhead and Dixon, 1986; Trenter and Warren, 1996). For example, limit equilibrium back-analyses of reactivated landslides, such as the Folkestone Warren Landslide, were carried out several times by different teams including Trenter and Warren (1996). Average residual internal friction angle of Gault clay at this site measured from ring shear and multiple reversal tests was 9.5° whereas back analyses of the main slip surface gave an average value of 10.7°. For the smaller slip surface, the field value at 13° was much larger. However, it was noted that a first-time movement at the hinge to the west of this slip would have influenced the results.

Decades earlier, Hamel (1973a, 1974, 1976, 1978a) also studied the differences between field and laboratory residual values of ϕ. In his experience field residual ϕ values appeared to be higher than laboratory residual ϕ values by up to 5°. Such differences could arise from factors such as the following: (1) Failure surface irregularities (asperities, waviness) in the field, (2) variability in material properties along the failure surface, (3) environmental and shearing conditions in the field being different from those in the laboratory, and (4) variable curvature of most failure surfaces in contrast to plane surfaces in specimens for laboratory tests.

The residual strength concept was originally proposed in terms of the drained condition for clay which is also referred to as the 'long-term' condition. Sometimes it may be necessary to refer to the undrained shear strength of clay subjected to large deformations as the residual strength, as has been done by Lo (1970) when discussing the operational strength of fissured clays. Residual strength of clay in undrained deformation has received comparatively little attention to date. Undrained behaviour may be plastic or brittle depending on the type of soil. For instance, sensitive clays and cemented soils show brittle behaviour in undrained shear. Undrained strength and its relationship to drained strength for saturated soils is considered in section 2.9.

The following are typical values of peak and residual shear strength parameters of mining spoil (unsaturated and saturated states) from Goonyella mine (Richards, 1982):

i   Unsaturated spoil in the "dry" areas (the upper part of the pile)

    Peak $c = 130$ kPa, $\phi = 32°$ (typical) but can be as high as 49° and as low as 20° (in consolidated areas after infiltration). The most important variable is the moisture constant which is related to the suction.

    Residual $c = 125$ kPa, $\phi = 15°$ (typical)

ii Saturated spoil in the basal zone along the pit floor, the spoil having been thoroughly remoulded by large shear strains associated with the dumping operations

    Peak $c = 50$ kPa, $\phi = 15°$

    Residual $c = 50$ kPa, $\phi = 3°$

2.4.8   Undrained strength of fissured clays

The measured undrained strength of fissured clays depends on the size of the sample tested in relation to the spacing of the fissures. Therefore care must be exercised in interpreting laboratory measurements for use in field problems (Skempton and La Rochelle, 1965; Morgenstern, 1977). The upper limit of strength approaches the strength of intact material and the lower limit approaches the strength along the fissures. The strength along discontinuities has been discussed by Skempton and Petley (1968). The operational strength may be significantly higher than the fissure strength and the following relationship between undrained strength and specimen size has been proposed by Lo (1970):

$$C = C_m + (C_0 - C_m)e^{-\alpha(a-a_0)^\beta} \qquad a > a_0 \tag{2.13}$$

where a is the area of the potential failure plane of the specimen, C is the undrained shear strength of the specimen having a potential failure plane of area a, C_0 is the intact strength, C_m is the operational strength of the soil mass $(a \to \infty)$, a_0 is the area of the potential failure plane at and below which value the intact strength is measured. α and β are parameters which define the strength-size relationship and depend on the intensity of fissuring of the clay. As α and β increase, the strength C approaches the strength C_m more rapidly.

For intact clays $\alpha = 0$ and $C = C_0$. Dividing both sides of Equation (2.13) by C_0 we have:

$$r = r_m + (1 - r_m)e^{-\alpha(a-a_0)^\beta} \tag{2.14}$$

where r is the ratio of strength of any size of sample to the intact strength and r_m is the ratio of operational strength to intact strength. A typical plot is shown in Figure 2.3.

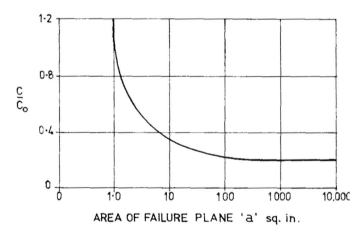

Figure 2.3 Typical strength-size relationship for fissured clay – plot of ratio of undrained strength for any size specimen to intact undrained strength (after Lo, 1970). With permission, see page 713, No 8.

For further discussion of undrained shear strength of stiff-fissured clay and its use in stability analysis the reader is directed to chapter 5.

The shear strength of a soil may vary with direction and it is of interest to investigate the influence of anisotropy on the stability of soil masses.

Equation (2.14) was found to be useful in relation to experimental data obtained from a number of stiff overconsolidated insensitive clays. As an example of typical values Lo (1970) found $\alpha = 0.6$ and $\beta = 0.28$ for brown London clay. He also found that 6 in. diameter triaxial specimens gave strength values for this clay closely approximating the operational strength.

2.5 MOHR-COULOMB CRITERION IN TERMS OF PRINCIPAL STRESSES AND STRESS PATH CONCEPT

2.5.1 Stress paths

It is often useful to express a failure criterion in terms of principal stresses at failure. Such a procedure facilitates plotting and interpretation of test results and also enables the use of the failure criterion in stress analysis type of calculations (e.g., using the finite element method as discussed in chapter 6). Note that in the following discussion effective stresses and corresponding strengths are implied. The Mohr-Coulomb criterion may be expressed in the following form:

$$(\sigma_1 - \sigma_3) = 2c \cos\phi + (\sigma_1 + \sigma_3)\sin\phi \tag{2.15}$$

This is illustrated by Figure 2.4 which shows a Mohr circle at failure and the failure envelope represented by Equation (2.15). This equation may be rearranged (so that σ_1 at failure is expressed in terms of σ_3 at failure) as follows:

$$\sigma_1 = \sigma_3 \tan^2(45° + \phi/2) + 2c \tan(45° + \phi/2) \tag{2.16}$$

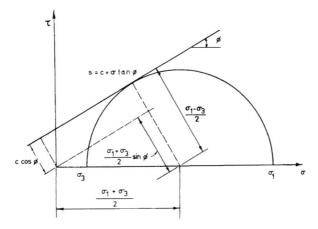

Figure 2.4 Relationship between principal effective stresses at failure – Mohr's circle of stress is tangent to the Coulomb envelope of strength.

These equations suggest alternative ways of plotting the results of triaxial compression tests or of other tests in which principal stresses are measured. For example a plot of $q = (\sigma_1 - \sigma_3)/2$ against $p = (\sigma_1 + \sigma_3)/2$ is a straight line with a slope of $\sin \phi$ and an intercept on the ordinate of $c \cos \phi$ (considering failure values of σ_1 and σ_3). If the principal stresses on any element or specimen from initial loading to failure are successively plotted on the same p-q diagram, a 'stress-path' is obtained which clearly shows the manner in which the state of failure was reached. A stress path graphically portrays the loading history of a soil sample or soil element. Thus it helps to gain insight into the stress-strain-time behaviour of a soil element. The stress path approach was developed over a number of years at MIT and is adequately discussed with useful examples by Lambe and Whitman (1969). Stress paths may be drawn in terms of total stresses as well as effective stresses. The end point of any effective stress path which goes to failure is a point on the failure envelope with slope $\sin \phi$ as shown in Figure 2.5 for isotropically consolidated drained test (CID or ICD) on a specimen. Different shapes of effective stress paths would result from different types of tests such as unconsolidated undrained test (UU), isotropically-consolidated undrained test (CIU or ICU), anisotropically-consolidated undrained test (CAU or ACU) and anisotropically consolidated drained test (CAD or ACD). Typically, an effective stress path in undrained deformation is curved in shape and tangent to the failure envelope at the end point.

Stress paths may also be plots of principal stress difference against the sum of the principal stresses rather than plots of halves of these quantities. Also some reported stress paths are plots of half the stress difference against the minor principal stress (Janbu, 1977).

Sometimes it may be useful to plot σ_1 at failure against σ_3 at failure. If the Coulomb failure criterion is obeyed, such a plot is a straight line with a slope of $\tan^2 (45° + \phi/2)$ and an intercept on the ordinate equal to $2c \tan (45° + \phi/2)$. This intercept represents the uniaxial compressive strength of the soil or rock material.

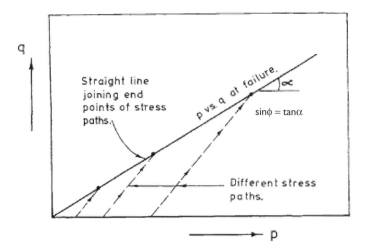

Figure 2.5 Stress paths for CID triaxial compression test – (corresponding to drained loading).

2.5.2 Failure plane inclination and intermediate principal stress

According to the Mohr-Coulomb theory the failure plane makes an angle $\theta = (45° + \phi/2)$ with direction of the minor principal stress, (where ϕ is the effective stress angle of shearing resistance). This inclination is the theoretical orientation of failure plane one should observe after failure of an ideal material in an ideal test. However, observed angles in shear tests are influenced by test limitations and departures of real from theoretical soil behaviour. Therefore, it would be unwise to infer values of ϕ from the inclination of failure planes in laboratory tests except perhaps in highly sophisticated tests for research purposes.

The Mohr-Coulomb theory is considered to be valid for the general case $\sigma_1 > \sigma_2 > \sigma_3$ and predicts that the failure plane passes through the direction of the principal stress σ_2. (However, the influence of the intermediate principal stress is not considered in the Mohr-Coulomb equation and this is discussed in the following paragraph). In order that the normal stress σ on any plane be always positive (compressive) it can be shown that the major principal stress must always be greater than half the uniaxial compressive strength, i.e.,

$$\sigma_1 > c \tan(45° + \phi/2) \tag{2.17}$$

In usual triaxial compression tests, two principal stresses (minor and intermediate) are equal. In extension tests, the major and intermediate principal stresses are equal. Apart from usual triaxial apparatus, tests may be carried out in plane strain compression apparatus so that strain is not allowed in one of the directions. These tests have been successfully carried out at many research centres in UK, USA and elsewhere. In these tests the intermediate principal stress has a magnitude which is determined by the soil properties and is not equal to either the major or the minor principal stress. Plane strain compression tests are better than triaxial compression tests in simulating deformation conditions in the field. The deformation of long soil structures, such as embankments, slopes, earth dams and retaining walls, is considered to approximate to plane strain. In all such cases, the strain in the direction of length or the axis is regarded as negligible or zero.

2.5.3 Coulomb failure criterion for compression and extension tests

It is useful to consider different magnitudes of the intermediate principal stress at failure in terms of the Mohr-Coulomb theory by comparing a triaxial compression test to a triaxial extension test.

In the former the axial stress σ_a is the major principal stress and the intermediate and minor principal stresses are equal to the radial stress σ_r whereas in the latter case the major and intermediate principal stresses are both equal to σ_r whereas the minor principal stress is σ_a. It is interesting to consider the ratio of the deviator stress q to the spherical stress p (or mean normal stress) in each case. (This definition of q and p is different from that used in discussing stress paths, e.g., Figure 2.5). Consider now, in turn, a compression test and an extension test.

Compression test

$$\frac{q}{p} = \frac{\sigma_a - \sigma_r}{(\sigma_a + 2\sigma_r)/3} \tag{2.18}$$

from Equation (2.15)

$$(\sigma_a - \sigma_r) = 2c \cos\phi + (\sigma_a + \sigma_r)\sin\phi \tag{2.19}$$

from Equations (2.18) and (2.19)

$$\frac{q}{p} = \frac{6\sigma_r \sin\phi + 6c \cos\phi}{\sigma_r(3 - \sin\phi) + 2c \cos\phi} \tag{2.20}$$

when $c = 0$,

$$\frac{q}{p} = \frac{6\sin\phi}{3 - \sin\phi} \tag{2.21}$$

when $\sigma_r = 0$,

$$\frac{q}{p} = 3 \tag{2.22}$$

This can also be checked directly from Equation (2.18) by putting $\sigma_r = 0$.

Extension test

Following the above steps:

$$\frac{q}{p} = \frac{6\sigma_a \sin\phi + 6c \cos\phi}{\sigma_a(3 + \sin\phi) + 4c \cos\phi} \tag{2.23}$$

when $c = 0$,

$$\frac{q}{p} = \frac{6\sin\phi}{3 + \sin\phi} \tag{2.24}$$

when $\sigma_a = 0$,

$$\frac{q}{p} = \frac{3}{2} \tag{2.25}$$

Summing up

Thus, for a material with a unique value of ϕ, the strength criterion predicts different ratios of spherical to deviatoric stress at failure for different kinds of test. For example when $c = 0$, it is easy to see that q/p at failure (which depends only on ϕ), is greater for compression than for extension. For unconfined compression and for extension with zero axial stress, the q/p ratio at failure is (a) independent of material properties and, again, (b) greater for compression than for extension. Note, however, that the major principal stress at failure is the same in both cases.

$$\sigma_a = 2c\tan(45° + \phi/2) - \frac{2c\cos\phi}{1 - \sin\phi}$$

$$\sigma_r = 2c\tan(45° + \phi/2) = \frac{2c\cos\phi}{1 - \sin\phi}$$

(2.26)

Similarly, from Equation (2.16) it is useful to note that for $c = 0$, the ratio of major to minor principal stress is the same. Thus:

$$\frac{\sigma_a}{\sigma_r} = \tan^2(45° + \phi/2) \quad \text{compression}$$

$$\frac{\sigma_r}{\sigma_a} = \tan^2(45° + \phi/2) \quad \text{extension}$$

(2.27)

Reference to the yield surface in three dimensions is made in section 2.7.

2.6   SHEAR STRENGTH OF ROCKS

2.6.1   A rock mass as a discontinuum

There are both similarities and differences between the mechanical behaviour of soils and rocks. Soils are particulate materials and rocks are often broken up by a network of discontinuities such as joints and faults into individual blocks or elements. Thus both soil and rock masses may be regarded as discontinua. However, rock elements are much larger in size in comparison to soil particles. The latter have a very large size range in comparison to the size range of rock elements. The properties of individual elements are often important in determining the properties of a rock mass. Also in the case of rocks the properties of discontinuities (e.g., joints and faults) are very important in relation to stability problems such as those concerning slopes. Distortion within a rock mass often occurs by sliding between elements which is analogous to slip between particles and particle groups in soils. However, the elements of a rock mass are frequently interlocked and large stress gradients may occur in rock elements.

In slope stability problems, the strength along discontinuity planes is of primary interest. It is usual to represent the shear strength in terms of the Mohr-Coulomb (or Terzaghi-Coulomb equation) relating shear stress at failure to the normal stress on the failure plane. However, the roughness of a discontinuity is extremely important and this is discussed separately in subsequent paragraphs. A discontinuity may not be continuous and attention then needs to be given to occurrence of failure partly through intact material. Further, a discontinuity may be filled by gouge material and the shear strength will be influenced by the nature and extent of filling (gouge material) in the discontinuities. Failure may also occur through closely fractured rock. In all these cases the strength envelope is generally non-linear, the shape being concave downwards. Therefore, great care must be exercised in extrapolating test data outside the stress range used for testing.

2.6.2 Example of the importance of discontinuities in rock – the occurrence of catastrophic landslides

Many catastrophic landslides involve the detachment of rock masses and their movement at high speeds and it is necessary to gain a good understanding of the mechanical behaviour of such masses and how adverse changes in stability are related to the strength and orientation of discontinuities, amongst other potential factors. For example, McSaveney (2002), while discussing four rock falls and rock avalanches in Mount Cook National Park, New Zealand, observed that all failures involved steep slopes of intensely fractured rock. The three largest were of cohesionless, anisotropic materials and had joints dipping parallel to the slope with dips steeper than the slope inclination. Initial failures were of limited extent and occurred at elevations well below the respective mountain peaks but each of these failures extended to the entire slope by a rapid process of retrogression. The basic causes of landsliding are complex and not easy to determine especially when there has been no obvious triggering agent. While acknowledging that the precise causes of these rock falls and avalanches are undetermined, McSaveney offers the following relevant indications of the sliding potential: "There is no part of the Southern Alps not under tectonic compressive and shear stresses; no slope within Mount Cook National Park that has not undergone rapid denudation and dissection; and there are few slopes not highly fractured. Given the few processes acting to denude snow-covered summits of the high Alps, perhaps all of the upper slopes are undergoing rock mass bulging and are thus subject to episodic collapse on a greater or lesser scale".

2.6.3 Griffith theory of rock fracture

For understanding the behaviour of a rock mass at a fundamental level, it is appropriate to refer to the theory proposed by Griffith (1921, 1924) concerning fracture of rock. This theory is based on the assumption that tensile fracture is initiated at stress concentrations at the ends of hypothetical flat elliptic cracks in rock and leads to the following equations:

$$(\sigma_1 - \sigma_3)^2 = C_0(\sigma_1 + \sigma_3) \quad \text{for } \sigma_1 + 3\sigma_3 > 0$$
$$\sigma_3 = \frac{-C_0}{8} \quad \text{for } \sigma_1 + 3\sigma_3 < 0$$

(2.28)

in which C_0 is the uniaxial compressive strength. The corresponding Mohr envelope has the following equation:

$$\tau^2 = \frac{C_0}{2}\left(\sigma + \frac{C_0}{8}\right)$$

(2.29)

It has been suggested that these equations are valid only if the 'Griffith cracks' remain open. Minute cracks in real rocks may close and reopen under polyaxial stresses depending on the magnitude of octahedral normal and shear stresses and Griffith's theory is, therefore, not strictly applicable. The validity of Equations (2.28) and (2.29) has also not been established by experimental evidence. Modifications to the theory of Griffith have been proposed from time to time (e.g., McClintock and Walsh, 1962). Attention has also been given to the generalisation of Equations (2.28) and (2.29) for a three-dimensional stress system.

Although Griffith's theory does not have a direct role to play in problems of slope stability, it has proved valuable as a basis for studying rock behaviour at a fundamental level. This theory may also contribute towards a better understanding of the processes involved in the formation of slip surfaces. Reference to the application of fracture mechanics and energy concepts in relation to the propagation of shear bands in slopes is made in chapter 8. Discussion of the stress-strain behaviour of intact rock under polyaxial stresses is outside the scope of this book. Stress-strain behaviour of rocks depends to a significant extent on rock type and stress level and it is not appropriate to make a general statement about the shapes of curves that may be obtained. Similarly changes in volume (including aspects such as dilatancy) under polyaxial stresses will depend on rock type, stress level and other factors.

2.6.4 Shear failure along rough discontinuity

As stated in the previous section, the shear strength along a planar discontinuity may be represented by the Coulomb equation. At any given normal stress, the curve of shear stress against shear deformation may show a peak and an ultimate or residual value. (For discontinuities, the two adjectives, 'ultimate' and 'residual', are sometimes used interchangeably and judgment is required to decide if this is justified.)

The residual strength is reached only after large deformations. The extent of difference between peak and residual values depends not only on the type of rock and rock discontinuity but also on the stress level. The Coulomb equation may be written for peak strength in terms of peak strength parameters and for residual strength in terms of residual strength parameters. If a discontinuity is smooth and the direction of shearing coincides with the direction of the discontinuity, then straight line Coulomb envelopes will generally be obtained. The friction angle resulting from such shear tests is referred to as the basic friction angle. Typical values of basic ϕ are $27°$ for shale, $25°$–$35°$ for sandstone, $27°$–$31°$ for siltstone, $33°$–$40°$ for limestone etc. (Barton, 1973).

Real discontinuities are almost always rough and the real friction angle is increased considerably above the basic friction angle depending on the inclination of asperities or projections relative to the direction of shearing. To understand this consider shearing along a smooth plane inclined at an angle i to the direction of shear. Neglecting any cohesion it is easy to show that the applied shear stress at failure is related to the applied normal stress (acting perpendicular to the direction of applied shear) by $\tan(\phi + i)$. Thus the friction angle is increased effectively by i. The presence of undulations, asperities or projections along a discontinuity has precisely this effect since the surface of each projection is inclined to the direction of shearing. Of course the value of i must be taken as an average one for all the projections. Figure 2.6 shows a definition of roughness angle i for shear along a wavy sliding surface or through stepped joints.

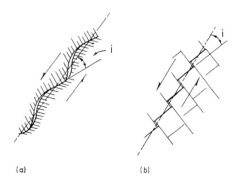

(a)   (b)

Figure 2.6 A definition of roughness angle corresponding to (a) sliding surface, (b) stepped joints.

Patton (1966) was the first to emphasise the importance of the roughness angle *i* and to demonstrate its practical significance. He measured average values of *i* from photographs of bedding plane traces in unstable limestone slopes and found that the inclination of a bedding plane trace was approximately equal to the sum of the average angle *i* and the basic friction angle ϕ measured from prepared smooth surfaces in the laboratory.

As long as the normal stresses are sufficiently low and none of the projections or undulations are sheared off, sliding over the undulations or projections is accompanied by dilation or an increase in total specimen volume. As the normal stress on the surface of sliding increases, shearing takes place through the material forming the projections or undulations and the effective roughness angle *i* is reduced. The value of *i* eventually becomes zero at some value of the normal stress. Testing a specimen at low normal stress may show a Coulomb envelope with zero cohesion and a friction angle equal to $(\phi + i)$ but testing at high normal stresses would show a high cohesion intercept and a reduced friction angle equal to ϕ. Thus an idealised bilinear failure envelope may be described by:

$$s = \sigma \tan(\phi + i), \quad \sigma < \sigma_0$$
$$s = c + \sigma \tan \phi, \quad \sigma > \sigma_0 \tag{2.30}$$

where σ is the effective normal stress (difference of total normal stress and pore water pressure) and it is easily shown that the limiting stress, σ_0 is given by:

$$\sigma_0 = \frac{c}{\tan(\phi + i) - \tan \phi} \tag{2.31}$$

In reality, abrupt change in the slope of the strength envelope at a specific normal stress seldom occurs and the strength envelope is curved. Several equations for curved envelopes have been proposed and reference to these is made subsequently.

The effect of undulations and projections was further clarified by Barton (1973) who suggested that second order irregularities on a discontinuity surface come into play at very low normal stresses. These second order projections (small bumps and ripples) have much higher i values than the first order projections corresponding to major undulations on a discontinuity. Large differences in i values are confirmed by Patton's (1966) measurements of both first order and second order projections. Barton (1973) compiled evidence to show that at low normal stresses (e.g., 0.21 kg/cm² for a shale and 1.5–3.5 kg/cm² for granite specimens) average i may be the order of 40° to 50°. As normal stress on a surface increases, second order projections are sheared off and first order projections come into play. With further increase in normal stress the first order projections are sheared off and progressively the effective friction angle is reduced to basic friction angle.

In terms of principal stresses, the Coulomb criterion of failure leads to the following condition for sliding on a single joint plane inclined at α to the major principal stress σ_1 (Jaeger, 1971):

$$\sigma_1 - \sigma_3 = \frac{c \cos\phi + \sigma_3 \sin\phi}{\cos(\phi + \alpha)\sin\alpha} \tag{2.32}$$

With a value of $\alpha = (45° - \phi/2)$, the theoretical inclination of failure plane for the Coulomb criterion Equation (2.32) reduces to the following familiar form of Coulomb equation discussed in section 2.5:

$$\sigma_1 = \sigma_3 \tan^2(45° + \phi/2) + 2c\tan(45° + \phi/2) \tag{2.16}$$

It is obvious from the previous discussion that values of c and ϕ for a particular rock to be used in Equation (2.32) would depend largely on the stress level under consideration.

2.6.5   Continuity of jointing and actual area of contact

The degree of continuity of joints is of considerable importance. Consider that 'a' is a fraction of the surface area of a joint which is open or filled and that a fraction '$1 - a$' consists of solid rock. The cohesion c for the whole surface may be estimated as follows

$$c = ac_j + (1-a)c_s \tag{2.33}$$

in which c_j is the cohesion of the joint and c_s the cohesion of the solid material. The application of this equation in practice presents many problems mainly because it is very difficult to determine the value of 'a' reliably (see also section 4.10).

Attention may also be given to the actual area of contact during sliding. If the actual area of contact is A_a and total area A, the shear strength may be a expressed in the form (Jaeger, 1971)

$$s = c_a(A_a/A) + \mu_a\sigma_n \tag{2.34}$$

in which c_a and μ_a are constants. At high normal stresses A_a/A approaches 1 and c_a may have very high values. For contact at low normal stresses A_a/A may be in small fraction (say 0.01) and values of cohesion may be quite small. Jaeger and Cook (1968) quote the following values for sliding of trachyte on trachyte with varying area of contact: $c_a = 10,000$ psi and $\mu_a = 0.32$ at high normal stresses and $c_a = 10$ p.s.i and $\mu_a = 0.48$ at low normal stresses. Byerlee (1967) quotes the following results concerning triaxial tests on granite $c_a = 9,000$ psi and $\mu_a = 0.6$ in the normal stress range 30,000 to 225,000 psi. At low normal stresses c_a was only of the order of 90 psi suggesting a value of A_a/A of the order of 0.01. In discussing applications to rock slope stability problems Jaeger (1971) suggested the use of high normal stresses in shear testing and the subsequent calculation of actual cohesion at low normal stress on the basis of the ratio A_a/A. However, he acknowledged serious practical difficulties in determining this ratio.

2.6.6   Curved strength envelopes

It is well known that shear strength envelopes for many rocks show a marked departure from linearity (Jaeger, 1971; Hoek, 1976). The envelopes are concave downwards and a number of non-linear relationships have been suggested e.g., Murrell (1965), Hobbs (1970). None of the many proposed empirical equations has accepted status and care must be exercised in interpretation of shear strength data. Alternative interpretations may lead to marked differences in calculated factors of safety of rock slopes. Reference to two striking examples is made in this regard in section 4.8. In section 2.4 mention was made of a linear relationship between zero cohesion peak friction angle and the logarithm of the effective normal stress for some soils and in one case for desert alluvium (which was like a soft rock). It would be of interest to investigate the validity of such a relationship for different types of rocks.

Curved strength envelopes for sliding along discontinuities are of special interest in rock slope stability problems. The gradual transition from dilation to shearing along a discontinuity was studied by Ladanyi and Archambault (1970, 1972) who proposed the following equation for peak shear strength:

$$s = \frac{(1-a_s)\,(\dot{v} + \tan \phi) + a_s s_s}{1 - (1-a_s)\dot{v}\,\tan \phi} \tag{2.35}$$

in which a_s is the proportion of discontinuity surface was which is sheared through projections of intact rock, $\dot{v}$ is the dilation rate at peak shear strength (the rate of dilation is the ratio of small incremental change in specimen normal displacement dv to small incremental change in shear displacement du i.e., dv/du), and s_s is the shear strength of intact rock material. At low normal stresses a_s is nearly zero, $\dot{v} = \tan i$ and Equation (2.35) reduces to the simple form $s = \sigma \tan(\phi + i)$ which is identical to the first of equation (2.30). Using a parabolic equation for the shear strength of material adjacent to the discontinuity in accordance with Fairhurst (1964) and empirical relationships for a_s and $\dot{v}$, Ladanyi and Archambault modified Equation (2.35) for possible practical use (see also Hoek and Bray, 1977). The resulting empirical equation is a relationship between s/C_j and σ/C_j involving only the parameters i (roughness angle) and ϕ (basic friction angle). C_j is the uniaxial compressive strength of the rock material adjacent to the discontinuity which may be lower than the strength of intact rock material due to weathering or loosening of the surface near the discontinuity. Barton (1973) proposed the following equation:

$$s = \sigma \tan\left(\phi + JRC \ \log_{10} \frac{C_i}{\sigma} \right) \tag{2.36}$$

where JRC is a joint roughness co-efficient which varies from 5 for smooth joints (planar shear joints, planar foliation, planar bedding) to 20 for rough undulating joints (tension joints, rough sheeting, rough bedding). When normal stresses are low and i (or JRC) is high the strength predicted by Ladanyi and Archambault's equation is in close agreement with that predicted by Barton's equation. The curves predicted by the two equations diverge considerably as normal stresses increase. Barton's equation is more conservative and reduces to $s = \sigma \tan \phi$ for σ/C_i approaching 1 whereas the equation of Ladanyi and Archambault reduces to $s = s_s$ i.e., the strength of intact rock which is much higher than $\sigma \tan \phi$ (ϕ being the basic friction angle for smooth surfaces here). Since Barton's studies were carried out at very low normal stresses, Hoek and Bray (1977) suggest that his equation is applicable in the range $\sigma/C_i = 0.01 - 0.3$. The stress levels in rock slope stability are often in this range and Barton's equation can be quite useful. Barton suggests that his equation be used only when the term within brackets in Equation (2.36) does not exceed 70°.

2.6.7   Strength of filled discontinuities

Discontinuities are often filled with some form of soft material which may be (a) gouge or detrital material resulting from previous shear movements, (b) material deposited in open joints due to water movement or other causes. The influence of filling material on the shear strength of a given discontinuity depends on the thickness of the filling. Goodman (1970) showed experimentally that (a) the shear strength reduces continuously with increase in filling thickness and (b) that once the filling thickness exceeds the amplitude of the surface projections, the strength of the joint is controlled by the strength of the filling material. Barton (1974) reviewed the strength of filled discontinuities and compiled tables of shear strength values. Filling of discontinuities with gouge material has a significant influence on the permeability. This is because the material often has a significant proportion of fine clayey material which has an extremely low permeability in comparison to that of a rock mass (with joints, fissures, etc.). Therefore, the presence of filling in discontinuities may hinder natural drainage and result in building up of pore water pressures. Thus stability is decreased due to two reasons (a) reduced strength along discontinuities due to presence of filling material, (b) high pore water pressures due to decreased natural drainage.

2.6.8   Shear strength of closely jointed or fractured rock

A hard rock mass may be closely jointed or fractured and its shear strength in this condition is often significantly different from that of a single discontinuity. Studies of jointed rock masses have been made by many research workers, e.g., John (1969), Brown (1970) and, Einstein and Hirschfeld (1973). In particular, the Hoek-Brown criterion (Hoek, 1990) for the strength of a rock mass has been proposed and is widely accepted; Mohr Coulomb friction and strength parameters may, of course, be estimated from the Hoek-Brown failure criterion (Hoek, 1990).

Individual blocks within a jointed mass may undergo deformations to a significant degree and the nature of these deformations varies from one jointed system to another. From model studies Ladanyi and Archambault (1970, 1972) found that three main types of failure can occur in jointed rock masses with two sets of discontinuities (1) shear along a failure plane inclined to both discontinuity sets, (2) formation of a narrow failure zone in which block rotation has occurred in addition to sliding and (3) formation of a kink band of rotated and separated columns of 3, 4 or 5 blocks. They proposed empirical equations for shear strength similar to those for a single discontinuity to which reference was made in an earlier paragraph. The values of empirical constants to be used with their equations are chosen according to the mode of failure which is considered relevant among the three possible modes listed above.

There are many similarities between the shear strength characteristics of jointed rock masses and those of rockfill. Deformation properties of rockfill have been discussed in many publications such as Wilkins (1970), Marachi et al. (1972) and Marsal (1973).

An interesting recent contribution to the strength theory of homogeneous jointed rock mass has been made by Wu and Wang (2001). They extended basic probability concepts concerning the strength of a brittle material and applid these to a rock mass which may be characterized by the Hoek-Brown criterion (Hoek, 1990). The failure criterion and failure probability of a set of cracks was proposed based on fracture mechanics and a statistical theory of rock mass structure. They concluded that the compressive strength of a rock block has a most probable value which usually differs from the average strength. The compressive strength and its variance show a strong scale effect. Also for the rock mass, composed of the rock material as well as joints, the compressive strength has strong scale and inter-angle effects.

2.6.9   Determination of shear strength

Before performing shear tests concerning rock strength, it is essential to obtain specimens which have suffered as little disturbance as possible. Joint surface materials should be retained on the joints to be tested. If gouge material is present, attempts should be made to avoid relative movement of the two halves of a specimen. It is also desirable to prevent changes in moisture content. Shear tests on poor quality samples may be quite misleading. Preliminary studies should be conducted to see if high quality shear tests on carefully procured samples are justified in terms of cost, time and the sensitivity of slope design to strength parameters in any particular problem. In some cases, it may be quite sufficient to use values of strength parameters based on past experience in a particular area or type of rock. In other cases, it may be possible to use empirical relationships which require only the determination of basic friction angle ϕ, average roughness angle i, and the uniaxial compressive strength. The latter may conveniently be determined from the simple point load index test, (Broch and Franklin, 1972) using empirical correlations which have been developed between point load index I_s and uniaxial compressive strength C_0 (e.g., Bieniawski, 1974):

$$C_0 = 24 I_s \tag{2.37}$$

The constant 24 is for a 54 mm core and is replaced by 17.5 for a 20 mm core, 19 for a 30 mm core, and 23 for a 50 mm core and so on. It should be noted that, due to weathering, loosening etc., the uniaxial compressive strength of material near a discontinuity C_j may be smaller than C_0 Barton (1973) states that weathering can reduce uniaxial compressive strength to as low as one quarter of that of intact unweathered material. The influence of weathering on compressive strength has also been discussed by Hamrol (1961), Fookes et al. (1971) and Franklin and Chandra (1972). Correlations between alteration index (weight of water absorbed by rock in a quick absorption test divided by dry weight of rock expressed as a percentage) and uniaxial compressive strength have been suggested on an empirical basis (e.g., Serafim, 1964). Such correlations show that there is a rapid fall of strength with first few percent increases in alteration index.

The basic friction angle ϕ may be determined by direct shear testing along surfaces prepared by means of a smooth diamond saw cut. A wide range of normal stresses should be used to give a linear relationship between normal stress and shear strength with zero cohesion intercept. The basic friction angle ϕ may also be determined from shear tests in which a specimen has been subjected to large displacements. Average values of roughness angle i may be determined from measurements of the surface profile of rough surfaces or inferred from tests at low normal stresses. For further details concerning measurements with regard to roughness, basic friction angle and compressive strength, the reader may refer to Hoek and Bray (1974, 1977). The reader should always bear in mind the pitfalls of using empirical strength equations without adequate appreciation of their limitations and of the assumptions on which they are based.

Where reliance cannot be placed on tabulated values or empirical correlations, shear tests should be carried out in the laboratory or field using appropriate apparatus. For useful details of in-situ direct shear tests, laboratory shear tests, portable shear machines etc., the reader may again refer to Jaeger (1971) and to Hoek and Bray (1974, 1977). Shear tests should be carried out as far as possible on undisturbed specimens and for a normal stress range appropriate to the type and size of slope stability problem which is to be solved. When residual strengths are required, the shear tests should be continued for large deformations or using multiple reversals of shear.

The differences between peak and residual (or ultimate) strength values may be large or small depending on factors such as nature of rock, nature of discontinuity etc. As an example, the measured values of strength parameters for different discontinuities in the limestone formations at the site of the Frank slide may be considered. This slide occurred in 1903 on the east face of the Turtle Mountain in the Crowsnest Pass area of the Canadian Rockies in South Western Alberta. Krahn and Morgenstern (1976) reported that the peak ϕ values were 32° for joints, 28° for flexural slip surfaces and 51.7° for bedding planes and ultimate values were 14° for joints, 15.6° for flexural slip surfaces and 32.3° for bedding planes. Peak cohesion values ranged from 172 to 262 kN/m^2 and ultimate cohesion values from 55 to 124 kN/m^2.

In some case studies, large differences in peak and ultimate (or residual) strength values have not been found. For example, in connection with a rock wedge stability problem Hamel (1976) reported residual friction angles of 25.5°–30° and peak friction angles of 29.5°–32.5° on remoulded specimens of joint gouge and bedding fault gouge material consisting mainly of silt and sand size argillite fragments. It is interesting that Krahn and Morgenstern (1976) used the term ultimate strength rather than residual strength throughout their paper. It may be that in some cases the deformations suffered by a rock mass have not been sufficient to reduce the strength to real residual values along an existing discontinuity. However, once a slide has occurred the strength would fall to a residual value on the slip surface. Therefore, residual strengths are of tremendous importance in connection with analysis of renewed slope movements along existing shear surfaces or slip planes.

Closely fractured rock material may be tested in large scale triaxial tests as described by Jaeger (1970). It is very difficult to get undisturbed specimens of closely fractured rock and Hoek and Bray (1977) recommend testing of compacted rockfill under conditions which simulate the jointed rock mass. Many studies of closely jointed rock masses have, in fact, been carried out by testing models made of artificial "rock". Once triaxial tests have been performed, data may be plotted in the form of Mohr circles at failure and a curved envelope to these circles drawn. Alternatively a curve is first drawn relating normal stress to shear stress on a 45° plane. This curve is the locus of tops of the Mohr circles. A set of idealised Mohr circles is then drawn at regular intervals of normal stress and finally an envelope to these circles is drawn (see Hoek and Bray, 1977).

2.7   PLASTICITY AND RELATED CONCEPTS

A material is considered to enter the plastic flow range, indicating continuous deformation at constant stress, when the stress intensity first reaches a critical value called the yield value. In order to maintain plastic flow the yield value must be maintained but cannot be exceeded. Such a material is said to exhibit perfect plasticity. For a complex stress state, an adequate yield criterion is required for this perfect plasticity condition. Coulomb's equation discussed previously is one form of yield criterion that may be used for soils. Tresca' yield criterion, which applies to ductile materials, corresponds to the particular case of Coulomb's yield criterion where there is no internal friction. With $\phi = 0$ in the Coulomb equation, c is the shear yield stress for a purely cohesive material. In fact, this criterion is applicable to metals. Often the term 'Tresca material' and 'cohesive soil' are used interchangeably in discussions of plasticity.

The Coulomb yield surface in three-dimensional representation is a right hexagonal pyramid equally inclined to the σ_1, σ_2, σ_3 axes. (Figure 2.7). The section of such a pyramid by a deviatoric plane is an irregular hexagon since the yield stress in tension is different from the yield stress in compression. A deviatoric plane has the following equation:

$$\sigma_1 + \sigma_2 + \sigma_3 = 0 \tag{2.38}$$

Tresca's yield criterion is represented by a right hexagonal cylinder. Drucker (1953) proposed an 'extended Tresca' yield surface which is a right hexagonal pyramid but contrasts with the Coulomb surface in that the section by the deviatoric plane is a regular hexagon which lies well within the Coulomb hexagon. In contrast to the original Tresca criterion, the extended Tresca criterion is dependent, like the Coulomb criterion, on the mean normal stress.

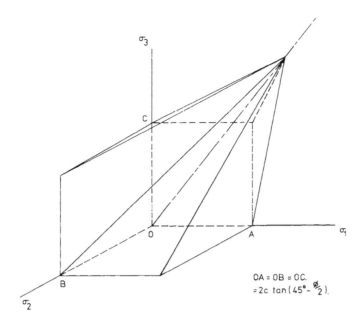

$OA = OB = OC.$
$= 2c \tan(45° - \frac{\phi}{2}).$

Figure 2.7 Coulomb yield surface in three-dimensional stress space.

Another well-known yield criterion is the Von Mises criterion. The Von Mises yield criterion gives a surface which is a circular cylinder inscribed in the Tresca prism and the equation is written as:

$$J_2 = \frac{1}{6}\{(\sigma_1 - \sigma_2)^2 + (\sigma_2 - \sigma_3)^2 + (\sigma_3 - \sigma_1)^2\} = k^2 \tag{2.39}$$

Drucker and Prager (1952) proposed the extended Von Mises criterion for soils so that yield would be dependent on the mean normal stress. The extended Von Mises surface is a right circular cone equally inclined to the three principal axes. The intersection of the deviatoric plane with this cone is a circle as shown in Figure 2.8. The extended Von Mises yield surface lies between two right circular cones obtained by inscribing and circumscribing the extended Tresca hexagon respectively. Drucker and Prager gave the following form of the yield function, using octahedral stresses Equation (2.1):

$$\alpha \sigma_{oct} + \sqrt{\frac{3}{2}}\, \tau_{oct} = k, \quad \text{or} \quad \alpha \sigma_{oct} + J_2^{\frac{1}{2}} = k \tag{2.40}$$

in which α and k are material parameters. ($\alpha = 0$) reduces Equation (2.40) to Von Mises criterion for metals. Comparison of Equation (2.40) with Coulomb's equation shows that, for plane strain:

$$\alpha = \frac{3\tan\phi}{\sqrt{9 + 12\tan^2\phi}}, \quad k = \frac{3c}{\sqrt{9 + 12\tan^2\phi}} \tag{2.41}$$

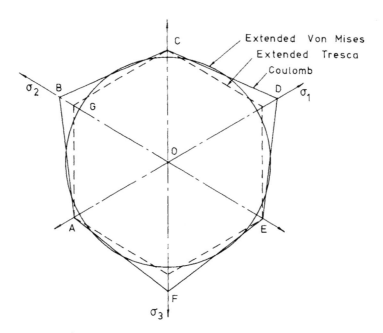

Figure 2.8 Various yield criteria projected on deviatoric plane.

The extended Tresca and extended Von Mises yield criteria may be considered as attempts to generalise the Coulomb rule to three dimensions. The correct yield surface for the Coulomb criteria is of course the one discussed first and is properly based on interpretation by the Mohr diagram. It has been shown for soils (Bishop, 1966) that the Mohr Coulomb criterion is in better agreement with experiment results than the others. For plane strain the extended Von Mises and extended Tresca criteria reduce to Coulomb rule in two dimensions. This has implications for their use in determining collapse loads in plane strain problems.

The theory of plasticity is concerned with the plastic deformation increments of a soil and the directions of these increments, and this involves the concept of a flow rule. The yield function (for the particular yield criterion) is considered as a plastic potential from which the stress and plastic strain increments can be determined by a condition which is known as the flow rule.

The requirement of coincidence of the principal axes of stress and strain increment gives the following ratio of principal strain increments:

$$\frac{\dot{\varepsilon}_1}{\dot{\varepsilon}_3} = \frac{\partial f / \partial \sigma_1}{\partial f / \partial \sigma_3} \tag{2.42}$$

in which f is the yield function which, for a Coulomb material, may be written from Equation (2.16) thus:

$$f = \sigma_1 - \sigma_3 \tan^2(45° + \phi/2) - 2c \tan(45° + \phi/2) \tag{2.43}$$

Consequently, from equation (2.42), the volumetric strain $\dot{\upsilon}$ and the distortional strain $\dot{\gamma}$ are obtained as follows:

$$\dot{\varepsilon}_1 = -\dot{\varepsilon}_3 \tan^2(45° + \phi/2)$$
$$\dot{\upsilon} = \dot{\varepsilon}_1 + \dot{\varepsilon}_3 = \dot{\varepsilon}_3\{2\sin\phi/(1+\sin\phi)\}$$
$$\dot{\gamma} = \dot{\varepsilon}_1 - \dot{\varepsilon}_3 = \dot{\varepsilon}_3\{-2/(1+\sin\phi)\}$$

$$\frac{\dot{\upsilon}}{\dot{\gamma}} = -\sin\phi$$

(2.44)

The angle of dilation v is defined as:

$$v = \sin^{-1}\left\{\frac{-\dot{\upsilon}}{\dot{\gamma}}\right\}$$

(2.45)

Therefore, from the last of Equations (2.44) and (2.45) we have:

$$v = \phi$$

(2.46)

Soils are observed to increase in volume (or dilate) at a rate considerably less than that given by Equation (2.46) above and this is one of the difficulties in the application of the theory of perfect plasticity if the associated flow rule is used.

The above flow rule implies that the plastic strain increment vector is normal to the yield surface at yield and is, therefore, called the normality condition of the theory of plasticity.

In chapter 8 of this book reference is made to the limit theorems (upper bound theorem and lower bound theorem) of the theory of plasticity which have been used in the solution of stability problems including slopes. In so far as the flow rule of perfect plasticity does not correspond with the variable dilation rates of real soils, it may be argued that these theorems have no relevance to these materials. Other techniques have sometimes been used to study deformation problems concerning soils (James and Bransby, 1971). On the other hand it is worth noting that non-associated flow rules which correspond with material behaviour have also been used in the theory of plasticity with some success and the corresponding theorems have, for instance, been given by Chen (1975).

In conventional plasticity, kinematic hardening is normally described with translation of yield surfaces in stress space. Thus a strain state can be updated knowing the changes in stresses. However, if a stress state has to be updated knowing changes in strain, theories based on strain space rather than stress space have some advantages. Alternatively, a hyperplasticity approach may be used as discussed by Puzrin and Houlsby (2001). Hyperplasticity is an approach that allows a compact development of plasticity theories based on thermo-mechanical principles so that laws of thermodynamics are obeyed.

The deformation behaviour of real soils is neither truly frictional nor perfectly plastic and involves many complexities. Drucker et al. (1957) introduced the strain-hardening theories of plasticity in order to bridge the gap between the perfectly plastic idealization and the behaviour of real soils. Many workers have since attempted to develop sophisticated theories for ideal soils. Notable progress in these directions has been made at Cambridge University, England (Roscoe et al., 1958; Schofield and Wroth, 1968).

2.8   EXCESS PORE WATER PRESSURES

The paramount importance of excess pore water pressures in soil mechanics problems was recognised as a consequence of an understanding of the principle of effective stress. Loading or unloading of soils results in pore water pressure changes which are of a transient nature. Low permeability of most soils causes a delay in the dissipation of these excess pore pressures which occurs with drainage and migration of pore water within a soil mass. While excess pore pressures have not been dissipated fully, effective or stresses increase or decrease depending on whether the pore pressure excess is a decrease or an increase respectively. Shear strength is controlled by effective stress and, therefore, excess pore pressures are extremely important in evaluating stability for short-term (end-of-construction) and long-term conditions. Excess pore water pressures may dissipate very quickly in soils of high permeability such as sands and gravels but the time required for pore pressure equilibrium to be reached increases as the permeability decreases and may be of the order of 50 years for some clays.

Field measurement of pore water pressure by means of piezometers is now a recognised practice in geotechnical engineering. Monitoring of pore water pressure before, during and after construction is extremely useful in analysis and design (e.g., Terzaghi and Peck, 1967, Art 68). Pore water pressure observations have enabled great advances to be made in applied soil and rock mechanics in the last few decades and their value cannot be over-emphasised. In situations where pore pressures have not been measured by reliable means, considerable uncertainty often exists concerning stability and performance of slopes inspite of the most refined methods of analysis that may be employed. Similarly back-analyses from an actual failure cannot be used to draw meaningful conclusions without knowledge of pore pressure conditions at the time of the failure. Measurement of pore pressures in earth and rockfill dams and their foundations is considered essential. Instrumentation of natural slopes is not always economically feasible but is often essential in large projects or in situations which are significant with regard to safety, economy, convenience or other factors.

Two distinct classes of problem may be considered in regard to excess pore pressures and both of these are concerned with slopes and their stability. The construction of an earth dam or embankment on a soft clay foundation results in positive excess pore water pressures in the foundation. Thus the immediate end-of-construction, pore water pressures are high and consequently the shear strength and factor of safety are low. With the passage of time the pore pressures will dissipate, the strength and factor of safety will increase as explained by Bishop and Bjerrum (1960). This is shown in Figure 2.9.

Consider, on the other hand, the excavation of a cut in a clay soil. This is equivalent to a release of stress and produces an immediate, end-of-excavation relief of pore

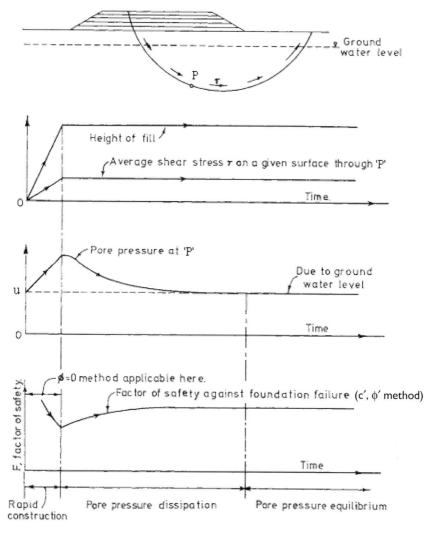

Figure 2.9 Changes in pore water pressure and factor of safety of an embankment on soft clay during and after construction (after Bishop and Bjerrum, 1960). With permission from ASCE, see page 713, No 9.

pressure. Consequently the shear strength and the factor of safety are high. With the passage of time pore pressure equilibrium is gradually attained and shear strength and factor of safety decrease. This is illustrated in Figure 2.10.

The changes in the shear stress, pore water pressure and factor of safety of an earth dam at various stages are shown in Figure 2.11. Note that different stages are critical for downstream and upstream slopes. For upstream slope, construction phase and rapid draw down are often critical. For the downstream slope the impounding of reservoir and subsequent steady seepage condition reduce the factor of safety considerably in comparison to that of the upstream slope.

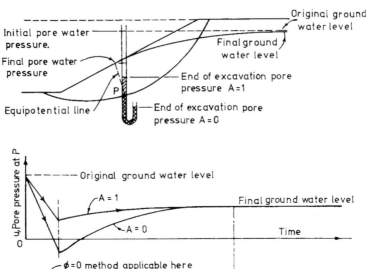

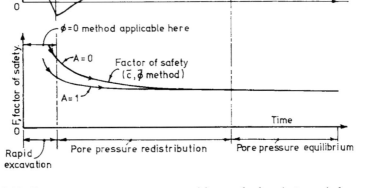

Figure 2.10 Changes in pore water pressure and factor of safety during and after excavation in clay (after Bishop and Bjerrum, 1960). With permission from ASCE,
see page 713, No 9.

These principles are not generally applicable to the stability of rock masses for
several reasons. In the first place the bond or cementation between particles must
be considered. The effective area of interparticle contact is significant in comparison to that for soils. Again the degree of saturation would seldom be 100%. The
compressibility of the solid phase is not negligible in comparison to the compressibility of the rock mass as in the case of soils. Thirdly, rock masses usually have
a high secondary permeability due to fissures, joints and other discontinuities. In
principle, it would be possible to extend the above concepts to rock masses using
Skempton's modified effective stress equations for rock and concrete. However, in
reality the role of excess pore water pressures due to loading or unloading of rocks
is insignificant.

Estimation of excess pore water pressures, based on the type and magnitude of
stress increments and on soil properties, is an important problem in soil mechanics.
The most well known approach is based on the concept of pore pressure coefficients *A*
and *B*, first proposed by Skempton (1954). Considering increments in principal

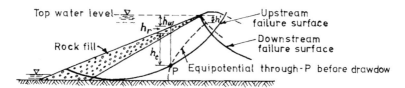

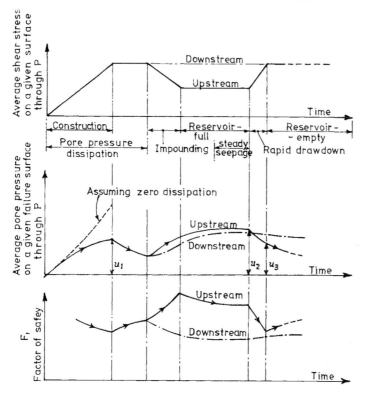

Figure 2.11 Changes in shear stress, pore pressure and safety factor during and after construction of earth dam (after Bishop and Bjerrum, 1960). With permission from ASCE, see page 713, No 9.

stresses $\Delta\sigma_3$ and $\Delta\sigma_1$ during an undrained triaxial compression test, he proposed the following equation for the excess pore pressure*:

$$\Delta u = B\left[\Delta\sigma_3 + A(\Delta\sigma_1 - \Delta\sigma_3)\right] \tag{2.47}$$

---

* The stress difference or deviator stress in the second term may work out negative for a soil element subjected to unloading (one or both principal stress increments being negative). This will depend on how the major principal stress increment is defined. However, the Equation (2.47) is valid only when a positive value of the stress difference is used. [Refer to chapter 7, (Section 7.2), where the application of the pore pressure equation to a case study of an excavation is considered. Moreover, a generalized form of the pore pressure equation is also presented in Section 7.2.]

For saturated soils, B approaches unity but its value decreases drastically with decrease in the degree of saturation. The value of A depends on the type of soil and also varies with stress level and other factors. The values of A at failure are significantly different from those at stress levels well below failure. Lambe and Whitman (1969) state that the value of A is significantly influenced by the following factors (a) the level to which the soil has previously been strained, (b) the initial stress system in the soil, (c) the stress history of the soil and (d) the type of total stress path to which the soil is subjected or the type of stress change e.g., loading or unloading.

The concept of pore pressure coefficients has many applications in soil mechanics relating both to deformation and stability problems. Some applications are not immediately obvious. For example, the concept of pore pressure coefficients can be used to estimate draw-down pore pressures in an initially submerged slope and hence to assess slope stability during rapid draw-down. Such an approach is developed in detail in chapter 4 of this book.

The original form of Equation (2.47) and its generalisation to a three-dimensional stress system are discussed in chapter 7 [see equations (7.5a) and (7.16)]. Typical values of pore pressure coefficient A are given in Table 7.1.

Henkel (1960) proposed the following equation for excess pore pressure in saturated soil in terms of increments of octahedral normal and shear stresses:

$$\Delta u = \Delta \sigma_{oct} + a \Delta \tau_{oct}^{k}$$

(2.47a)

where a and k are pore pressure parameters. This equation is suitable for a general three-dimensional stress system and it separates contributions due to increments in hydrostatic stress and increments in shear stress. It is interesting that adoption of zero values for both a and k giving $\Delta u = \Delta \sigma_{oct}$ has led to acceptable pore pressure predictions in some situations (Hoeg et al., 1969; D'Appolonia et al., 1971; Foott and Ladd, 1977). Obviously, no generalised conclusion about all clays can be drawn from such limited experience.

2.9   RELATIONSHIPS BETWEEN DRAINED AND UNDRAINED STRENGTH OF COHESIVE SOILS

2.9.1   Unique w-$\bar{p}$-q relationships at peak and ultimate strength

In section 2.4 a brief reference was made to undrained shear strength of cohesive soils and its importance. At that stage the importance of excess pore water pressures had not been discussed. Having considered the development of excess pore water pressures during undrained loading, it is possible to explore relationships between undrained shear strength, pore water pressure and drained shear strength parameters. Meaningful relationships have been established only for saturated fine-grained (cohesive) soils and, therefore, the following discussion does not apply to unsaturated soils.

In simple terms, water content w decreases with increasing effective mean normal stress $\bar{p}$ during drained loading and shear strength or deviator stress at failure q increases with decreasing water content. This is the basis of the concept of a unique relationship between the values of w, $\bar{p}$ and q at failure. The values of these parameters will go on changing continuously from initial loading to failure in a drained test on a specimen or on an element of soil in the field. (On the other hand, during undrained loading of a saturated soil element, water content w remains unchanged while the values of pore pressure u, $\bar{p}$ and q go on changing).

In reality a truly unique relationship between the values of q, $\bar{p}$ and w at failure (drained loading and peak strength) does not exist because the soil element or soil sample may have different degrees of preconsolidation (or overconsolidation) to begin with. However, having determined the relationship for a given degree of overconsolidation, it is possible to determine the strength for any type of loading as shown by Lambe and Whitman (1969) with illustrative examples.

In contrast to failure values (or peak values) of q, $\bar{p}$ and w, the values of these quantities at ultimate strength are uniquely related for any given cohesive soil. This is because the degree of preconsolidation has no influence on the ultimate strength. Ideally, ultimate strength of both dense (overconsolidated) and loose (normally consolidated) specimens of the same soil is identical at a given mean normal stress and both types of specimens have the same water content in the ultimate condition which is reached after large strains.

The established conclusions stated above indicate some similarities in the strength behaviour of sands and clays. In both types of soils initial void ratio or initial water content (which depends on stress history or preconsolidation and other factors) controls the peak shear strength at a given effective normal stress. In both types of soil ultimate strength at given normal stress and ultimate void ratio or water content are independent of initial void ratio, water content or stress history. In both types of soil shear strength increases with increasing effective normal stress for given initial conditions. The main difference lies in the fact that application of stress is effective in altering the void ratio and water content of clay but vibration or cyclic loading is required to achieve significant densification of sands. Further, the densification of clay under static pressure can only occur slowly as drainage of water must occur if void spaces in a saturated soil are to be reduced. Drainage occurs slowly because the permeability of clays is usually extremely low.

2.9.2 Undrained strength and pore pressure parameter at failure

For a given clay with a given stress history, any relationship between values of q, $\bar{p}$ and w at failure is the same whether specimens have been subjected to drained shear or undrained shear. Regardless of how the soil is sheared, the relationship between strength and effective stress is the same for the same soil with the same stress history. This does not mean that two identical specimens consolidated under the same effective normal stress will have the same strength if one is tested in drained shear and the other in undrained shear. The strength will be different in the two cases because pore water pressures will be developed in the specimen which is tested undrained and thus the effective stress at failure will be different from that of the specimen tested in drained shear. If the developed pore water pressure is quantified in terms of pore pressure coefficient A at failure, i.e., A_f, the following relationship may be developed between undrained shear strength c_u and initial consolidation stress $\bar{p}_0$ (See Lambe and Whitman, 1969);

$$c_u = \frac{c \cos\phi + (\bar{p}_0 - 2 A_f c_u) \sin\phi}{1 - \sin\phi} \tag{2.48}$$

in which c and ϕ are effective stress parameters of strength. A_f, c and ϕ are all functions of stress history. The effective stress path and undrained strength depend only on the conditions just before the start of shearing. It is of interest for the reader to consider simple forms of Equation (2.48) for $c = 0$, or $A = 0.5$, 1 etc.

2.9.3   Relative magnitude of drained and undrained strength

It is difficult to formulate simple rules to determine whether drained or undrained strength may be greater for a particular soil. The relative magnitude depends on the stress history and the stress path followed by a soil element and it is necessary to consider water content changes as well as effective stresses at failure.

As a guide, Lambe & Whitman (1969) suggest that (1) for triaxial compression loading (σ_1 increasing, with σ_3 constant) CD strengths are greater than CU strengths for normally consolidated clay (N.C.), but CD strengths are approximately equal to CU strengths for heavily overconsolidated clay (O.C.); (2) for triaxial compression unloading (σ_1 constant with σ_3 decreasing) CU strengths are approximately equal to CD strengths for N.C. clays and CU strengths are much greater than CD strengths for O.C. clays.

2.9.4   "$\phi = 0$" concept

Undrained strength of a saturated soil is unaffected by changes in total stress unless accompanied by a change in water content (implying a change in volume). Therefore such a soil behaves in undrained shear as if it has a value of $\phi = 0$, i.e., the total stress Mohr-Coulomb envelope is horizontal. Stated another way, the concept implies that a number of unconsolidated-undrained tests (UU tests) on identical samples of the same saturated soil would give the same undrained shear strength c_u regardless of the level of stresses used for testing. (Note that c_u is half the difference of total principal stresses or effective principal stresses at failure and is independent of developed pore pressure). The validity of a "$\phi = 0$" concept rests on the assumption of no volume change or change in water content during loading or unloading. Such conditions are prevalent immediately after loading or unloading of saturated soft clays whose permeability is often extremely low. Therefore, the $\phi = 0$ concept is of considerable importance in the analysis of slopes of saturated cohesive soils for short-term or end-of-construction stability.

The use of a "$\phi = 0$" concept for short-term stability problems in normally consolidated and lightly overconsolidated soils is widely accepted. However, if the overconsolidation ratio is higher than about 4 to 8, the volume of the soils tends to increase significantly during shear with consequent decrease of pore water pressure. Thus the undrained strength exceeds the drained strength but high negative pore pressures tend to draw water into the soil with consequent swelling and reduction of strength. Therefore the undrained strength cannot be relied upon and its use in stability analysis would lead to results on the unsafe side. On the other hand, for normally loaded or lightly overconsolidated soils, the tendency to decrease in volume implies that strength would increase with time and thus use of undrained strengths would lead to results on the safe side. According to Terzaghi and Peck (1967), the "$\phi = 0$" concept should not be used for clays with overconsolidation ratios higher than about 2 to 4.

For a normally consolidated clay, the following relationship for undrained strength has been suggested (Terzaghi and Peck, 1967):

$$\frac{c_u}{p_3} = \frac{\sin \phi_{cu}}{1 - \sin \phi_{cu}} \tag{2.49}$$

in which p_3 is the minor principal stress (consolidation stress) and ϕ_{cu} is the consolidated-undrained value of shearing resistance (inclination of line drawn from the origin and tangent to the total stress Mohr circle for consolidated-undrained test, consolidation stress being p_3). This equation led Skempton (1957) to suggest that a constant ratio should exist between undrained strength of normally loaded natural deposits and the effective overburden pressure at depths corresponding to the strength tests (which may be unconfined compression or shear vane test). In fact a large number of undrained strength measurements confirmed that the ratio of c_u and the effective overburden pressure $\bar{p}$ is indeed constant for a given deposit. A useful statistical relationship was proposed by Skempton (1957), relating the ratio of undrained shear strength to effective overburden stress on the one hand to plasticity index (PI) of normally-consolidated natural deposits on the other. The proposed relationship is:

$$\frac{c_u}{\bar{p}} = 0.11 + 0.0037 \, PI \tag{2.49a}$$

2.9.5   Anisotropy of shear strength

The mechanical properties of soil and rock masses are often anisotropic and consideration must be given in analytical studies to the possibility that one or more parameters may vary with direction. In stability problems such as those concerning slopes, shear strength anisotropy is of the greatest interest just as 'elastic' anisotropy is of paramount concern in problems of settlement. Casagrande and Carrillo (1944) suggested the following relationship for the anisotropic shear strength of a cohesive soil:

$$s = s_h \cos^2 \theta + s_v \sin^2 \theta \tag{2.50}$$

in which s_h and s_v are the shear strengths in the horizontal and vertical directions respectively. They did not give any theoretical or experimental grounds for the equation. However, it has been found acceptable in many studies concerning undrained strengths of cohesive soil.

At this stage it is important to differentiate between 'inherent anisotropy' and 'induced anisotropy'. If a soil is inherently anisotropic with principal directions of shear strength in the horizontal and vertical directions, then the above equation gives the inherent strength in any direction. Therefore, in the ideal case s_h, s_v and s may be regarded as independent of the principal stress directions and any other factors. For instance s_h may be considered to be the shear strength of a vertical specimen in a shear box, s_v the strength of a horizontal specimen (or the vertical specimen rotated through 90°) and s that of a specimen cut at an angle θ to horizontal.

However, it is well known that the orientation of principal stresses may have a significant influence on the measured shear strength. If this influence exists for a particular soil, the change of strength with change in orientation of principal stresses may be called 'induced anisotropy'. (This term may of course be defined in other ways depending on the nature of the problem under consideration). For the ideal case of 'induced anisotropy' as defined here, s_v represents the shear strength of a triaxial specimen in which the major principal stress at failure acts in the vertical direction, s_h represents the strength in which this stress acts in a horizontal direction. Therefore, s is the shear strength when the major principal stress makes an angle θ with the horizontal. Lo (1965) considered this concept of anisotropy and his experimental work concerning undrained shear strength of a clay appeared to support Equation (2.50). He made use of the concept of anisotropy induced by change in stress orientation in slope stability analysis and this is explained later. It is obvious that both factors contribute to anisotropy and, in fact, it is doubtful if shear strength tests mentioned (shear box and triaxial) can isolate anisotropy due to only one of the two significant factors. Matthai and Ranganatham (1968) appear to have interpreted Equation (2.50) as relevant to inherent anisotropy which may be considered to apply to the general case of a soil with cohesion and friction. Assuming the Coulomb's shear strength equation to apply in each direction and substituting for s_h and s_v in terms of the corresponding parameters c and ϕ, Equation (2.50) yields:

$$s = (c_h + \sigma_v \tan \phi_h)\cos^2 \theta + (c_v + \sigma_h \tan \phi_v)\sin^2 \theta \tag{2.51}$$

For soils only anisotropy in cohesion is likely to be significant and anisotropy in ϕ to be of minor consequence. Therefore, if $\phi_h = \phi_v = \phi$, Equation (2.51) becomes:

$$s = (c_h \cos^2 \theta + c_v \sin^2 \theta) + \tan \phi \, (\sigma_v \cos^2 \theta + \sigma_h \sin^2 \theta) \tag{2.52}$$

For undrained failure of saturated cohesive soils, "$\phi = 0$" concept may be considered as valid, and the expression for shear strength in any direction becomes from Equation (2.52):

$$s = c = c_h \cos^2 \theta + c_v \sin^2 \theta \tag{2.53}$$

Duncan and Seed (1966a, b) investigated anisotropy and stress reorientation in clay and found that shear strength parameters in effective stress terms are practically independent of stress orientation. Anisotropically consolidated clays were found to be anisotropic with respect to undrained strength. The pore pressure coefficient at failure A_f (which represents, for saturated soil, the ratio of excess pore water pressure to the increment in deviator stress which caused it) showed significant variation with orientation of the failure plane. Thus undrained strength anisotropy could be explained in terms of anisotropy in A_f. An expression derived by Hansen and Gibson (1949) expressed the undrained strength in terms of effective stress parameters of shear strength (Hvorslev parameters c_e and ϕ_e), the co-efficient of earth pressure at rest and a parameter λ. This parameter λ is related to pore pressure parameter A_f.

Thus there is a theoretical basis for the existence of undrained anisotropy even when c and ϕ are isotropic, provided A_f is anisotropic.

In conclusion, it is obvious that inherent anisotropy may exist due to previous consolidation and stress history and that reorientation of principal stresses during loading to failure may also cause anisotropy. Separation of the two effects is not easy with usual testing techniques. If anisotropy is to be included in stability analysis, θ in Equation (2.50) is the angle made by any plane with respect to the horizontal directions for inherent anisotropy. (Other relationships are possible and there is no suggestion that this equation is universally applicable. For instance Hansen (1952) assumed sinusoidal variation of shear strength with the angle between failure plane and the horizontal). Alternatively if stress re-orientation is the basis for using Equation (2.50), θ is the angle between the horizontal and the direction of the major principal stress. Note that in any soil mass the direction of principal stresses at failure will vary from point to point.

The assumption of a slip surface does not necessarily mean that stability analysis will predict failure. In many cases a factor of safety higher than one will be obtained. Therefore, it may be inaccurate to consider the local slip surface direction to be the failure plane direction. If the principal stress directions can be found independently, it is not necessary to consider the potential slip surface to be a failure plane. Thus a stress analysis by finite element technique would be necessary (see chapter 6).

Lo (1965) considered the assumed slip surface to be a failure plane and then found the orientation of principal stresses by assuming the angle f between the minor principal stress and the failure plane to be constant. While classical theories support this, he also found experimental evidence for the independence of angle f with change in orientation of principal stresses. The angle θ between the major principal stress and the horizontal is given by:

$$\theta = 90° - f + \alpha \tag{2.54}$$

in which α is the inclination of the slip surface to the horizontal at that point. The theoretical value of f may be used and then we have:

$$\theta = 45° - \phi/2 + \alpha \tag{2.54a}$$

in which ϕ is the effective angle of shearing resistance. If Equation (2.50) is considered to represent only inherent anisotropy unaffected by stress reorientation, then we have:

$$\theta = \alpha \tag{2.55}$$

2.10   PROGRESSIVE FAILURE OF SLOPES

Landslides seldom occur abruptly and it is doubtful if shear failure occurs simultaneously along the entire slip surface except perhaps in very small slides. Moreover, many large slides are a succession of small individual slides. First a small slide occurs and as a consequence of the movement of this mass, other adjacent masses become unstable. This process may then be repeated so that landslide grows during its movement. For example, Kjellman (1955) discussed the mechanics of two recognised forms of successive landslides in Sweden, viz. progressive slides and retrogressive slides. A slide that grows in the direction of its motion was termed a progressive slide and one that grows in the opposite direction is called a retrogressive slide. Retrogressive Swedish clay slides consist of a series of simple circular-cylindrical slides. Each slide removes the support of the adjacent ground behind it leading to the next slide. Often such slides spread over long distances and involve slopes which are quite flat. Progressive slides in Swedish sensitive clay do not involve rotational movements, and are propagated over nearly horizontal ground by motions which are essentially translations. Such movements occur frequently in these quick (extra-sensitive) clays which lose their strength dramatically during remoulding. It is obvious that 'removal of support' does not occur in the manner of retrogressive slides and therefore a simple explanation of such slides cannot be given except by a consideration of 'progressive' as distinct from 'simultaneous' failure.

Progressive failure in single simple slides or in successive slides is often a consequence of non-uniform stress and strain conditions. Failure occurs first at those points which are overstressed in relation to the strength of the soil or where excessive deformations have occurred. The adjacent points are then overstressed so that conditions are created for the zone of failure to increase. Thus failure may progress within a soil mass from one end of a slip surface to the other. Taylor (1948) compared the phenomenon of progressive failure to the tearing of a piece of paper. He pointed out those stress-strain curves obtained from laboratory tests are also influenced by non-uniform conditions of stress and strain to which the tested samples are subjected by most forms of testing equipment. The degree to which progressive action occurs in such tests is represented by the difference between stresses at peak points of (1) the ideal curve which would be obtained under uniform conditions of stress and strain, and (2) the actual experimental curve. The latter has a lower peak than the former and the difference is predominantly influenced by the difference between peak and ultimate points of the ideal curve.

While progressive action occurs both in laboratory tests and actual failures, the mode and extent of progressive action is often very different in the two cases. Bishop (1967) made an important contribution to an understanding of the mechanism of progressive failure by carefully examining the question of non-uniform stress distribution in cut slopes and embankments. He considered available analytical and experimental data on stresses within slopes (Bishop, 1952; La Rochelle, 1960; Turnbull and Hvorslev, 1967) which clearly show that the stress-distribution in slopes is often far from uniform and that the zone of overstress varies in location and extent for different types of slopes. (The zone of overstress may be regarded as the zone in which stresses are in excess of the average). For example in the case of an homogeneous embankment the shear stress at the ends of a potential slip surface is very low in comparison to the shear stress in the interior. Thus short-term failure in saturated clay may commence within the soil mass and progress towards the ends because strength is then independent of the normal stress and is likely to lie well below the shear stress in the overstressed zone somewhere in the interior. On the other hand the ratio of maximum shear stress to normal stress has high values at the ends and low values in the middle of a potential slip surface. As shear strength increases with effective normal stress when long-term drained conditions are approached, the likelihood of failure starting in the middle is remote under such conditions. In the interior the normal stresses are high since there is a greater depth of material above points on the slip surface. At the ends the maximum shear stresses are high in relation to the very low normal stresses which imply a low shear strength under drained conditions. Therefore failure is most likely to progress from one or both ends of a potential slip surface. Decrease of shear strength along this surface as failure progresses is considered separately in the next section. Reduction in strength due to pore pressure changes may initiate local failure during the construction of a slope or at any time thereafter. At any point, local shear strength may be adequate in relation to existing local shear stress under one set of conditions. When the conditions are altered, failure may develop and then progress outwards.

In natural and cut slopes, studies of stress-distribution must take into consideration the initial stress field. The stress changes due to slope formation should be superimposed on the original stresses. It has often been assumed that failures in natural and cut slopes begin at the toe (or the bottom of a potential failure surface). This assumption is a consequence of the fact that, in many such slopes, stress concentration is likely to be the highest at the toe. However, failure may not initiate only at the toe of a slope and sometimes it may initiate at its crest. This conclusion is inescapable from an interesting paper of Peck (1967) in which he discussed significant results concerning the effect of stress level and strain on the shear strength of cohesive soil obtained by Conlon (no reference was cited).

While it is wrong to argue that failure always initiates in the upper parts of a natural or cut slope, Peck's (1967) paper does cast serious doubt on the widely held belief about failure always initiating and progressing from the toe. In many cases the first sign of impending slope failure in slopes of cohesive soil is the opening of tension cracks at the crest of a slope. This phenomenon has been frequently observed and commented upon and is widely accepted. In the light of the above discussion it is, therefore, appropriate to regard the appearance of such cracks at the crest of a slope as evidence of failure of a 'progressive' nature. Similarly the widening of open joints at the crest of a rock slope which is frequently observed may be regarded as a sign of progressive failure. There is support for this view in the work of Barton (1971) who found that the opening of cracks was a consequence of the initiation of shear failure. Hoek and Bray (1977, p. 164) are also of the view that cracks are an evidence of the initiation of progressive failure.

However, a potential failure mass may already have suffered a significant extent of deformation before cracks open up. In fact, such deformations must often occur in soil and rock masses, their magnitudes depending upon soil or rock mass stiffness and other relevant factors. The occurrence of such initial deformations is in no way inconsistent with the concept of 'progressive', as opposed to 'simultaneous' failure. Little attention has so far been given, in developing slope analysis methods, to failure mass stiffness except to some extent in the shear band approach (see chapter 8).

Geological details (both major and minor) may contribute significantly to the development of progressive failure in the field. For example, failure may start as a consequence of local yield in a weak zone, near a fault, within a shear zone etc. An interesting case history of progressive failure due to the presence of a fault zone has been described by Hamel (1971) who also suggested a simple procedure for analysing such a problem by the sliding block method. (For a discussion of the sliding block or wedge method, see chapter 4). The influence of geological details on slope failure is frequently discussed by geotechnical experts. However, there are relatively few direct references to the role of geological details in failures of progressive nature. Progressive slope failures following liquefaction of isolated silt and sand lenses during earthquakes have been described by Seed (1968) and are briefly discussed in chapter 9.

In connection with progressive failure, attention also needs to be given to factors such as (1) the nature of any disturbance or trigger mechanism, (2) the extent of disturbance and the rate at which it occurs, e.g., pore pressure may increase slowly or rapidly, excavation may be rapid or slow, (3) the location of disturbing agent with respect to a slope e.g., stream erosion may occur at the toe of a slope, ponding may occur at the crest etc. These and other factors may govern the time scale of progressive action and the speed with which complete failure occurs.

2.11　RESIDUAL STRENGTH AND OTHER FACTORS IN PROGRESSIVE FAILURE

From time to time efforts have been made to collect evidence concerning the development of failure in soil masses, and non-uniform stress distribution is now considered to be only one of many possible reasons for the development of progressive failure. Traditional as well as sophisticated methods of numerical analysis such as the finite element method (see chapter 6) have increasingly been used to simulate slope behaviour in order to gain a better understanding of the factors that contribute to progressive and/or delayed failure (Cooper, 1988; Dounias et al., 1996, Potts et al., 1997). Observations associated with a full scale field experiment, when properly interpreted, can also contribute to knowledge and understanding of these phenomena (Cooper et al., 1998). Several concepts of progressive failure have, in fact, been proposed and these may be applicable under different conditions.

The decrease of shear strength at large deformations from a peak value to a residual value provides a very favourable condition for progressive failure. Thus nonuniform strain distribution has a special significance in slope stability problems. It is easy to envisage a situation in which the shear strength reduces to residual values gradually along a potential failure surface. In this connection Skempton (1964) proposed the term residual factor R to denote the proportion of a slip surface in a slope along which the strength has fallen to a residual value.

R is given by the following:

$$R = \frac{s_p - s}{s_p - s_r}, \quad \text{or,} \quad s = R s_r + (1 - R) s_p \tag{2.56}$$

in which s is the average shear stress along a slip surface at failure, s_p and s_r are the peak and residual shear strength respectively.

Skempton (1970) found that some first-time slope failures, especially those in intact overconsolidated clays, correspond to a residual factor close to zero. This means that these failures occur at the peak strength or very close to it. However, a residual factor of zero has also been interpreted as simultaneous failure or absence of progressive failure. Therefore, the use of the term 'progressive failure' may mean different things in different contexts. On the other hand, Skempton found that first-time slides in fissured overconsolidated clays correspond to a residual factor between zero and one. These failures occur at an average shear stress lower than the peak but considerably higher than the residual strength. In London clay, these failures seem to correspond closely to the fully softened strength of that clay. Skempton's 1970 paper was, therefore, an important revision of his 1964 paper (his Rankine Lecture paper) in which he suggested that the strength falls to the residual along parts of the slip surface. Failures along existing slip surfaces (in contrast to first-time slides in unfailed material) generally correspond to a residual factor R of one. This is not surprising since the strength would have fallen to residual values during previous deformations and movements. (As discussed in chapter 1, it is necessary to consider the direction of potential sliding or new movements relative to the direction of past movements along a given failure surface.)

In his original contribution, Skempton (1964) presented an interesting correlation between the residual factor and the time to failure of slopes. However, in his later work he found that the delay in failure, sometimes of the order of fifty or more years, was primarily due to the delay in the rise of pore water pressures to equilibrium values after a cutting had been made (Skempton, 1977). Originally it was believed that, in these fissured clays, the mass permeability would be high and the rise to equilibrium pore water pressures would take little time after the initial cutting had been completed. However, field measurements in failed and unfailed slopes showed that the delay in rise of pore water pressures was indeed very large and of the same order as the delay in actual failures. Softening or loss of cohesion is still considered to be valid but is believed to occur very rapidly in comparison to the rise of pore water pressures to equilibrium values. Softening, however, may be a progressive phenomenon itself. There is, as yet, incomplete evidence concerning the actual rate of softening of stiff-fissured clays (see also Chandler, 1974; Morgenstern, 1977).

Bjerrum (1967) discussed the progressive failure of overconsolidated clays and clay-shales in considerable detail and postulated a number of requirements for the development of progressive failure in such soils. He emphasised that there was a link between recoverable strain energy and the potential for progressive failure and asserted that weathering increases this potential by destruction of diagenetic bonds in clays and clay-shales. Originally these clays may have a low potential for progressive failure because of locked-in strain energy. He considered the following ratios to be of paramount importance in both weathered and unweathered clays and clay-shales: (i) ratio of lateral internal stress to peak shear strength p_H/s_p (ii) ratio of lateral internal strain due to recoverable strain energy to peak strain $\varepsilon_H/\varepsilon_p$ (iii) ratio of peak strength to residual strength s_p/s_r. Table 2.1 shows the comparative potential for progressive failure of clays with different values of these ratios. Bishop et al. (1971) drew attention to the importance of brittleness index I_B in relation to progressive failure of overconsolidated clays, the index being defined as follows:

$$I_B = \frac{s_p - s_r}{s_p} \tag{2.57}$$

They referred to evidence which suggests that high brittleness index leads to progressive failure (residual factor R greater than zero). This is somewhat similar to the third criterion suggested by Bjerrum (1967).

Table 2.1 Potential for progressive failure (after Bjerrm, 1967). With permission from ASCE, see page 713, No 10.

	Overconsolidated plastic clay with weak bonds		Overconsolidated plastic clay with strong bonds		Overconsolidated clay with low plasticity
	Unweathered	*Weathered*	*Unweathered*	*Weathered*	
p_H/s_{peak}	2	3	0–1	3	1
$\varepsilon_H/\varepsilon_{peak}$	2	2	1	3	0–1
s_{peak}/s_{res}	2	1	3	2	0–1
Relative danger of progressive failure	high	high	low	very high	very low

Potential for progressive failure of various types of clay, based on an evolution of the degree to which the three significant ratios are fulfilled.

Notations used:

0	fulfilment not pronounced	p_H	lateral internal stress
1	fulfilment less pronounced	ε_H	lateral strain due to stored recoverable strain energy
2	fulfilment pronounced		
3	fulfilment very pronounced	ε_{peak}	failure strain at peak

Brittleness index is a function of the effective normal stress. Assuming straight line peak and residual strength envelopes, the latter passing through the origin (zero residual cohesion), it is easy to see that brittleness index decreases with increasing normal stress. Therefore relatively shallow slides have a significant tendency for progressive failure because of associated low normal stresses. In the same material, the tendency for progressive failure along a deep-seated surface may be relatively low, since the brittleness index is low at high normal stress. It is important to note, however, that strain-softening (and hence brittleness) is only one of many factors that influence the tendency for progressive failure.

There has also been some discussion concerning the possibility that the mobilised shear strength at the time of a slide or slip may vary in an arbitrary manner between the peak and residual values (Bishop, 1971). Skempton's (1964) estimation of a residual factor R was interpreted by him as the proportion of the slip surface along which strength had fallen to the residual value. The remaining part of the slip surface was considered to be at the peak strength and no transition zone was considered. It appears more logical that there is a continuous variation of the mobilised shear strength between peak and residual values along at least part of the slip surface. This would correspond with non-uniform strains and deformations which may be expected in real problems.

A local residual factor R_l may be defined at any point (rather than for the whole slip surface) thus:

$$R_\ell = \frac{s_l - s_r}{s_p - s_r} \tag{2.58}$$

in which s_l is the mobilised shear strength at the point under consideration.

It is always important to make a distinction between progressive failure and delayed failure. Firstly, failure may be progressive in the sense that it does not occur simultaneously along the whole of a slip surface or within the entire potential failure zone. However, the mechanism involved in this process and the nature of soil and other features of the problem may be such that failure is a 'delayed' one. In overconsolidated clays, for instance, delays of the order of 50 years or more have been found in many slope failures. Secondly, time dependent weakening of clay soils due to loss of cohesion may also lead to a delayed failure. Such weakening may occur simultaneously within the whole mass, and in that sense failure may occur simultaneously along the entire slip surface. The term 'progressive failure' is sometimes considered appropriate even in these cases because it is a 'long-term' failure. James (1971a) used the term progressive failure to mean a time-dependent but simultaneous decay in c and ϕ and not a time-dependent decay in c alone. Thirdly, consider a short-term or immediate failure of an excavated slope or an embankment slope. Such a failure could be considered either a simultaneous one or a progressive one, depending on the mechanism involved, although there was no significant element of delay in it. For instance stress concentrations and local yield may provide conditions favourable to the progressive propagation of a continuous failure surface resulting in rapid failure. Fourthly, delayed failure may result primarily due to increase of pore water pressures to equilibrium values after a lapse of time in the case of cuttings as discussed earlier in this section and in the section 2.8 on excess pore water pressures. There may also be environmental factors leading to changes in water table, pore water pressures or creating other conditions which endanger stability with time. Bishop (1967) referred to weathering and its effects on strength and permeability, delayed release of strain energy, and rheological decrease in shear strength.

In many cases eventual failure cannot be explained fully without considering some final trigger mechanism. There are many case histories in which the nature of the trigger mechanisms has not been fully understood and remains a matter of speculation. Two prominent examples are the Frank slide (Krahn and Morgenstern, 1976) and the 1963 Vaiont slide in Italy (Muller, 1964). For a discussion of the latter slide and alternative interpretations concerning its occurrence refer to chapter 7.

A simple application of progressive failure concepts to excavated slopes in jointed rock has been considered by Barton (1972). The overstressing of joints as a result of excavation was simulated leading to a multi-linear failure mode with a stepped portion of the failure surface along which reduction of strength to residual was considered appropriate. The concept was explained with reference to a weakening mechanism which is a function of time and displacement.

Discussions of progressive failure invariably involve considerations of stability in terms of effective stresses and effective stress parameters. This is a consequence of the fact that concepts of progressive failure have provided useful answers to otherwise puzzling problems posed by delayed or long-term failures in which effective stress analyses alone are valid. The choice between 'total stress' and 'effective stress' methods of analysis in problems of undrained failure has been discussed in detail by Lambe and Whitman (1969), and a discussion of their merits in different types of problem follows in chapter 5.

2.12   PROGRESSIVE FAILURE AND THE STRESS FIELD

Regardless of the manner in which failure may progress, it is of interest to consider the changes in the stress field within a slope during progressive failure. All concepts discussed in the previous section are primarily concerned with changes in shear strength due to decrease of the parameters c or ϕ or the increase of pore water pressure. Stress concentration and local yield are of course accepted as contributing factors and Bjerrum (1967) did emphasise the importance of the initial lateral stress. Yet, he did not consider changes in the magnitude or orientation of stresses during the process of progressive failure. The transformation of a slope from an initial stress field (with a given magnitude and orientation of principal stresses) to one consistent with the conditions at the time of failure is discussed further in chapter 7.

It is interesting to note that conventional methods of stability analysis (which are introduced in chapters 4 and 5 of this book) are based on the concept of limit equilibrium. Thus each of these methods is concerned with one and only one state of stress along a given slip surface or failure surface, regardless of the original stresses in the slope under consideration. This state of stress is one which is consistent with the assumption that the potential sliding mass is in a state of limit equilibrium. (This state should not be confused with critical equilibrium which corresponds to real incipient failure and is reached when a slope has a real factor of safety $F = 1$). The calculated stresses on an assumed slip surface depend on the individual limit equilibrium method of analysis which is used. Each method is based on different assumptions as will become clear in chapters 4 and 5. The factor of safety F itself may be defined in different ways e.g., (a) as the ratio of moments due to resisting and disturbing forces, or, (b) as the ratio of available to mobilised unit shear strength at any point along the slip surface. These matters are discussed fully in subsequent chapters.

A comprehensive approach for simulating progressive slope failure requires sophisticated stress-deformation analysis (see chapter 6). However, an interesting but simple approach for simulating localized failures, stress redistribution and progressive slope failure, within the framework of limit equilibrium, is outlined in chapter 5.

2.13   NUMERICAL EXAMPLES

EXAMPLE 2.1

Effective shear strength parameters of cohesive soil from a slope have been estimated based on results of shear tests on intact (undisturbed) samples under drained conditions. The values are $c' = 15 \text{ kN/m}^2$ and $\phi' = 27°$.

A potential slip surface within the slope has been divided into several segments. On one of the segments the total normal stress has been estimated as $\sigma = 300$ kPa and the pore water pressure $u = 95$ kPa. What is the shear strength along the segment? State any assumptions made.

Solution
Effective normal stress = total normal stress – pore water pressure

$$\sigma' = \sigma - u = 300 - 95 = 205 \text{ kN/m}^2$$

Shear strength based on the Mohr-Coulomb equation

$$s = c' + \sigma' \tan \phi' = 15 + 205 \tan 27° = 119 \text{ kN/m}^2$$

Assumptions

1 The shear strength is for long-term drained conditions.
2 The soil at the particular location is intact and undisturbed.
3 The segment is not coinciding with an existing slip surface which may have been formed during a previous failure.

EXAMPLE 2.2

In a sloping area, which is being assessed for development, the soil conditions are found to be non-uniform. Although the soil materials are generally similar, some zones are highly fissured and jointed. Moreover, failure of slopes by sliding has occurred at some locations. Stability studies would, therefore, include consideration of potential first-time slides as well as reactivation of previous slides along existing slip surfaces.

Drained shear tests have been performed on intact (undisturbed) samples as well as remoulded samples. Multiple reversal shear tests, tests on pre-cut samples and ring shear tests have also been carried out in order to determine residual shear strength. The following shear strength parameters have been estimated as average values:

Intact (undisturbed) soil:	$c' = 10 \text{ kN/m}^2, \phi' = 22°$
Remoulded soil:	$c' = 0, \phi' = 20°$
Residual shear strength:	$c'_r = 0, \phi'_r = 12°$

Consider a segment of a potential slip surface with a total normal stress of 250 kN/m², shear stress of 45 kN/m² and pore water pressure of 80 kN/m². What is the shear strength along this slip surface segment if

(i) the segment is located in intact soil?
(ii) the segment is located in fissured and jointed soil?
(iii) he segment is part of a pre-existing slip surface?

Solution

(i) Peak shear strength values apply and these relate to test results from intact samples.
   Hence, $c' = 10 \text{ kN/m}^2, \phi' = 22°$
   Effective normal stress $\sigma' = 250 - 80 = 170 \text{ kN/m}^2$
   Peak shear strength $s_p = c' + \sigma' \tan \phi' = 10 + 170 \tan 22° = 79 \text{ kN/m}^2$
(ii) Fully softened shear strength values apply and these relate to test results from remoulded samples.
   Hence, $c' = 0, \phi' = 20°$
   $s = c' + \sigma' \tan \phi' = 170 \tan 20° = 62 \text{ kN/m}^2$
(iii) Residual shear strength values apply
   Hence, $c'_r = 0, \phi'_r = 12°$
   Shear strength $s_r = c'_r + \sigma' \tan \phi'_r = 170 \tan 12° = 36 \text{ kN/m}^2$

EXAMPLE 2.3

The local factor of safety at any point along a potential slip surface in a slope may be defined as the ratio of shear strength to shear stress at that point. Estimate the local factor of safety in the three cases of Example 2.2, noting that the shear stress at the particular location was 45 kPa. Comment on the results.

Solution
Denote the local factor of safety by F_ℓ

Case (i) $F_\ell = \dfrac{s_p}{\tau} = \dfrac{79}{45} = 1.76$

Case (ii) $F_\ell = \dfrac{s}{\tau} = \dfrac{62}{45} = 1.38$

Case (iii) $F_\ell = \dfrac{s_\tau}{\tau} = \dfrac{36}{45} = 0.8$

(Note that the shear stress is unaffected by pore water pressure whereas effective normal stress is obtained by deducting pore water pressure from the total normal stress. The latter follows directly from the principle of effective stress. The former is evident from the fact that water carries no shear stress.)

Comments on the above results for local factor of safety

1   These values of local factor of safety do not reflect on the stability of the slope as a whole. In order to estimate the overall stability the sum of the shear strengths of all the segments along a potential slip surface would have to be estimated and also the sum of the shear stresses along all the segments. Based on these, the equilibrium of the slope would then be analysed. (Chapters 4 and 5 deal with several methods of limit equilibrium analysis.)

2   If at all the local factor of safety represented average conditions along the whole slip surface then for the above three cases one would conclude

Case (i)   The factor of safety is well above 1 and hence the slope is safe to a high degree of reliability.

Case (ii)   The factor of safety is again greater than 1 and hence the slope is safe although the reliability is less then that in the first Case (i).

Case (iii) The factor of safety is below 1 which is the threshold for critical equilibrium. Thus the slope is expected to fail unless suitable remedial measures are taken. For example, pore water pressure could be reduced by drainage and thus effective normal stress could be increased.

EXAMPLE 2.4

For Case (iii) of Examples 2.2 and 2.3, calculate

•   the pore water pressure at which local factor of safety becomes 1; this may be referred to as the 'critical' pore water pressure.

- the pore water pressure which should not be exceeded if the local factor of safety has to be kept to a value not less than 1.1.

Solution

(a) To calculate the critical pore water pressure, set $F_\ell = 1 = s_r/\tau$, and $\tau = 45$ kN/m².
   Hence, $s_r = 45$ kN/m²
   $c'_r + \sigma'$ tan $\phi'_r = 45$
   i.e., $0 + (250 - u)$ tan $12° = 45$, thus, $u = 39$ kN/m²
   Thus, drainage would have to ensure reduction of pore water pressure from 80 kN/m² to 39 kN/m².

(b) Pore water pressure for $F_\ell = 1.1$,
   If $F_\ell = 1.1$, $s_r = 1.1 \times 45 = 49.4$
   i.e., $0 + (250 - u)$ tan $12° = 49.5$, thus, $u = 17$ kN/m²
   Thus drainage would have to ensure reduction of pore water pressure from 80 kN/m² to 17 kN/m².

EXAMPLE 2.5

At a level site, a temporary slope has to be excavated and the soil is cohesive and saturated with shear strength parameters $c' = 5$ kPa and $\phi' = 32°$. The undrained shear strength increases with depth linearly from $c_u = 5$ kN/m² at the ground surface to $c_u = 65$ kN/m² at a depth of 30 m.

The inclination of the slope to be excavated has been set at 1:1 or 45°. Consider the segment of a potential slip surface 20 m below original ground level and 15 m below the excavated surface. The total normal stress on this segment is estimated to be 200 kN/m² and the pore water pressure after the excavation is 40 kN/m². Calculate the effective normal stress on the segment and its shear strength for short-term conditions.

Solution

(i) Effective normal stress $\sigma' = \sigma - u = 200 - 40 = 160$ kN/m²
(ii) Shear strength applicable to this temporary slope is the undrained shear strength (short-term "undrained" conditions apply for a temporary slope). At a depth of 20 m below ground level the undrained shear strength is

$$c_u = 5 + \frac{20}{30}(65 - 5) = 45 \text{ kN/m}^2$$

Comment

1   If shear strength is calculated on the basis of effective shear strength parameters

$$s = c' + \sigma' \tan \phi' = 5 + (200 - 40) \tan 32° = 105 \text{ kN/m}^2$$

This is much higher than the calculated undrained shear strength at that location but it is only applicable for long-term conditions. However, the pore water pressures in the long-term would be different from short term values. Therefore the above calculated value would change anyway.

2   In this example, a saturated cohesive slope was considered without submergence. However, excavations may be carried in submerged areas as well. If this site was submerged, the calculated undrained shear strength would still apply for excavating a temporary slope. However, the slope as a whole would be more stable because of the buoyancy effect. (This will be considered in the following chapters dealing with limit equilibrium methods).

EXAMPLE 2.6

In the previous example consider that the site is submerged and that excavation will be carried out under water. Assume that the soil has a saturated unit weight of 20 kN/m³. Consider a potential slip surface divided into segments. The effective normal and shear stresses on any segment of the slip surface have to be estimated for the following two cases:

(i) the slip surface segment is horizontal
(ii) the slip surface segment is inclined at 35.2° to the horizontal

Solution

The effective stresses in submerged soil due to gravitational forces may be estimated based on submerged (or buoyant) unit weight γ' which is the difference between saturated unit weight and unit weight of water $\gamma' = (\gamma_{sat} - \gamma_w)$.

The effective normal stress on a plane inclined at angle β to the horizontal and located at depth z below ground surface (the final surface after a slope has been excavated)

$$\sigma' = \gamma' z \cos^2 \beta = (\gamma_{sat} - \gamma_w) \cos^2 \beta \qquad (E2.1)$$

The shear stress under submerged conditions is given by

$$\tau = \gamma' z \sin \beta \cos \beta = (\gamma_{sat} - \gamma_w) \sin \beta \cos \beta \qquad (E2.2)$$

The derivation of these equations is left to the student reader who will encounter these equations again in Chapter 4. The corresponding equations for a slope under seepage conditions (rather than submerged conditions) are

$$\sigma' = \gamma z \cos^2 \beta - u \qquad (E2.3)$$

$$\tau = \gamma z \sin \beta \cos \beta \qquad (E2.4)$$

where γ is the bulk unit weight, the saturated unit weight for fully saturated soil, and u is the pore water pressure based on actual seepage conditions. If there is no seepage, pore pressure may be zero. For a dry slope γ would be the dry unit weight and pore water pressure would be zero.

Numerical Solution

(i) $\gamma' = 20 - 9.81 \approx 10$ kN/m³, $z = 15$ m (depth below finished slope surface after excavation)

$\beta = 0°$, thus, $\cos^2 \beta = 1$ and, $\sin \beta \cos \beta = 0$
$\sigma' = \gamma'z \cos^2 \beta = 10 \times 15 = 150$ kN/m²
$\tau = \gamma'z \sin \beta \cos \beta = 0$

(ii) $\beta = 35.2°$
$\sigma' = \gamma'z \cos^2 \beta = 150 \cos^2 35.2° = 100.16$ kN/m²
$\tau = \gamma'z \sin \beta \cos \beta = 10 \times 15 \times \sin 35.2° \cos 35.2° = 70.65$ kN/m²

Note

The calculated values above apply only to submerged case. For general case of seepage, the seepage pore pressures are calculated first and the effective normal stress obtained by deducting pore pressure from total normal stress. The shear stress is based on bulk unit weight as per equation given earlier.

Hint concerning derivation of normal and shear stresses under submerged conditions

Effective normal stress and shear stress
Consider a soil element with its top and bottom surfaces parallel to the ground surface and with both of its sides vertical. The net force due to water pressure acts vertically upwards. This can be shown by considering the horizontal and vertical equilibrium of all water forces. The magnitude of this resultant water force is also obtained in the process.

Next, consider the weight of the soil element acting downwards and the resultant water force acting upwards and resolve both into components along and normal to the base of the element. These are the effective normal and shear forces on the base. Divide them by the length of the base to get effective shear and normal stresses in terms of the submerged (buoyant) unit weight of soil. These are the equations given earlier.

Pore water pressure and total normal stress
At any point within a slope, located at depth z below the slope surface and depth $(z + h)$ below the free water level (the submergence level), the pore water pressure is

$$u = (z + h)\gamma_w \tag{E2.5}$$

The total normal stress on a plane through the point parallel to the ground surface is

$$\sigma = \gamma z \cos^2 \beta + \gamma_w (h + z \sin^2 \beta) \tag{E2.6}$$

While these two stresses include both h and z, the effective normal and shear stresses are independent of h.

Knowledge of total stress could be important. For example, if draw-down occurs, the change in total stress must be calculated (see the relevant example in chapter 4, Example 4.6).

The derivation of the equation (E2.6) is left to the student reader.

EXAMPLE 2.7

When a slope failure occurs, the location of the slip surface may be investigated in the field. Also, analysis can be carried out to estimate the normal and shear stresses along the slip surface at the time of failure. The average shear strength can then be compared to the peak and residual strengths. Calculate the residual factor R for the following cases involving long-term slope failures in which effective shear strength parameters are relevant.

(i) Peak shear strength calculated by using the average normal effective stress and peak strength parameters c' and ϕ': $s_p = 85$ kN/m².
Residual shear strength calculated by using again the average normal effective stress but with residual strength parameters c'_r and ϕ'_r: $s_r = 60$ kN/m².
Shear stress at failure as given by back-analysis of the actual slope failure: $s = 72$ kN/m².
(ii) $s_p = 105$ kN/m², $s_r = 69$ kN/m², $s = 100$ kN/m².
(iii) $s_p = 93$ kN/m², $s_r = 55$ kN/m², $s = 58$ kN/m².

Solution

The residual factor is defined as $R = (s_p - s)/(s_p - s_r)$ [Equation (2.56)] and it is an indication of the proportion of slip surface on which shear strength has fallen to the residual value.

For the three cases here:

(i) $R = \dfrac{85 - 72}{85 - 60} = \dfrac{13}{25} = 0.52$

Nearly fifty percent of slip surface has fallen to the residual shear strength at failure assuming that the soil is perfectly brittle.

(ii) $R = \dfrac{105 - 100}{105 - 69} = \dfrac{5}{36} = 0.14$

Thus only about 14% of slip surface has fallen to residual strength at failure.

(iii) $R = \dfrac{93 - 58}{93 - 55} = \dfrac{35}{38} = 0.92$

Thus 92% of the slip surface has residual shear strength at failure. This may indicate that failure has occurred along a pre-existing slip surface from an earlier failure of the slope.

Notes

1   The above approach may also be applied to short-term failures of clay slopes under undrained conditions. However, the peak strength would be the average

peak undrained strength, c_u (peak) and the residual shear strength would be the average residual undrained strength, c_u (residual). The effective normal stresses would not be relevant. The shear stress at failure would be from a total stress analysis rather than an effective stress analysis. The distinction between effective stress and total stress analysis is explored fully in Chapters 4 and 5.

2   One may also evaluate the local residual factor at any point along a slip surface. Consider any segment of a slip surface which has been investigated after a slope failure has occurred. The shear and normal stress on the particular segment would be estimated from an analysis of the failure. Thus the local residual factor for that segment can be estimated based on either effective stress parameters (long-term or drained failure conditions) or undrained strength parameters (short-term or undrained conditions for saturated slopes in cohesive soil).

The only difference is that we consider normal and shear stresses for the particular segment rather than the average normal and shear stresses for the whole slip surface.

The local residual factor may be denoted by R_l to distinguish it from the average residual factor R.

The local residual factor does not represent the proportion of slip surface at the residual strength. It represents only the extent to which shear strength at a particular location has fallen to residual strength. Thus $R_l = 1$ means that the particular segment is at residual strength and $R_l = 0$ means that the particular segment is at peak strength.

EXAMPLE 2.8

The peak and residual shear strength values at a particular location are

$$s_p = 80 \text{ kN/m}^2 \quad \text{and} \quad s_r = 50 \text{ kN/m}^2$$

What is the brittleness index?

Solution

$$\text{Brittleness index } I_B = \frac{s_p - s_r}{s_p} \tag{2.57}$$

In this case, $I_B = (80 - 50)/80 = 0.375$

Notes
1   In this case, brittleness index is not based on average values along a slip surface but relates to a specific location in the soil and to the shear strength parameters of the soil at that location.
2   Brittleness index is not related to analysis of a failed slope.
3   High Brittleness index may be a contributing factor to progressive failure.
4   Brittleness index may also be calculated based on undrained peak and residual shear strengths where undrained behaviour is relevant.

Chapter 3

Performance indicators and basic probability concepts

3.1 INTRODUCTION AND SCOPE

3.1.1 Preliminary decisions concerning type of analysis

Before outlining and discussing methods of analysis, an overview of performance indicators will be useful. In the first chapter we have already referred, in general terms, to the conventional, site-specific approach of the geotechnical engineer involving mechanics (analysis of forces, stresses, strains), on the one hand, and the empirical or statistical regional approach of the geoscientist based on analysis and synthesis of observational data, on the other. Similarities and differences between these broad approaches, their strengths and limitations must be recognized. The need for an interdisciplinary approach for slope engineering which includes geotechnical slope analysis has also been emphasized. Thus it is always useful to consider a site specific analysis within the context of a regional analysis. Also, geological input is very useful in developing a geotechnical model for a slope analysis problem.

3.1.2 Choice of performance indicators

Having done the modeling and chosen a particular method of analysis, it is important to relate the outcomes of such an analysis to the performance of the particular slope or earth structure. There are two broad approaches for geotechnical slope analysis, deterministic and probabilistic. Performance indicators suitable to each approach must be selected and defined.

Within each framework there are, of course, methods based on different concepts. Within a deterministic framework, for example, it is important to distinguish between limit equilibrium methods and stress-deformation methods. In general, for each group of methods, different performance indicators would be required. Even within each group of methods there may be a choice of performance indicators. For example, within a limit equilibrium framework, one may use the concept of a 'factor of safety' or, alternatively, the concept of a 'critical seismic coefficient' as explained in sub-sections 3.2.1 and 2. Within a probabilistic framework it is important to define reliability index, probability of failure and probability of success. It is also important to introduce the concepts of hazard and risk as also to consider briefly the concept of progressive failure as different from simultaneous failure. Similarly, it is sometimes necessary to consider the slope or earth structure as a system. Finally, it is important to give consideration to the threshold value of a performance indicator, a value which indicates a slope at 'critical equilibrium' or which marks the boundary between acceptable and unacceptable performance of a slope.

3.1.3   Contents of this chapter

The main text of this chapter is covered in the first seventeen pages. The remaining pages consist of three appendices to this chapter. These are concerned with basic probability concepts including nine simple numerical examples. The reader will find this introduction to probability concepts very useful before reading chapter 10 which deals with the different aspects of the application of probabilistic approach in slope stability analysis.

Performance indicators, deterministic and probabilistic, are covered in sections 3.2 to 3.7. Geotechnical uncertainties, basic statistical parameters and variability of soil properties are considered very briefly in sections 3.8 and 3.9. A brief discussion of the requirements and limitations for using probabilistic analysis is included in section 3.10. Some conclusions from two case studies during the early phase of development of probabilistic applications in geotechnical engineering are also included. Appendix I summarises basic concepts of probability with nine numerical examples. Appendix II summarises the equations for a capacity-demand model. Appendix III reproduces a table of probability values corresponding to a Standard Normal Distribution.

3.2   DETERMINISTIC APPROACH

3.2.1   Global and local factors of safety

Firstly, there is the conventional deterministic approach which still dominates professional practice. A 'safety factor' or 'factor of safety', often denoted by F, is the well known performance indicator in limit equilibrium studies and is the most important part of the output of a geotechnical analysis. According to the "limit equilibrium" concept, F may be defined as the factor by which the average shear strength along a 'slip surface' within a slope must be reduced so that it is equal to the average applied shear stress. The "limit equilibrium" concept is considered in more detail in chapters 4 and 5.

Alternatively, F may be defined as the ratio of available shear strength to the applied shear stress along a slip surface. A value of $F = 1$ represents 'critical equilibrium' or 'limiting equilibrium' and implies that a slope is on the verge of collapse or sliding or complete failure. A value of $F > 1$ represents stability and a value of $F < 1$ represents instability.

There may be several possible slip surfaces which can be considered for assessing the potential for failure of a given slope. The particular slip surface of interest is the 'critical slip surface'. In other words, such a slip surface should yield the lowest value of factor of safety F for that slope under the specified conditions. Methods of analysis for evaluating the value of F, based on the limit equilibrium concept, are discussed in chapters 4 and 5.

The factor of safety F is a function of various parameters or variables related to the geotechnical model, such as geometrical parameters, shear strength parameters and pore water pressures. Thus it is appropriate to refer to the relationship between F and the various parameters or variables as a 'performance function'. The numerical value of F for a specific set of variables or parameters may be called a 'performance indicator'. Different ways to define this performance function are considered in the following chapters. Uncertainties of different types are not included in a deterministic analysis. For example, the variability of geotechnical parameters, such as shear strength parameters and pore water pressures are not considered for inclusion in a deterministic analysis. In contrast, the inclusion of the variability of each important parameter is an important aspect of a probabilistic approach introduced separately below.

A calculated factor of safety is based on a balance of disturbing and resisting forces (or moments or both) for the whole slope and, as such, may be termed a 'global factor of safety'. The calculation is based on a potential mechanism of failure and is often associated with a potential slip surface (also called 'sliding surface' or 'rupture surface'). As stated above, there may be many potential slip surfaces. The particular slip surface which leads to the minimum factor of safety is the 'critical slip surface'.

One may also calculate the factor of safety at a particular location along the slope or along any potential slip surface. This may be defined as a ratio of the local shear strength to the local shear stress (or the mobilized shear strength) and may be called a 'local factor of safety'. Obviously, a local factor of safety will, in general, vary spatially along any slip surface.

3.2.2   Critical seismic coefficient as alternative to factor of safety

Consider a slope subjected to a horizontal seismic acceleration kg in addition to gravitational body forces, where k is a seismic coefficient and g is the acceleration due to gravity. As the value of k increases, the stability of the slope decreases. At a critical value of $k = k_c$, called the 'critical seismic coefficient', the slope will reach a state of critical equilibrium and will be on the verge of sliding along a slip surface. A value of $k_c = 0$ represents $F = 1$ or critical equilibrium under static conditions. A value of $k_c > 0$ for a slope indicates stability under static conditions. The higher the magnitude of k_c, the greater the stability and, therefore, higher the value of F under static conditions. Thus for any slope, there is a direct, one to one relationship between k_c on the one hand and F on the other. Conversely, a value of $k_c < 0$ represents an unstable slope. Consequently, k_c can be considered as a performance indicator in slope stability analysis as an alternative to F. As mentioned in chapter 5, some methods of static limit equilibrium analysis are based on k_c as the performance function rather than F. Seismic stability analysis of slopes often includes the determination of k_c. The relevant concepts and methods are considered in some detail in chapter 9 of this book.

3.2.3   Progressive failure and system aspects

The calculation of a global factor of safety is based on an assumption of simultaneous failure all along a slip surface. In reality, failure is progressive in character. Therefore, considering a progressive failure mechanism may yield a different result. In other words, the global factor of safety based on an assumption of simultaneous failure may be different in magnitude from that based on a mechanism of progressive failure. The concept of stress redistribution and progressive failure within the framework of limit equilibrium is explained further in chapter 5. An illustrative example shows that there may be a significant decrease in F if a progressive rather than simultaneous failure mechanism is invoked.

One should also refer to problems of system failure. A slope may need to be considered as part of a system consisting of different site features or elements. For example, there may be several slopes of varying inclination so that the performance of one slope is likely to be influenced by the performance of others. In such a case, it may be important to assess the system factor of safety rather than just the individual values for the component slopes. Even a single slope with several failure mechanisms (or just several potential surfaces) may be considered as a system. This concept is considered further in chapter 10 within a probabilistic framework and illustrative examples are given.

3.2.4   Performance indicators for stress-deformation analyses

The factor of safety concept is most appropriate to limit equilibrium approaches. However, we may have to carry out stress-deformation studies as well. So, what indicators of performance are appropriate for such studies? Obviously the magnitudes of deformations at selected locations of the slope are the most important indicators. However, the distribution of shear stresses can also be useful. Also useful are the local ratios of shear strength and shear stress, which represent local factors of safety based on stress-deformation analysis. The spatial variation of local factor of safety based on a stress-deformation analysis will, in general, be different from that based on a limit equilibrium analysis. Stress-deformation analysis is particularly important for slopes and soil structures whose successful performance requires limits to the magnitude of displacement or deformation that occurs during the design life. The basis for stress-deformation studies and the various approaches and methods for carrying out such studies are considered in chapter 6 of this book.

3.2.5   Threshold or allowable values of factor of safety

The threshold for successful performance must be established on the basis of experience or assumed on the basis of engineering judgment. Although nominally the threshold for factor of safety is considered as unity ($F = 1$) indicating safe status of stability, in reality the allowable safety factor is significantly greater than unity. Guidelines for magnitudes of acceptable values of factor of safety may vary from country to country and from one organization to another in the same city. Interpretation of computed values of factor of safety may vary depending on method of analysis used, the particular application and the judgment of the concerned expert [see chapter 5, sections 5.14.4, 5 and 6].

What are the typical minimum values of factor of safety for natural slopes or for landslide management?

It is probably misleading to specify typical values as such. However, it is best to refer to experts from geotechnical practice.

As an example, Cornforth (2005) has suggested values of factor of safety ranging from 1.15 to 1.5 specifically for landslide management depending on details such as size of landslide, extent of investigation (no. of boreholes), speed of landslide movement and consequences of failure in general terms. Because of the great importance of the consequences of failure (threat to human life, safety as well as threat of economic loss), specific attention must be given to the particular location and function of a slope. For example, an allowable factor of safety of, say, 1.1 or 1.2 may be considered reasonable for a natural slope, the failure of which is considered unlikely to have adverse consequences. On the other hand, a higher factor of safety (say 1.5 to 2) may be required for an engineered slope adjacent to a railway line so that deformations are below the level that might cause derailment. For water-retaining structures such as earth dams, factors of safety as high as 2 or even 3 may be considered necessary (see below).

What are the typical minimum values of factor of safety for design of built-up slopes?

Again, it may be misleading to specify typical values representing worldwide application and it is best to refer to the opinion of an expert based on considerable experience.

For constructed slopes, obviously the required factors of safety would have to be higher than those for natural slopes and for landslide management, all other conditions being the same. Duncan (1992) mentions typical minimum values: $F = 1.5$ (long-term), $F = 1.3$ (end-of-construction and multi-stage loading) and $F = 1$ to 1.2 (rapid draw-down). Consideration has, of course, to be given to the level of uncertainties and to the consequences of a potential failure. The greater the level of uncertainty, the higher the required or acceptable value of F one would adopt. Similarly, the greater the adverse consequences of potential slope failure, the higher the acceptable value of F one would adopt. However, very high uncertainty and very high potential consequences of failure should not be allowed to occur together. In such a case, measures must be taken to decrease the level of uncertainty (e.g., more investigation) or/and decrease the potential consequences of failure (e.g., reducing the number of elements at risk or their vulnerability, or both). Merely choosing a higher value of F is not the answer. The reader should also refer to chapter 5, section 5.14.4, 5 and 6 for a comprehensive discussion of the meaning or interpretation of computed values of F.

What about limits to deformation?

Where an assessment of the magnitude of deformation is important, a limit equilibrium analysis alone would be insufficient. In such cases, stress-deformation analyses must be carried out. Alternatively, observation and monitoring of deformations must be carried out to supplement limit equilibrium or other analyses. For example, the design factor of safety of an earth dam or a high embankment may have to be as high as $F = 3$ in order that deformations are within the permissible limits. The factor of safety of a slope near a railway line under critical conditions (such as exceptional rainstorms) may need to be increased from say, $F = 1.3$ to a higher value, say, $F = 1.5$ in order to limit the magnitude of lateral deformation below a pre-determined threshold and thus reduce the probability of train derailment.

The first-time movement of a natural or engineered slope should be differentiated from pre-existing conditions such as a slow-moving landslide. The recognition of continuing movement at a sloping site is an important part of the investigations which precede slope analysis. In regions where rainfall-triggered landslides predominate, stick-slip movements of relatively small magnitude in some areas are not uncommon. However slow the movement, one is often dealing with an existing landslide and that fact will have a great bearing on the scope and goals of analysis. Landslide movements of the order of millimeters per year, (in the slow to extremely slow range), are very difficult to detect at first and require local knowledge and careful investigation such as a study of aerial photographs and search for subtle local effects such as minor cracking. Monitoring with subsurface instrumentation (for example, use of inclinometers) is often necessary under such circumstances (see chapter 11).

3.3   PROBABILISTIC APPROACH

3.3.1   Uncertainties and the probabilistic framework

Recognition and assessment of uncertainties in geotechnical engineering is of paramount importance. This process facilitates the assessment of a performance indicator which include the influence of key uncertainties. Moreover, using a probabilistic framework and using basic probability theory, one can calculate a performance indicator in probabilistic terms. This approach has received increasing recognition and acceptance within geotechnical practice. The profession also finds it useful for dealing with geoscientists and others who use the language of statistics and probability in dealing with spatial and temporal phenomena which are characterized by uncertainty and variability. Moreover, stakeholders in geotechnical projects such as owners, public officials and the general public require to know about the likelihood of alternative outcomes. This again requires the assessment of probabilities. Probabilities of failure may be calculated from an analysis of the performance function such as F, based on a geotechnical model, provided data concerning the geotechnical parameters is available. Alternatively, if enough observational and historical data concerning the occurrence of actual failures is available, probabilities of failure may be calculated directly from an interpretation of such data.

However, probabilities calculated by applying basic probability theory to a performance function may not correspond well with probabilities derived directly from observed data concerning the occurrence of failures. Therefore, one should always state clearly how the stated probabilities have been estimated. Often the relative probabilities are much more important than the absolute probability values which cannot be obtained accurately because of the complexities of geotechnical problems. In any case, the language of probability and probabilistic analysis are important for assessment of performance and its sound communication to stakeholders.

3.3.2   Systematic uncertainties and natural variability of geotechnical parameters

There are several types of uncertainty and a recent review has been presented by Christian (2004). A geotechnical engineer must deal with two main types of uncertainty: (1) natural variability of geotechnical parameters and (2) systematic uncertainties. After recognising the types of geotechnical uncertainties to be dealt with in a specific project, and after assembling the data on geotechnical and other relevant parameters, it is important to decide which amongst these parameters are the most important. Systematic uncertainty results from the limited extent of site investigation and testing that can be performed for a project. It may also result from imperfections in the geotechnical model. Natural variability of geotechnical parameters is the most obvious source of uncertainty. As a consequence of the uncertainties in the influencing factors and parameters, uncertainty is associated with the calculated value of F, the conventional or deterministic safety factor which is, after all, based on single values of the input variables such as shear strength parameters and pore water pressures. Consequently, it is important to analyse the data and calculate, for each geotechnical parameter, its mean value μ, and the standard deviation σ which represents the variability of the parameter. For definitions of these terms refer to sub-section 3.8.2 and to Appendix I at the end of this chapter.

The coefficient of variation, which is the ratio of standard deviation to the mean value of a parameter, may be used as an indicator of parameter variability. Data on even the most important geotechnical parameters are often limited. While the mean values of each parameter may be estimated with confidence, estimating the standard deviation may not be easy. In this regard, Duncan (2000) has suggested using a characteristic of the Gaussian or normal probability distribution, the three sigma rule, to estimate the standard deviation of a variable or parameter. It can be shown that 99.73% of all values of a normally distributed variable (parameter) are contained within three standard deviations on either side of the mean. Therefore, a geotechnical engineer may estimate the highest conceivable value of a particular parameter (HCV) and its lowest conceivable value (LCV) and then estimate the standard deviation as $\sigma = (\text{HCV} - \text{LCV})/6$.

Some geotechnical parameters often vary with depth below ground level (e.g., vertical effective normal stress of normally consolidated soil), others increase with increasing normal effective stress (e.g., shear strength). For such parameters both the mean and standard deviation will vary with depth. Duncan has, therefore, suggested a graphical version of the three sigma rule approach for estimating the standard deviation in such cases.

3.4 RELIABILITY INDEX, PROBABILITY OF FAILURE AND PROBABILITY OF SUCCESS (RELIABILITY)

Analysis can be performed to calculate the two statistical parameters of the factor of safety, F: the mean (expectation) and the standard deviation. For definitions of these terms, the reader should refer to sub-section 3.8.2 and to Appendix I at the end of this chapter. In particular, moments of a random variable are defined in sub-section C3I.5 of that Appendix.

These statistical parameters of F are evaluated by an appropriate procedure by combining the respective statistical parameters of all random variables on which F, the performance function, depends. The details of such procedures are presented in chapter 10.

A performance indicator combining both the mean (expectation) and the standard deviation of F can now be introduced as a simple index of reliability or safety.

This is called the Reliability Index RI (often denoted by β), a ratio of the mean of safety margin, (mean of $F-1$) and the standard deviation of safety margin (S.D. of F), first defined by Cornell (1969) and expressed as in Equation (3.1).

$$RI = \beta = \frac{(\text{Mean of } F-1)}{\text{S.D. of } F} = \frac{\bar{F}-1}{\tilde{F}} = \frac{E[F]-1}{\sigma_F} \qquad (3.1)$$

Thus, even without performing a probabilistic analysis, one can obtain a more meaningful performance indicator than the conventional factor of safety. However, we need to go further and calculate the probability of failure p_F and its complement, the probability of successful performance $(1 - p_F)$, often called reliability. (For basics of Statistics and Probability, and computation of reliability, the reader may refer Appendices to this chapter and Chapter 10.)

In order to do that it is necessary to assume a probability distribution for the performance function which in this case is the factor of safety F. The Gaussian or normal distribution is often used in the absence of detailed information. (For very low probabilities, the Gaussian distribution is considered less useful than other distributions such as lognormal distribution.)

From the probability distribution of F (Figure 3.1), and knowing the mean and standard deviation of F, one can calculate the probability of failure p_F which is defined as the probability that F is less than 1.

$$p_F = P(F < 1) \qquad (3.2a)$$

Thus, reliability or probability of success is given by

$$p_S = P(F > 1) \qquad (3.2b)$$

The calculated values of β, p_F or p_S are derived from the same geotechnical model which is used in the conventional deterministic analysis. Thus, in a major sense, the

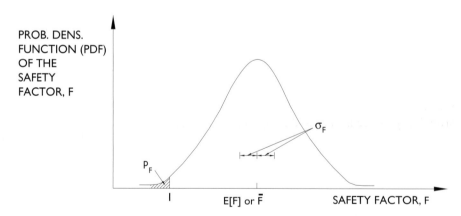

PROB. DENS. FUNCTION (PDF) OF THE SAFETY FACTOR, F

σ_F

P_F

1   E[F] or $\bar{F}$ SAFETY FACTOR, F

Figure 3.1 Probability density function of the safety factor F.

very basic probabilistic procedure described above is an extension of the deterministic approach; the two are complementary.

Basic concepts of probability are presented in three appendices at the end of this chapter. Simple illustrative examples are also provided. The above concepts and relevant applications are outlined in greater detail in Chapter 10.

It should be recognized that the probabilistic approach offers much more than the type of basic calculation of probability of failure or success derived from the performance function F. Therefore, it is important to try and develop new probabilistic perspectives and models. Reference to such developments are also made in chapter 10.

3.5 CONSIDERING THRESHOLDS – MINIMUM RELIABILITY INDEX, MAXIMUM PROBABILITY OF FAILURE

It is also important to consider thresholds for reliability and probability of failure as we did for the factor of safety above (section 3.2.5). Acceptable values of probability of failure may vary widely and there are no universal or even widely accepted guidelines. However, a table of suggested values for natural slopes has been published to generate discussion (Chowdhury and Flentje, 2003). This table considers minimum reliability index and maximum probability of failure for a specific type of slope, a potential failure mode, and potential consequences. Minimum reliability index varies from 1 to 3 and the corresponding maximum probability of failure varies from 0.15 to 0.001 in this table proposed for natural slopes located near urban areas or distant from such areas.

3.6 SPATIAL, TEMPORAL AND SYSTEM ASPECTS

So far we have considered the probability of failure at a particular slope and at a particular time. A regional study requires consideration of a range of slopes of different inclination and with different characteristics. Therefore, the probability of failure will vary spatially. There will also be differences in the performance of two identical slopes located in different environments within the region. Thus, prediction of performance during a causative or triggering event (rainstorm, earthquake etc.) is difficult. Even if we are able to predict that landslides will occur, it will be difficult to predict where they will occur. Therefore, it is useful to consider the outcome in terms of likelihood or probability of occurrence and its spatial variability.

Again, it is one thing to say that failure at a site will occur; but the information is only useful if one has a good understanding of the likely time-frame concerning the occurrence of such a failure. Therefore, particular attention must be given to temporal aspects of probabilistic assessment. Moreover, from a practical perspective, if the failure is likely to occur within the life of the project, the engineering significance is high. The failures of slopes are often triggered by external events such as rainstorms or earthquakes. Thus the temporal aspects of performance of a slope is often intimately linked with the frequency of occurrence of a triggering event with a certain threshold magnitude or intensity.

There is often significant uncertainty associated with the frequency of occurrence of natural events such as a landslide-triggering rainstorm or a landslide-triggering earthquake. Consequently, probabilistic assessment may be much more appropriate than deterministic assessment. Probabilistic modeling of spatially variable and time-dependent processes is, of course, much more complex than the simple calculations considered above which are based on a simple limit equilibrium model. Sophisticated probabilistic models have been developed for both static and dynamic geotechnical problems. The relevance of such models must be considered in relation to the availability of input data as well as the likelihood of validation in practice.

There are other special probability models required in different circumstances such as the assessment of the performance of geotechnical systems. For example, appropriate probabilistic models have been developed for calculating geotechnical systems reliability, for modeling the probability of progressive failure of a slope, and for updating the reliability of a slope when additional data become available. More discussion of such modeling is provided in chapter 10.

The concepts of failure susceptibility, hazard and risk are of particular relevance to slope analysis considering the spatial and temporal aspects mentioned above.

3.7 SUSCEPTIBILITY, HAZARD AND RISK

One can find isolated references to geotechnical risk in some research papers written more than half a century back by pioneers of modern geotechnical engineering. Terms such as 'calculated risk' were applied to particular strategies for relating design to the observed performance of a geotechnical project before its initiation, during its progress and after its completion. Decades later, with the development of probabilistic geotechnical analysis, there was a better understanding of the key elements required for defining geotechnical risk. By now there is a growing appreciation of geotechnical risk as a measure of the intersection between hazard and consequence. In relation to slope stability and landslides, the meaning of susceptibility, hazard and risk should be clearly understood. These terms are particularly important in communication within inter-disciplinary teams and also in communicating with those outside the teams. Moreover, these terms are very useful in relating site-specific studies, qualitative or quantitative, to regional studies, qualitative or quantitative.

Definitions of these terms can vary widely and can be detailed or concise. The following is an attempt to provide concise definitions directly relevant to slope analysis.

Susceptibility is the probability of occurrence of failure or the probability of landsliding. One must specify whether the value of the performance indicator (probability of failure) with reference to a particular type of event such as a slide or a debris-flow etc. Susceptibility is often expressed in relative terms especially if the assessment is qualitative. For example, one may refer to one site or one area as having high landslide susceptibility and another site or area as having low landslide susceptibility. However, it may also be expressed quantitatively.

Hazard relates to a threat from an event and thus, in addition to the probability of occurrence of the event (landsliding), information on factors such as speed (for example very fast, fast or slow), magnitude (volume) and frequency is appropriate. Assessing and specifying the annual probability of landsliding or the return period would provide information about the frequency of the event.

Risk is a product of the magnitude of the hazard and its consequences (to individuals, society, and environment, as appropriate). Alternatively one may refer to the intersection of hazard and consequence rather than the product. In order to assess consequences, one must identify the elements threatened by the hazard and how vulnerable those elements are. Thus vulnerability is an important aspect of assessing risk. A comprehensive discussion of the concepts and methods for the evaluation of geotechnical risk was presented by Whitman (1984).

3.8   FURTHER COMMENTS ON GEOTECHNICAL UNCERTAINTIES

3.8.1   Introduction

As stated earlier there may be significant uncertainties with regard to the data that are used for analysis, or with regard to the mechanism of failure or even with regard to the suitability of a method of analysis itself. Given that a method of analysis is suitable and that the mechanism of failure is fully understood, one still has to contend with uncertainty in material parameters, pore water pressures and other field data. Soils and rocks of which slopes are formed are natural materials with acknowledged spatial variability. They are seldom homogeneous and isotropic and samples obtained from the ground are always disturbed to some degree. In particulate materials like soils, samples are often not truly representative of the bulk or mass of soil especially when the soil is fissured or jointed or exhibits sensitivity. To a large extent this is also true of fissured and jointed rock masses.

Uncertainties with regard to material parameters and applied loads cannot be included in conventional approaches based on a deterministic concept of analysis. A rational approach would be to resort to methods of statistical inference so that meaningful conclusions can be drawn about available data and their characteristics. Based on significant characteristics such as the mean, the standard deviation and the co-efficient of variation, it is then possible and useful to apply concepts from the theory of probability to specific problems.

3.8.2   Basic statistical parameters

Often an engineer is interested in the central tendency of data and its variability. If estimates are to be made directly from data, the mean or sample mean is an indicator of the average or the central tendency of the data and the standard deviation is an indicator of the deviation from the mean and hence of the variability. On the other hand, if estimates are to be made from an assumed probability distribution, the estimates are based on the first and second moments of that distribution.

3.8.2.1   Estimates based on collected sampling data

The mean or arithmetic mean is the well known simple average of a collection of data and shows the central tendency of such data. For a collection of data x which is N in number the mean $\bar{x}$ is simply given by:

$$\bar{x} = \frac{\sum_{j=1}^{N} x_j}{N} \tag{3.3}$$

Now, the deviation of any value of x from the mean $\bar{x}$ is simply their difference. The mean of the squares of these deviations is called the variance and the square root of the variance is called the standard deviation S which is given as follows:

$$S = \sqrt{\frac{\sum_{j=1}^{N} (x_j - \bar{x})^2}{N-1}} \tag{3.4}$$

provided each value of x occurs with the same frequency; otherwise the equation must be suitably modified. The relevant equations can be looked up in any text book on statistics. For a simple example of calculating the sample mean and standard deviation from a set of data, the reader may refer to Ang and Tang (2007), Example 6.1, pp. 250–251.

The variance is simply the square of the standard deviation i.e., S^2 and may be designated as $V[x]$. The co-efficient of variation V_x is the ratio of the standard deviation and the mean and is often expressed as a percentage thus:

$$V_x = \left\{ \frac{S}{\bar{x}} \right\} \times 100 \tag{3.5}$$

3.8.2.2   Estimates from an assumed probability distribution

In probability applications, it is often necessary to determine the moments of the assumed probability distribution representing the variable under consideration. The 'first moment' or the 'mathematical expectation' of a probability distribution corresponds to the mean or average of the variable whereas the second moment is a measure of the dispersion of the variable and corresponds to the variance. Thus the square root of the second moment corresponds to the standard deviation. These terms and corresponding equations are further explained in sub-section C3I.5 of Appendix I to this chapter. The reader may also refer to Ang and Tang (2007), pp. 88–93, for relevant definitions and numerical examples. In sub-section C3I.4 of Appendix I to this chapter, the reader will find an outline of the concept of a random variable and reference to probability distributions together with some numerical examples.

3.8.3   Variability of soil properties and errors

Harr (1977) has compiled a number of tables concerning statistical variation in soil properties such as void ratio, porosity, degree of saturation, unit weight, compressibility characteristics and strength parameters. These tables reveal significant differences in the variability of different types of soils with regard to comparable or significant properties or parameters. For example, available information shows the friction angle of gravel to have a co-efficient of variation of only 6%. On the other hand the co-efficient of variation of the unconfined compressive strength of clay at a depth of 10 feet is shown to be 40.9% and for clay shale between 37% and 51%.

Wu and Kraft (1970) examined published data concerning errors due to various sources in undrained shear strength of clay with special reference to slope analysis for short-term conditions. The errors in per cent were found to be of the following order (a) −28 to 0 due to anisotropy, (b) −10 to 0 due to progressive failure, (c) 0 to 30 due to sampling effects, and (d) −5 to +5 due to plane strain nature of problems being ignored by use of data from triaxial compression test. Thus the sum of all these errors ranges in per cent from −43 to +35. Similarly it was found that errors in calculated shear stress ranged in per cent from (a) −5 to +15 due to slip surface shape being different from circular (as usually assumed) and (b) −10 to 0 due to end restraint which exists in the field but is ignored in a conventional two-dimensional analysis. Thus the sum of errors in calculated shear stress ranged in per cent from −15 to +15.

3.9   VARIANCE OF F FOR SIMPLE SLOPE PROBLEMS

Variability of data and errors of different kinds influence the calculation of the factor of safety and it is of interest to consider this for simple cases. For a cohesionless slope of inclination β the factor of safety is a ratio of tan ϕ and tan β. However, there is no uncertainty about the slope angle β which is given. Therefore, the variance of the factor of safety $V[F]$ is shown by definition to be related to the variance of the tangent of the friction angle $V[\tan \phi]$ as follows:

$$V[F] = \left\{ \frac{1}{\tan \beta} \right\}^2 V[\tan \phi] \tag{3.6}$$

The expected value of the factor of safety or its mean value $\overline{F}$ is given as follows:

$$\overline{F} = \left\{ \frac{1}{\tan \beta} \right\} \overline{\tan \phi} \tag{3.7}$$

where $\overline{\tan \phi}$ is the mean value of tan ϕ.

Thus the co-efficient of variation of the factor of safety, V_F, is the same as that of tan ϕ i.e., $V_{\tan \phi}$. This is obvious when we take the square root of the equation (3.6) to obtain the standard deviation and divide it by the mean value from equation (3.7). Therefore, for cohesionless soil:

$$V_F = V_{\tan \phi} \tag{3.8}$$

Now consider a situation in which only the cohesion parameter is relevant e.g., a "$\phi = 0$" analysis (which is valid for undrained failure of a slope in soft saturated clay). Only the unit undrained cohesion c determines the shearing resistance and in terms of the stability factor N_s, the critical height H is given

$$H = c\left(\frac{N_s}{\gamma}\right)$$

(3.9)

If the strength parameter c is the only random variable and the term within bracket can be regarded as a constant, then it is again easy to show that the co-efficient of variation of the critical height is the same as the co-efficient of variation of the undrained cohesion i.e.,

$$V_H = V_c$$

(3.10)

Consequently it is valid to state that the co-efficient of variation of the factor of safety with respect to height is the same as the co-efficient of variation of the undrained cohesion i.e.,

$$V_F = V_c$$

(3.10a)

The undrained cohesion is half the unconfined compressive strength. According to available information the latter may have a co-efficient of variation $V = 40\%$. Thus the factor of safety or critical height may have a similar variability. On the other hand, factors of safety for cohesionless soil will have a low value of V because ϕ (and hence, tan ϕ) has a low value of V as mentioned earlier. This gives us some idea of the relative degree of uncertainty in the two cases.

Next consider the situation in which both c and ϕ parameters are relevant. For example, taking the end-of-construction case in a partially saturated fill, non-zero values of c and ϕ are relevant to a stability analysis. The degree of uncertainty in the factor of safety or the critical height would now be due to the corresponding uncertainty in both c and ϕ. Therefore, the co-efficient of variation V_F or V_H is greater than the co-efficient of variation V_c i.e.,

$$V_H > V_c \quad \text{and} \quad V_F > V_c$$

(3.11)

3.10   USING PROBABILISTIC ANALYSIS

3.10.1   Requirements and limitations: discussions during early phase of development

There are many ways in which the theory of probability can be applied to stability problems. Deterministic approaches rely almost completely on the conventional 'F' value as a measure of safety and do not consider the fact that many of the quantities which are used in its calculation are random variables. The probability of failure or the degree of reliability associated with a specific calculated value of F is not known. These matters can be given due consideration by using the theory of probability.

It is necessary to start with the probability distribution or the probability density function (PDF) of each random variable (Figure 3.1). To obtain such a distribution, statistical data concerning a variable over a wide range of conditions is required. Such data are rarely available and in the absence of adequate information it is usual to make assumptions with regard to the probability distribution e.g., normal (Gaussian), log normal etc. Observed data may fit different distributions almost equally well but it must be recognised that the range of such data is often very limited. It is interesting and, of course, extremely important that computed probabilities at very small risk can vary by several orders of magnitude depending on the probability distribution of variables assumed for the calculations (Borges and Castenheta, 1971; Ang and Cornell, 1974). In view of this wide divergence care is required in the use of probability theory based on assumed extreme value probability density functions. Lack of information concerning different variables clearly limits our capacity to make probabilistic calculations. In this connection it is useful to consider the relationship between analysis and design (or vice versa) in geotechnical engineering. In his Rankine lecture concerned with design decisions of significance to embankment dams, De Mello (1977) emphasised the difference between statistics of averages and the statistics of extreme values. The settlement of an embankment may be regarded as a condition for the application of the statistics of averages since it is due to the cumulative effect of a large number of soil elements. On the other hand failure due to piping and tensile cracking in dams may be considered as problems in which the application of extreme value statistics and probability is relevant.

In view of the difficulties associated with extreme value analysis, it would be a desirable choice to change the 'statistical universe' by taking design decisions which exclude failure by extreme value events such as piping or tensile cracking in the example mentioned above. As a consequence of such a choice, the theory of probability can be applied with confidence and meaningful predictions made on the basis of computations relevant to the 'statistical universe' of averages. There are many problems of geotechnical engineering in which design decisions can be made in this manner. For example the risk of liquefaction failure of saturated sand due to an earthquake may be eliminated by driving compaction and drainage piles of crushed rock (De Mello, 1977). Other examples given by De Mello include full interceptor filter-drainage inclined into upstream zone of earth dams and use of grout buffer to homogenise a zone of foundations exhibiting extreme dispersions of pervious discontinuities. On the other hand it is quite valid to argue that extreme value conditions cannot always be foreseen and hence their effects cannot be avoided by taking design decisions even in the case of man-made structures such as embankments and dams. In natural slopes, it may be particularly difficult and frustrating to ensure that extreme value conditions are not relevant for stability analysis. There will be continued attempts at successful application of probability theory for extreme value conditions, i.e., attempts at computing probabilities for very low risk based on assumed probability density functions. Whether one is inclined to agree with De Mello's design philosophy or not, it is necessary to emphasise that results of computations for very low risk may be fallacious unless the assumed PDF happens to be very close to the actual PDF for each random variable. These introductory remarks must always be borne in mind while considering probabilistic approaches outlined below.

3.10.2   Example of a probabilistic slope study, De Mello (1977)

In section 3.9 reference was made to a relationship between the co-efficient of variation of the factor of safety and that of cohesion or friction parameters for two simple cases. In the same way it is easy to show that the co-efficient of variation of the factor of safety is significantly influenced by variations of other parameters. For example the co-efficient of variation of the pore water pressure would be extremely important in many problems of slope stability.

Two slopes in different materials and with different pore pressure conditions may have the same factor of safety determined on the basis of conventional limit equilibrium analyses. Yet they would generally show a significant difference in the probability of failure. Conversely, if the two slopes were to have the same probability of failure, their conventional factors of safety would have to be significantly different.

De Mello (1977) illustrated this difference by comparing a rockfill slope with an inclination of 1.4:1 and an earth slope with an inclination of 2.5:1. In both cases a slip circle of the same radius and maximum depth was considered and the mean factor of safety from effective stress analyses was chosen to be nearly the same (i.e., about 1.5, the rockfill slope having a standard deviation S of 0.0408 and the earth slope a value of S of 0.1669). Based on detailed geotechnical data and using the Monte Carlo simulation technique, frequency distribution curves of the factor of safety were generated. As may be expected the distribution curve for rockfill was narrower with a lower spread in comparison to that for earth which was flat and with a relatively large spread. These differences in shape reflect the differences in variability of the parameters of the two materials. Both distributions were, of course, symmetrical about the mean value of 1.5 chosen for the example. In order to obtain the same probability of failure the curve for rockfill was moved laterally so that the area under both curves to the left of $F = 1$ (i.e., safety margin of zero) was the same. In this position the curve for rockfill showed a mean or central value of $F = 1.12$ against $F = 1.5$ for earth slope with probability of failure $p_F = 1/625$ in both cases. This example is another way of illustrating that a given numerical value of the factor of safety F does not reflect the same degree of safety or reliability for different slopes or for the same slope under different conditions. In fact it may be advisable to develop other criteria to replace F values, and De Mello (1977) suggests 'Satisfaction Indices' based on mean and standard deviation of material parameters or of average behaviour represented by deformations, stresses etc.

3.10.3   Errors and probability of failure, Wu and Kraft (1970)

Wu and Kraft (1970) considered the conditional probability distribution of the safety margin for an excavation in clay (for a given value of undrained shear strength s) to be normal and plotted the probability of failure for various values of the safety factor for the following different cases (considering errors mentioned in sub-section 3.8.3): (A) variation in soil strength and no error in analysis, (B) variation in soil strength as well as errors of analysis, (C) same as case B but only 10 specimens tested as compared to 30 in case B, and (D) a very conservative case showing the upper limit of the probability of failure. For a given value of the safety factor (defined as ratio of shear strength to shear stress) the probability of failure increased from case A to case D as expected. The number of samples tested did not have a significant influence on the probability of failure. On the other hand the errors of analysis had marked influence on the failure probability.

The relationship between computed and actual safety factor may be derived in terms of the errors. Let s be the mean shear strength along a potential failure surface, Δs the errors in strength due to inaccuracies in measurement and analysis, τ the calculated shear stress and $\Delta \tau$ the errors in shear stress due to inaccuracies in analysis. The calculated factor of safety F_c and actual factor of safety F_a are:

$$F_c = \frac{s}{\tau}, \quad F_a = \frac{s + \Delta s}{\tau + \Delta \tau} \tag{3.12}$$

Assume that the errors in shear strength due to various sources are proportional to s and the errors in shear stress are proportional to τ, i.e.,

$$\Delta s = s k_i, \quad \Delta \tau = \tau \ell_i \tag{3.13}$$

in which $k_i = k_1 + k_2 + k_3 + \cdots$, $\ell_i = \ell_1 + \ell_2 + \ell_3 + \cdots$
where $k_1, k_2, k_3, \ldots$ and $\ell_1, \ell_2, \ell_3, \ldots$ are the constants of proportionality for various segments into which the potential slip surface is subdivided.

Substituting for the errors by using this equation in the second of Equation (3.12):

$$F_a = F_c \frac{(1 + k_i)}{(1 + \ell_i)} \tag{3.14}$$

For a failure which has already occurred the actual factor of safety is usually taken as unity and the computed factor of safety is thus given as follows:

$$F_c = \frac{(1 + \ell_i)}{(1 + k_i)} \tag{3.15}$$

From this equation the distribution of the computed factor of safety may be calculated based on known or assumed distribution functions of various errors. Considering the errors mentioned in section 3.8 and different distribution functions, Wu and Kraft (1970) obtained ranges of the computed probability of failure for different values of the computed safety factor. They then plotted points on the same graph representing known cases of undrained failure. The selected case studies included those listed in Table 5.5 of chapter 5 except the Bradwell failure together with four other case records. There was qualitative agreement between the calculated range and actual cases. This exercise was made to demonstrate with the help of probability theory that differences between computed and actual factors of safety may be explained on the basis of various errors associated with usual stability calculations.

APPENDICES TO THIS CHAPTER

Three appendices to this chapter follow:

APPENDIX I – Basic probability concepts with 9 numerical examples
APPENDIX II – Equations for a Capacity – Demand model
APPENDIX III – Table of Standard Normal Distribution

APPENDIX I TO CHAPTER 3

C3I.1   Axioms and rules of probability

There is some probability for every event E in a sample space S and it is either zero or a positive quantity but never negative, i.e.,

$$P(E) \geq 0 \tag{C3I.1}$$

The probability of an event E cannot be greater than one since a certain event S has a unit or 100% probability $P(S)$

$$P(S) = 1.0$$
$$0 \leq P(E) \leq 1.0 \tag{C3I.2}$$

The following expression refers to the probability of the union of two mutually exclusive events E_1 and E_2.

$$P(E_1 \cup E_2) = P(E_1) + P(E_2) \tag{C3I.3}$$

It follows that, for complementary event $\bar{E}$,

$$P(E \cup \bar{E}) = P(E) + P(\bar{E}) \tag{C3I.4}$$

However, we have, by definition of a certain event, that the sample space S will be taken up fully by the complementary events E and $\bar{E}$. Thus,

$$E \cup \bar{E} = S \tag{C3I.5}$$

and this leads to

$$P(E \cup \bar{E}) = P(S) = 1.0 \tag{C3I.6}$$

It follows that

$$P(\bar{E}) = 1 - P(E) \tag{C3I.7}$$

If E_1 and E_2 are not mutually exclusive, it can be shown that:

$$P(F_1 \cup E_2) = P(E_1) + P(E_2) - P(E_1 E_2) \tag{C3I.8}$$

Similarly one can show for three events E_1, E_2, E_3 which are not mutually exclusive that

$$\begin{aligned} P(E_1 \cup E_2 \cup E_3) = P(E_1) + P(E_2) + P(E_3) - P(E_1 E_2) \\ - P(E_1 E_3) - P(E_2 E_3) + P(E_1 E_2 E_3) \end{aligned} \tag{C3I.9}$$

For a large number of events, say n, use of de Morgan's rule leads to the following:

$$P(E_1 \cup E_2 \cup E_3 \ldots \cup E_n) = -1 - P\,(\bar{E}_1 \bar{E}_2 \bar{E}_3 \ldots \bar{E}_n) \tag{C3I.10}$$

For mutually exclusive events n in number

$$P(E_1 \cup E_2 \cup E_3 \ldots \cup E_n) = P(E_1) + P(E_2) + \cdots P(E_n) = \sum_{i=1}^{n} P(E_i) \tag{C3I.3a}$$

EXAMPLE C3I.I

Consider a single span bridge both abutments of which are founded on clay soil. A geotechnical engineer is concerned with the probability of excessive settlement of these abutments. Denote the event of excessive settlement of the left abutment by A and that of the right abutment by B and the event of both having excessive settlement by AB. Let $P(A) = 0.01$ and $P(B) = 0.02$ and $P(AB) = 0.009$. Then the probability that at least one of the abutments will have excessive settlement is given by

$$P(A \cup B) = 0.03 - 0.009 = 0.021$$

Note that A and B are not mutually exclusive events. (If A and B were mutually exclusive $P(AB) = 0$ and values of $P(A)$ and $P(B)$ would be different from above.)

C3I.2   Conditional probability and statistical independence

An important and useful concept is that of conditional probability. The probability of an event may depend on the occurrence of another event B and this is the conditional probability $P(A/B)$. In other words, this refers to the probability of an event A in the new or reconstituted sample space B. The following expressions relate the conditional probability to the probability of individual and joint occurrence of two events A and B:

$$P(A/B) = \frac{P(AB)}{P(B)}$$

$$P(B/A) = \frac{P(AB)}{P(A)} \tag{C3I.11}$$

From these one can write

$$P(AB) = P(A/B) \cdot P(B) + P(B/A) \cdot P(A) \tag{C3I.12}$$

Now A and B may be statistically independent. In that case the probability of A is independent of the probability of B, and vice versa. Therefore

$$P(A/B) = P(A) \text{ and } P(B/A) = P(B) \tag{C3I.13}$$

and, from Equation (C3I.12),

$$P(AB) = P(A) \cdot P(B) \tag{C3I.14}$$

Equation (C3I.13) will also apply if A and B are mutually exclusive rather than statistically independent events. However, in that case, the right hand side of equation (C3I.14) is zero, i.e., $P(AB) = 0$.

The complements of statistically independent events are also statistically independent. Thus, one can write:

$$P(\overline{AB}) = P(\overline{A})\,P(\overline{B}) \tag{C3I.15}$$

The probability equation for the union on two events A and B given event E is similar to union without any condition:

$$P(A \cup B/E) = P(A/E) + P(B/E) - (PAB/E) \tag{C3I.16}$$

The probability of intersection may similarly be written:

$$P(AB/E) = P[(A/B)/E]\,P[B/E] \tag{C3I.17}$$

or,

$$P[(A/B)/E] = \frac{P(AB/E)}{P(B/E)} \tag{C3I.18}$$

The conditional probability equation for more than two events is an extension of the equation for two events. For example, considering three events A, B, C, the joint probability of their occurrence is the product of three quantities as below:

$$P(ABC) = P(A/BC)\ P(B/C)\ P(C) \tag{C3I.19}$$

For independent events A, B, C,

$$P(ABC) = P(A)\ P(B)\ P(C) \tag{C3I.19a}$$

EXAMPLE C3I.2

From example C3I.1, consider the conditional probability of excessive settlement of one abutment given the excessive settlement of the other abutment. Here there are two possibilities:

- Considering excessive settlement of right abutment as given, i.e., given B

$$P(A/B) = \frac{P(AB)}{P(B)} = \frac{0.009}{0.02} = 0.45 \text{ or } 45\%$$

- Considering excessive settlement of left abutment as given, i.e., given A

$$P(B/A) = \frac{P(AB)}{P(A)} = \frac{0.009}{0.01} = 0.9 \text{ or } 90\%$$

We note a dramatic increase in the probability in both situations in comparison to the independent probability. We also note that the two conditional probabilities are markedly different.

However, if A and B are mutually exclusive, or, if A and B are statistically independent,

$$P(A/B) = P(A) = 0.01 \text{ or } 1\%$$

$$P(B/A) = P(B) = 0.02 \text{ or } 2\%$$

EXAMPLE C3I.3

From example C3I.1, consider the probability that at least one abutment will have excessive settlement, given that A and B are statistically independent. In this case,

$$P(AB) = P(A) \cdot P(B) = 0.01 \times 0.02 = 0.0002$$

Therefore

$$P(A \cup B) = P(A) + P(B) - P(AB)$$
$$= 0.03 - 0.0002 \approx 0.03$$

This result happens to be very close to the case where A and B are mutually exclusive. In that case $P(AB) = 0$ and, $P(A \cup B) = P(A) + P(B) = 0.03$.

C31.3   Total probability and Bayes' theorem

The theorem of total probability of an event E is written as follows:

$$P(E) = P(E/A_1) \, P(A_1) + P(E/A_2) \, P(A_2) \, P(E/A_3) \, P(A_3)$$
$$+ \cdots + P(E/A_n) \, P(A_n) \tag{C31.20}$$

in which the events A_1, A_2 ..., A_n are other events which accompany the occurrence of event E; these n events are mutually exclusive and collectively exhaustive.

This theorem is useful in problems in which the probability of an event E cannot be determined directly whereas the probabilities of events A_1, A_2 ..., A_n can be determined.

Bayes' theorem combines the conditional probability equation with the total probability theorem and seeks to determine the probability that an event A_1 or A_2 or A_3 ... or A_i occurred, given the occurrence of event E. Considering the joint event EA_i one can obtain the following statement of Bayes' theorem from the equation of conditional probability

$$P(A_i/E) = \frac{P(E/A_i) \, P(A_i)}{P(E)} \tag{C31.21}$$

Using the total probability theorem one can replace the denominator on the right hand side by a summation term:

$$P(A_i/E) = \frac{P(E/A_i) \, P(A_i)}{\sum_{j=1}^{n} P(E/A_j) \, P(A_j)} \tag{C31.21a}$$

EXAMPLE C31.4

An earth dam may fail due to one of three causes, namely: (a) overtopping; (b) slope failure; (c) piping and subsurface erosion. The probabilities of failure due to these causes are respectively 0.7, 0.1 and 0.2. The probability that overtopping will occur within the life of the dam is 10^{-5}, the probability that slope failure will take place is 10^{-4} and the probability that piping and subsurface erosion will occur is 10^{-3}. What is the probability of failure of the dam, assuming that there are no other phenomena which can cause failure?

Solution

Denoting the event of failure of dams by E, the events likely to cause failure by A_1, A_2, A_3 and using the total probability theorem:

$$P(E) = P(E/A_1)P(A_1) + P(E/A_2)P(A_2) + P(E/A_3)P(A_3)$$
$$P(E) = (0.7 \times 10^{-5}) + (0.1 \times 10^{-4}) + (0.2 \times 10^{-3})$$
$$= 0.217 \times 10^{-3}$$

EXAMPLE C31.5

Solution

In the above example, suppose that failure of the dam occurred, what is the probability that failure was accompanied by (or caused by) (a) overtopping, (b) slope failure, (c) piping and subsurface erosion?

(a) The probability that overtopping occurred given that the dam failed is $P(A_1/E)$. Using Bayes' theorem

$$P(A_1/E) = \frac{P(E/A_1) \, P(A_1)}{P(E)}$$
$$= \frac{0.7 \times 10^{-5}}{0.217 \times 10^{-3}} = 3.23 \times 10^{-2}$$

(b) Similarly the probability that slope failure occurred is

$$P(A_2/E) = \frac{P(E/A_2) \, P(A_2)}{P(E)}$$
$$= \frac{0.1 \times 10^{-4}}{0.217 \times 10^{-3}} = 4.61 \times 10^{-2}$$

(c) The probability that piping and subsurface erosion occurred is

$$P(A_3/E) = \frac{0.2 \times 10^{-3}}{0.217 \times 10^{-3}} = 0.92 \text{ or } 92\%$$

C31.4 Random variables and probability distributions

To use probability or a probabilistic model for formulating and solving a given problem, one accepts the view that the problem is concerned with a random phenomenon or phenomena. Significant parameters influencing the problem are random variables or are regarded as such. A random variable is a function of the value(s) which identify an outcome or an event. A random variable may be discrete or continuous or a combination of the two. Each numerical value of a random variable is associated with a probability measure. For example, if A is a discrete random variable with values 1, 2 and 3 then a value of $A = 1$ may have a probability of 0.2 a value of $A = 2$ may have a probability of 0.3 and a value of $A = 3$ would have a probability 0.5. (Note that the sum of these probabilities is unity.)

A random variable is usually denoted by a capital letter and its numerical value by a small letter although this distinction is not always considered necessary in the following sections. The rule for describing the probability measures associate with all possible values of a random variable is a probability law or distribution.

For a continuous random variable X, probabilities are associated with intervals on the real line (abscissa). At a specific value of X (say $X = x$) only the density of the probability is defined. The probability law or probability distribution is therefore defined in terms of a probability density function denoted by 'PDF'. Let $f_X(x)$ be the 'PDF' of X, then the probability of X in the interval (a, b) is

$$P(a < X \leq b) = \int_a^b f_X(x)dx$$

(C3I.22)

However, the probability distribution can also be defined by a cumulative distribution function denoted by CDF which is

$$F_X(x) \equiv P(X \leq x)$$

(C3I.23)

The CDF is extremely useful as we obtain a measure of probability directly, whereas to obtain the probability measure from the PDF the area under the PDF has to be calculated. For the continuous random variable we can write:

$$F_X(x) = \int_{-\infty}^x f_X(x)dx$$

(C3I.24)

Assuming that $F_X(x)$ has a first derivative,

$$f_X(x) = \frac{dF_X(x)}{dx}$$

(C3I.25)

The probability that the values of X lie in the interval $\{x, (x + dx)\}$, is given by $f_X(x)dx$, i.e.,

$$P(x < X \leq x + dx) = f_X(x)dx = dF_X(x)$$

(C3I.26)

Figure C3I.1 shows an example of a continuous random variable with PDF and CDF.

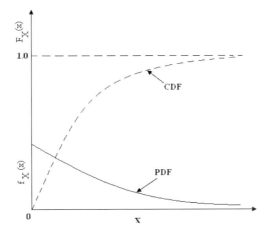

Figure C31.1 A continuous random variable X showing PDF and CDF.

A function used to describe a probability distribution must be positive and the probabilities associated with all possible values of the random variable must add up to unity. Therefore,

$$F_X(-\infty) = 0, \quad F_X(+\infty) = 1, \quad F_X(x) \geq 0 \tag{C31.27}$$

Note also that $F_X(x)$ will never decrease with increasing x and that it is continuous with x. Obviously the CDF is a continuous curve, the magnitude of the ordinate at the end of the curve being unity. This represents the total are under PDF which is also unity, the total probability associated with associated random variable.

Consider now the corresponding terms with respect to a discrete random variable. The CDF has the same meaning as for a continuous variable and the same equation applies. However, instead of the PDF, the alternative to CDF is a probability mass function denoted by PMF. The PMF gives the probability of the random variable for all its discrete values (as stated for the variable A earlier in this section).

Let X be a discrete random variable with PMF $p_X(x_i) \equiv p(X = x_i)$ in which x_i represents all the discrete values of X, that is, x_1, x_2, x_3 etc. Then, its CDF, $F_X(x)$ is given by

$$F_X(x) = P(X \leq x) = \Sigma p(X = x_i) = \sum_{\text{all } x_i \leq x} p_X(x_i) \tag{C31.28}$$

It is easy to show that in interval $a < X \leq b$

$$P(a < X \leq b) = F_X(b) - F_X(a) \tag{C31.29}$$

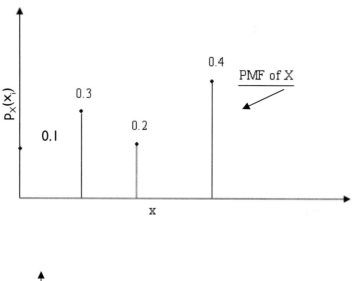

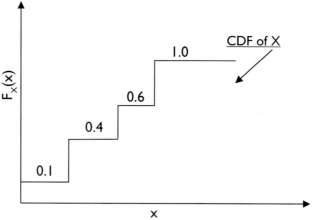

Figure C31.2 A discrete random variable X showing PMF and CDF.

The PMF is not a curve but a series of vertical lines (see Figure C31.2) or ordinates with heights representing probability measures (not probability density as in the case of continuous case, i.e. PDF). The sum of the ordinates must be n unity. A bona fide cumulative distribution function for the discrete case must satisfy the same conditions as in the case of the continuous random variable. Thus the CDF is a continuous curve and is non-decreasing with increasing x.

The simplest continuous distribution is a uniform distribution, that is, a line parallel to the horizontal or abscissaw as shown in Figure C31.3. Another relatively simple distribution is a triangular distributions. A modification of the triangular distribution is a trapezoidal distribution. It is useful to consider some of these as examples before proceeding to well known and widely used distributions such as the normal (or Gaussian) distribution and the lognormal distribution.

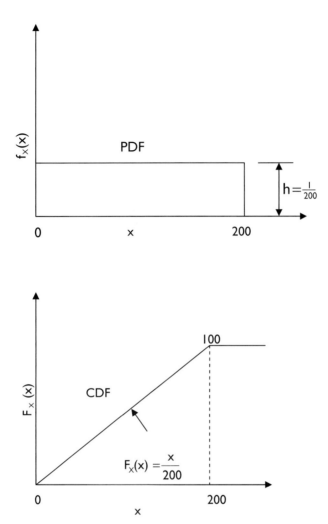

Figure C31.3 An Example of a uniform probability density function with associated CDF.

EXAMPLE C31.6

The undrained shear strength c_u of a stratum of clay has a uniform probability distribution, the maximum and minimum values of the distribution being 50 kN/m² and 25 kN/m² respectively. What is the probability that the undrained shear strength has a magnitude (a) less than 40 kN/m², (b) less than 30 kN/m², (c) less than 10 kN/m², (d) greater than 55 kN/m²?

Solution

The area under the probability density function must be unity. In this case the abscissa or the base of the rectangle (Figure C31.3) is $(50 - 25) = 25$. Therefore, the height of the rectangle (i.e., the uniform probability density, p_{cu}) is given by equating the area to 1, that is:

$$p_{cu} \times 25 = 1, \quad \therefore p_{cu} = \frac{1}{25}$$

We use this value as follows:

(a) $p_1 = P(c_u \leq 40)$
This probability is the area of the rectangle between the ordinates at $c_u = 25$ (minimum value) and $c_u = 40$.

$$\therefore p_1 = (40 - 25) \times \frac{1}{25} = 0.6$$

(b) $p_2 = P(c_u \leq 30) = (30 - 25) \times \frac{1}{25} = 0.2$

(c) 10 kN/m² is outside the range 25–50. Accordingly,
$p_3 = P(c_u \leq 10) = 0$
(d) 55 kN/m² is outside the range 25–50. Accordingly,
$p_4 = P(c_u > 55) = 0$.

C31.5 Moments of a random variable

Before proceeding to more sophisticated distributions, it is necessary to consider important descriptors of a distribution. A random variable may be described in terms of its mean value called 'mean' and a measure of variability called 'variance'. (The 'standard deviation', which is the square root of the variance, is often used instead of the variance.) The use of these parameters with a known or assumed distribution is very convenient. The mean and the standard deviation are generally the main descriptors of a random variable; however, other parameters may have to be used to describe a distribution properly. Reference is made later to another descriptor or parameter of a distribution called the skewness. Often a distribution is not known but estimate of the mean and the standard derivation (or the variance) can be made. It is then possible to solve problems on the basis of an appropriate assumption concerning the distribution. In other words, one tries to fit a distribution to the known values of these descriptors.

The mean value is a central value which presents the weighted average of the values of the random variable where the weight for each value is its probability density for a continuous distribution and its probability for a discrete distribution. The mean value is called an expected value and it is also referred to as the 'first central moment' or, simply, 'the first moment' of a random variable. The mean value of X is denoted by $E(X)$ or $\bar{x}$ or μ_x. For a continuous random variable with PDF $f_X(x)$ we have

$$\bar{x} = E(X) = \int_{-\infty}^{\infty} x \, f_X(x) \, dx$$

(C31.30)

For a discrete random variable with PMF, $p_X(x_i)$

$$\bar{x} = E(X) = \sum_{\text{all } x_i} x_i p_X(x_i)$$

(C3I.30a)

Other descriptors such as the 'mode' and the 'median' may also be used to designate the central value of a random variable. The mode is the most probable value of a random variable and the median is the value of the random variable at which the cumulative probability is 0.50 or 50%. For a symmetric PDF with a single 'mode' the mean, the median and the mode are identical. But, in general, the values of all three may be different from one another.

The variance of a random variable is a measure of its dispersion and is defined as follows for a continuous random variable

$$V(X) = \int_{-\infty}^{\infty} (x - \bar{x})^2 f_X(x) \, dx$$

(C3I.31)

Noting the form of the expression, the variance is also called the 'second central moment' or, simply, the 'second moment' of a random variable as it is the expectation of $(x - \bar{x})^2$ or $E(x - \bar{x})^2$. By expanding the right-hand side of Equation (C3I.31), it can be shown that

$$V(X) = E(X^2) - \bar{x}^2 = E(X^2) - \{E(X)\}^2$$

(C3I.32)

In practice, the standard deviation S_x (also denoted by σ_x) of a random variable is used in preference to the variance primarily because it has the same units as the mean. We recall that:

$$S_X = \sqrt{V(X)}$$

(C3I.33)

A relative measure of dispersion of a random variable is its coefficient of variation V_x which is the ratio of the standard deviation to the mean, that is:

$$V_X = \frac{S_x}{\bar{x}}$$

(C3I.34)

The coefficient of variation is a good parameter for comparing different random variables as to their spread or dispersion. In other words it is useful for comparing the variability or uncertainty associated with different quantities.

The 'third central moment' or, simply, the 'third moment' of a random variable is a measure of the asymmetry or skewness of its distribution. Its value is zero for a symmetrical distribution: otherwise, it may be negative or positive. For a continuous random variable, the expression is

$$E(x - \bar{x})^3 = \int_{-\infty}^{\infty} (x - \bar{x})^3 f_X(x) dx$$

(C3I.35)

The skewness coefficient θ is the ratio of skewness to the cube of the standard deviation.

C31.6   The normal distribution

C31.6.1   The standard normal variate

The normal or Gaussian distribution is represented by a continuous and symmetric PDF given by the following equation (Figure C31.4):

$$f_X(x) = \frac{1}{S_x\sqrt{2\pi}} \exp\left[-\frac{1}{2}\left(\frac{x-\bar{x}}{S_x}\right)^2\right] \quad -\infty < x < \infty \tag{C31.36}$$

A short notation $N(\bar{x}, S_x)$ is often used for a normal distribution.

A very useful form of the distribution is one with a zero mean and unit standard deviation and is referred to as the 'standard' normal distribution. Thus if S is the standard normal random variable (or simply variate), its PDF (Figure C31.5) is

$$f_S(s) = \frac{1}{\sqrt{2\pi}} \exp\left[-\frac{1}{2}s^2\right], \quad -\infty < s < \infty \tag{C31.37}$$

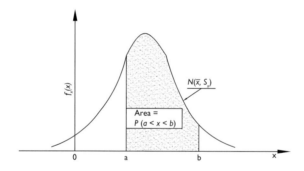

Figure C31.4 A normal distribution of random variable X with mean $\bar{x}$ and standard deviation S_x.

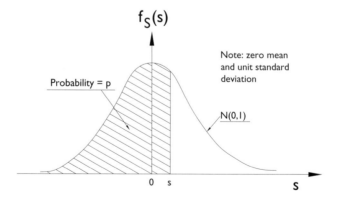

Figure C31.5 A standard normal distribution.

This is also denoted by $N(0, 1)$ and is symmetrical about zero. Its cumulative distribution function or CDF is often denoted by $\Phi(s)$, that is:

$$\Phi(s) = F_s(s) = p \tag{C3I.38}$$

where p is the probability $p = P(S \le s)$. This probability p represents the area under the standard normal distribution to the left of s, that is, form $\propto$ to s. This distribution is available in tables and often values are given only for positive values of the standard normal variate. Thus, values will start from 0.5 for $s = 0$ and approach unity for increasing positive values of s.

For negative values of s the probability is obtained by subtraction from unity (the total area under the distribution being unity). Hence, we have

$$\Phi(-s) = 1 - \Phi(s) \tag{C3I.38a}$$

This is obviously correct because the standard distribution is symmetrical about $s = 0$.

The reverse calculation, that is, determination of the value of the variate s for a given cumulative probability p is often important and one may write

$$s = \Phi^{-1}(p) \tag{C3I.39}$$

Tables of CDF of the standard normal distribution $N(0, 1)$ are widely available in text books concerned with probability and its applications. Consequently, calculation of probability associated with normal distribution can be made without the necessity of performing integrations of the PDF. For accurate work, however, it is advisable to use a computer program for numerical integration of the PDF, that is, for calculation of the area under the PDF. Standard computer programs are widely available for this type of numerical calculation. The table of cumulative normal distribution of the standard normal variate is included as Appendix III to chapter 3.

Returning to tabulated values, as noted earlier, the tables usually contain the CDF for positive values of the variate, s. Because of symmetry the CDF for negative values of s can be simply obtained using Equation (C3I.39). Positive values of the variate s are associated with CDF > 0.5 or $p > 0.5$. For values of $p < 0.5$, the variate s is given by:

$$s = \Phi^{-1}(p) = -\Phi^{-1}(1 - p) \tag{C3I.39a}$$

(Note: In some tables the values of cumulative probability start from zero even though only positive values of the variate are considered. In such cases the users should add 0.5 to the tabulated value for the left symmetrical half of the area below the probability distribution curve.)

C31.6.2   Application of standard normal variate

The first step is to obtain the standard variable s from the given mean and standard derivation of the random variable x. The relationship between x and s is obvious from the corresponding expressions for PDF and we have

$$s = \frac{x - \bar{x}}{S_x} \tag{C31.40}$$

The probability that the random variable X lies between two limits a and b is given by the probability that the standard normal variate lies between s_1 and s_2, and we have:

$$P(a \le X \le b) = \Phi(s_2) - \Phi(s_1)$$
$$= \Phi\left(\frac{b - \bar{x}}{S_x}\right) - \Phi\left(\frac{a - \bar{x}}{S_x}\right) \tag{C31.41}$$

EXAMPLE C31.7

The mean and coefficient of variation of the angle of the angle of internal friction, ϕ, of a soil supporting a multi-storeyed structure are $\bar{\phi} = 20°$ and $V_\phi = 30\%$. What is the probability that ϕ will be less than (a) 16°, (b) 10°, (c) 5°? Assume that ϕ has a normal distribution.

Solution

(a) $V_\phi = \dfrac{S_\phi}{\phi} = 0.3$

$\therefore S_\phi = 0.3 \times 20° = 6°$

$$s = \frac{\phi - \bar{\phi}}{S_\phi} = \frac{16 - 20}{6} = \frac{-4}{6} = -0.666$$

$\Phi(-s) = 1 - \Phi(s) = 1 - \Phi(0.666)$

where $\Phi(\bullet)$ is obtained from tabulated values (Appendix III to Chapter 3)

$\therefore P(s \le 16°) = 0.253$

(b) $s = \dfrac{10 - 20}{6} = -\dfrac{5}{3} = -1.666$

$\Phi(-1.666) = 1 - \Phi(1.666) = 1 - 0.952 = 0.048$

$\therefore P(s \le 10°) = 0.048 = 0.48 \times 10^{-1}$

(c) $s = \dfrac{5 - 20}{6} = \dfrac{-15}{6} = \dfrac{-5}{2} = -2.5$

$\therefore \Phi(-2.5) = 1 - \Phi(2.5) = 1 - 0.994 = 0.006 = 6 \times 10^{-3}$

It should be noted that ϕ denotes the friction angle and $\Phi(s)$ is the cumulative probability of the standard normal variates.

C31.7 Logarithmic normal distribution

Consider a random variable X which does not follow a normal distribution but whose natural logarithm (ℓnX) has a normal distribution. The variable X is then said to have a logarithmic normal or lognormal probability distribution and its density function is given by

$$f_X = \frac{1}{\sqrt{2\pi}\beta x} \exp\left[-\frac{1}{2}\left(\frac{\ell nx - \alpha}{\beta}\right)^2\right], \quad 0 \le x < \infty \tag{C31.42}$$

in which

$$\alpha = E\,(\ell nX) = \overline{\ell nX}$$

and

$$\beta = \sqrt{Var(\ell nX)} = S_{\ell nX}$$

are respectively the mean and standard derivation of ℓnX and are the parameters of the distribution.

Assumption of a lognormal distribution is often preferred to the assumption of a normal distribution for random variables which must have a positive value. For instance the factor of safety F is, by definition, a positive quantity. Therefore, it appears desirable to adopt F as a lognormal variate than as a normal variate. Figure (C31.6) shows a typical lognormal distribution.

It is easy to show that the tabulated values of the CDF of a standard normal distribution can be used for a lognormal distribution as well. The probability of X being in the interval (a, b) is

$$P(a < X \le b) = \Phi\left(\frac{\ell n\,b - \alpha}{\beta}\right) - \Phi\left(\frac{\ell n\,a - \alpha}{\beta}\right) \tag{C31.43}$$

The probability of X being less than or equal to unity is given by:

$$P(X \le 1) = \Phi\left(\frac{\ell n\,1 - \alpha}{\beta}\right) = \Phi\left(\frac{-\alpha}{\beta}\right) \tag{C31.44}$$

It can be shown that in terms of $\bar{x}$ ad S_x, α and β are as follows:

$$\beta^2 = \ell n\left(1 + \frac{S_x^2}{\bar{x}^2}\right), \quad \text{and} \quad \alpha = \ell n(\bar{x}) - \frac{1}{2}\beta^2 \tag{C31.44a}$$

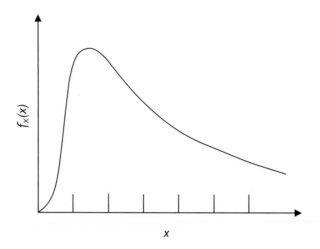

Figure C31.6 Lognormal distribution showing typical shape of PDF.

For

$$\frac{S_x}{\overline{x}} \le 0.3, \quad \beta \simeq \frac{S_x}{\overline{x}} = V_x$$

(C31.44b)

C31.8   Joint distribution, covariance and correlation

If X and Y are two random variables, then probabilities associated with any pair of values x and y may be described by a joint distribution function. e.g.,

$$F_{X,Y}(x,y) = P(X \le x, Y \le y)$$

(C31.45)

For discrete random variable the joint PMF may be used

$$p_{X,Y}(x,y) = P(X = x, Y = y)$$

(C31.46)

For a continuous random variable the joint PDF (Figure C31.7b) may be defined by:

$$f_{X,Y}(x,y)\, dx\, dy = P(x < X \le x + dx,\ y < Y \le y + dy)$$

(C31.47)

Appling the total probability theorem, the marginal density functions of this joint distribution are:

$$f_X(x) = \int_{-\infty}^{\infty} f_{X,Y}(x,y)dy$$

$$f_Y(y) = \int_{-\infty}^{\infty} f_{X,Y}(x,y)dx$$

(C31.48)

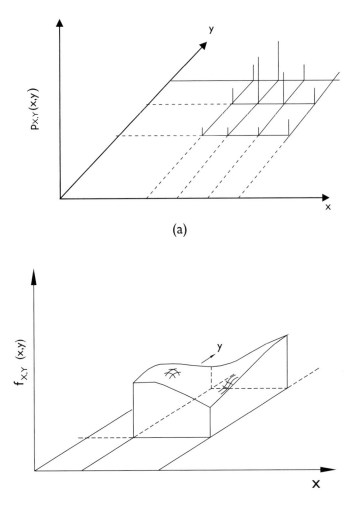

Figure C31.7 (a) Joint PMF of X and Y, (b) joint PDF of X and Y.

The CDF is given by the volume under the surface $f_{X,Y}(x, y)$ and is given by

$$F_{X,Y}(x,y) = \int_{-\infty}^{x}\int_{-\infty}^{y} f_{X,Y}(u,v)dv\ du$$

$$(C31.49)$$

Description of a joint distribution of two random variables requires five statistical parameters, namely, the mean and standard deviation of each variable and the correlation coefficient between them. This coefficient is denoted by ρ and is the ratio of the covariance denoted by cov(x, y) and the product of the standard deviations.

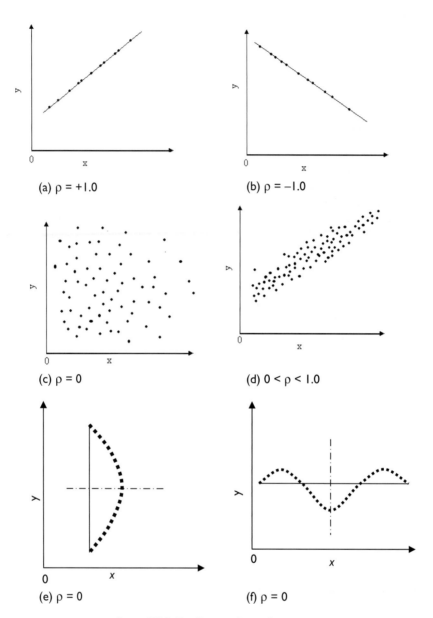

Figure C31.8 Coefficient of correlation ρ.

$$\rho_{X,Y} = \frac{\text{cov}(x,y)}{S_x S_y}$$

(C31.50)

The covariance itself is defined as the joint central second moment, that is, the expectation of the product $(X - \bar{x})(Y - \bar{y})$ and hence

$$\begin{aligned} \text{cov}(X, Y) &= E[(X - \bar{x})(Y - \bar{y})] \\ &= E(XY) - E(X)E(Y) \end{aligned} \tag{C3I.51}$$

If X and Y are statistically independent, then

$$E(XY) = E(X)E(Y) \quad \text{and} \quad \text{cov}(X, Y) = 0 \tag{C3I.52}$$

If two variables are statistically independent then the variables are uncorrelated. However, the reverse is not true. If the variables are uncorrelated, they may not be statistically independent.

The correlation coefficient ρ may vary from -1 to $+1$ and may be regarded as a normalized covariance. It is a measure of the linear relationship between the two random variables (Figure C3I.8). For further discussion of concept of joint probability distribution, see Ang Tang (2007).

C3I.9   Moments of functions of random variables

C3I.9.1   Sum of variates x_1, x_2 etc.

Consider a function Y which is dependent on two random variables X_1 and X_2. Thus (a_1 and a_2 are constants),

$$Y = a_1 X_1 + a_2 X_2$$

Then, it can be shown that

$$\bar{y} = E(Y) = a_1 \bar{x}_1 + a_2 \bar{x}_2$$

and

$$V(y) = a_1^2 V(x_1) + a_2^2 V(x_2) + 2a_1 a_2 \text{ cov } (x_1, x_2) \tag{C3I.53}$$

Now, if $Y = a_1 X_1 - a_2 X_2$,

$$\bar{y} = a_1 \bar{x}_1 - a_2 \bar{x}_2$$

and

$$V(y) = a_1^2 V(x_1) + a_2^2 V(x_2) - 2a_1 a_2 \text{ cov}(x_1, x_2) \tag{C3I.54}$$

In general, if

$$Y = \sum_{i=1}^{n} a_i X_i, \qquad \bar{y} = \sum_{i=1}^{n} a_i \bar{x}_i$$

$$V(y) = \sum_{i=1}^{n} a_i^2 V(x_i) + \sum_{i}^{n} \sum_{j}^{n} a_i a_j \ \text{cov}(x_i, x_j) \qquad \text{(C3I.55)}$$

Suppose Z is another function of random variable X, i.e.,

$$Z = \sum_{i=1}^{m} b_i X_i$$

$$\text{cov}(Y, Z) = \sum_{i=1}^{n} a_i b_i \ V(x_i) + \sum_{i \neq j}^{n} \sum_{}^{n} a_i a_j \ \text{cov}(x_i, x_j) \qquad \text{(C3I.56)}$$

C3I.9.2   Product of independent variates x_1, x_2, x_3, etc.

If $Z = X_1 X_2 X_3 \dots X_n$

$\bar{Z} = E(Z) = \bar{x}_1 \bar{x}_2 \bar{x}_3 \dots \bar{x}_n$

$S_Z^2 = E(X_1^2)E(X_2^2) \dots E(X_n^2) - (\bar{x}_1 \bar{x}_2 \dots \bar{x}_n)^2$

(C-3I-57)

C3I.9.3   First order approximation for general functions

Let $Y = g(X)$

Then, by expanding $g(X)$ in a Taylor series about the mean value $\bar{x}$, the following first-order approximation can be made

$$\bar{y} = E(Y) \simeq g(\bar{x}) + \tfrac{1}{2} V(x) \frac{d^2 g}{dx^2}$$

$$V(y) \simeq V(x) \left(\frac{dg}{dx} \right)^2 \qquad \text{(C3I.58)}$$

Good approximation of exact moment is obtained if $g(X)$ is approximately linear for the entire range of values of X (even if the second term in the expression for the mean is neglected; this is generally done).

Now if Y is function of several variables X_1, X_2, X_3 etc.

$$Y = g(X_1, X_2, X_3, \dots, X_n)$$

the corresponding first order approximations are

$$\bar{y} = E(Y) \simeq g(\bar{x}_1, \bar{x}_2, \ldots, \bar{x}_n)$$

$$+ \frac{1}{2} \sum_{i=1}^{n} \sum_{j=1}^{n} \left(\frac{d^2 g}{dx_i dx_j} \right) \mathrm{cov}(x_i, x_j)$$

$$V(y) \simeq \sum_{i=1}^{n} c_i^2 V(x_i) + \sum_{i=j}^{n} \sum_{j}^{n} c_i c_j \, \mathrm{cov}(x_i, x_j)$$

(C3I.59)

where c_i and c_j are the partials derivatives $(\partial g / \partial x_i)$ and $(\partial g / \partial x_j)$ evaluated at $\bar{x}_1, \bar{x}_2, \bar{x}_3, \ldots, \bar{x}_n$.

The second term of the first equation is generally omitted. The second term of the second equation is not omitted but will vanish if x_1, x_2, $x_3, \ldots, x_n$ are uncorrelated or statistically independent.

An alternative approach for approximate calculation of the first and second moments of a general function of several random variables has been proposed by Rosenblueth (1975). This method is called the Point Estimate Method (PEM) and is extremely useful in practice because the partial derivatives of the function are not required. Often it is not possible to find the derivatives and, therefore, Rosenblueth's method is convenient to use. Moreover, it generally gives the same order of accuracy as the method based on first order approximation of the function expanded as a Taylor series.

EXAMPLE C3I.8

The mean of value of the tangent of the angle of internal friction, $\tan \phi$, of a soil is 0.364 and its coefficient of variation $V_{\tan\phi}$ is 10%. The mean value of the cohesion $\bar{c}$ of the same soil is 15 kN/m² and its coefficient of variation, V_c is 35%. What is the coefficient of variation of the shearing resistance along a plane with a normal stress σ of (a) 100 kN/m² and (b) 10 kN/m²? Assume c and $\tan \phi$ to be statistically independent.

Solution
(a) The shearing resistance is derived from $\tau = c + \sigma \tan \phi$. The partial derivatives evaluated at the means are $\partial \tau / \partial c = 1$ and $\partial \tau / \partial \tan \phi = 100$. (The second derivatives are zero). Now, using first order approximation,

$$\bar{\tau} = 15 + (100 \times 0.364) = 51.4 \text{ kN/m}^2$$

$$V(\tau) = (1^2)V_c + (100)^2 V_{\tan\phi} + 0 \times \mathrm{cov} \, (c, \tan \phi)$$

$$V_c = S_c^2 = (0.35 \times 15)^2 = (5.25)^2 = 27.56$$

$$V_{\tan\phi} = S_{\tan\phi}^2 = (0.1 \times 0.364)^2 = 1.32 \times 10^{-3}$$

$$\therefore \quad V(\tau) = 27.56 + 100^2 \times 1.32 \times 10^{-3} = 40.76$$

$$\text{and, } S_\tau = \sqrt{40.76} = 6.384$$

$$V_\tau = \frac{6.384}{51.4} \times 100\% = 12.41\%$$

(b) $\bar{\tau} = 15 + (10 \times 0.364) = 18.64 \text{ kN/m}^2$

$V(\tau) = 27.56 + 10^2 \times 1.32 \times 10^{-3} = 27.692$

$S_\tau = \sqrt{27.692} = 5.26$

$V_\tau = \dfrac{5.26}{18.64} \times 100\% = 28.23\%$

Note that the coefficient of variation is much higher in this case because the shear strength is predominantly cohesive compared to the first case and because cohesion has a high coefficient of variation.

EXAMPLE C31.9

In Example C31.8, c and $\tan \phi$ are correlated with a coefficient of correlation of -0.2. What is the change in the values of the mean and the standard deviation of the shearing resistance? Repeat this exercise if the correlation coefficient is $+0.2$.

Solution

(i) $\rho = -0.2$ (negative correlation coefficient)

The shear strength is a linear function of both random variables. Therefore, instead of using first order approximation, exact equations may be used for the mean and the variance, that is,

$\bar{\tau} = \bar{c} + \sigma \overline{\tan \phi}$ (same as in first order approx.)

$V(\tau) = V_c + \sigma^2 V_{\tan \phi} + 2 \times 1 \times \sigma \times \text{cov} (c, \tan \phi)$

In Example C31.8(a),

$\text{cov} (c, \tan \phi) = -0.2 \ S_c \ S_{\tan \phi} = -0.2 \times 5.25 \times 0.0364 = -0.0382$

$V(\tau) = 27.56 + (100)^2 \times 1.32 \times 10^{-3} + 2 \times 1 \times 100 \ (-0.0382) = 40.76 - 7.64$

$\qquad = 33.12$

$\therefore S_\tau = \sqrt{33.12} = 5.75$ [decrease of 9.9% from Example C31.8(a)]

In Example C31.8(b),

$\text{cov} (c, \tan \phi) = -0.2 \times 5.25 \times 0.0364 = -0.0382$

$V(\tau) = 27.56 + (10)^2 \times 1.32 \times 10^{-3} + 2 \times 1 \times 10 \ (-0.0382) = 27.69 - 0.764$

$\qquad = 26.93$

$\therefore S_\tau = 5.19$ [decrease of 1.33% from Example C31.8(b)]

(ii) $\rho = +0.2$ (positive correlation coefficient)

In Example C31.8(a),

$V(\tau) = 40.76 + 7.64 = 48.4$
$\therefore S_\tau = 6.96$ (increase of 9.02% from Example C3I.8(a))

In example C3I.8(b),

$V(\tau) = 27.69 + 0.764 = 28.45$
$\therefore S_\tau = 5.33$ [increase of 1.33% from Example C3I.8(b)]

APPENDIX II TO CHAPTER 3

C3II.1 Equations for a capacity – demand model (after Harr, 1977)

C3II.1.1 Safety margin and factor of safety

We may begin with the definition of factor of safety, safety margin and central factor of safety within the framework of probability. Often a standard normal distribution is assumed for various random variables which are then called normal variates. For example in the analysis of a slope the disturbing moments (or forces) and the resisting moments (or forces) may be treated as normal variates. Following Harr (1977), denote the latter by C (capacity) and the former by D (demand). The distributions of C and D are shown in Figure C3II.1(a). In a deterministic approach single estimated values $\hat{C}$ and $\hat{D}$ would be used for each of these random variables to calculate the conventional factor of safety F [see Figure C3II.1(a)]. The safety margin SM may be defined as the difference between capacity and demand and it is also a random variable. The central factor of safety CFS is defined as a ratio of expected capacity to expected demand. Often the expected values are considered to be mean values $\overline{C}$ and $\overline{D}$ (Figure C3II.1(a)) which are unique for given distributions. Thus we have:

$$F = \frac{\hat{C}}{\hat{D}}, \quad SM = C - D, \quad \text{and} \quad CFS = \frac{\overline{C}}{\overline{D}} \tag{C3II.1}$$

When the safety margin is less than zero, failure can be expected. This is applicable to the shaded area of the probability density function for the safety margin SM shown in Figure C3II.1(b).

C3II.1.2 Defining probability of failure and reliability

The area under the probability density function between given limits represents the cumulative density function. The proportion of the total area under the curve to the left of a given value represents the probability that the random variable will have a value less than or equal to that value. Therefore, the cumulative density function has values between 0 and 1. Note that it is usual to take the total area under the curve as unity. Therefore the area under the curve between two ordinates directly gives the proportion of the total area.

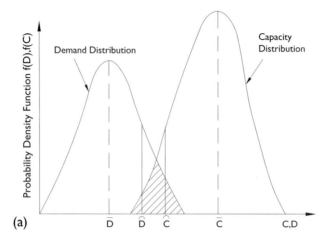

(a)

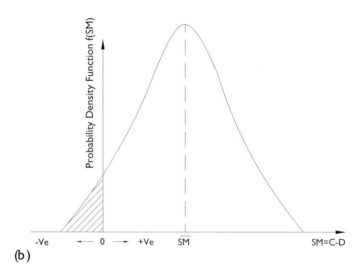

(b)

Figure C3II.1 (a) Distribution of capacity *C* and demand *D*, both considered as random variables. (b) Distribution of safety margin *SM* considered as a random variable.

The probability of failure P_f is denoted as follows as the probability that $(C-D)$ is less than or equal to zero:

$$p_F = P[(C - D) \leq 0] = P(SM \leq 0) \tag{C3II.2}$$

It is axiomatic that the probability of an outcome ranges between zero and unity, i.e.,

$$0 \le p_F \le 1 \tag{C3II.3}$$

Therefore the reliability R is given by:

$$R = 1 - p_F \tag{C3II.4}$$

C3II.1.3   Probability of failure with normal distribution

In accordance with our assumption that both the capacity and demand have a normal distribution, their probability density functions are expressed in terms of their means $(\bar{C}, \bar{D})$ and standard deviations (S_C, S_D) as follows:

$$f_C(C) = \frac{1}{S_C \sqrt{2\pi}} \exp\left\{ -\frac{1}{2}\left(\frac{C - \bar{C}}{S_C} \right)^2 \right\} \tag{C3II.5}$$

$$f_D(D) = \frac{1}{S_D \sqrt{2\pi}} \exp\left\{ -\frac{1}{2}\left(\frac{D - \bar{D}}{S_D} \right)^2 \right\} \tag{C3II.6}$$

It is known mathematically that the difference between variables which have a normal distribution is also normally distributed. Therefore, the probability density function of the safety margin has the same form as above. The mean and standard deviation of the safety margin are:

$$\overline{SM} = \bar{C} - \bar{D} \quad \text{and} \quad S_{SM} = \sqrt{S_C^{\,2} + S_D^{\,2}} \tag{C3II.7}$$

Therefore, the probability density function for SM is

$$f_{SM}(SM) = \frac{1}{S_{SM} \sqrt{2\pi}} \exp\left\{ -\frac{1}{2}\left(\frac{SM - \overline{SM}}{S_{SM}} \right)^2 \right\} \tag{C3II.8}$$

In order to calculate the probability of failure we need the cumulative probability function of the standard normal distribution associated with $SM \le 0$. Tables are widely available from which the cumulative probability function for the standard normal variate can be read for given limits. The probability of failure may be expressed in the following form:

$$p_F = \frac{1}{2} - \psi\left(\frac{\bar{C} - \bar{D}}{\sqrt{S_C^{\,2} + S_D^{\,2}}} \right) \tag{C3II.9}$$

where ψ is read from tables for the particular value in brackets and gives the area under the PDF or frequency curve between the line of symmetry and any other ordinate ($SM = 0$ in this case). This equation may also be written in terms of the central factor of safety CFS as follows:

$$P_F = \frac{1}{2} - \psi \left[\frac{CFS - 1}{\sqrt{(CFS)^2\, V_C^2 + V_D^2}} \right] \tag{C3II.10}$$

The use of these equations for determining the value of p_F in slope stability problems is quite straightforward and many examples have been solved by Harr (1977).

It may be of interest to determine the probability that the capacity C is less than a certain level of demand D_1. This probability is the product of two quantities i.e., (1) the probability that the level of demand is D_1 and (2) the probability that the failure occurs at level of demand D_1. After integrating to account for all possible values of demand the following is obtained (Harr, 1977):

$$p_F = \int_{-\infty}^{\infty} \left[\int_{-\infty}^{D} f_C(C)\,dc \right] f_D(D)\, dD \quad \text{or} \tag{C3II.11}$$

$$p_F = \int_{-\infty}^{\infty} F_C(D)\, f_D(D)\, dD \tag{C3II.12}$$

in which $F_C(\bullet)$ is the cumulative distribution function of capacity C.

C3II.1.4   Probability of failure with lognormal distribution

Probability distribution functions other than normal may be used. The lognormal distribution is found to be particularly useful since negative values of the variable are not possible (such negative values may be unacceptable in some situations). Such a distribution is obtained by substituting in the normal distribution for variable x another variable y such that $x = \ln(y)$.

Suppose both capacity and demand are lognormal variates; it can be shown that the probability of failure is given by:

$$p_F = \frac{1}{2} - \psi \left[\frac{\ln\left\{ \left(\frac{\bar{C}}{\bar{D}}\right) \sqrt{1 + \frac{V_D^2}{V_C^2}} \right\}}{\sqrt{\ln\, (1 + V_D^2)\,(1 + V_C^2)}} \right] \tag{C3II.13}$$

Simplification of (C3II.13) results when the co-efficient of variation is less than or equal to 30%, and the following expression gives a close approximation to p_F (Harr, 1977):

$$p_F = \frac{1}{2} - \psi \left[\frac{\ln\left(\frac{\bar{C}}{\bar{D}}\right) - \frac{1}{2}(V_C^2 - V_D^2)}{\sqrt{V_C^2 + V_D^2}} \right] \tag{C3II.14}$$

C3II.1.5 Safety margin required for given reliability

It may be desired to have a safety margin which is associated with a given probability of failure p_F so that reliability $(1 - p_F)$ is indicated. Then we have from equation (C3II.9) the following expressions for the capacity and the safety margin:

$$\bar{C} \geq \bar{D} + \psi^{-1} \left(\frac{1}{2} - p_F \right) \sqrt{S_C^2 + S_D^2}$$

$$\overline{SM} \geq \psi^{-1} \left(\frac{1}{2} - p_F \right) \sqrt{S_C^2 + S_D^2} \tag{C3II.15}$$

or,

$$\overline{SM} \geq \psi^{-1} \left(\frac{1}{2} - p_F \right) S_{SM} \tag{C3II.16}$$

Here ψ^{-1} function is obtained from the same tables from which ψ is obtained. The last equation for safety margin states that the mean value of the safety margin is ψ^{-1} times standard deviations of the safety margin above zero.

It is also useful to consider the theorem called the Chebyshev inequality. If x is a random variable with expectation $\bar{x}$ and a finite standard deviation S_x, then the Chebyshev inequality is:

$$P[(\bar{x} - hS_x) \leq x \leq (\bar{x} + hS_x)] \geq 1 - \frac{1}{h^2} \tag{C3II.17}$$

or,

$$P([x - \bar{x}] > hS_x) \leq \frac{1}{h^2} \tag{C3II.18}$$

Thus, accordingly to the Chebyshev inequality, the probability that the random variable x is outside the interval $\bar{x} - hS_x$ to $\bar{x} + hS_x$ is not greater than $(1/h^2)$ and the reliability is $(1 - 1/h^2)$.

These inequalities may be used to determine a factor of safety with a specified reliability. Suppose it is required to calculate the value F_1 of the factor of safety which has a reliability R_1 per cent when the expectation of the factor of safety is $\bar{F}$ and the standard deviation is S_f. The expectation could be the conventional value of the factor of safety say from limit equilibrium analysis. Now equating $(1 - 1/h^2)$ to $(R_1 / 100)$ we get the value of h. The required minimum factor of safety which gives reliability R_1 is given by:

$$F_1 = \bar{F} + h S_f \tag{C3II.19}$$

Once the value of factor of safety F_1 is known, the required height and inclination of the slope can be decided upon by conventional procedures.

APPENDIX III TO CHAPTER 3

Table C3III.1 Table of Standard Normal Probability $\Phi(x) = \frac{1}{\sqrt{2\pi}} \int_{-\infty}^{x} \exp\left(-\frac{1}{2}\xi^2\right)d\xi$. With permission, see page 713, No 11.

x	$\Phi(x)$	x	$\Phi(x)$	x	$\Phi(x)$
0.0	0.500000	0.50	0.691463	1.00	0.841345
0.01	0.503989	0.51	0.694975	1.01	0.843752
0.02	0.507978	0.52	0.698468	1.02	0.846136
0.03	0.511966	0.53	0.701944	1.03	0.848495
0.04	0.515954	0.54	0.705401	1.04	0.850830
0.05	0.519939	0.55	0.708840	1.05	0.853141
0.06	0.523922	0.56	0.712260	1.06	0.855428
0.07	0.527904	0.57	0.715661	1.07	0.857690
0.08	0.531882	0.58	0.719043	1.08	0.859929
0.09	0.535857	0.59	0.722405	1.09	0.862143
0.10	0.539828	0.60	0.725747	1.10	0.864334
0.11	0.543796	0.61	0.729069	1.11	0.866500
0.12	0.547759	0.62	0.732371	1.12	0.868643
0.13	0.551717	0.63	0.735653	1.13	0.870762
0.14	0.555671	0.64	0.738914	1.14	0.872857
0.15	0.559618	0.65	0.742154	1.15	0.874928
0.16	0.563560	0.66	0.745374	1.16	0.876976
0.17	0.567494	0.67	0.748572	1.17	0.878999
0.18	0.571423	0.68	0.751748	1.18	0.881000
0.19	0.575345	0.69	0.754903	1.19	0.882977
0.20	0.579260	0.70	0.758036	1.20	0.884930
0.21	0.583166	0.71	0.761148	1.21	0.886860
0.22	0.587064	0.72	0.764238	1.22	0.888767
0.23	0.590954	0.73	0.767305	1.23	0.890651
0.24	0.594835	0.74	0.770350	1.24	0.892512
0.25	0.598706	0.75	0.773373	1.25	0.894350
0.26	0.602568	0.76	0.776373	1.26	0.896165
0.27	0.606420	0.77	0.779350	1.27	0.897958
0.28	0.610262	0.78	0.782305	1.28	0.899727
0.29	0.614092	0.79	0.785236	1.29	0.901475
0.30	0.617912	0.80	0.788145	1.30	0.903199
0.31	0.621720	0.81	0.791030	1.31	0.904902
0.32	0.625517	0.82	0.793892	1.32	0.906583
0.33	0.629301	0.83	0.796731	1.33	0.908241
0.34	0.633072	0.84	0.799546	1.34	0.909877
0.35	0.636831	0.85	0.802337	1.35	0.911492
0.36	0.640576	0.86	0.805105	1.36	0.913085
0.37	0.644309	0.87	0.807850	1.37	0.914656
0.38	0.648027	0.88	0.810570	1.38	0.916207
0.39	0.651732	0.89	0.813267	1.39	0.917735
0.40	0.655422	0.90	0.815940	1.40	0.919243
0.41	0.659097	0.91	0.818589	1.41	0.920730
0.42	0.662757	0.92	0.821214	1.42	0.922196

(Continued)

Table C3III.1 (Continued).

x	Φ(x)	x	Φ(x)	x	Φ(x)
0.43	0.666402	0.93	0.823815	1.43	0.923641
0.44	0.670032	0.94	0.826391	1.44	0.925066
0.45	0.673645	0.95	0.828944	1.45	0.926471
0.46	0.677242	0.96	0.831473	1.46	0.927855
0.47	0.680823	0.97	0.833977	1.47	0.929219
0.48	0.684387	0.98	0.836457	1.48	0.930563
0.49	0.687933	0.99	0.838913	1.49	0.931888
1.50	0.933193	2.00	0.977250	2.50	0.993790
1.51	0.934478	2.01	0.977784	2.51	0.993963
1.52	0.935744	2.02	0.978308	2.52	0.994132
1.53	0.936992	2.03	0.978822	2.53	0.994297
1.54	0.938220	2.04	0.979325	2.54	0.994457
1.55	0.939429	2.05	0.979818	2.55	0.994614
1.56	0.940620	2.06	0.980301	2.56	0.994766
1.57	0.941792	2.07	0.980774	2.57	0.994915
1.58	0.942947	2.08	0.981237	2.58	0.995060
1.59	0.944083	2.09	0.981691	2.59	0.995201
1.60	0.945201	2.10	0.982136	2.60	0.995339
1.61	0.946301	2.11	0.982571	2.61	0.995473
1.62	0.947384	2.12	0.982997	2.62	0.995604
1.63	0.948449	2.13	0.983414	2.63	0.995731
1.64	0.949497	2.14	0.983823	2.64	0.995855
1.65	0.950529	2.15	0.984223	2.65	0.995975
1.66	0.951543	2.16	0.984614	2.66	0.996093
1.67	0.952540	2.17	0.984997	2.67	0.996207
1.68	0.953521	2.18	0.985371	2.68	0.996319
1.69	0.954486	2.19	0.985738	2.69	0.996427
1.70	0.955435	2.20	0.986097	2.70	0.996533
1.71	0.956367	2.21	0.986447	2.71	0.996636
1.72	0.957284	2.22	0.986791	2.72	0.996736
1.73	0.958185	2.23	0.987126	2.73	0.996833
1.74	0.959071	2.24	0.987455	2.74	0.996928
1.75	0.959941	2.25	0.987776	2.75	0.997020
1.76	0.960796	2.26	0.988089	2.76	0.997110
1.77	0.961636	2.27	0.988396	2.77	0.997197
1.78	0.962462	2.28	0.988696	2.78	0.997282
1.79	0.963273	2.29	0.988989	2.79	0.997365
1.80	0.964070	2.30	0.989276	2.80	0.997445
1.81	0.964852	2.31	0.989556	2.81	0.997523
1.82	0.965621	2.32	0.989830	2.82	0.997599
1.83	0.966375	2.33	0.990097	2.83	0.997673
1.84	0.967116	2.34	0.990358	2.84	0.997744
1.85	0.967843	2.35	0.990613	2.85	0.997814
1.86	0.968557	2.26	0.990863	2.86	0.997882
1.87	0.969258	2.37	0.991106	2.87	0.997948
1.88	0.969946	2.38	0.991344	2.88	0.998012

(Continued)

Table C3III.1 (Continued).

x	Φ(x)	x	Φ(x)	x	Φ(x)
1.89	0.970621	2.39	0.991576	2.89	0.998074
1.90	0.971284	2.40	0.991802	2.90	0.998134
1.91	0.971933	2.41	0.992024	2.91	0.998193
1.92	0.972571	2.42	0.992240	2.92	0.998250
1.93	0.973197	2.43	0.992451	2.93	0.998305
1.94	0.973810	2.44	0.992656	2.94	0.998359
1.95	0.974412	2.45	0.992857	2.95	0.998411
1.96	0.975002	2.46	0.993053	2.96	0.998462
1.97	0.975581	2.47	0.993244	2.97	0.998511
1.98	0.976148	2.48	0.993431	2.98	0.998559
1.99	0.976705	2.49	0.993613	2.99	0.998605
3.00	0.998650	3.50	0.999767	4.00	0.316712E-04
3.01	0.998694	3.51	0.999776	4.05	0.256088E-04
3.02	0.998736	3.52	0.999784	4.10	0.206575E-04
3.03	0.998777	3.53	0.999792	4.15	0.166238E-04
3.04	0.998817	3.54	0.999800	4.20	0.133458E-04
3.05	0.998856	3.55	0.999807	4.25	0.106885E-04
3.06	0.998893	3.56	0.999815	4.30	0.853906E-05
3.07	0.998930	3.57	0.999821	4.35	0.680688E-05
3.08	0.998965	3.58	0.999828	4.40	0.541254E-05
3.09	0.998999	3.59	0.999835	4.45	0.429351E-05
3.10	0.999032	3.60	0.999841	4.50	0.339767E-05
3.11	0.999065	3.61	0.999847	4.55	0.268230E-05
3.12	0.999096	3.62	0.999853	4.60	0.211245E-05
3.13	0.999126	3.63	0.999858	4.65	0.165968E-05
3.14	0.999155	3.64	0.999864	4.70	0.130081E-05
3.15	0.999184	3.65	0.999869	4.75	0.101708E-05
3.16	0.999211	3.66	0.999874	4.80	0.793328E-06
3.17	0.999238	3.67	0.999879	4.85	0.617307E-06
3.18	0.999264	3.68	0.999883	4.90	0.479183E-06
3.19	0.999289	3.69	0.999888	4.95	0.371067E-06
3.20	0.999313	3.70	0.999892	5.00	0.286652E-06
3.21	0.999336	3.71	0.999896	5.10	0.169827E-06
3.22	0.999359	3.72	0.999900	5.20	0.996443E-07
3.23	0.999381	3.73	0.999904	5.30	0.579013E-07
3.24	0.999402	3.74	0.999908	5.40	0.333204E-07
3.25	0.999423	3.75	0.999912	5.50	0.189896E-07
3.26	0.999443	3.76	0.999915	5.60	0.107176E-07
3.27	0.999462	3.77	0.999918	5.70	0.599037E-08
3.28	0.999481	3.78	0.999922	5.80	0.331575E-08
3.29	0.999499	3.79	0.999925	5.90	0.181751E-08
3.30	0.999516	3.80	0.999928	6.00	0.986588E-09
3.31	0.999533	3.81	0.999931	6.10	0.530343E-09
3.32	0.999550	3.82	0.999933	6.20	0.282316E-06
3.33	0.999566	3.83	0.999936	6.30	0.148823E-09
3.34	0.999581	3.84	0.999938	6.40	0.77688 E-10

(Continued)

Table C3!!!.1 (Continued).

x	$\Phi(x)$	x	$\Phi(x)$	x	$\Phi(x)$
3.35	0.999596	3.85	0.999941	6.50	0.40160 E-10
3.36	0.999610	3.86	0.999943	6.66	0.20558 E-10
3.37	0.999624	3.87	0.999946	6.70	0.10421 E-10
3.38	0.999637	3.88	0.999948	6.80	0.5231 E-11
3.39	0.999650	3.89	0.999950	6.90	0.260 E-11
3.40	0.999663	3.90	0.999952	7.00	0.128 E-11
3.41	0.999675	3.91	0.999954	7.10	0.624 E-12
3.42	0.999687	3.92	0.999956	7.20	0.301 E-12
3.43	0.999698	3.93	0.999958	7.30	0.144 E-12
3.44	0.999709	3.94	0.999959	7.40	0.68 E-13
3.45	0.999720	3.95	0.999961	7.50	0.32 E-13
3.46	0.999730	3.96	0.999963	7.60	0.15 E-13
3.47	0.999740	3.97	0.999964	7.70	0.70 E-14
3.48	0.999749	3.98	0.999966	7.80	0.30 E-14
3.49	0.999758	3.99	0.999967	7.90	0.15 E-14

(reproduced from the book "Probability Concepts In Engineering Planning And Design" Vol. 1, by Alfred H.S. Ang and Wilson H. Tang (1975), pp. 380–382.)

Chapter 4

Limit equilibrium methods I – planar failure surfaces

4.1 INTRODUCTION TO LIMIT EQUILIBRIUM METHODS

4.1.1 Methods considered in chapters 4 and 5

It is useful to distinguish between two classes of conventional limit equilibrium methods on the basis of the shape of potential slip surfaces: (1) Methods in which the surface is assumed to consist of one or more plane segments, such as considered in this chapter and, (2) methods in which the slip surface may be of curved, composite or arbitrary shape, such as considered in the next chapter.

Planar failure surfaces have special relevance to stability problems concerning hard rock slopes in which failures often occur along discontinuities. Failures along curved slip surfaces are common in most slopes of cohesive soil. Such failures may also occur in some soft rocks (Hoek and Bray, 1974, 1977). Composite failure surfaces often occur in non-homogeneous slopes consisting of different types of soil or rock or both.

The reader will find that much of the material covered in chapter 4 is useful mainly in connection with rock slopes and similarly most of the material in chapter 5 is useful for slopes of cohesive soil. Nevertheless there are important sections in both chapters which are equally relevant to both soil and rock slopes.

In each of chapters 4 and 5 attention is primarily directed towards problems which are two-dimensional in character. Idealisation of real problems of three-dimensional nature is essential if two-dimensional methods are to be used. In order that conventional methods are used successfully, experience is required in idealisation of real problems. In recent years there has been a growing realisation of the need for three-dimensional analyses. Several useful approaches have in fact been proposed to tackle specific types of three-dimensional problems. These approaches are briefly discussed towards the ends of chapters 4 and 5.

Recommendations concerning the choice of a method of analysis for different situations are given in chapter 5. Comparative advantages of 'total stress' and 'effective stress' methods of analysis are also discussed in chapter 5.

4.1.2 Scope of limit equilibrium studies

The aim of limit equilibrium studies is to analyse the stability of any mass of soil or rock assuming incipient failure along a potential slip surface. This approach often enables the solution of many problems by simple statics provided some simplifying assumptions are made. In general, a failure surface of simple shape is assumed and the material above this surface is considered to be a 'free body'. The disturbing and resisting forces are estimated enabling the formulation of equations concerning force equilibrium or moment equilibrium (or both) of the potential sliding mass. The solution of these equations provides quantitative information concerning the stability of a slope. However, this information is relevant only to the assumed slip surface and it is, therefore, customary to repeat the calculations for a number of trial slip surfaces to find the critical (potential) slip surface. Even when there is a well-defined discontinuity, surface of weakness or old slip surface, along which part of the potential slip surface may be located, trials are still necessary because the complete potential slip surface is rarely known in advance. However, the number of trials is considerably reduced when geological discontinuities and surfaces of weakness have been identified. After a number of trials have been performed, it is possible to locate the most dangerous position for the potential slip surface. This surface is one which gives the minimum factor of safety for the slope in conventional terms, and is theoretically the critical slip surface. If failure actually occurs, the actual slip surface may differ considerably from the theoretical 'critical' surface, depending on how accurately the real slope problem has been idealised and on the assumptions that have been made in the analytical procedures. For homogeneous slopes without discontinuities of any kind, it is usual to assume the shape of the slip surface before trials are conducted, e.g., circular, log-spiral etc. (See chapter 5). A procedure based on variational calculus has been used for the determination of the critical slip surface in a homogeneous slope without discontinuities and in this approach no prior assumption is necessary with regard to the shape of the slip surface. This approach (Revilla and Castillo, 1977) is briefly discussed towards the end of chapter 5. Over the last three decades, approaches based on variational calculus have been developed further. Such solutions are valuable contributions to analytical soil mechanics although they are not used widely in practice.

In this connection it is appropriate to mention that sometimes possible shapes of slip surfaces have been interpreted on the basis of theoretical inclination of failure plane at a point relative to principal stress direction determined from stress analysis (Brown and King, 1966, Resendiz, 1974, see chapter 6). However such procedures have not been adopted in practice.

Often the problem of slope stability is statically indeterminate, the number of unknowns being greater than the number of available equations. This is almost always the case for continuously curved slip surfaces which are considered in chapter 5. However, the problem of static indeterminacy may arise even when the failure surface is composed of several plane segments. One of the main difficulties concerns the magnitude, position and direction of frictional forces acting along the slip surface. Suitable assumptions are made in almost all the methods to overcome this difficulty. (Other problems which arise in the popular method of slices are discussed in chapter 5). In the simpler methods, the assumptions lead to somewhat inaccurate results. In the so-called 'rigorous' methods, the assumptions are more refined and greater confidence can be placed on the results under a variety of conditions. Using a single method, different assumptions may be made to furnish lower and upper 'bounds' to the factor of safety. Such bounds can be useful in practice and may help towards decisions concerning the effects of construction or slope alteration on the stability.

Conceptually a major shortcoming of limit-equilibrium methods is that incipient failure is assumed which is justified only for a real factor of safety of one. Yet these methods are most frequently, if not always, used in problems in which the calculated factor of safety is greater than one. Moreover, a calculated factor of safety equal to one will most often not correspond to a state of incipient failure for the real slope. The real factor of safety is strongly influenced by many variables associated with geological details, material parameters, pore water pressures and stress-deformation characteristics of the mass of soil or rock. It may also be influenced by factors such as initial stresses, stress and strain distribution, discontinuities, stress level and, of course, progressive failure. On the other hand, the calculated factor of safety is based on a number of simplifying assumptions and it is often difficult to quantify the influence of these assumptions on the calculations. It is, therefore often desirable to perform sensitivity analyses in which the influence of changes in significant variables on the factor of safety is studied. In fact, such studies are frequently made in practice particularly when precise data are not available. Such studies would also be useful when the nature and extent of any progressive cannot be clearly identified. The concept of a resistance envelope is also useful in this regard and this is explained in sub-section 5.1.6.

4.1.3 The concept of slip surfaces

Limit equilibrium methods are generally not concerned with stress distribution at every point above or below the assumed slip surface nor do they seek to satisfy the equations of stress equilibrium at every point within the potential failure mass. The assumption of a discontinuity in the form of a slip surface is an important one for these methods. Such a surface may be considered as a hypothetical one separating two rigid bodies. Observations on slides have confirmed the existence of slip surfaces in reality. However, whereas limit equilibrium methods are concerned with the main bounding surface of failure, there may be other slip surfaces within a potential failure mass. It is thus possible that shearing resistance is mobilised along these other surfaces as well as the main slip surface. Therefore it is preferable to define the customary slip surface as the one which describes the outer boundary to which instability extends. In respect of clay slopes, Janbu (1977) referred to a case history in which the resistance envelope was close to the strength envelope over a wide range of average normal stress indicating near failure conditions in a broad zone of the slope. (For explanation of resistance envelope concept, see section 5.1.)

A limit equilibrium approach is not a precise one in the mathematical sense and is different from approaches based on the theory of plasticity which are briefly discussed in chapter 8. Yet the results obtained by limit equilibrium and plasticity analyses show remarkably close agreement. A number of such comparisons have been made by Chen (1975) who used the limit analysis technique of plasticity. Reference to these comparisons for isotropic soils is made in chapter 8 and for anisotropic soils in the Appendix to chapter 8. Because of their basic simplicity and versatility in handling non-homogeneous and non-uniform slopes, limit equilibrium methods continue to be popular. As will be shown in chapter 5, the methods are adaptable for considerations of progressive failure. Plasticity solutions also have a useful role to play but plasticity theory may not be applicable to all types of soil and its value for rock slopes is questionable.

Attention requires to be given to an understanding of the formation or propagation of slip surfaces. It is obvious that failure must be preceded by the formation of one or more discontinuities resulting perhaps from concentrated strains and large deformations. Research workers are becoming increasingly interested in aspects of slope studies concerned with propagation of failure. Because of the scale effect, it has been found difficult to study the development of failure surfaces in centrifuge model tests, which have become popular in many research centres around the world. Over the last few decades centrifuge modeling has been developed further and many limitations have been overcome. It has been a useful research tool for the study of earthquake effects on slopes and the behavior of soils under offshore conditions. The development of large strains at increasing loads can be studied adequately by subjecting small models of slopes to high centrifugal forces to simulate slopes of different heights. However, the development of complete failure presents difficulties (e.g., see Frydman and Beasley, 1976) and the correspondence between model and prototype is no longer valid when the existence of a shear band or discontinuity is considered. This has been discussed by Palmer and Rice (1973) who proposed an energy approach based on fracture mechanics concepts to study the growth of shear bands, i.e., planar slip surfaces. This approach is discussed in chapter 8 and suggestions are made for its further development to include arbitrary variation of shear resistance along a shear band and failure surfaces of arbitrary inclinations. Little progress has so far been made concerning a study of the manner in which curved slip surfaces are propagated in slopes. The value of such theoretical studies would be greatly enhanced by full-scale field studies in which the effects of disturbance (e.g., surcharging, excavation, increase of pore pressure etc.) could be studied. The role of slope instrumentation (e.g., to measure surface and subsurface displacements and pore water pressures) is of paramount importance in this regard. [Reference is made in chapter 8 (see section 8.12) to one case history where the performance of an excavated slope was monitored (Burland, 1973; Burland et al., 1977) and the propagation of a slip surface inferred from precision measurements.] For a discussion of the role and limitations of centrifuge model tests the reader may also refer to Palmer (1973a, pp. 259–62, 290–96, 310).

4.1.4 Defining factor of safety as per concept of limit equilibrium

There are many different ways in which a 'factor of safety' may be defined in conventional limit equilibrium methods. It is thus necessary to explore different meanings of this term since a definition adopted in the context of a proposed method of analysis may be quite different from that for another method. Often there is a tendency to assume a uniform meaning for the term and this can lead to incorrect interpretation of results from different methods. Particular care is necessary when comparisons between different approaches are made.

Firstly let us consider the common definition of 'factor of safety' as the ratio of available unit shear strength s to required unit shear strength s_m, also referred to as the 'mobilised shear strength'. The required shear strength is of course equal to the actual in-situ shear stress which is generally estimated from calculations. Available shear strength depends on the real properties of the soil which are measured from laboratory or field tests. In the case of embankments or earth dams or other man-made structures it is to some extent possible to vary or select the available shear strength but this is not possible in the case of natural soils or rock deposits. Assume that the available shear strength is such that the factor of safety is F. Using Coulomb's equation for shear strength in terms of effective stress, we have the following ratio in terms of a particular effective normal stress σ':

$$F = \frac{s}{s_m} = \frac{c + \sigma' \tan \phi}{c_m + \sigma' \tan \phi_m} \tag{4.1}$$

in which c and ϕ are available shear strength parameters and, c_m and ϕ_m are required or mobilised shear strength parameters. Rearranging Equation (4.1) we have:

$$\frac{c}{F} + \sigma' \frac{\tan \phi}{F} = c_m + \sigma' \tan \phi_m \tag{4.2}$$

We may define $F = c/c_m = \tan\phi/\tan\phi_m$. Such an assumption implies that the factor of safety with respect to the cohesion parameter is the same as that with respect to the friction parameter. However, this is just one alternative.

It is often desirable to have different factors of safety with respect to cohesion and friction components of shear strength. There are several reasons for this. It is usually easier to measure or infer ϕ values with greater confidence than c values (considering effective stress parameters). In many cases, less reliance can be placed on c values because of decrease of the effective cohesion parameter with time due to various processes such as softening mentioned in chapter 2. It has often been suggested that there is a far greater variability in the cohesion parameter than in the friction parameter. For example the coefficient of variation of the friction angle for a cohesionless material may be as low as 6% whereas the coefficient of variation of undrained cohesion or undrained shear strength may be as high as 40% according to values presented by Harr (1977). In rock masses also there is much greater uncertainty with respect to cohesion parameter in comparison to the friction parameter. There are many pertinent references in relation to relative magnitudes of factor of safety with respect to friction and cohesion, e.g., Morgenstern (1968), Rocha (1964), Londe (1973), Hoek and Londe (1974) and Rocha (1974).

Let the factor of safety with respect to cohesion be F_c and that with respect to friction be F_ϕ. The overall of factor of safety is then given as follows:

$$F = \frac{c + \sigma' \tan \phi}{c/F_c + \sigma' \tan \phi/F_\phi} \tag{4.3}$$

For a given value of effective normal stress, a number of variations of F_c and F_ϕ can be found which give the same overall F (and $F_c = F_\phi = F$ is only one such combination). If $F_\phi = 1$, indicating that friction is fully mobilised, the factor of safety with respect to cohesion F_c has a special meaning. This is because the cohesion required for stability is directly proportional to the height of a simple homogeneous slope of given geometry and inclination. Therefore Taylor (1937, 1948) used the term 'factor of safety with respect to height' F_H for F based on mobilised cohesion. Thus with friction fully mobilised, $F_c = F_H$ and we have:

$$F_H = \frac{c}{c_m}, \quad s_m = \frac{c}{F_H} + \sigma' \tan \phi \tag{4.4}$$

F_H gives an indication of the ratio between the critical height and actual height of a slope in which friction is always fully mobilised. Selection of F_c different from F_ϕ is justified in situations when greater reliance can be placed on the available value of one parameter relative to another or when one parameter is likely to suffer some reduction with time and the other remains unaltered. In order to investigate the effects of variation of one or other parameter on the overall factor of safety, it is often convenient to use the concept of a resistance envelope. This concept is discussed in section 5.1.6.

Let us now consider another definition of factor of safety which is common in problems involving planar failure surfaces. In many of these methods F is defined as the ratio of total resisting to total disturbing forces. F may also be defined as the ratio of total resisting to total disturbing moments as in the case of circular slip surfaces. It should be noted that the values of F obtained on this basis are, in general, not identical with values obtained on the basis of definition as ratio of available to mobilised unit shear strength. In the former case, we can avoid defining factor of safety at a point.

In almost all conventional limit equilibrium methods, the factor of safety is considered as, or implied to be, a constant all along the failure surface. This is a very important simplifying assumption even for homogeneous isotropic slopes noting that the stress distribution along a potential failure surface, whether calculated by a stress analysis or limit equilibrium technique, is always non-uniform. A local factor of safety may be defined at each point along the surface as the ratio of shear strength to shear stress assuming both normal and shear stresses on the surface are known. Such local factors of safety quite often show a great deal of variation over the length of the slip surface. Further attention is given to this aspect in chapter 6.

Another possible way of defining a factor of safety against overall failure is to average local factors of safety (based on the ratio of local available shear strength and mobilised shear strength or shear stress) over a potential failure surface. Again such a procedure does not, in general, give the same value for the overall factor of safety as that based on the other definitions. (See chapters 6 and 7.) Averaging of local factors of safety is only possible if an approach based on stress analysis (chapter 6) is used either separately or in combination with a limit equilibrium method. For two-dimensional problems, a two-dimensional stress analysis would ordinarily suffice. However, where failures of a marked three-dimensional character are to be analysed, it would be necessary to conduct three-dimensional stress analyses using a versatile technique such as one based on the finite element method. Reference to the factor of safety in practice is made in chapter 5 (see section 5.14.5).

4.1.5 *Alternatives to conventional safety factor*

Adoption of some value for the conventional safety factor may have little meaning with respect to strains or deformations that can be tolerated within an embankment or slope. It is usually difficult to establish any realistic relationship between the factor of safety and actual performance, and incipient failure rarely corresponds to a calculated safety factor of one. The importance of strains and deformations in problems of geotechnical engineering (and especially in soil mechanics problems) has been recognised for a long time both at a fundamental and a practical level. Increasing recognition of the fundamental importance of strains is reflected in the work of Roscoe (1970). In the early stages of development of soil mechanics, few solutions for stresses and deformations were available. It is useful to recall that Bishop's (1952) relaxation solution for stresses due to an idealised embankment became possible due to the development of the finite-difference technique. Bishop's solution showed that significant variations from average stress could occur within an embankment and that a conventional limit equilibrium solution could not provide such vital information concerning the stress conditions within a slope.

During the last four decades, rapid advances have been made in the development of powerful numerical techniques, and high speed computing facilities have become available for applying these methods to geotechnical problems. For instance, the versatile finite element techniques can handle problems involving non-homogeneity, anisotropy, complex construction history, arbitrary boundary conditions as well as non-linear and stress-dependent material behaviour (e.g., see Zienkiewicz, 1971, Clough and Woodward, 1967). At the same time geotechnical engineers have developed confidence in the value of field measurements concerning stresses, strains, deformations and pore water pressures. Advances in instrumentation techniques have enhanced the reliability and effectiveness of performance monitoring systems. Performance observations are not merely a means for checking a design or for detecting early signs of failure. The value of such observations also lies in providing a basis for continuing improvement in analysis and design during construction and in the lifetime of a project or facility.

In view of these developments it may seem surprising that no widely accepted alternatives to the conventional safety factor have been established. It would appear desirable to base analysis and design on limiting strains and deformations within soil and rock masses. This could be done by specifying a number of criteria concerning localised deformations, strains etc. within embankments or cut slopes. An interesting discussion of criteria called 'satisfaction indices' can be found in the paper by De Mello (1977) concerning design decisions related to embankment dams.

Over the last few decades, there is an increasing trend to consider concepts of safety and reliability within a probabilistic framework as discussed in chapters 3 and 10.

4.1.6   Saturated and unsaturated soil slopes

4.1.6.1   Saturated soil slopes

Many slope stability situations concern saturated soil zones (region below the water table or phreatic surface), often with seepage occurring through these saturated zones. Consequently the shear strength equation for saturated soil is used for modeling the stability and for developing appropriate equations and procedures for analysis. The assumption of a fully saturated soil medium is justified when a potential slip surface is located almost entirely within the saturated zone. The factor of safety F decreases as the pore water pressure increases. Slope failure is associated with $F = 1$ corresponding to a critical value of the average pore water pressure along a potential slip surface. Thus it is important to determine the pore water pressures associated with seepage through slopes. The assumption of steady seepage is often justified for slope stability problems. For several practical situations, analytical (closed-form) or numerical solutions of seepage, modeled as a one-dimensional (1-D) or two-dimensional (2-D) process, are easy to develop. Geotechnical engineers find the use of flow-nets very rewarding even with the increasing availability of computer-based solutions. For complex situations involving non-homogeneity or anisotropy (with respect to permeability) or other factors, sophisticated numerical solutions may be required. Computer-based methods and software utilising such methods have become widely available. In particular, seepage solutions based on the finite-element method (FEM) have been in use for several decades.

In summary, there are two main requirements for analysis of slope stability in saturated slopes.

1 The shear strength equation for saturated soil must be used.
2 Distribution of positive pore water pressures must be determined corresponding to the situation of interest. In most cases, simple seepage solutions based on steady seepage assumption will be sufficient. In this chapter simplest cases of seepage are considered. Special cases such as submergence of a slope and sudden draw-down are also considered. Due to geological constraints, artesian pore water pressures may be relevant for some natural slopes. In those cases, it would be incorrect to estimate pore pressures on the basis of a seepage solution. Field evidence or measurement can be useful in such cases (see chapter 11). Where data from field measurements are available, analytical and numerical seepage solutions can also be validated.

4.1.6.2 Unsaturated soil slopes

Potential stability above the water table requires consideration of the characteristics of unsaturated soil. Modelling and analysis based on the assumption of saturated or dry soil can be very misleading. Thus it is necessary to use the shear strength equation for unsaturated soil in the stability model; otherwise shear strength and, therefore, the factor of safety will be underestimated. The first question to ask is the following: "For what situations is it necessary to consider slope stability above the water table?"

Generally, the need for considering stability above the water table arises for soil slopes of steep inclination which have large unsaturated zones. Such slopes, formed in residual soils, are encountered in many tropical countries. For example, many residual soil slopes in Hong Kong are steep and have deep water tables. Apart from natural slopes of unsaturated soil, there may be steep fill slopes and embankments which require consideration of their unsaturated soil characteristics.

The next question is the following: "Under what circumstances may slope failures occur in these unsaturated soil slopes?"

During dry weather, such a slope is stable because the factor of safety is well above 1 for any potential slip surface located in the unsaturated zone. This is due to the additional component of shear strength related to suction (negative pore water pressure). Following significant rainfall, as infiltration of water occurs through the unsaturated zone of a slope, the suctions are progressively eliminated. Consequently the shear strength is reduced, and a slope may fail if the reduction in suction reaches a critical value corresponding to $F = 1$. Modelling of rainfall infiltration through unsaturated soil requires consideration of transient or unsteady seepage as the conditions governing the flow of water will change progressively with time. For example, the permeability of unsaturated soil is related to the magnitude of suction which, in turn, changes with time as infiltration proceeds.

As regards the progressive decrease in suctions, some important points may be noted.

Firstly, the decrease of suction following rainfall infiltration is generally only partial and will depend on the intensity and duration of rainfall. Even with a significant rainstorm, complete elimination of suctions may not occur. (Except in that part of a slope where a temporary saturated band may develop or a part that may become flooded after a rainstorm. Such situations are more likely to occur in non-homogeneous slopes.)

Secondly, slope failures in unsaturated residual soil associated with rainfall infiltration are generally not associated with the development of saturated soil zones after rainfall. Following some significant landslides in Hong Kong, slide debris did not show evidence of saturated or seepage conditions (Lumb, 1975).

Some discussions associated with modelling of unsaturated soil behaviour refer to the concept of a 'wetting front' developing in a homogeneous slope as rainfall infiltration progresses. However, such a concept requires to be validated by field studies. Field validation is necessary for an understanding of the circumstances under which a wetting front may develop.

Thirdly, it has been noted that failures occur well after the end of the peak intensity period of a rainfall event (Lumb, 1975). Such a time lag can be understood in terms of the process of unsteady seepage which is further complicated by soil variability and geological complexity. In general, both the maximum intensity and the antecedent rainfall influence the likelihood of slope failure. Consideration of the magnitude of one day rainfall combined with the magnitude of preceding 15 days was suggested by Lumb (1975) for assessing rainfall thresholds for slope failures in Hong Kong.

The main requirements for analysis of slope stability in unsaturated soil are:

(1) The shear strength equation for unsaturated soil must be used. This means that the additional shear strength parameter representing the rate of increase of strength with suction must be determined.
(2) The distribution of suction (negative pore water pressure) within the unsaturated zone must be estimated. The suction values may be based on analysis or on values measured in the field. For preliminary studies,

   (a) the initial suction may be considered hydrostatic, and
   (b) for decreased suctions after a rainstorm, worst-case distribution may be assumed based on judgment. Alternatively, the simulation of transient suctions (change of suctions with time) may be based on one-dimensional infiltration analysis. The distribution of suctions along a potential slip surface would be obtained as a function of time. For simplified assessment, only the initial and worst-case distributions of suction along the potential slip surface may be estimated.

A more systematic or rigorous approach for step 2 above would require unsaturated seepage modelling combined with integrated seepage analysis for the saturated and unsaturated zones within a slope. Modelling requires the development of the governing equation for seepage in terms of the coefficient of permeability of unsaturated soil as a function of the saturated permeability and matric suction. Fredlund and Barbour (1992) computed the permeability functions for colluvium and decomposed granite in Hong Kong. As suction increases by two orders of magnitude from about 10 kPa to about 1000 kPa, the coefficient of permeability decreases by about 5 orders of magnitude from 10^{-6} m/sec to about 10^{-11} m/sec. Corresponding to steps 2(a) and 2(b) above, the estimation of initial and transient suctions involves the following:

> For 2(a): The initial suction at a point will depend not only on the location of a point above the water table but also on the conditions of recharge at the given location. Applying the average annual rainfall rate as a steady state flux or surface recharge, analysis may be carried out to determine the initial or ambient suctions. For Hong Kong, Fredlund and Barbour (1992) applied the flux as 2050 mm/year. From a review of literature, they reported that slopes of decomposed granites in Hong Kong are in a condition of recharge even in the dry season and that the simulated pore-water pressures correspond well with values measured in the field (suction head increasing in the range 0.1–0.3 meter per meter elevation above the water table).

> For 2(b): Distribution of suctions with time after the start of a rainstorm would require a transient analysis. In general, such an analysis would be an integrated or saturated-unsaturated seepage analyses. For example, Fredlund and Barbour (1992) carried out two sets of analyses for a steep cut slope in Hong Kong. The first set was for a very high intensity rainfall case (119 mm/hour) for two hours and the second set was for a low intensity rainfall case (variable rainfall over 5 days, the rate on each day in mm/hr being 1.04, 0.42, 7.7, 1.25 and 1.04). Fredlund and Barbour (1992) used the FEM method with appropriate boundary conditions for these integrated seepage analyses.

The distribution of suctions along a potential slip surface would be obtained as a function of time. It is also useful to note that commercial software for integrated (saturated-unsaturated) seepage analyses are now available.

(3) After the above two steps have been carried out, choice of a suitable limit equilibrium method may be made amongst those described in this and the next chapter. Of course, the potential failure mechanism and the shape of the potential slip surface would be taken into consideration in selecting the particular method of analysis. The factor safety at several discrete intervals of time after the start of a rainfall event may then be estimated. Alternatively, only the initial and worst-case values of the factor of safety may be estimated.

4.2   INFINITE SLOPES IN COHESIONLESS SOILS

4.2.1   Dry cohesionless soil

Consider a long natural or man-made slope formed of cohesionless material like sand of bulk unit weight γ. Such a slope will remain stable if it is flat enough in relation to its angle of shearing resistance ϕ. If the inclination β equals the angle of shearing resistance ϕ (When the sand is in a loose state, this angle is often referred to as the angle of repose.), the slope is at limit equilibrium and is said to have a factor of safety F equal to one, where F is defined as follows:

$$F = \frac{\tan \phi}{\tan \beta} \qquad (4.5)$$

When $\beta < \phi$, the slope is stable with factor of safety greater than one, and when $\beta > \phi$, the slope is unstable with a factor of safety less than one. In the latter case stability is restored only when β becomes equal to or less than ϕ.

The factor of safety F may also be defined by analysing an element of soil as shown in Figure 4.1 which is acted upon by the weight $W = \gamma bz$, and normal and tangential forces (a) on the sides of the element and (b) on the base of the element. For an 'infinite' slope (A very long slope is often referred to as an 'infinite' slope in geotechnical engineering literature.) with uniform inclination, the forces on the sides of the element exactly balance each other. Hence, equilibrium gives the following relationship between tangential force $T = \gamma bz \sin \beta$ and normal force $N = \gamma bz \cos \beta$ on the base of the slice:

$$T = N \tan \beta \qquad (4.6)$$

Dividing both sides by the length l of the base of the element and noting that $l = b \sec \beta$, and assuming unit length perpendicular to the plane of paper, the following relationship is obtained between shear stress τ and normal stress σ on the base of the element:

$$\tau = \sigma \tan \beta \qquad (4.7)$$

in which

$$\sigma = \gamma z \cos^2 \beta \quad \text{and} \quad \tau = \gamma z \sin \beta \cos \beta \qquad (4.8)$$

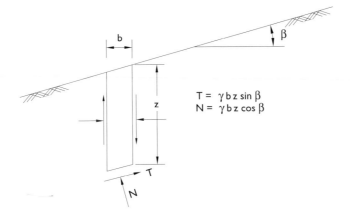

Figure 4.1 Element in a long cohesionless slope.

Here γ is the bulk unit weight for dry soil. However, the same equations are valid for wet soil, fully or partially saturated, provided γ denotes the corresponding bulk unit weight.

The full shear strength s on the base of the slice is given by

$$s = \sigma \tan \phi \tag{4.9}$$

Assuming that the factor of safety is F, the mobilised shear strength is s/F and is equal to the shear stress τ required for equilibrium given by Equation (4.7) and we have:

$$\tau = \frac{s}{F}, \quad \text{or,} \quad F = \frac{s}{\tau} = \frac{\tan \phi}{\tan \beta} \tag{4.10}$$

4.2.2 Submerged cohesionless soil

Consider a submerged slope of sand (Figure 4.2) so that the element of soil under consideration is at a depth z below the ground surface and the water table is h above the ground surface. Submergence reduces the unit weight to $\gamma' = \gamma_{sat} - \gamma_w$ (where γ_{sat} is the saturated unit weight and γ' is the submerged or buoyant unit weight) and the normal effective and shear stresses on the base of the slice are:

$$\sigma' = \gamma' z \cos^2 \beta$$
$$\tau = \gamma' z \sin \beta \cos \beta \tag{4.11}$$

Assuming a factor of safety F, the mobilised shear strength is

$$\frac{s}{F} = \sigma' \frac{\tan \phi}{F} = \gamma' z \cos^2 \beta \frac{\tan \phi}{F} \tag{4.12}$$

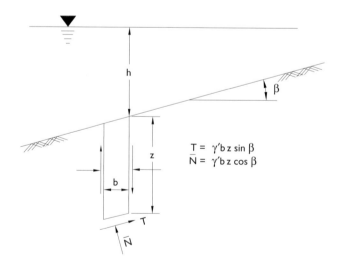

Figure 4.2 Element in a long submerged cohesionless slope.

Equating the mobilised shear strength to the shear stress, we have

$$F = \frac{\tan\phi}{\tan\beta} \qquad (4.13)$$

Therefore, the factor of safety is the same for a dry or submerged slope assuming that the value of the effective angle of friction ϕ remains unaltered.

4.2.3   Cohesionless soil with seepage parallel to slope

The most usual practical case concerns a slope in which seepage of water is occurring (Figure 4.3). Assuming that seepage is parallel to the ground surface and is occurring throughout the slope, it can be shown that the pore water pressure u on the base of a slice at depth z is given by

$$u = \gamma_w\, z\cos^2\beta \qquad (4.14)$$

The effective normal and shear stresses on the base of a slice are

$$\sigma' = \sigma - u = z\,(\gamma_{sat} - \gamma_w)\cos^2\beta = \gamma'z\cos^2\beta$$
$$\tau = \gamma_{sat}z\,\sin\beta\cos\beta \qquad (4.15)$$

Again, for the mobilised shear strength we have

$$\frac{s}{F} = \gamma'z\cos^2\beta\,\frac{\tan\phi}{F} \qquad (4.16)$$

Equating the shear stress to the mobilised shear strength

$$F = \frac{\gamma'}{\gamma_{sat}}\,\frac{\tan\phi}{\tan\beta} \qquad (4.17)$$

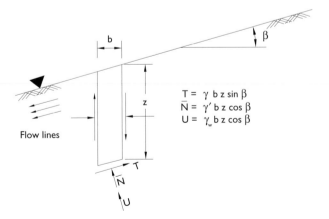

$$T = \gamma\,b\,z\,\sin\beta$$
$$\bar{N} = \gamma'\,b\,z\,\cos\beta$$
$$U = \gamma_w\,b\,z\,\cos\beta$$

Flow lines

Figure 4.3 Element in a long cohesionless slope with seepage parallel to ground surface.

Typically γ'/γ_{sat} may have a value of 1/2 and the factor of safety is reduced by this factor if seepage is occurring throughout the slope. In the case of a submerged infinite slope, no decrease of F occurs because the weight itself is decreased so that both shear stress and normal stress are reduced by the same factor. For a rigorous proof the reader may refer to Lambe and Whitman (1969).

It is also of interest to consider the situation when seepage is occurring within only part of a slope. Let the top seepage line be parallel to the surface of slope and at depth z_1 below it. The factor of safety above the top seepage line is given by $F = \tan \phi / \tan \beta$ as for a dry slope. Below the seepage line we have

$$\sigma' = \{\gamma_1 z_1 + \gamma'(z - z_1)\} \cos^2 \beta$$
$$\tau = \{\gamma_1 z_1 + \gamma_{sat}(z - z_1)\} \sin \beta \cos \beta \qquad (4.18)$$
$$F = \frac{\frac{z_1}{z-z_1}\gamma_1 + \gamma'}{\frac{z_1}{z-z_1}\gamma_1 + \gamma_{sat}} \frac{\tan \phi}{\tan \beta}$$

in which γ_1 and γ_{sat} are the bulk unit weights of soil above and below the top seepage line respectively. When z_1 approaches zero or z becomes very large, this equation approaches Equation (4.17).

4.2.4 Rapid drawdown of water level in a slope of cohesionless soil

'Rapid' drawdown condition is important for the stability analysis of slopes which are initially submerged. Consider the situation when external water level of a submerged slope falls or is lowered. If the rate of lowering is faster than the rate at which drainage can occur through the soil, the factor of safety, F, will decrease from its value during submergence. This is because the pore water pressures may continue to remain relatively high due to delay in drainage while the stabilizing effect of submergence has been removed as a consequence of drawdown of the external water level.

Most cohesionless soils have relatively high permeability. Therefore, drainage may occur even faster than the rate of drawdown. This would constitute a 'slow' rather than 'rapid' drawdown. Thus factor of safety may not decrease at all or not decrease significantly. However, it is useful to check the soil parameters and drainage conditions on a case by case basis. Seepage pore water pressure for drawdown conditions must be estimated. For example, a flow net with appropriate boundary conditions can be used to estimate drawdown pore pressures within a slope. Then the factor of safety can be calculated using the appropriate equation in terms of effective stress.

For an 'infinite slope', a very conservative estimate of the factor of safety after 'rapid' drawdown may be obtained on the assumption that the highest pore water pressures on the potential slip surface will correspond to the full seepage condition (section 4.2.3). Thus the value of F will be given by Equation (4.17). This value is approximately 50% lower than the value for dry or submerged cohesive soil. However, the value of the factor of safety will rise again after first falling immediately after rapid drawdown. In fact, after the pore water pressures have dissipated fully, the value of F will be the same as it was during submergence [Equation (4.13)].

Notes

Finite slope with partial submergence

During a 'slow' drawdown, one would expect the factor of safety to remain unchanged in an infinite slope of cohesionless soil. However, according to recent study based on the limit analysis method of plasticity (Michalowski, 2009), this is not correct for partially submerged, finite slopes of cohesionless soil. The factor of safety is a few percent smaller than that given by Equation (4.13). The critical failure mechanism was found to be associated with a slip surface of log spiral shape rather than one of planar shape parallel to the surface of the slope. On this basis, it was argued that failures of cohesionless slopes under partial submergence may not be just surficial maintenance problems. Instability may be deeper and more significant. More research backed by case studies will be needed to establish the validity of such claims.

On cohesive soil

The rapid drawdown condition is much more significant for slopes of cohesive soil. In particular, it can be a critical condition for the stability of the upstream face of any earth dam or earth-rockfill dam. It may also be important for checking the stability of natural slopes and existing landslides located on the rims of reservoirs such as those formed after the construction of earth or gravity dams. The reader may refer back to Figure 2.11 for a general representation of the changes in stability which occur during and after construction of an earth or earth-rock dam including reservoir filling and drawdown.

The simplified drawdown case of an infinite slope of cohesive soil is considered in some detail in section 4.3.2 below. The analysis requires consideration of soil characteristics in a more comprehensive way than in the case of cohesionless soil considered briefly above.

4.3   INFINITE SLOPES IN COHESIVE SOIL

4.3.1   Seepage through a slope – simple cases

Following a procedure similar to that adopted in the previous section and assuming the slope material to be cohesive (with shear strength given by the linear Mohr-Coulomb equation), it is easy to obtain equations for factors of safety for different slope conditions. Distinction should be made between total stress and effective stress parameters of shear strength, depending on the type of problem. Since long natural slopes are considered here, the discussion relates to natural, long-term stability. Thus drained, effective stress parameters of shear strength are implied. However, the equations could be used without much alteration for other conditions of interest. The general equation for mobilised shear strength may be written as follows:

$$\frac{s}{F} = \frac{(c' + \sigma'\tan\phi')}{F} \tag{4.19}$$

By equating this to the shear stress τ,

$$F = \frac{c' + \sigma' \tan \phi'}{\tau} \tag{4.19a}$$

(i) For the case of no seepage and no pore water pressure (neutral pressure)

$$\sigma' = \gamma z \cos^2 \beta \quad \text{and} \quad \tau = \gamma z \sin \beta \cos \beta \tag{4.8}$$

Thus, from Equation (4.19a)

$$F = \frac{c'}{\gamma z \sin \beta \cos \beta} + \frac{\tan \phi'}{\tan \beta} \tag{4.20}$$

(ii) When the slope is submerged, substituting σ' and τ from Equation (4.11),

$$F = \frac{c'}{\gamma' z \sin \beta \cos \beta} + \frac{\tan \phi'}{\tan \beta} \tag{4.21}$$

(iii) When seepage is occurring parallel to the slope with the top flow line at the surface, substituting σ' and τ from Equation (4.15),

$$F = \frac{c'}{\gamma_{sat} z \sin \beta \cos \beta} + \frac{\gamma'}{\gamma_{sat}} \frac{\tan \phi'}{\tan \beta} \tag{4.22}$$

(iv) Assuming that the top seepage line is at depth z_1 below the surface, substituting σ' and τ from Equation (4.18),

$$F = \frac{c'}{\{\gamma_1 z_1 + \gamma_{sat}(z - z_1)\} \sin \beta \cos \beta} + \frac{\frac{z_1}{z - z_1} \gamma_1 + \gamma'}{\frac{z_1}{z - z_1} \gamma_1 + \gamma_{sat}} \frac{\tan \phi'}{\tan \beta} \tag{4.23}$$

In a homogeneous layer of soil saturated above the top seepage line, $\gamma_1 = \gamma_{sat}$, leading to some simplification of the above equation.

Based on the above approach the critical depth $z = H_c$ of a layer of cohesive soil may be calculated by setting $F = 1$. For example with seepage occurring throughout the slope, the following is obtained from Equation (4.22):

$$(z)_{F=1} = H_c = \frac{c'}{\cos^2 \beta} \frac{1}{\gamma_{sat} \tan \beta - \gamma' \tan \phi'} \tag{4.24}$$

Similar equations for the critical depth of a layer of cohesive soil may be obtained for other conditions of seepage. Such equations are especially useful when a stratum of soil overlies a rock surface at shallow depth. As the value of effective cohesion c' increases, the maximum thickness of soil layer which is stable also increases. These equations are meaningful only for inclinations β above a certain value. For example, Equation (4.24) shows that any depth of soil is theoretically stable if $\gamma_{sat} \tan \beta > \gamma'$ $\tan \phi'$, however small the value of c'.

If the soil unit weight and shear strength parameters vary with depth, the factor of safety must be calculated at various depths and its minimum value found. In most situations the critical factor of safety will occur at a time when seepage is occurring throughout the slope. This may occur after heavy rainfall. In some slopes, there may be higher pore water pressures due to artesian conditions. In terms of arbitrary pore water pressure u, the factor of safety is easily shown to be:

$$F = \frac{c' + (\gamma z \cos^2 \beta - u) \tan \phi'}{\gamma z \sin \beta \cos \beta} \tag{4.25}$$

For a fully submerged slope, replace γ by γ' and set $u = 0$. For a total stress analysis, set $u = 0$ and instead of effective stress parameters, use total stress parameters of shear strength appropriate to the soil and site conditions.

For full seepage parallel to the slope (top flow line at the ground surface), Equation (4.25) is the same as Equation (4.22), and may also be written as follows:

$$F = \frac{c' + \gamma' z \cos^2 \beta \tan \phi'}{\gamma_{sat} z \sin \beta \cos \beta} \tag{4.25a}$$

Setting $F = 1$, in Equation (4.25) the critical depth of a layer of cohesive soil may be obtained:

$$(z)_{F=1} = H_c = \frac{c' - u \tan \phi'}{\gamma_{sat} \cos^2 \beta (\tan \beta - \tan \phi')} \tag{4.26}$$

A different form of expression is obtained in terms of dimensionless pore pressure ratio $r_u = u / \gamma_{sat} z$:

$$(z)_{F=1} = H_c = \frac{c'}{\gamma_{sat} \{\sin \beta \cos \beta - \tan \phi' (\cos^2 \beta - r_u)\}} \tag{4.26a}$$

If the pore pressure corresponds to seepage throughout the slope, $u = \gamma_w z \cos^2 \beta$ and $r_u = \gamma_w \cos^2 \beta / \gamma_{sat}$, and Equation (4.26a) reduces to Equation (4.24) as expected.

When the direction of seepage is not parallel to the ground surface, a seepage face may develop. The pore water pressure u at depth z below the point of intersection of the top flow line and the surface of the slope is given by (Chowdhury, 1975):

$$u = \gamma_w z \frac{\cot \beta}{\tan \theta + \cot \beta} \tag{4.27}$$

in which θ is the inclination of the top flow line to the horizontal. When $\theta = 0$, $u = \gamma_w z$, as expected and when $\theta = \beta$, $u = \gamma_w z \cos^2 \beta$, as expected from Equation (4.14). The stability of a seepage face in a natural or excavated slope may be investigated using Equation (4.27) for pore water pressure and this is shown in section 4.13.

4.3.2   Rapid drawdown of water level in a slope of cohesive soil

4.3.2.1   Effective stress analysis: proposed new approach

Cohesive soils such as clays have coefficients of permeability several orders of magnitude lower than cohesionless soils. In contrast to cohesionless soils, the reduced factor of safety after rapid drawdown may persist for considerable time. Several factors influence shear strength of cohesive soils under undrained conditions. The response of cohesive soils to stress changes is determined by factors such as soil permeability, drainage conditions and dilatancy characteristics. "Excess" pore pressures will be generated under undrained conditions due to stress changes as shown by Skempton's equation using two pore pressure coefficients A and B. [Section 2.8 and Equation (2.47).] Here we will consider stress changes caused by rapid drawdown. Such stress changes will result in the generation of "excess" pore water pressures.

At any point within a slope, the total pore water pressure after rapid drawdown is, therefore, the sum of the pore water pressure due to water level or seepage u_0 and the estimated excess pore water pressure Δu.

$$u = u_0 + \Delta u \qquad\qquad (4.28)$$

The excess pore pressure may be positive or negative depending on the type of soil and its stress history. Positive excess pore pressures are associated with a saturated soil which tends to contract during undrained shear while negative excess pore pressures may develop in a dilatant soil, such as overconsolidated clay, which expands during undrained shear. The higher the overconsolidation ratio of a clay, the greater the dilatancy effect or the tendency to expand. The pore pressure coefficient A in Skempton's equation has relatively higher values for contractant soils and relatively lower values, including negative values, for dilatant soils. Lambe and Whitman (1969) have tabulated values of A for different types of soil considering both stress conditions at failure and stress conditions applicable to foundation settlement.

Since the excess pore pressure can be either positive or negative, the total pore pressure in a cohesive soil immediately after rapid drawdown can be either lower or higher than the estimate based on hydrostatic conditions alone. It will be higher if the soil is contractant and the value of A is relatively high. It will be lower if the soil is dilatant and A is relatively low. The latter effect will be marked if the value of A is negative.

Accordingly, the calculation of factor of safety F after rapid drawdown requires a reliable estimation of the total pore water pressure along the potential slip surface. The initial pore water pressure can be estimated, for example, by drawing a flow-net with boundary conditions corresponding to the instant of drawdown. The estimation of the excess pore water pressure requires calculation of major and minor principal stress increments during rapid drawdown and the use of Skempton's pore pressure coefficients A and B [Equation (2.47)].

$$\Delta u = B[\Delta\sigma_3 + A(\Delta\sigma_1 - \Delta_3)]$$ (2.47)

Bishop (1954) did follow Skempton (1954) in order to use the approach based on pore pressure coefficients A and B. He suggested an approximate solution for pore water pressure after drawdown of the water level on the upstream face of an earth-rockfill dam. This approximate solution is presented in Appendix II at the end of the book. Although Bishop's approximate solution may work well for the particular application considered and under the various assumptions made, some of those assumptions are of questionable merit or validity. For example, the vertical overburden stress is taken as the major principal stress (for conditions both before and after drawdown). Secondly, the minor principal stress is not estimated at all. Stress changes which can produce volume change during drained deformation can produce excess pore water pressure during undrained deformation. Estimation of both the effective principal stress increments due to drawdown is essential for the correct use of the Skempton's equation as explained below.

Consider a point on a potential slip surface which has an inclination β at that point. Let the effective normal stress and the shear stress at this point be σ' and τ respectively. These are the stresses under working conditions (local $F > 1$) and not at critical equilibrium (local $F = 1$). Without additional information, the principal stresses cannot be estimated. For stress conditions at failure, the direction of principal stresses relative to the failure plane is known and hence the principal stresses can be estimated in terms of shear strength parameters. In particular, this may be done easily from the geometry of the Mohr circle at failure.

Assume that the principal stresses for the general non-failure case (local $F > 1$) have the same orientation as the principal stresses at failure. Then a specific Mohr circle can be drawn through the point representing the combination of σ' and τ. Consequently, it is easy to derive the following two equations for minor and major principal stresses in terms of σ', τ and the internal friction angle ϕ'.

$$\sigma'_3 = \sigma' + \tau\left(\frac{\sin\phi' - 1}{\cos\phi'}\right)$$ (4.29)

$$\sigma'_1 = \phi' + \tau\left(\frac{\sin\sigma' + 1}{\cos\sigma'}\right)$$ (4.30)

Consider now the stress changes at a point on the slip surface in an 'infinite slope' which is submerged. The slip surface is at depth z below the ground surface and parallel to it (inclined at angle β), and the free water level is h above the ground surface (Figure 4.2). Thus the point on the slip surface is located $(h + z)$ below free water level.

The effective normal stress and shear stress before drawdown are

$$\sigma' = \gamma' z \cos^2 \beta, \quad \tau = \gamma' z \sin \beta \cos \beta \tag{4.11}$$

In which γ' is the submerged (buoyant) unit weight of the soil.

Immediately after drawdown, the effective normal stress does not change (because drainage cannot occur rapidly enough in a cohesive soil) but the shear stress increases due to removal of submergence effect. Thus the stresses are

$$\sigma' = \gamma' z \cos^2 \beta, \quad \tau = \gamma z \sin \beta \cos \beta \tag{4.31}$$

in which γ is the saturated (bulk) unit weight of the soil.

Applying equation (4.29) for minor principal effective stress before and after drawdown [Equations (4.11) and (4.31)], the change due to drawdown is the difference of the two, i.e.,

$$\Delta\sigma'_3 = \gamma_w z \sin 2\beta \left(\frac{\sin\phi' - 1}{2\cos\phi'} \right) \tag{4.32}$$

Similarly, using Equation (4.30) with Equations (4.11) and (4.31), the change in major principal stress is

$$\Delta\sigma'_1 = \gamma_w z \sin 2\beta \left(\frac{\sin\phi' + 1}{2\cos\phi'} \right) \tag{4.33}$$

From Equations (4.32) and (4.33), the difference of principal stress increments is

$$(\Delta\sigma'_1 - \Delta\sigma'_3) = \frac{\gamma_w z \sin 2\beta}{\cos\phi'} \tag{4.34}$$

So far, we have considered effective stress increments. However, Skempton's equation requires the total stress increments for estimation of the "excess" pore pressure under undrained conditions. Therefore, let us also consider what changes occurred in the applied pore water pressure as a consequence of drawdown. The pore pressure at the point under consideration changes from $\gamma_w (h + z)$ at submergence to $\gamma_w z$ immediately after sudden drawdrown. Thus the change is $-\gamma_w h$.

It might thus be argued that, in order to obtain the total principal stress increments, this term must be added to both the effective principal stress increments. However, the difference of total principal stress increments will remain the same as the difference of effective principal stress increments.

$$(\Delta\sigma_1 - \Delta\sigma_3) = (\Delta\sigma'_1 - \Delta\sigma'_3) \tag{4.35}$$

Thus the second term of Skempton's equation [Equation (2.47)] is unaffected by the change in hydrostatic water pressure.

What about the first term? Should the total minor principal stress increment be the sum of two terms as below?

$$\Delta\sigma_3 = \Delta\sigma_3' - \gamma_w h \qquad (4.36)$$

The answer to this is "No" for the following reason. A change in the free water level h cannot produce volume change during drained deformation. Accordingly, such a change cannot produce "excess" pore water pressure during undrained deformation.

Therefore, in this particular case it is quite valid to use the effective principal stress increments in the Skempton equation in order to calculate the 'excess' pore water pressure.

For saturated soil, the value of pore pressure coefficient $B = 1$. Therefore, the use of Skempton's equation gives

$$\Delta u = \frac{\gamma_w z \sin 2\beta}{\cos\phi'}\left[\frac{\sin\phi' - 1}{2} + A\right] \qquad (4.37)$$

The first term of this equation will always be negative. The second term can be positive, zero or negative depending on the value of pore pressure coefficient A. The sum of the two terms can, therefore, be positive or negative.

The pore pressure increment or excess pore pressure given by Equation (4.37) is the second term of Equation (4.28). In the absence of a flow net or a numerical solution, we may use the following very conservative approximation for the first term

$$u_0 = \gamma_w z \qquad (4.38a)$$

In fact, this follows also from Bishop's simplified solution (see also, Morgenstern, 1963) (for drawdown pore pressure within an earth dam) to which reference was made earlier.

Alternatively, one may assume seepage parallel to the slope with the top flow line at the ground surface. This provides a less conservative but more realistic value of hydrostatic pore water pressure immediately after drawdown, as follows:

$$u_0 = \gamma_w z \cos^2\beta \qquad (4.38b)$$

Having thus estimated the pore pressure immediately after rapid drawdown, the factor of safety, F, of the slope can be calculated by using the basic equation for infinite slope analysis.

For a soil with $c' = 0$, it is easy to show that the value of F is independent of the depth z of the slip surface provided all other parameters are constant with depth and that includes pore pressure coefficient A.

4.3.2.2 Total stress analysis

Duncan and Wright (2005) proposed the use of total stress analysis and undrained shear strength for cohesive soil slopes during rapid drawdown. Considering a slip surface in an infinite slope analysis, the factor of safety F is calculated as the ratio of undrained shear strength at the appropriate effective normal stress to the appropriate shear stress. There is no need to estimate the pore pressure on the potential slip surface immediately after rapid drawdown. The undrained shear strength may be estimated as follows.

From undrained tests carried out on a soil which has previously been consolidated under isotropic stresses (ICU or CIU tests), a shear strength envelope is obtained with a cohesion intercept d and an inclination ψ. This envelope corresponds to consolidation principal effective stress ratio $K = 1$. Thus the undrained shear strength corresponding to any effective normal consolidation stress σ' is given by

$$\tau_{fu} = d + \sigma' \tan \psi \tag{4.39}$$

This must be corrected because the consolidation stresses in the field are anisotropic with a principal effective stress ratio $K = K_{An}$.

Alternatively, undrained shear strength could be obtained from tests in which the consolidation is carried out under anisotropic stresses before undrained loading (ACU or CAU tests). However, that approach might be very cumbersome. Therefore, Duncan and Wright (2005) suggest adjustment based on interpolation between two known shear strength values corresponding to two different effective principal stress ratios which are also known.

Duncan and Wright (2005) also made the assumption that the orientation of principal stresses is the same during consolidation as it would be for stress conditions at failure.

Accordingly, for the infinite slope problem, the consolidation principal effective stress ratio for any combination of effective normal and shear stresses can be estimated from Equations (4.29) and (4.30) as follows:

$$K = K_{An} = \frac{\sigma_1'}{\sigma_3'} = \frac{\cos \beta \cos \phi' + \sin \beta \, (\sin \phi' + 1)}{\cos \beta \cos \phi' + \sin \beta \, (\sin \phi' - 1)} \tag{4.40}$$

The principal effective stress ratio for stress conditions at failure can easily be derived from the effective stress failure envelope and the corresponding Mohr circle as follows:

$$K_f = \frac{\sigma_1'}{\sigma_3'} = \frac{\sigma' + c' \cos \phi'}{\sigma' - c' \cos \phi'} \times \frac{(1 + \sin \phi')}{(1 - \sin \phi')} \tag{4.41}$$

For $c' = 0$, this gives the well known result

$$K_f = \frac{1 + \sin \phi'}{1 - \sin \phi'} = \tan^2 \left(45° + \frac{\phi'}{2} \right) \tag{4.41a}$$

For the appropriate normal effective stress (immediately after rapid drawdown) the undrained shear strength corresponding to $K = 1$ is known from the undrained strength envelope mentioned earlier [Equation (4.39)] and the shear strength corresponding to $K = K_f$ is known from the effective stress strength envelope. From these two values, the shear strength for $K = K_{An}$ may, therefore, be estimated approximately by using linear interpolation.

This would be the appropriate undrained shear strength to be used in total stress analysis, according to Duncan and Wright (2005).

Dividing this shear strength by the shear stress after rapid drawdown, the value of F based on total stress analysis may thus be estimated.

Notes

Finite slope with partial submergence

The stability of cohesionless slopes during partial submergence has been considered, among others, by Baker et al. (2005). A recent study based on the limit analysis method of plasticity has come to the conclusion that, for a partially submerged finite slope of cohesive soil, the factor of safety during 'slow' drawdown depends on the extent of drawdown (Viratjandr and Michalowsky, 2006), and that there is a critical pool level associated with the lowest factor of safety. For one set of parameters, the critical level was about a third of the slope height above the base. For 'rapid' drawdown, on the other hand, the critical condition (lowest factor of safety) was associated with full (complete) drawdown.

EXAMPLE 4.1*

Effective stress approach

A long slope, initially submerged under water, has an inclination of 1 vertical to 3 horizontal ($\beta = 18.417°$). There is a potential slip surface parallel to the ground surface at a vertical depth of $z = 9.15$ m.

The soil parameters are:

Saturated bulk unit weight, $\gamma_{sat} = 19.65$ kN/m³
Shear strength parameters (effective stress parameters) $c' = 0$, $\phi' = 40°$
Using an effective stress approach, calculate

(a) the factor of safety during submergence.
(b) the approximate factor of safety after rapid and complete drawdown.
(c) a more realistic value of factor of safety after rapid drawdown given the following alternative values of the pore pressure coefficient A.

   (i) $A = -0.5$ (ii) $A = 0$ (iii) $A = +0.5$

(d) Repeat the solution for a potential slip surface at a depth $z = 1.52$ m, all other data remaining the same.

* This is an example problem from Duncan and Wright (2005) who advocated a total stress approach. The imperial units are converted here to SI units. The solution presented here is based on the proposed new effective stress approach. The answers are quite different from those based on the total stress approach. For comparison and completeness, the total stress solution is summarized in the next example.

Solution

(a) Submerged slope (before drawdown) [Equation (4.13) or (4.21)]

$$F = \frac{\tan \phi'}{\tan \beta} = \frac{0.839}{0.333} = 2.52$$

(b) After complete drawdown and assuming full seepage parallel to the slope [Equation (4.17) or (4.22)]

$$F = \frac{\gamma' \tan \phi'}{\gamma_{sat} \tan \beta} = \left(\frac{9.84}{19.65}\right)(2.52) = 1.26$$

This value does not take into consideration the excess pore water pressure that will be generated in the slope by the stress changes associated with rapid drawdown under undrained conditions

(c) Using Equations (4.37), (4.38b) and Equation (4.28),

   (i) For $A = -0.5$, $\Delta u = -12.53$, $u_0 = 80.78$, $u = 68.25$
   (ii) For $A = 0.0$, $\Delta u = -47.62$, $u_0 = 80.78$, $u = 33.16$
   (iii) For $A = +0.5$, $\Delta u = 22.55$, $u_0 = 80.78$, $u = 103.33$

The factor of safety in each case may be estimated from equation (4.25):

$$F = \frac{(\gamma z \cos^2 \beta - u)\tan \phi'}{\gamma z \sin \beta \cos \beta}$$

The values of calculated F are as follows:

   For $A = -0.5$, $F = 2.00$
   For $A = 0.0$, $F = 1.46$
   For $A = +0.5$, $F = 0.92$

Thus it may be noted that the approximate solution in (b) above can be conservative or unconservative depending on the type of soil which, in the present approach, is reflected in the value of pore pressure coefficient A for the soil forming the slope and, more precisely, for the soil along the potential slip surface.

(d) The reader may now repeat the calculations assuming $z = 1.52$ m. It will be found that all values of F in (a) and (b) are the same as the corresponding values for $z = 9.15$ m.

EXAMPLE 4.2

Total stress approach
For the above example the total stress analysis results of Duncan and Wright (2005) are summarized below. The additional data related to the undrained shear strength (ICU) envelope are as follows:

$$d = 95.76 \text{ kN/m}^2 \quad \text{and,} \quad \psi = 20°$$

(Moreover, depth of submergence is given as $h = 30.48$ m but it is stated, quite correctly, that this depth has no influence on the factor of safety after drawdown).

The factor of safety is estimated for two potential slip surfaces with $z = 1.52$ m and $z = 9.15$ m respectively.

Results

For both values of z, the principal effective stress ratio for consolidation is estimated to be $K_{An} = 2$. The principal effective stress ratio at failure in both cases is estimated to be $K_f = 4.6$. These values can be checked from the equations presented in the text [Equation (4.40) and (4.41a)].

(i) *For slip surface with $z = 1.52$ m*

The effective normal stress after drawdown is 13.5 kN/m².
The undrained shear strength is calculated as 100.7 kN/m² and corresponds to $K = 1$.
This is adjusted for the anisotropic consolidation ($K_{An} = 2$) by interpolation between the above value at $K = 1$ and the shear strength at $K_f = 4.6$ (from effective stress strength envelope) as explained in the text.
The adjusted undrained strength is 75.9 kN/m².
The shear stress immediately after rapid drawdown is 8.95 kN/m².
Therefore, based on total stress approach, $F = 75.9/8.95 = 8.48$.
This is indeed a very high value of F!

It is interesting, however, that Duncan and Wright (2005) adopted $F = 2.52$ as the answer for the rapid drawdown condition in this case. That value corresponds to the stage when pore pressures have been fully dissipated after drawdown. However, this value cannot be justified immediately after rapid drawdown in a cohesive soil of very low permeability.

(ii) *For slip surface with $z = 9.15$ m*

The effective normal stress after drawdown is 81.0 kN/m².
The undrained shear strength is calculated as 125.2 kN/m² and corresponds to $K = 1$.
This is adjusted for the anisotropic consolidation ($K_{An} = 2$) by interpolation between the above value at $K = 1$ and the shear strength at $K_f = 4.6$.
The adjusted undrained strength is 109.3 kN/m².
The shear stress immediately after rapid drawdown is 53.77 kN/m².
Therefore, based on total stress approach, $F = 109.3/53.77 = 2.03$.
This value was adopted as the answer by Duncan and Wright (2005).

Final comments

(1) While the procedure for estimation of undrained shear strength is reasonable, there is a serious discrepancy in the values of F based on the total stress approach.
(2) It is difficult to accept that the factor of safety of a submerged slope can increase after rapid drawdown from $F = 2.52$ (submerged) to $F = 8.48$ (after rapid drawdown) for the case when $z = 1.52$ m.
(3) For the case when $z = 9.15$ m, the decrease in F from 2.52 to 2.03 is reasonable but, in arriving at this value, the soil dilatancy has not been considered.

(4) For the slip surface at $z = 1.52$ m, the adopted value of $F = 2.52$ immediately after rapid drawdown is questionable. The value of F should decrease from the value at submergence. The exact value will depend on the type of soil as explained in the text and in the effective stress solution to this numerical example.

After all the pore pressures have been dissipated, the value of F will increase again to 2.52.

(5) The reason for a significant discrepancy between total stress and effective stress solutions has not been explored by Duncan and Wright (2005).

(6) Excess pore pressures developed during undrained loading associated with rapid drawdown cannot be taken into consideration in the total stress approach. Thus soil dilatancy cannot be taken into consideration.

4.4   ULTIMATE INCLINATION OF NATURAL SLOPES

The preceding analysis of infinite slopes shows that long-term stability is controlled by slope inclination, pore water pressure and effective shear strength parameters. The shear strength of a soil may decrease with time through weathering and geological processes. In particular, large deformations tend to reduce the shear strength to a residual value. In many cohesive soils the effective residual cohesion c_r is usually negligible and the value of residual shear strength is thus predominantly dependent on the effective residual friction angle ϕ_r. The value of ϕ_r is dependent on the percentage of clay in the soil, the type of clay-minerals present and the pore-fluid composition (Kenney, 1967b, 1977). High values of the plasticity index PI and clay fraction CF are associated with low values of ϕ_r and vice versa. Correlations between PI and CF on the one hand and ϕ_r on the other have been suggested (e.g., Voight, 1973). However, these cannot always be relied upon because there are many exceptions from such statistical relationships. The residual shear strength may also be influenced by other factors such as the shapes and sizes of the particles in the non-clay fraction and the preferred particle orientation.

Knowing the values of c_r and ϕ_r, and assuming seepage throughout the slope, the ultimate stable depth H_c of a cohesive layer may be determined. Alternatively, noting that c_r is often negligible in clay slopes, the ultimate stable angle β_{cr} of a natural slope may be determined from Equation (4.17) by setting $F = 1$, giving

$$\tan \beta_{cr} = \frac{\gamma'}{\gamma_{sat}} \tan \phi_r \qquad (4.42)$$

Since γ'/γ_{sat} is typically about 1/2 and ϕ_r is usually small for clays, it has often been suggested that:

$$\beta_{cr} = \frac{1}{2} \phi_r \qquad (4.42a)$$

In this discussion attention has been restricted to possible failure along planes parallel to the slope and other planes have not been considered. This has resulted in considerable simplification of the equations for normal and shear stress on an assumed failure plane. The stress state within soil and rock masses is dependent not only on the unit weight of the soil but also on the stress history, tectonic stresses and other possible factors. Such 'initial' stresses may have a considerable influence on the problem of stability and this is examined in chapter 7. Consequently these stresses also influence the postulate of an ultimate stable angle of natural slopes.

Apart from considerations of initial stresses, it is also necessary to consider the role of natural and other processes in altering slope form and hence the slope angle. It is a gross oversimplification of the problem to ignore the many complex factors which continuously alter the conditions controlling the stability, form, and behaviour of natural slopes. The equations discussed in this chapter are concerned only with gravitational forces, pore water pressures and shear strength at any particular instant. They do not reflect the interaction of a slope with various natural processes or particular events such as flooding, erosion, earthquakes etc. Man's activities resulting in increased loads, loss of support, increased pore water pressures, altered drainage conditions etc. can also upset the stability of a slope and alter the slope inclination.

Even if the problem may be merely one of intermittent slipping under gravitational forces, the dynamics of such failures would have a considerable influence on the slope angles after failure. Therefore, it may be misleading to refer to the ultimate 'stable' angles of a natural slope. Lastly, however flat a finite natural slope, it is possible to envisage exceptional conditions under which instability may occur.

NUMERICAL EXAMPLES OF INFINITE SLOPE ANALYSIS

EXAMPLE 4.3

Stress Strain curves were plotted from triaxial compression tests on a clean sand in relatively loose and dense states. From those curves, the following results were obtained for peak and ultimate angles of internal friction for the sand.

Dense specimen (initial void ratio $e_0 = 0.55$):	Peak friction angle, Ultimate friction angle,	$\phi_p = 43°$ $\phi_{ult} = 33°$
Loose specimen (initial void ratio $e_0 = 0.79$):	Peak friction angle, Ultimate friction angle,	$\phi_p = 33°$ $\phi_{ult} = 32°$

Suggest the design inclination for a temporary slope in this sand considering dry and full seepage conditions if (a) the sand is poorly compacted, and (b) if the sand is compacted to a void ratio of 0.67.

Solution
(a) *Loose or poorly compacted slope*

(i) A dry slope in the poorly compacted state should have an inclination no steeper than the angle of repose which approximates to the ultimate friction angle of 32°.

(ii) With full seepage throughout the slope, assuming direction of seepage parallel to the ground surface, the stable angle will be approximately half that of the dry slope. Thus the slope inclination should be no steeper than about 16°.

(b) *Slope compacted to a void ratio of 0.67*

One may estimate the peak friction angle at a void ratio of 0.67 by interpolation of the peak friction angles at void ratios of 0.55 and 0.79. Assume that the variation follows a linear relationship. The peak friction angle falls by $10°$ as the void ratio increases by 0.24. Thus linear interpolation gives, at $e_0 = 0.67$, a Peak friction angle, $\phi_p = 33 + [(43 - 33)/(0.79 - 0.55)] \times (0.67 - 0.55) = 38°$.

   (i) The slope angle of dry sand in this compacted state should not exceed $38°$.
   (ii) With full seepage the slope angle should not exceed $0.5 \times 38 = 19°$.

EXAMPLE 4.4

Calculate the factor of safety of a natural soil slope with an inclination of $20°$ in which the potential slip surface is located at a vertical depth, $z = 2.1$ m. This surface is an interface of the upper soil layer with the underlying, relatively firm stratum. The slip surface is planar and approximately parallel to the ground surface. The saturated bulk unit weight of the soil is $\gamma_{sat} = 19.62$ kN/m³; the effective shear strength parameters are cohesion $c' = 4$ kN/m² and internal friction angle, $\phi' = 18°$.

Consider the following cases:

(a) Soil is saturated but the pore water pressure at the slip surface is negligible
(b) Full seepage, i.e., seepage throughout the slip surface in a direction parallel to ground surface
(c) If the factor of safety for full seepage is less than 1, what is the critical pore water pressure or the critical position of the top flow line in relation to the slip surface and the ground surface?
(d) The slope is submerged with water level well above the slope
(e) If from an initially submerged condition sudden draw-down of water level occurs, how can the changed factor of safety be estimated? In the absence of more information, provide an approximate estimate of the change in F.

Solution

The 'infinite slope' model is clearly appropriate in this case and Equation (4.25) applies for an effective stress analysis.

(a) *No pore pressure on the slip surface*

From Equation (4.25) with pore water pressure $u = 0$ all along the slip surface, $F = 1.2$

(b) *Slope with full seepage*

With full seepage parallel to the slope i.e., the top flow line is at the ground surface, $(z_w = z)$, the pore water pressure all along the slip surface, $u = 9.81 \times 2.1 \times (\cos^2 20°) = 18.19$ kN/m².

Using Equation (4.25), $F = 0.75$.

Clearly, the slope would have failed at a much lower magnitude of pore water pressure since $F = 1$ corresponds to critical equilibrium.

(c) *Critical pore water pressure*

The critical pore water pressure may be calculated by setting $F = 1$ in Equation (4.25) and calculating u. This gives $u = 7.95$ kN/m², and thus one can calculate the critical position above the slip surface of the top flow line, $z_w = 0.92$ m. Thus depth of top flow line below ground surface is $2.1 - 0.92 = 1.18$ m.

To prevent failure the water level or top flow line location should be below this level.

(d) *Submerged slope*

Regardless of how high the water level is in a submerged slope, the effective normal and shear stresses are simply obtained by substituting submerged (buoyant) unit weight, γ', for bulk unit weight, γ, in the corresponding equations for saturated soil slope [Equation (4.11)].

Thus, in order to represent submerged or buoyant conditions, replace in Equation (4.25), in both numerator and denominator, the bulk unit weight by the submerged unit weight which, in this case, is $\gamma' = (19.62 - 9.81) = 9.81$ kN/m³ and also set $u = 0$ in the numerator.

Using Equation (4.25) with these changes, we get, $F = 1.50$. This is greater than $F = 1.2$ calculated for no pore water pressure along the slip surface as in (a) above. Alternatively, using Equation (4.21), $F = 0.6 + 0.9 = 1.5$. Thus submergence increases the factor of safety significantly for a cohesive soil slope due to the stabilizing effect of external (lateral) water pressure on a submerged slope.

(e) *Effective stress analysis for sudden draw-down (refer to section 4.3.2)*

Let us consider that from full submergence a sudden and complete draw-down of water level occurs. The shear stress on the slip surface will increase significantly because the buoyancy effect will no longer be present. Hence, in the denominator of the factor of safety equation, buoyant (submerged) unit weight will be replaced by saturated bulk unit weight. So shear stress will be the same as in the case (a) above. The shear strength (numerator of equation for F) will depend on the pore water pressure after sudden draw-down.

(i) If the material is free draining and pore water pressure is reduced to zero, the shear strength will be the same as in case (a) above. Thus the factor of safety will be $F = 1.2$. However, this answer is unrealistic because the assumption of free drainage for a cohesive soil is incorrect. Even in a cohesionless soil, there will be some delay before pore pressure can reduce to zero.

(ii) Thus pore pressure after sudden draw-down must be estimated. A simple approach for a cohesionless soil would be based on flow-net for appropriate boundary conditions. For a cohesive soil, the use of Skempton's pore pressure coefficients A and B [refer Equation (2.47)] is appropriate as the pore water pressure is developed under undrained conditions because of changes in total stresses during draw-down. Thus a knowledge of pore pressure coefficient A for the particular soil deposit is required (Pore pressure coefficient $B = 1$ for saturated soil).

Details of this approach have been presented in section 4.3.2.1 and illustrated with an example (Example 4.1). The reader should follow that procedure after assuming alternative values for pore pressure coefficient A.

An approximate estimate

An approximate estimate may be made by assuming a worst case scenario. Assume that, immediately after sudden draw down, seepage will occur within the slope in a direction parallel to slip surface. On this basis, the factor of safety will fall to 1 if the top seepage line is 1.18 m below the slope surface [see cases (c) and (d) above]. This implies pore water pressure on the slip surface corresponding to $z_w = 0.92$ m. If pore pressure during draw-down is any greater than that, the slope will fail. This is also the conclusion if estimate of pore pressure is based on Equation AII.11 in Appendix II at the end of this book.

The alternative is a total stress analysis

The alternative is to carry out a total stress analysis for this clay slope under the undrained conditions which apply after sudden draw-down. For that type of analysis we do not need to estimate the pore water pressure. However, we need the undrained shear strength along the slip surface. The strength should correspond to an undrained test on a specimen initially consolidated to the effective normal stress in the slope before undrained loading occurs. The procedure has been summarised in section 4.3.2.2. Moreover, reference is made to a published example (Example 4.2).

EXAMPLE 4.5

Estimate the critical height of a long, natural soil slope inclined at $\beta = 20°$ to the horizontal considering the soil layer to be above a rock surface with approximately the same inclination as the ground surface. Consider that seepage will occur throughout the soil slope in a direction parallel to the ground surface. The effective shear strength parameters are $c' = 4$ kN/m^2 and $\phi' = 18°$ and the soil unit weight is $\gamma_{sat} = 20$ kN/m^3.

Solution

Once again, the "infinite slope" model is appropriate. In order to estimate the critical height H_c, put factor of safety $F = 1$ and $z = H_c$ in Equation (4.25) and substitute the values of c', ϕ' and γ_{sat} and express $u = \gamma_w H_c \cos^2 \beta$. Alternatively, Equation (4.24) can be used directly.

Thus we obtain, the estimate of critical soil depth, $H_c = 1.14$ m.

If soil depth is smaller, factor of safety is greater than 1. If soil depth is greater, the slope will fail unless pore water pressure is less than that at full seepage.

EXAMPLE 4.6

The stability of a very long natural slope is to be estimated. The ground surface may be assumed to have a uniform inclination $\beta = 11°$. The potential slip surface is located at a vertical depth of $z = 2.1$ m below the ground surface. The effective shear strength parameters are $c' = 2$ kN/m^2 and $\phi' = 16°$ and the bulk unit weight of soil is $\gamma_{sat} = 19.62$ kN/m^3.

Seepage occurs in this slope to varying depths and the following measurements of the height of phreatic surface (top seepage line) above the slip surface level have been made at 6 nearly equidistant points along the length of the slope: $z_w = 1.9$ m, 1.7 m, 1.4 m, 1.1 m, 0.8 m and 0.3 m.

(a) Calculate the local values of factor of safety obtained from individual measurements of z_w and then the simple average value of F.
(b) Calculate the factor of safety F based on average z_w value.
(c) Comment on the pitfalls in the use of an average factor of safety for the whole slope.

Solution

(a) *Local factors of safety in different stretches of long slope*
Using Equation (4.25) as before, with $u = \gamma_w z_w \cos^2 \beta$ [or Equation (4.23) directly] the local factors of safety are as in Table E4.1.
Simple average value, $F = 1.31$.
We might also base these calculations on the individual values of pore pressure ratio r_u which is a dimensionless parameter defined in Equation (4.26a). The answers would still be the same.

(b) *Alternative calculation based on the average value of z_w*
The simple average of z_w values is 1.2 m.
Based on this value Equation (4.25) gives average $F = 1.31$, the same as calculated in (a) above.
Instead of using the average z_w value, an average pore water pressure ratio r_u (average) could also be used. The answer would be the same. However, for general two-dimensional problems, such correspondence cannot be assumed (see Note below).

(c) *Comment on the pitfalls in the use of an average factor of safety for the whole slope*
Whether we take average of the calculated local F values directly or we average z_w values and then calculate an average F value, the answer is the same. However, that answer is not sufficient by itself and relying only on the average value of F is unwise when F values at individual locations can be obtained easily and reliably as in this case. These can be regarded as F values for different parts or segments considered along the length of the slope. *Thus the spatial variability of the factor of safety must be highlighted.*

It is best to make decisions on the full range of local F values. We note that one part of the slope is close to critical equilibrium ($F = 1.07$ is close to $F = 1$) while, for other segments, the value of F is greater than 1 to different extents. Given some uncertainties in data, the likelihood of instability at one of the locations cannot be

Table E4.1 Results of analysis (Example 4.6).

z_w(m)	1.9	1.7	1.4	1.1	0.8	0.3
F		1.07	1.14	1.24	1.35	1.45	1.63

ruled out. This knowledge is important so that adequate preventive measures could be considered as appropriate.

Moreover, if the uppermost part of a long slope is at critical equilibrium, the implications may be different than if the section at critical equilibrium is the lowest part of the slope. One should consider the likelihood of failure progressing from one part of the slope to adjacent parts. It is also important to realize that there may be adverse consequences for structures/elements at risk which are located close to the parts of the slope most likely to fail. Therefore the locations of low factor of safety are important in addition to the average factor of safety.

Even if a probabilistic approach was to be used in this case, it would be desirable to consider different sections along the length of the slope separately and then, for each section, to calculate the reliability index and probability of failure (as defined in chapter 3 and considered in more detail in chapter 10). For such an analysis, any variability associated with each value of z_w would be considered along with any variability associated with depth z and the shear strength parameters for each section along the slope length.

Note

Extending the above comments to 2-D analyses

The "infinite slope" model is a very simple model. Although it is extremely useful for understanding slope stability concepts and their application, it is only a one-dimensional model. For two-dimensional problems, the pore water pressure along the slip surface within a single cross section is spatially variable (for example seepage with a curved top flow line within a cross section is often encountered). Thus it is often convenient to estimate an average pore water pressure ratio for the cross section. A procedure for the calculation of average r_u values for an earth dam or slope was first proposed by Bishop and Morgenstern (1960). Also it is often important to study how the value of the factor of safety F changes when the pore pressure ratio is varied.

While such studies are useful, the calculated factor of safety based on a given pore water pressure distribution along the slip surface may be different from the value of F calculated on the basis of an average pore water pressure ratio estimated from the real pore water pressure variation. This fact should not be ignored when evaluating the results of analyses and making decisions relevant to slope stability and reliability.

EXAMPLE 4.7

Two natural slope failures have occurred in the same soil which has a unit weight of $\gamma = 20$ kN/m³. The ground surface slope was about $\beta = 12°$ in both failures. One failure occurred with full seepage parallel to the ground surface. The slip surface was at a depth of 0.8 m below the ground surface. Thus the top flow line was close to the ground surface. The second failure occurred with slip surface at 1.5 m below the ground surface. Failure occurred when the top flow line was at 1.2 m below the ground surface. In both cases, "infinite slope" analysis is considered appropriate.

(a) Considering each failure separately for back-analysis, estimate the angle of internal friction assuming cohesion to be negligible.
(b) Considering the two failures together, estimate both the effective shear strength parameters for the soil; cohesion and angle of internal friction.

Solution
(a) *Considering each failure separately for back-analysis*
Setting $F = 1$ in Equation (4.25) and using Equation (4.14) for pore water pressure, a linear equation linking c' and $\tan \phi'$ is obtained.
Substituting $c' = 0$ and the values of unit weight γ, depth z and slope inclination β, the following results are obtained

For $(z = 1.5$ m, $z_w = 1.2$ m, $c' = 0$, $F = 1$), $\phi' = 19.28°$
For $(z = 0.8$ m, $z_w = 0.8$ m, $c' = 0$, $F = 1$), $\phi' = 22.64°$

(b) *Considering the two failures together*
If we consider both failures together, setting $F = 1$ in each case, we obtain two linear equations with two unknowns, c' and $\tan \phi'$.
Solving these as two simultaneous equations, we obtain: $c' = 0.95$ kN/m^2 and $\phi' = 16.45°$.
This example shows the extent of error in estimated (back-calculated) value of ϕ' if cohesion, however small, is ignored. Of course, there may be cases where cohesion is zero or negligible but it is important to establish if that indeed is the case.

Note
In some failure cases, pore water pressure at the time of failure may be unknown while one or both of the shear strength parameters are known. In such cases, back-analysis can be used to estimate the pore water pressure on the slip surface at the time of failure.

4.5 VERTICAL CUTS IN COHESIVE MATERIAL

4.5.1 *Unsupported height of a vertical cut and tension crack depth*

In contrast to the problems discussed in the previous section the stability of a vertical cut in cohesive material is essentially one involving short-term failure. This corresponds to undrained failure in cohesive soils especially when completely saturated. Therefore total stress or undrained shear strength parameters are implied in the following discussion. Terzaghi and Peck (1967, p. 197) note that the equations given below would also apply at least crudely to dry or moist cohesive soil located above the water table.

The relationship between major and minor principal stresses at the time of failure is obtained in terms of the Mohr-Coulomb theory as follows:

$$\sigma_1 = \sigma_3 \tan^2(45° + \phi/2) + 2c \tan(45° + \phi/2) \tag{2.14}$$

in which the shear strength parameters, based on undrained conditions, are 'total stress' parameters.

The excavation of a cut corresponds to the active Rankine state in which the vertical normal stress is the major principal stress ($\sigma_1 = \sigma_v = \gamma z$) and the lateral stress corresponds to the minor principal stress ($\sigma_3 = \sigma_h$). Therefore from Equation (2.14),

$$\sigma_h = \frac{\gamma z}{\tan^2(45° + \phi/2)} - \frac{2c}{\tan(45° + \phi/2)} \tag{4.43}$$

Thus the lateral stresses vary with depth and are negative or tensile up to a depth z_c (Figure 4.4) which is the value of z when σ_h is zero and is given by:

$$z_c = \frac{2c}{\gamma}\tan(45° + \phi/2) \tag{4.44}$$

Cracks open in a cohesive soil due to its low tensile strength and Equation (4.44) gives the theoretical depth of these cracks due to a cut in cohesive soil. The question of tension crack depth to be used in a stability analysis is considered in a subsequent paragraph of this section.

Integrating Equation (4.43) over the full depth H of a cut, the total lateral force is given by:

$$P_A = \frac{\gamma H^2}{2\tan^2(45° + \phi/2)} - \frac{2cH}{\tan(45° + \phi/2)} \tag{4.45}$$

when $P_A = 0$,

$$H = H_c = \frac{4c}{\gamma}\tan(45° + \phi/2) = 2z_c \tag{4.46}$$

This is the theoretical critical depth to which a vertical cut may be made safely within a cohesive soil (assuming the original ground surface to be horizontal). Such a cut would be stable in the short-term assuming there is no external disturbing force, erosion, flooding etc. (Note that this discussion is not relevant to long-term stability of a vertical cut.)

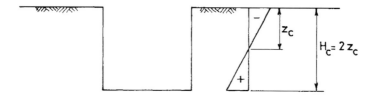

Figure 4.4 Vertical cut in cohesive soil: active Rankine state.

For saturated clays short-term stability involves consideration of undrained failure with no volume change. Thus a '$\phi = 0$' concept is implied and values of z_c and H_c are given by:

$$z_c = \frac{2c}{\gamma}, \quad H_c = \frac{4c}{\gamma} \tag{4.47}$$

It is worth repeating that c in this section is the undrained unit cohesion or shear strength of the material, and not the effective unit cohesion.

In the above treatment, an unsupported vertical bank is considered equivalent to a vertical section through a soil mass on the verge of failure. In reality the stresses are zero on the surface of the cut but stresses vary linearly with depth from negative to positive in the case of the assumed vertical section. This has some influence on the critical height H_c. Assuming a curved surface of sliding of circular shape, Fellenius (1927) found that $H_c = 3.85c/\gamma$, a value only 5% smaller than the value obtained on the basis of the simple assumption of a Rankine active state. (The latter gives identical results to those obtained by assuming a plane surface of sliding through the toe of a cut and considering the stability of the triangular wedge.)

When a vertical bank has been weakened by tension cracks, the critical height is reduced considerably to H'_c given by (Terzaghi, 1943):

$$H'_c = H_c - z = \frac{4c}{\gamma}\tan(45° + \phi/2) - z \tag{4.48}$$

in which z is the depth at which a tension crack intersects the plane surface of sliding inclined at critical angle $(45° + \phi/2)$ to the horizontal. Assuming $z = H'_c/2$, and $\phi = 0$ conditions:

$$H'_c = 2.67\frac{c}{\gamma} \tag{4.49}$$

A bank with height H_c may be expected to remain stable for a considerable time unless the conditions are altered in some way such as the accumulation of surface water in open tension cracks, decrease of shear strength, application of surcharge loads etc. It has been shown that there is no danger of base failure of an unsupported vertical cohesive bank of height H_c. The minimum value of the critical height H_f at which base failure can occur is given by (Terzaghi, 1943):

$$H_f = 5.14\frac{c}{\gamma} \tag{4.50}$$

This value is considerably greater than the value H'_c based on slope failure. According to Terzaghi and Peck (1967), the actual depth of tension cracks lies between the values z_c and H_c given by Equations (4.44) and (4.46) respectively. Reference is made in a subsequent chapter (chapter 8) to a comparison between the simple solutions given above and those obtained by the limit analysis approach of plasticity.

4.5.2   Tension crack depth for use in stability analysis

4.5.2.1   Computed depth of tension crack

The existence of tension cracks is likely to increase the tendency of a soil or rock slope to fail. Firstly the length of failure surface along which shear strength can be mobilised is reduced. Secondly, a crack may fill with water (e.g., due to rainfall) and an additional force due to water pressure increases the tendency for a slip to occur (see section 4.7). It is therefore often necessary to estimate the depth of tension cracks for use in stability analysis. Use of equations (4.44) and (4.46) is, of course, valid for a 'total stress' analysis concerned with undrained or short-term slope failure in cohesive soil (e.g., Lambe and Whitman, 1969, p. 464). The question arises as to the validity of Equation (4.44) for calculating z_c to be used in an effective stress analysis since it contains total stress parameters of shear strength. Before answering this question one must distinguish between (1) embankments and undisturbed natural slopes on the one hand and (2) excavated cuts on the other. In the former case (1) it would be logical to use effective stress parameters of strength in Equation (4.44) to calculate z_c, since an undrained condition due to sudden removal of lateral support has not arisen. For example, Spencer (1973) used an equation similar to Equation (4.44) based on zero lateral effective stress for embankment stability analysis in terms of effective stresses. His equation in terms of mobilised effective stress parameters and the pore pressure ratio $r_u = u/\gamma z$ is:

$$z_c = \frac{2c'_m}{\gamma(1-r_u)} \tan(45° + \phi'_m/2) \tag{4.44a}$$

When the pore pressure ratio is zero, Equations (4.44) and (4.44a) are identical except that one is expressed in terms of total stress parameters and the other in terms of mobilised effective stress parameters. A similar equation would be valid for analysis of undisturbed natural slopes for long-term stability. Again, if lateral earth pressure on a wall is to be calculated on an effective stress basis a form similar to Eq. (4.44a) is to be used. (See Lambe and Whitman, 1969, p. 342.)

In the latter case (2) concerning an excavated slope the use of c' and ϕ' may not be logical or safe. Tension crack depth based on c' and ϕ' is likely to be much less than that based on c and ϕ noting that c' is often much smaller than c. Yet tension cracks would be formed in the short-term after a cut is excavated and their depth could not decrease thereafter. Consequently the value of z_c given by use of c and ϕ in Equation (4.44) should be adopted even for effective stress analysis concerned with long-term conditions of an excavated slope unless the use of c' and ϕ' results in a higher value of z_c than the use of c and ϕ.

The importance of tension cracks and their effect on stability (particularly when filled with water) is not always duly emphasised in soil mechanics. This may be due, in part, to conclusions reached by some workers that the effect of tension cracks on factor of safety of embankments is negligible (e.g., Spencer, 1968, 1973). Such conclusions must be understood in terms of the small depth of tension cracks predicted by using c and ϕ [in Equation (4.44)]. In cut slopes, tension cracks could extend to considerable depth and exert a significant influence on the value of F as in the case of the slips at Bradwell (Skempton and La Rochelle, 1965).

Quite apart from the effect of tension cracks on a conventional limit equilibrium analysis, there is the important question of progressive failure. As was pointed out in chapter 2, tension cracks may be a consequence of the initiation of progressive shear failure. As such the existence of tension cracks deserves careful attention.

4.5.2.2   Observation of tension cracks

While tension cracks are frequently observed near both failed and unfailed slopes, observations may not include details such as depth of cracks. In some cases these depths can be significant. For example, from investigation of failed slopes in weathered rock, ranging in height from 20.8 m to 30.5 m, Sancio and Goodman (1979) reported tension crack depths in the range 2.11 m–5.84 m. It is interesting to note that including an open, dry crack in stability analysis showed insignificant influence on the computed value of factor of safety, F. They computed value of F based on an impending crack (with some tensile strength) and compared with the value of F based on open dry crack. The differences for the cases studied were negligible and more details will be given in chapter 5 (see Example 5.1). No general conclusions should be drawn from this on the significance of tension cracks based on this result concerning inclusion of dry cracks in analysis. Even in the cases studied by Sancio and Goodman, the critical slip surface location and shape in each case was obviously influenced by the tension cracks. When dry cracks are filled with water, the adverse influence on stability can be significant and computed values for those conditions will show that effect.

4.5.2.3   Effect of a gap or crack under exceptional circumstances

In exceptional cases, the formation of a deep gap or crack may have catastrophic consequences Attention was drawn in sections 1.2 and 1.7 to catastrophic failures of levees associated with Hurricane Katrina (Katrina, 2008). While some breaches were the result of erosion following overtopping of levees, others occurred due to an unusual mechanism of shear failure. In these sections the I-walls had been used with the levees as part of the Hurricane Protection System. At many locations the formation of a deep gap was observed along the I-wall on the flood side. This was due to the deflection of the I-wall under the load of the storm surge. The formation of the gap reduces the factor of safety to a significant extent (Brandon et al., 2008; Duncan et al., 2008). For further discussion the reader may refer to sections 1.2, 1.7 and 5.1.4 and to the 'important note' following example 5.3 in chapter 5.

4.6   PLANE FAILURE IN ROCK SLOPES

Failure may occur in hard rock slopes along clearly defined planar discontinuities such as joints or bedding planes which strike approximately parallel to the slope and dip from the slope to daylight in the slope face. In order to establish whether a basis for slope failure along a planar discontinuity exists, it is thus necessary to consider the direction of its dip and strike in relation to the slope. Dip is the maximum inclination of a discontinuity plane and dip direction is the direction of the horizontal trace of the line of dip measured clockwise from the North. Strike is the trace of the intersection of an oblique discontinuity plane with a horizontal reference plane and it is at right angles to the dip and dip direction of the oblique plane. It is usually sufficient to define a plane by its dip and strike or by its dip and dip direction. In considering the two-dimensional problem of plane failure in rock, it is assumed that resistance at the ends of the potential sliding mass is negligible, i.e., release surfaces exist at the ends. There may be situations in which some resistance is offered at the ends. Such resistance must, of course, be included in an analysis.

Consider a slope of inclination i and height H and a potential failure plane of inclination β as shown in Figure 4.5. For simplicity assume the ground surface to be horizontal first. Considering the forces acting on the rigid block of rock ABC above the failure plane AB, the following equation for the factor of safety F is obtained simply by solution of the force equilibrium equations or by equating available strength to shear stress along the failure plane AB (the force triangle is shown in Figure 4.5).

$$F = \frac{2c \sin i}{\gamma H \sin(i - \beta) \sin \beta} + \frac{\tan \phi}{\tan \beta} \tag{4.51}$$

Critical equilibrium corresponds theoretically to a value of $F = 1$. For this value Equation (4.51) may be written in terms of the dimensionless parameter $\gamma H/c$ as follows

$$\frac{\gamma H}{c} = \frac{2 \sin i \cos \phi}{\sin(i - \beta) \sin(\beta - \phi)} \tag{4.52}$$

When F is not equal to one, a more general form of Equation (4.52) in terms of mobilised shear strength parameters may be written as follows:

$$\frac{\gamma H}{c_m} = \frac{2 \sin i \cos \phi_m}{\sin(i - \beta) \sin(\beta - \phi_m)} \tag{4.52a}$$

So far we have assumed that plane failure occurs along an existing discontinuity. This is certainly the usual case in rock slopes. However, it may sometimes be required

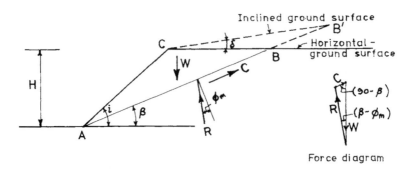

Figure 4.5 Failure along a plane surface in jointed rock.

to consider the possibility of plane failure which does not coincide with a single major discontinuity or plane of weakness. This possibility may occur in steep rock slopes where an actual slip surface can be approximated by a plane (Hoek, 1970; Hoek and Bray, 1974, 1977). Moreover, in some cases geological investigation may fail to reveal a dominant thorough-going discontinuity but may reveal a number of intersecting joints. Thus failure may occur on a composite planar surface which can be approximated by a single plane the critical inclination of which is not known in advance (see p. 153, Hoek and Bray, 1974 or p. 165, Hoek and Bray, 1977). It is, therefore, of interest to investigate the critical inclination of the failure plane on a theoretical basis. This may be done by minimising Equation (4.52a) with respect to β. Differentiating the right hand side with respect to this angle and equating to zero, the following equation is obtained for the critical failure plane:

$$\beta_{cr} = \frac{1}{2}(i + \phi_m)$$
(4.53)

Substituting this value in Equation (4.52a) the critical value of the dimensionless parameter $\gamma H / c_m$ is obtained as follows:

$$\left(\frac{\gamma H}{c_m}\right)_{cr} = \frac{4 \sin i \cos \phi_m}{1 - \cos(i - \phi_m)}$$
(4.54)

For a vertical slope $i = 90°$, and we get

$$\beta_{cr} = (45° + \phi_m / 2)$$
(4.53a)

This result corresponds to the one obtained for the theoretical inclination of the failure plane considering Rankine active state of failure, a general state of plastic failure for which it is justified to assume $F = 1$, $c = c_m$ and $\phi = \phi_m$. Similarly, substituting $i = 90°$ in Equation (4.54) yields the equation derived earlier for the critical height of a vertical cut:

$$H_c = \frac{4c}{\gamma}\frac{\cos \phi}{1 - \sin \phi} = \frac{4c}{\gamma} \tan(45° + \phi/2)$$
(4.46)

To find the location of the critical plane of failure, minimisation was made with respect to the dimensionless parameter $\gamma H / c_m$ leading to an expression for the critical failure plane dependent only on mobilised ϕ and slope inclination. It is common practice in most limit equilibrium methods to find a minimum F. Therefore, it is interesting to note that minimisation of F given by Equation (4.51) does not lead to the same result as minimisation of $\gamma H / c_m$ given by Equation (4.52a). The former gives a failure plane inclination which is dependent on c, γ, H and ϕ or simply the dimensionless parameters $c/\gamma H$ and ϕ. It is misleading to assume that critical value of the failure plane will be given as $1/2 (i + \phi)$ by minimising with respect to F. With known available parameters, the critical value of failure plane inclination to give minimum F may be obtained simply by trial and error.

Now consider the general case of plane failure with the ground surface inclined at an angle δ to the horizontal. The factor of safety may be obtained by considering the equilibrium of the assumed failure wedge $AB'C$ (Figure 4.5) or alternatively by taking the ratio of available to mobilised shear strength along the assumed failure plane AB'. It is interesting to note that the expression for F is identical to Equation (4.51) and, therefore, independent of the ground surface inclination. Consequently, when there is no known discontinuity and it is required to find the critical failure plane, its inclination is still given by Equation (4.53a). The critical value of the dimensionless parameter $(\gamma H/c_m)$ is still given by Equation (4.54). The fact that F is independent of ground surface inclination was first pointed out by Taylor (1948) and is a consequence of the assumption of plane failure which is not generally valid in a soil or rock slope which is without a dominant discontinuity. Where failure occurs along a curved slip surface the ground surface inclination will no doubt influence the value of F. It is also necessary to point out that when a given water table location is assumed the factor of safety will, in general, be dependent on the ground surface inclination since the similitude associated with plane failure without water pressure is no longer retained.

The dimensionless parameter $\gamma H/c_m$ is known as a stability factor and this parameter or its inverse have been used widely in the preparation of slope stability charts since Taylor (1937, 1948) first demonstrated their use. Reference to his charts for failure surfaces of circular shape will be made in the next chapter. The stability factor is extremely useful because it reduces the number of variables to be considered in preparing stability charts. Consequently the number of charts is also reduced and relevant information can be presented in an economical and convenient manner. Irrespective of differences in slope height, unit weight and unit cohesion, two slopes of same inclination (and similar geometry) have the same factor of safety if they have the same values of $\gamma H/c_m$ and ϕ and all other conditions are identical. Such slopes may be considered as similar slopes in relation to stability analysis.

Hoek (1970) prepared charts for plane failure in rock slopes using the slope height function Y and slope angle function X given below:

$$X = 2\sqrt{(i - \beta)(\beta - \phi)}, \quad Y = \frac{\gamma H}{c} \tag{4.55}$$

He found an approximately unique relationship between X and Y for ϕ values between $10°$ and $40°$. For values of ϕ less than $5°$ he found that serious errors would result if the derived approximate relationship was used. The factor of safety depends on the parameters in Equation (4.55) as well as on the seepage conditions and the depth of tension cracks thus:

$$F = f\left(\frac{\gamma H}{c}, i, \beta, \frac{z_c}{H}, \frac{H_w}{H}\right) \tag{4.56}$$

in which z_c is the depth of tension cracks and H_w the height of water table from the toe of the slope. Following Janbu (1954b), Hoek modified X and Y to take into consideration these other dimensionless parameters so that his charts would be applicable to a variety of conditions e.g., water-filled tension crack, normal draw-down, horizontal seepage etc. In later publications (Hoek and Bray, 1974, 1977) this approach was discarded because of errors as suggested in the book review (E.T.B., 1977). However, the reader may use alternative charts for plane failure given in Hoek and Bray (1974, 1977).

Slope stability charts should be used only after carefully establishing their validity for particular problems and after understanding their limitations. Charts are devised for specific slope geometries and pore water pressure conditions. For problems in which the ground or slope surface is of irregular shape or surcharge loading is included, use of charts can only be made on an approximate basis for initial calculations. Average slope inclination and average strength parameters may be used when slope conditions are non-uniform and the accuracy of such initial cal-culations can only improve with experience. Finally results must often be obtained by more accurate analytical or graphical means where time and resources permit. Sometimes a non-linear strength envelope may have to be used for stability analysis in place of the Coulomb or linear strength envelope. In such cases, charts based on the linear envelope may not be of much use and an appropriate equation for the factor of safety should be derived. For failure along single planes this should not present any difficulty. The manner in which strength data is interpreted may have a significant influence on the calculated factor of safety and this is shown in section 4.8.

4.7 PLANE FAILURE WITH WATER IN TENSION CRACK

4.7.1 Conventional analysis

Tension cracks or open joints are often found at the crest of a soil or rock slope and their influence on stability can be significant particularly when the cracks are filled with water. Let the crack have a depth of z and let the depth of water be z_w. Figure 4.6 shows the failure plane joining the bottom of the crack with the toe of the slope. Due to the pressure of water in the crack, there will be water pressure acting on the slip surface. The distribution of this pressure drops linearly from the value $\gamma_w z_w$ to zero (above atmospheric) at the toe of the slope where the water finds an exit after seeping through the discontinuity. In fact a more dangerous water pressure distribution can exist particularly if drainage from the slope is partially or completely blocked. Let W be the weight of the potential sliding wedge. The factor of safety F may be found as the ratio of total resisting force along the sliding surface of length L and the total disturbing force. Taking components of all the forces in the direction of the sliding surface we have:

$$F = \frac{cL + (W \cos\beta - U - V \sin\beta) \tan\phi}{W \sin\beta + V \cos\beta} \tag{4.57}$$

in which $L = (H - z)\operatorname{cosec}\beta$

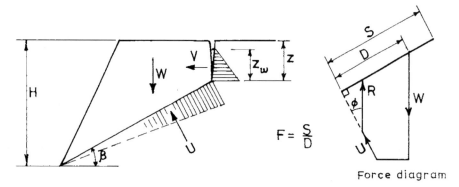

Force diagram

Figure 4.6 Planar slip surface with water pressure in tension crack. The tension crack shown here in
the crest could also be in the slope face itself. Also, other water pressure distributions on
slip surface could exist depending on seepage conditions. In the force polygon horizontal
line joining W and U forces is the force V due to water pressure in the tension crack.

$$U = \frac{1}{2}\gamma_w z_w (H - z) \operatorname{cosec} \beta$$

$$\tag{4.58}$$

$$V = \frac{1}{2}\gamma_w z_w^2$$

The expression remains unchanged even when the tension crack with water is in the
slope face rather than in the crest of the slope. Only the shape and weight of the sliding
wedge are modified. It may be useful to study the influence of variations in z and z_w on
F since z is not always accurately known. Such sensitivity studies may be conveniently
made by rewriting F in terms of dimensionless parameters $c/\gamma H$ and ϕ. Naturally the
critical tension crack depth will vary with the inclination of the failure plane.

Graphical analysis is also quite convenient. A force polygon is constructed by
drawing W, V and U to scale. The line representing U is then extended and a line
perpendicular to it drawn from the starting point of the line representing W. This is
the closing line of the force polygon and represents the required or mobilised shear
strength. The factor of safety is obtained as a ratio of available to mobilised shear
strength. For the available shear strength the normal force on the failure plane is equal
to the extended part of the U vector in the force polygon. The procedure for finding
F graphically is shown in Figure 4.6.

If the rock mass is dry and impermeable, the force U in the expression for F may
be neglected. However, tension crack may get filled with water after heavy rainfall
and the V force can be included as appropriate.

On the other hand the rock mass may be heavily fractured and relatively permeable and there may be a given ground water flow pattern in the slope. The most critical
condition is generally occurs after prolonged rainfall when the whole slope is saturated
with seeping water. The pore pressures may be reasonably approximated by assuming a
water filled tension crack and a linear distribution of water pressure along the slip surface. For greater accuracy the pressure of water at each point should be determined after

drawing a flow net for the critical seepage condition. The intersection of the slip surface with equipotential lines directly gives the pore water pressure at each point of intersection. (Sometimes the pore water pressure is taken simply on the basis of the depth of any point on the slip surface below the top seepage line. Such a procedure can only be regarded as an approximate one in comparison to one based on the use of a flow net.)

It is easy to study the influence of remedial or preventive measures for rock slopes involving potential sliding along plane surfaces. For example the effect of drainage measures (drainage galleries, horizontal drainage holes, etc.) can be studied by suitably varying the forces U and V. The installation of rock bolts or cables or rock anchors which are anchored into the rock mass behind the possible failure plane can be studied by including another force in the equation for factor of safety. Let P be the external force applied through the rock anchor or rock bolt which has an inclination θ to the normal to the failure plane. We have:

$$F = \frac{cL + (W\cos\beta - U - V\sin\beta + P\cos\theta)\tan\phi}{W\sin\beta + V\cos\beta - P\sin\theta} \tag{4.59}$$

This expression is based on P as the design force or allowable load in the anchor or bolt, and fully mobilized shear strength along the discontinuity. However, if P is considered to be the ultimate load in the rock bolt or anchor, a factor of safety may be applied to P. (Note that 'load factor' would be a more appropriate term than 'factor of safety'.)

The above expression will change if a factor is applied to force P. The reader may carry out this simple exercise to write down the revised expression for F if a factor on P is applied on the right hand side of Equation (4.59).

Since uncertainties related to shear strength parameters are different from those associated with the reinforcing force P, the factor of safety (load factor) on P may be different from the allowable factor of safety relevant to the shear strength parameters. Moreover, the allowable factor of safety may be chosen differently for cohesion and friction parameters in the manner of Equation (4.3).

A slope may be undercut during mining operations either intentionally or by accident. Undercutting may also occur by the action of waves for coastal slopes or due to weathering of weak bed under strong bed. By modifying the weight of the sliding wedge suitably, the basic equation given in this section for F may be used in practical problems of this nature. Of course, it would be necessary to model or simulate the manner and extent of undercutting before such calculations could be made.

4.7.2 Alternative ways of defining F

Considerable attention has been given to the concept of a factor of safety F in relation to analytical methods. Emphasis has been given to the fact that F may be defined in a number of ways whether a limit equilibrium or stress analysis approach is used for analysis. Several alternative definitions are possible on the basis of limit equilibrium. Let us consider another simple example of how F may be defined in alternative ways for a problem in which possible failure of a rock along a single plane is considered. The factor of safety for a reinforced rock slope was defined by Equation (4.59) as a ratio of resisting forces and disturbing forces. The disturbing forces are reduced by the reinforcing cables or rock anchors to the extent of $P \sin \theta$. Thus we may write F as follows:

$$F = \frac{X}{Y - P \sin \theta} \tag{4.60a}$$

It has been suggested by Hoek and Bray (1977) that F may be defined in an alternative way if $P \sin \theta$ is considered to be an increase in the resisting forces rather than a decrease in the disturbing forces. This leads to the following equation for F:

$$F = \frac{X + P \sin \theta}{Y} \tag{4.60b}$$

Different values of F would result from these alternative expressions, the extent of difference being mainly dependent on the magnitude of P in relation to the magnitudes of X and Y. In other words, for a given value of required F, the difference in force P (required from anchor cables) predicted by the two equations increases as the magnitude of F increases. The use of Equation (4.60a) would be justified where P is active force in the sense that the reinforcing cables are tensional before any movement of the rock block or wedge has taken place. However Equation (4.60b) was considered more appropriate if P is a force applied by untensioned bars or cables since the resisting force can only be developed after some movement has taken place. The choice between the two equations is an arbitrary one if, as is often the case, the sequence of loading and movement in a slope is unknown. By giving careful attention to site conditions and field observations it may be possible to make a wise choice between the two alternative definitions of F.

Other uncertainties may also arise in relation to reinforced rock slopes. For example, the development of frictional and cohesive components of shear strength requires some deformation. The extent of required deformation may not be compatible with the magnitude of force P due to reinforcing cables. It may, therefore, not be correct to assume that the two components of shear strength are mobilised fully at the same time. Thus it may be advisable to use different values of F for cohesion and friction even if both these components of strength are known with the same degree of confidence. The use of F_c different from F_ϕ where c and ϕ are not known with the same degree of confidence has already been discussed earlier in this chapter.

4.8   INTERPRETATION OF STRENGTH DATA FOR USE IN STABILITY CALCULATIONS

The simple analysis discussed in the previous section is based on the Coulomb equation for shear strength. Reference has already been made in the previous chapter to the fact that envelopes of strength of many rocks and rock discontinuities are concave downwards. Attention has also been drawn to the necessity for care in the interpretation of measured data relating to the shear strength of rocks. Jaeger (1971) demonstrated the drastic influence of strength interpretation on calculated factors of safety by the following two examples.

EXAMPLE 4.8

Slope height $H = 700$ ft. unit weight $\gamma = 160$ lb/ft³, slope inclination $i = 55°$, failure plane angle $\beta = 45°$, shear strength is given by power law of the form:

$$s = k\sigma^m \tag{4.61}$$

where σ is the normal stress. Based on this law the factor of safety is given by:

$$F = k\left\{\frac{1}{2}\gamma H \sin{(i - \beta)} \cos\beta \operatorname{cosec} i\right\}^{m-1} \cot\beta \tag{4.62}$$

On this basis the factor of safety F has a value of 1.5 with $m = 0.7$ and $k = 5.2$.

Jaeger fitted Coulomb's law to values given by the power law at two points σ_0 and $a\sigma_0$ and chose a value for 'a' of 2. He found the factor of safety using Coulomb's law to be strongly dependent on σ_0 as shown in Table E4.2.

(1 ft = 0.3048 m; 1 lb/ft³ = 0.157 kN/m³)

EXAMPLE 4.9

A set of experimental results of shear strength were considered and found to be approximated by:

(1) $s = 20 + 0.65\sigma$, $\sigma < 1,000$ psi
(2) $s = 150 + 0.47\sigma$, σ between 1000–5000 psi

Note: 1 psi = 6.895 kN/m²

The results could also be approximated by the following expressions corresponding respectively to a power law or an exponential law:

(3) $s = 1.2\,\sigma^{0.9}$
(4) $s = 270\,\{1 - \exp{(-0.0015\,\sigma)}\} + 0.41\,\sigma$

Table E4.2 Values of factors of safety, (after Jaeger, 1971). With permission, see page 713, No 12.

	100	200	300
σ_0 (psi)	100	200	300
F based on Coulomb's law	1.61	1.96	2.31
Actual factor of safety based on power law for strength = 1.5			

Note: 1 psi = 6.895 kN/m².

Table E4.3 Values of factors of safety, (after Jaeger, 1971). With permission, see page 713, No 12.

H ft	γ pcf	β deg.	i deg.	σ psi	F (1)	F (2)	F (3)	F (4)
1000	160	35	45	112	1.07	1.12	1.18	2.58
100	160	35	75	30	1.22	1.15	1.88	7.81

Note: 1 psi = 6.895 kN/m²; 1 pcf = 0.157 kN/m³.

Table E4.3 shows the values of F calculated using the four different equations for two different slopes.

An important lesson may be drawn from these examples. For any given problem estimates can be made of the level or range of stresses for which test results are required. It is in this range of stresses that the actual measured strength should be made to correspond to that used in the calculations. Indiscriminate use of shear strength data or its incorrect interpretation may lead to results which are very misleading.

Selection of design values of strength parameters is a matter requiring judgment based on experience especially when the material is heterogeneous. Some guidance concerning empirical rules has been given by Sowers and Sowers (1970) and Hoek (1976).

4.9   TWO-DIMENSIONAL SLIDING ALONG ONE OF TWO JOINT SETS

Figure 4.7 shows two conjugate sets of joints in a rock mass at angles α and α_1 to the horizontal such that sliding occurs on the α joints while the α_1 joints dilate. The joints are assumed to be equally spaced for simplicity and OB is drawn at an angle β so that OAB represents the volume of material associated with potential sliding.

The determination of spacing and inclination of joints is often difficult in practice. The following equation can be useful only when reliable geological data are available. Using the Coulomb's equation for shear strength the factor of safety F is given by:

$$F = \frac{2c \sin i \, \sin(\alpha_1 - \beta)}{\gamma H \, \sin(i - \beta) \, \sin(\alpha_1 - \alpha) \, \sin \alpha} + \frac{\tan \phi}{\tan \beta} \tag{4.63}$$

Note that when $\alpha = \beta$, Equation (4.63) reduces to familiar form Equation (4.51). Using the power law Equation (4.61) the factor of safety is given by:

$$F = \frac{k \left(\frac{\gamma H}{2} \right)^{m-1}}{\tan \alpha} \left\{ \frac{\sin(i - \beta) \cos \alpha \, \sin(\alpha_1 - \alpha)^{m-1}}{\sin i \, \sin(\alpha_1 - \beta)} \right\} \tag{4.64}$$

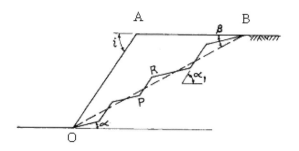

Figure 4.7 Sliding in rock involving two sets of joints.

When fracture spreads between joints of one system by tensile failure normal to them (i.e., $\alpha_1 = \pi/2 + \alpha$), the factor of safety depends on the tensile strength T_0 since the force acting across any α_1 joint like PR is the product of T_0 and PR. Based on Coulomb's equation of shear strength the following expression is obtained for F:

$$F = \frac{2\{c\cos(\beta-\alpha)+T_0\sin(\beta-\alpha)\}\sin i}{\gamma H \sin(i-\beta)\sin\alpha} + \frac{\tan\phi}{\tan\alpha} \tag{4.65}$$

The presence of the term containing T_0 represents an increase in the factor of safety due to the fact that tensile strength is mobilised against sliding. For $(\beta-\alpha)$ of the order of 10°, it represents an increase in c of the order of $T_0/5$ according to Jaeger (1971) who considered the above conditions and originally gave the accompanying derivations.

4.10 CONTINUITY OF JOINTING

Jennings (1970) considered the situation in unweathered rocks when failure tends to take place partly along pre-existing joint surfaces and partly through intact rock. On the basis of a simple model (Figure 4.8), he proposed a coefficient of continuity of the joints k defined as:

$$k = \frac{\Sigma a}{\Sigma a + \Sigma b} \tag{4.66}$$

The resisting force RF along AB is given by:

$$\begin{aligned}RF &= AB\,(c_a + \sigma_n \tan\phi_a) \\ &= b\,(c_m + \sigma_n \tan\phi_m) + a(c_j + \sigma_n \tan\phi_j)\end{aligned} \tag{4.67}$$

where c_a and ϕ_a are strength parameters corresponding to a hypothetical material a equivalent to the real one; c_m and ϕ_m correspond to the intact rock; c_j and ϕ_j to the joint surface. Substituting $AB = \Sigma a + \Sigma b$ and using Equation (4.66):

$$c_a = (1-k)s_m + kc_j, \quad \tan\phi_a = k\tan\phi_j \tag{4.68}$$

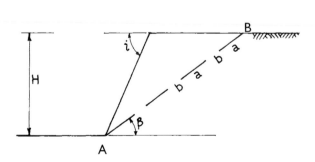

Figure 4.8 Shear plane in jointed rock passing through joints (a) and intact material (b).

in which s_m is the mean shear strength of the intact rock on the plane of failure (considered by Jennings to be predominantly dependent on c_m). Following the above concepts Jennings tackled the problem involving two joint sets discussed in the previous section. The equations derived are too cumbersome to reproduce here. Based on information from joint surveys, Jennings (1970) found some support for his approach in which failure is considered to occur partly along joints and partly along intact material. His theory can be useful only when reliable geological data about details of jointing (continuity, spacing etc.) are available. The collection and interpretation of such data is often a formidable task.

4.11   WEDGE METHOD OR SLIDING BLOCK METHOD OF TWO-DIMENSIONAL ANALYSIS

A two-dimensional analysis involving sliding along a surface consisting of two or three planes is often performed by the so called 'wedge method' or sliding block method. It is noteworthy that such sliding surfaces are realistic and have been observed in many slope failures (see Figure 4.9). Hence there is considerable incentive for using an approach based on equilibrium of wedges above a bi-planar or tri-planar failure surface.

4.11.1   Bi-planar slip surface

The potential sliding mass is separated into two wedges by a vertical line as *AB* shown in Figure 4.9(a) and the conditions for force equilibrium are considered for each wedge in turn. The forces are the weights W_1 and W_2, uplift forces due to water pressures U_1 and U_2, shearing forces T_1 and T_2, and normal forces N_1 and N_2 on the sliding surface, the water pressure U_{12} acting normal to the separation line *AB* and the effective force P_{12} between wedges acting at an inclination α to the normal. An assumption requires to be made as to the value of α. Assuming a value for the factor of safety F (=1 say) and considering the equilibrium of the first wedge, the value of the interface force P_{12} is obtained. Knowing this force, the equilibrium of the second wedge is then checked. If the forces on this wedge are not in equilibrium, the assumed value of F is incorrect and the analysis is repeated with new assumed value of F. When both wedges are in equilibrium the value of F is considered to be correct. However, the value of F is often sensitive to the assumed inclination α of the force P_{12}, particularly when the basal surface is nearly horizontal or at a steep inclination to the ground surface and also if there is high pore water pressure acting on the failure surface combined with a water-filled tension crack at the rear of the failure mass. If α is assumed to equal zero, the factor of safety F is underestimated since no shear force is assumed to be mobilised along *AB*. In short deep failure masses with high pore water pressures, this underestimate may be as much as 30%. (See also section 5.9 where reference is made to work of Hamel et al., 1976.) On the other hand, F is overestimated if α is assumed to equal the friction angle implying full mobilisation of shear force along the interface.

It is obvious that failure across the whole of the interface is not necessary to permit motion along the slip surface. For a comparison it may be useful to perform analyses with different values of α. Note that the shear strength within the sliding

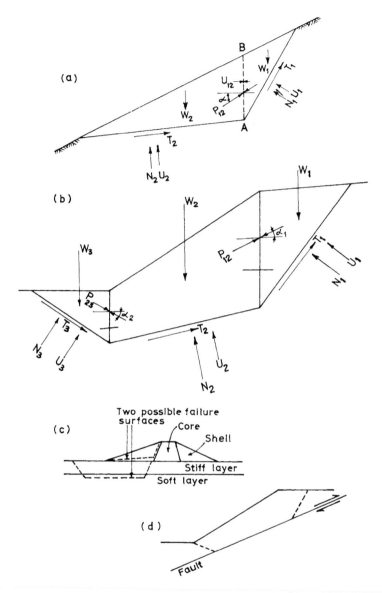

Figure 4.9 Sliding block or wedge method showing forces in (a) bi-planar (b) triplanar cases, and typical triplanar failure surfaces in (c) earth dam and (d) cut slope above a major discontinuity (a geological fault). (After J.V. Hamel, unpublished notes for continuing education short course, 1974, University of Pittsburgh, U.S.A.).

mass and hence along AB may be considerably different from that along the basal failure surface especially when the latter follows a geological discontinuity or a weak layer in the slope.

It is usual to use a graphical procedure for the wedge analysis described above. Force polygons are drawn for the two wedges with varying values of F till they both close. For any trial $T_1 = cL_1/F + N_1 \tan\phi/F$, in which L_1 is the length of the failure plane forming the base of the first wedge. Only the magnitudes of N_1 and P_{12} are unknown since values of α and F are assumed. These magnitudes are easily determined using either a graphical or an analytical procedure. Knowing P_{12} it is then possible to check the equilibrium of the second wedge in which $T_2 = cL_2/F + N_2 \tan\phi/F$. Again, either a graphical or an analytical approach may be used.

More than two wedges can be used for the solution of a problem and the procedure still remains the same as for two wedges. The equilibrium of successive wedges is analysed with different values of F. The imaginary interface line AB is usually assumed to be vertical only for convenience. Inclined interface has been used in some cases. Sultan and Seed (1967) made model studies in connection with the end-of-construction stability of a sloping core zoned earth dam. Their studies were useful not only in understanding the mechanism of failure but also in establishing the accuracy of sliding block or wedge analysis procedures (Seed and Sultan, 1967). In their studies the use of an inclined interface between wedges gave lower factor of safety (upto 8%) than the use of a vertical interface. It is not possible to say whether an overestimate of F of this order results in all cases of wedge analysis with vertical inter-wedge boundary.

4.11.2   Tri-planar slip surface

We now give some attention to a tri-planar failure surface. Three blocks or wedges may be considered as shown in Figure 4.9(b). The potential failure mass consists of an upper or active wedge, a central or neutral wedge and a lower or passive wedge. Such situations often arise e.g., when potential failure is expected through a weak layer underlying a strong layer in the foundation of an embankment or an earth dam as in Figure 4.9(c), and when potential failure is expected predominantly along discontinuities such as a joint or a fault in a natural or cut slope as shown in Figure 4.9(d). The procedure for analysis is summarized below:

Assume inter-wedge friction angles α_1 and α_2 and factor of safely F. Ordinarily F is assumed to be the same for different blocks but the circumstance may arise in which it is considered advisable to choose different values of F for different blocks. Consider the first wedge and determine P_{12} (either by solution of the two equations or by use of force polygon). Consider this force and all other relevant forces on second wedge and determine P_{23}. With this force and other known forces acting on the third wedge check the equilibrium of the third wedge. If equilibrium is not satisfied (force polygon does not close), repeat the whole procedure with a new assumed value of F until equilibrium of all wedges is satisfied. The quickest way to achieve this is to note in each trial the closing error in the force polygon, plot F versus this closing error and interpolate the value of F for zero closing error.

In any study either the whole of the slip surface location or significant parts of it may be unknown. Therefore several probable failure surfaces are analysed to determine the minimum value of F.

Recommendations for the selection of values for inter-wedge friction angles have been made by Seed and Sultan (1967) and U.S. Army Corps of Engineers (1970) in relation to the analysis of earth and rockfill dams. The latter recommendations express the mobilised friction angles at an inter-wedge boundary in terms of side slope inclination of an embankment or dam, slope material (e.g., sand, silt or clay), the depth of wedge being analysed etc. These recommendations are a good guide to the practitioner who must also exercise judgment based on past experience, sensitivity analyses and comparison with other methods of analysis.

4.12   FAILURE OF THREE-DIMENSIONAL WEDGE

It may sometimes be necessary to consider the sliding of tetrahedral blocks on a pair of surfaces. According to Jennings (1970), such failures are very common on single benches but relatively uncommon in slopes which embrace many benches. These failures are mainly associated with planes which are continuous over lengths at least equal to the height of the slope or slope segment involved. Generally the factor of safety calculated from analysis of the three-dimensional wedge is higher than that from a two-dimensional analysis considering the critical orientation. This is not surprising because in a failure involving a three-dimensional wedge, resistance to sliding will develop over a surface area of relatively greater extent in comparison to the surface area that would be considered in a two-dimensional analysis. (All boundary planes of the rock wedge may, however, not remain in contact to develop shear resistance to sliding.) During the last few decades three-dimensional wedge analysis has received a great deal of attention in connection with the possibility of failure of large blocks in dam abutments. Such studies are further complicated by the actual restrictions to movement and the thrust due to the dam itself. John (1968) and Londe et al. (1969) used the method of stereographic projection while Wittke (1965) and Goodman and Taylor (1967) used a Vector approach. Reference to work of Hoek and Bray (1974, 1977) is made in subsequent paragraphs.

In this section attention is restricted to the slope stability problem. Paulding (1970) and Jaeger (1971) considered the problem shown in Figure 4.10 and the latter obtained the equations which follow. OP_1Q and OP_2Q are the two planes of sliding which intersect along OQ with an inclination α to the horizontal. The Z direction is chosen along OQ. The coordinate axes and the angles viewed from the Z direction are shown in the figure, ψ_1 and ψ_2 being the inclination of the planes OP_1 and OP_2 to the vertical plane through OZ. Let W be the weight of the block, N_1 and N_2 the normal reactions on the planes OP_1 and OP_2, A_1 and A_2 their respective areas and S_1 and S_2 the shear resistances mobilised along them. Consider the simple case of a slope of height H and inclination i with a flat (horizontal) top and let the direction of sliding OQ be parallel to P_1P_2. Let δ_1, δ_2 be the dips and w_1, w_2, the strikes of the planes OP_1Q and OP_2Q respectively. The factor of safety against sliding is given by (Jaeger, 1971):

$$F = \left\{ \tan\phi \,(\cos\psi_1 + \cos\psi_2) + \frac{3c \,\sin i(\cos\psi_1 + \cos\psi_2)}{\gamma H \,\cos\alpha \,\sin(i-\alpha)} \right\} \cot\alpha \,\operatorname{cosec}(\psi_1 + \psi_2)$$

$$(4.69)$$

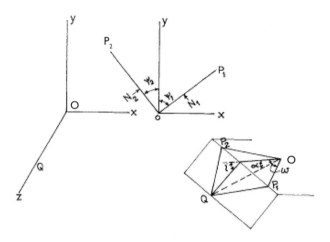

Figure 4.10 Three dimensional wedge failure.

For a symmetrical wedge, $\psi_1 = \psi_2$ and

$$F = \left\{ \tan \phi + \frac{3c \, \sin i}{\gamma \, H \, \cos \alpha \, \sin(i - \alpha)} \right\} \cot \alpha \, \mathrm{cosec} \, \psi_1 \qquad (4.69a)$$

It is interesting to note the similarity in form between Equations (4.69a) and (4.51) for a two dimensional case (α here corresponds to β in the latter equation). The factor of safety for the three dimensional case is greater since $2c$ is increased to $3c$ and there is a multiplying factor of cosec ψ_1.

The following equation applies to the general unsymmetrical case when $\psi_1 \neq \psi_2$ and where the shear strength parameters are different for the two planes (c_1, ϕ_1 and c_2, ϕ_2 respectively):

$$F = \left\{ (\tan \phi_1 \, \cos \psi_2 + \tan \phi_2 \, \cos \psi_1) + \frac{3 \, (c_1 \cos \psi_2 + c_2 \cos \psi_1) \sin i}{\gamma \, H \, \cos \alpha \, \sin(i - \alpha)} \right\}$$
$$\times \cot \alpha \, \mathrm{cosec} \, (\psi_1 + \psi_2) \qquad (4.69b)$$

Hoek and Bray (1974, 1977) outlined a general analysis of the three-dimensional wedge problem by including (a) an inclined top surface (b) a water-filled tension crack (c) water pressure along the two intersecting discontinuities, i.e., planes of sliding and (d) an external force applied by cable anchors or rock bolts. In order to minimise errors that might arise due to the cumbersome nature of the equations, tabular data sheets were proposed by them for computations. Two alternatives to the analytical solution were also explained, viz. an engineering graphics solution and a solution based on spherical projections.

The problem considered in Figure 4.10 was one in which there were two free surfaces, the surface of the slope QP_1P_2 and the horizontal top surface OP_1P_2. The situation is more complex when a tetrahedral block has only one free surface i.e., the slope face. Further, it has been assumed that sliding along both faces is the mode of failure. It may be that during the application of an external load contact is lost along one of the discontinuities so that sliding can occur only on the other plane. Also there may be a rotational mode of failure or one which involves combined sliding and rotation. The problem of stability analysis therefore requires a consideration of all these matters. A systematic and concise vector approach has been outlined by Goodman and Taylor (1967) to check the kinematics of sliding and rotation and to consider the degree of safety during sliding, and combined sliding and rotation. Jaeger and Cook (1968) also considered the restrictions on the movement of a tetrahedral wedge. (See also Hoek and Bray, 1974, 1977.)

For practical purposes the following steps may be followed in analysing three-dimensional wedge stability problems:

(1) Determine kinematically possible modes of failure considering (a) sliding on one plane (b) sliding on two planes (c) rotation or toppling. This is achieved by stereographic projection or vector analysis. (2) Use available charts (e.g., Hoek and Bray, 1974, 1977). This can lead to results of sufficient accuracy considering the numerous uncertainties in geometry, geology, shear strength, water pressures etc. (3) For more detailed or accurate analysis, one may use equations and data sheets given by Hoek and Bray (1974, 1977) or procedures outlined by Hendron (1971). In the last three decades, geotechnical software development, including rock slope stability software, has progressed a great deal. Several software products are available commercially. The reader will find the work of Goodman (1976) an excellent early reference for detailed discussion of three-dimensional stability analyses in rock.

For a review and discussion on three-dimensional aspects of slope stability problems, the reader should turn to section 5.11 of this book. That review is relevant to both soil and rock slopes.

4.13   LAYERED NATURAL DEPOSITS AND THE EFFECT OF WATER PRESSURE

4.13.1   Interbedded sand and clay layers

The importance of local geology to an understanding of slope behaviour was mentioned briefly in chapter 1. Soils are far from homogeneous and geological conditions may be quite complex. Most interesting practical situations arise when there is interbedding of permeable and impermeable strong and weak layers. Interbedded sand and clay layers or sandstone and shale beds are quite common. Let us first consider a sand layer on an impermeable clay layer whose surface makes an inclination α with the horizontal. Critical conditions will arise when seepage occurs through the sand layer. The critical angle of stability (the critical value of β) of the sand layer may be determined by equating the shear strength and shear stress at the base of an element, the base being parallel to the surface of the sand layer. The total normal stress and the shear stress on the base is (see Figure 4.11):

$$\sigma = \gamma z \cos^2 \beta, \qquad \tau = \gamma z \cos \beta \sin \beta \qquad (4.70)$$

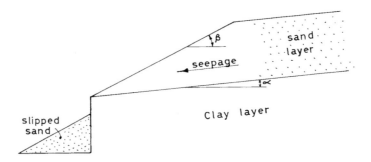

Figure 4.11 Sand layer on inclined clay layer with seepage parallel to top of clay layer.

The pore water pressure u is given by Equation (4.27) when the top flow line is inclined at angle θ to the horizontal. Critical conditions may be expected when seepage is parallel to the top of the clay layer i.e., $\theta = \alpha$. Therefore we have, from Equation (4.27):

$$u = \frac{\gamma_w z \cot \beta}{\tan \alpha + \cot \beta} \tag{4.71}$$

Equating the shearing resistance with the shear stress we have the following expression for the maximum stable angle of the sand layer, assuming ϕ to be the effective angle of shearing resistance of the sand layer:

$$\tan \beta = \left(1 - \frac{\gamma_w}{\gamma} \frac{1}{\sin \beta \cos \beta} \cdot \frac{1}{\tan \alpha + \cot \beta}\right) \tan \phi \tag{4.72}$$

When the clay layer has a horizontal surface, Equation (4.72) reduces to:

$$\tan \beta = \left(1 - \frac{\gamma_w}{\gamma} \frac{1}{\cos^2 \beta}\right) \tan \phi \tag{4.72a}$$

Considering a typical value of γ_w/γ to be 1/2, Equation (4.72a), gives $\beta = 1/2\phi$. This applies only when the top of the clay layer is horizontal. If it dips towards the slope surface, stable angle of sand increases, otherwise it decreases from the value it will have with a horizontal clay surface. In each case, erosion will reduce the angle of the sand (particularly in the lower parts) from the value given by the equation.

Henkel (1967) obtained Equation (4.72) in a different form and also considered the case when the sand layer is in between two clay layers (Figure 4.12a) and due to loss of support part of the top clay layer has fallen over the sand layer, blocking drainage. In this situation sliding of this sand-clay debris may occur on the top of the clay layer due to the water pressures even when the clay layer has a horizontal surface. The forces acting on the soil mass are shown in Figure 4.12b. Equilibrium requires that:

$$(W \cos \alpha - U_b) \tan \phi_c = W \sin \alpha + (U_u - U_d) \tag{4.73}$$

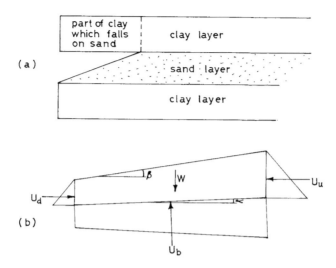

Figure 4.12 (a) Interbedded sand and clay layers (b) Forces acting when drainage has been prevented by fallen debris (after Henkel, 1967). With permission from ASCE, see page 713, No 13.

in which ϕ_c is the equivalent effective angle of friction of the clay. This angle may be obtained as follows: On the stress diagram, join the stress origin to the point where the vertical line corresponding to the effective stress in the clay layer joins the 'failure' envelope or 'failure' line. The inclination of this line is the assumed equivalent angle of friction.

Instead of using ϕ_c, it would be more precise to use directly the effective c and ϕ for the clay. Here ϕ_c is used for simplicity in explaining the concept of a stable slope angle. After substituting the values of the various water pressures, the following expression is obtained for the maximum stable angle β of the debris:

$$\tan \beta = \frac{(\tan \phi_c - \tan \alpha)\left(1 - \frac{\gamma_w}{\gamma}\right)}{\frac{\gamma_w}{\gamma}\left(1 + \tan \alpha \tan \phi_c\right) - \tan \alpha\left(\tan \phi_c - \tan \alpha\right)} \tag{4.74}$$

The value of β is maximum when $\alpha = 0$ and is equal to ϕ_c for $\gamma_w/\gamma = 1/2$. The minimum value occurs when $\alpha = \beta$ and is nearly $\frac{1}{2}\phi_c$ for $\gamma_w/\gamma = 1/2$. Therefore sliding will occur for values of β between $\frac{1}{2}\phi_c$ and ϕ_c depending on the magnitude of α. It should be noted that seepage parallel to the top of clay layer has been assumed.

The relative angles of shearing resistance of sand and clay will determine the actual slope angle considering the two mechanisms analysed above. The ϕ values for typical sands may be almost twice the ϕ_c value for clay. When the dip of the beds is towards the slope surface, the maximum stable angle in sand alone will exceed the angle required for failure in clay. Therefore failure will occur in the clay. In many cases, the supply of water may not be sufficient to maintain flow parallel to the top of the clay layer and flow may not even occur throughout the debris. Therefore, much steeper slopes may be stable for temporary periods. However, the most important conclusion is that failure at the clay-sand interface may occur even when the interface is horizontal, provided water pressures build up as explained above. It is clear from Equation (4.73) that if there is no water pressure, sliding cannot occur when $\alpha = 0$. (See section 7.10 for initial stress approach.)

4.13.2   Interbedded sandstones and shales

The behaviour of interbedded shales and sandstones is also worthy of study. Principles similar to those in the previous paragraph will, in general, apply. However, sandstones are not cohesionless like sand and, therefore, retain their form under the influence of gravitational forces and seepage. Often there may be vertical cracks and joints along the direction of strike and these will accumulate water. The pressure of water in these joints has a significant influence on the stability and determines the extent of the material likely to slide.

Consider the situation in Figure 4.13(a) which shows a layer of sandstone exposed by the erosion of the top layer of clay-shale. It is assumed that seepage is occurring in the sandstone layer parallel to the strata. Let W be the weight of the sandstone block upto a certain distance x from the exposed vertical face, U_b the total pressure due to pore water in the open joints or cracks, and U_b the total water pressure on the base. From equilibrium consideration:

$$(W \cos \beta - U_b - U_b \sin \beta) \tan \phi_c = W \sin \beta + U_b \cos \beta \qquad (4.75)$$

in which β is the dip of the strata and ϕ_c is the equivalent angle of shearing resistance of the shale as defined before. (Note that sandstones generally have higher strength and failure will usually occur in the clay shales).

In Equation (4.75) all the terms depend on x. As x increases ϕ_c required for equilibrium decreases and vice versa (Figure 4.13b). Therefore, if a value of available ϕ_c is

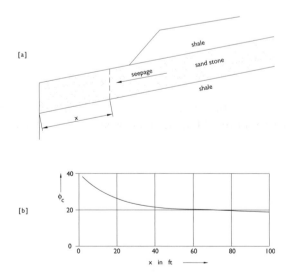

Figure 4.13 (a) Interbedded sandstones and shale. (b) Increase of failure length with decrease of ϕ_c (after Henkel, 1967). With permission from ASCE, see page 713, No 13.

known, the extent x of the sandstones which is likely to slip can be found. In Henkel's example $\beta = 10°$ and ϕ_c value of $22°$ gives failure length of 45 feet while ϕ_c value of $30°$ gives a failure length of only 13 feet. The influence of water pressure in the joints is obvious from this discussion.

Movement opens up the cracks further with consequent lowering of the water levels and slowing down or stoppage of further movement unless sufficient water is available to increase the water levels in the cracks to the original level. With permeability of the order of 10^{-6} cm per sec.(1 ft./year) and a hydraulic gradient of 0.18 for a $10°$ slope, Henkel calculated a water flow velocity of $2\frac{1}{4}$ in. per year and concluded that the total movement of the slide would be of this order unless surface water increased the water levels. Catastrophic movements would occur only if very large supplies of surface water were available at a time when critical conditions with regard to stability had already been reached. Of course, large movements could also result from decrease of shear strength e.g., due to softening or other causes discussed in chapter 2.

4.14   EARTH DAMS – PLANE FAILURE ANALYSES

4.14.1   Introduction

In general any slope stability failure associated with an earth dam would be expected to occur along a curved surface of sliding or a slip surface of arbitrary shape. The relevant methods for analysis of slope stability along slip surfaces of general shape are outlined in chapter 5. Stability charts for circular failure surfaces are often applicable for homogeneous earth dams. However, care must be exercised in selecting the seepage and pore pressure conditions, noting in particular that upstream and downstream slopes may have their lowest factor of safety at different stages. In most cases, the stability of downstream slope is critical at full reservoir when the top flow line is at its highest level and steady seepage is occurring. On the other hand, the upstream slope may have its critical factor of safety at end of construction or after rapid draw down (fall of reservoir level). These conditions were graphically illustrated in Figure 2.11.

If an earth dam has a shearing strength greater than that of its foundation it may be necessary to investigate the stability along a surface of sliding passing through the foundation of the dam in addition to the usual studies for possible failure within the dam itself. A predominantly planar failure surface develops if the weak foundation layer is relatively thin. Therefore stability may be analysed by a sliding block approach discussed briefly below in (b). Many dam cross sections are far from homogeneous and usually there is a core of material different from the shell. Thus a bi-planar or tri-planar wedge failure may take place and the method outlined in section 4.11 can be used to great advantage. Comprehensive investigations of this type have been made by Sultan and Seed (1967) and Seed and Sultan (1967). Where a weak layer occurs between strong layers the failure surface must be located predominantly in the weak layer whether it occurs in the dam or the foundation.

During a strong earthquake, a loose, cohesionless soil layer may undergo liquefaction leading to a catastrophic failure of an earth structure. (Refer to chapter 9 for earthquake effects and seismic slope analysis.) The danger of liquefaction failures in dams of granular material must be eliminated by avoiding void ratios greater than the critical. This is achieved by proper site selection followed by adequate compaction control of the fill material and adoption of soil stabilisation procedures where necessary. The higher the relative density, the lower the danger of a liquefaction failure. It should, however, be noted that the critical void ratio of any material depends on a number of factors such as stress level, stress path, strain level and rate of strain. A dam may be of the hydraulic fill type in which case a different approach must be used and this is discussed below in section 4.14.3.

It should be noted that the following simple analyses are included mainly for completeness. The reader will appreciate that real situations concerning dams are seldom so simple and it is often necessary to use more versatile procedures concerning slip surfaces of curved and composite shape as discussed in chapter 5. In general, it is best to avoid the construction of hydraulic fill dams. Yet, in spite of the associated hazards, such structures are perhaps unavoidable in connection with mine tailings dams. Even for these dams it would be advisable and often necessary to use more elaborate procedures of analysis and control. Nevertheless, simple procedures of analysis are of both academic and historical interest. Therefore a brief outline is considered appropriate here.

4.14.2   *Simple sliding block analysis*

The forces acting on a downstream sliding wedge with a vertical side and a horizontal base passing through a weak stratum are shown in Figure 4.14. Force Q represents the passive resistance of the weak soil against movement of the wedge ABC under the action of effective force P. The latter is determined from active pressure considerations since the sliding wedge is moving away from the upstream part of the dam exerting the pressure. The water pressure U also acts in the same direction as P. In addition to Q, movement is resisted by shearing resistance S along the length L of the horizontal failure surface. The weight W, vertical force V and total vertical reaction R (which includes water pressure on the base) and the vertical component of the passive pressure must balance each other and need not be considered here. Balancing the horizontal forces:

$$P + U = s_m L + Q_b \tag{4.76}$$

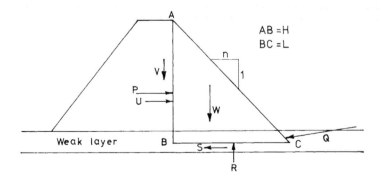

Figure 4.14 Simple sliding block analysis of earth dam with weak layer in foundation.

in which s_m is the mobilised unit shearing resistance and Q_h is the horizontal component of the passive resistance. The left hand side may be expressed as the product of an average pressure p and dam height AB. For a thin layer of weak material, Q can be ignored. L may be expressed as product of downstream slope inclination n and H. Therefore we have Taylor's (1948) expression

$$p = s_m n \tag{4.77}$$

Hence we can write:

$$p = \left(\frac{s}{F}\right)n; \quad \text{therefore,} \quad F = \left(\frac{s}{p}\right)n \tag{4.77a}$$

In this simple expression it is also assumed that the shearing resistance is independent of the normal pressure. This assumption is on the safe side but may, in fact, be too conservative.

In a realistic analysis, the passive resistance Q must not be ignored and the correct shearing resistance must be used for the weak layer. When the weak layer has considerable thickness, the failure plane must be assumed at different depths to find its critical location which gives the lowest factor of safety or highest required strength. It is also necessary to investigate the stability considering different positions of the face AB of the sliding wedge. Also AB may not be vertical. A position of AB other than that shown in the figure may be critical. Sliding block action may involve other complexities depending on the type and details of the dam cross-section (which is usually non-homogeneous), method of compaction used in the dam, consolidation and swelling characteristics of the material in the dam and foundation, erodibility of these materials, exit gradients etc.

A general limit equilibrium analysis for slip surface of arbitrary shape, or a general wedge type analysis can be used for a dam with several soil zones (and thus with complex cross sections). These methods are outlined and discussed in chapter 5.

4.14.3 Hydraulic fill dam

The critical condition for the stability of a hydraulic fill dam is generally that occurring at the end of construction when the core is still practically a viscous fluid. The method of construction using rapidly flowing mixture of soil and water is such that coarser material is deposited in the outer sections forming the shell and there is a zone of transition between the core fluid and the shell. This transition zone has somewhat finer material than the shell but much coarser than that in the core fluid. The strength of the core develops as consolidation progresses with lapse of time after construction. At the end of construction it has practically no shear strength and exerts a 'fluid' pressure P on the shell acting normal to the core shell interface (Figure 4.15). This may be calculated from the density γ_c of the core fluid. A trial failure plane BC may be assumed in the shell. There is practically no water pressure acting on this plane because the transition material along AB is so much finer than the shell material that all the head is dissipated in the transition material. The reaction R acting at an obliquity α to the assumed failure plane and the weight W of the potential failure wedge are the forces which tend to balance the core fluid pressure P. The weight W may be determined from the saturated density γ_s of the shell. Therefore, a total stress analysis

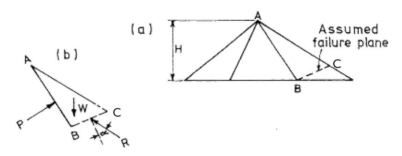

Figure 4.15 Simple stability analysis—hydraulic fill dam.

requires that forces P, W and R balance. The critical failure plane may be determined from trial and error as the one which gives the highest value for obliquity α. In each trial the magnitude and direction of reaction R can be determined graphically (from a triangle of forces) or analytically. If the maximum value of α for any failure plane is less than the angle of shearing resistance ϕ, the dam is safe and no failure can be expected at the end of construction.

Based on passive resistance considerations, Gilboy (1934) determined the ratio of the core fluid and shell densities for stability. Note that the shell offers passive resistance and P is analogous to a passive pressure which will be developed at incipient failure. Gilboy's formula derived on the basis of Coulomb's passive wedge analysis is given below:

$$\sqrt{\frac{\gamma_c}{\gamma_s}} = \frac{(n-m)\sqrt{1-\cot^2\phi}+\sqrt{n-m}\sqrt{n-\cot\phi}\sqrt{1+m^2}}{(1+n^2)-(n-m)(n-\cot\phi)} \tag{4.78}$$

in which n is the cotangent of the outer slope angle and m is the cotangent of the core slope angle. From this formula the value of γ_c which would just cause failure can be determined. The factor of safety F with respect to core fluid pressure is given by:

$$F = \frac{\gamma_c \text{ required to cause failure}}{\gamma_c \text{ actual}} \tag{4.79}$$

4.15   SLURRY TRENCH STABILITY

4.15.1   Cohesionless soil

The practice of using clay slurries to support trenches is well known. The slurry or mud is usually a bentonite suspension which forms an impermeable layer on the exposed surfaces of the soil in the walls of the trench. The slurry does not, therefore, penetrate the soil and exerts a hydrostatic pressure on the excavated faces which aids their stability. The greater the density of the slurry the greater the stability. The disturbing force is the weight of any potential sliding mass and the stabilising forces are provided by this external slurry pressure and the cohesion and friction of the soil along the assumed failure plane. The critical case is that of a cohesionless soil. Assume a plane failure surface at inclination β [(Figure 4.16(a)]. Let H be the height of the trench, mH the height of water table in soil, nH the height of drilling mud in trench, γ the bulk unit weight of soil, γ_s the bulk unit weight of slurry. Consideration of force equilibrium gives the following relationship

$$n^2 \frac{\gamma_s}{\gamma_w} = \frac{\frac{\gamma}{\gamma_w}\cot\beta\,(\sin\beta - \cos\beta\tan\phi) + m^2\,\mathrm{cosec}\,\beta\tan\phi}{\cos\beta + \sin\beta\tan\phi} \tag{4.80}$$

in which γ_w is the unit weight of water and ϕ the friction angle of the soil. This equation gives the bulk unit weight of the slurry required for assumed value of the failure plane inclination β. The maximum required density or critical density is obtained by varying β. The actual slurry density must always be greater than this critical one. The initial density of a slurry suspension is often quite low (e.g., a concentration of 4% bentonite may give 1025 kg/m³) and would not explain the stability of slurry trenches in many cases. However, cuttings from the trench often remain in suspension and increase the slurry density to higher values (say 1300 kg/m³). This was explained by Morgenstern and Tahmasseb (1965) who studied several case histories. Any slurry that is used has quite a low strength (say 0.04 lb/ft² for a 4% suspension) which does not aid the stability of the trench directly. However, this strength does explain how even sand-sized particles can remain in suspension. Morgenstern and Tabmasseb also note that if calcium montmorillonite were used in making the slurry an increased concentration would be required since it does not form an impermeable membrane as well as does sodium montmorillonite (bentonite).

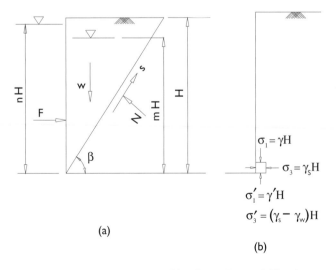

(a)

(b)

Figure 4.16 Slurry trench stability in (a) cohesionless soil (b) cohesive soil.

4.15.2   Cohesive soil – soft clay

In this case analysis may be made in terms of total or effective stresses. First consider the total stresses at the bottom of the trench side [Figure 4.16(b)]. The major principal stress is vertical and equal to γH where γ is the bulk density and the minor principal stress is $\gamma_s H$. Therefore the maximum shear stress is half the difference of principal stresses i.e., $\frac{1}{2}(\gamma - \gamma_s)H$. Equating this maximum shear stress to the undrained shear strength c we obtain:

$$\gamma_s = \gamma - \frac{2c}{H} \tag{4.81}$$

This gives a simple expression for the determination of slurry unit weight γ_s required to prevent failure. A factor of safety would, of course, be required for design.

Now consider the principal effective stresses for a soil element at the bottom of the side of the excavation. Assuming ground water level at the surface the major principal effective stress is $\gamma'H$ acting vertically and the minor principal effective stress is again horizontal and equal to $(\gamma_s - \gamma_w) H$. These are related at failure by the Terzaghi-Coulomb shear strength equation. (Excavation usually results in temporary negative excess pore pressures which are ignored here.) Therefore the following relationship is obtained:

$$\gamma_s = \gamma_w + \frac{\gamma'}{N_\phi} - \frac{2c}{H\sqrt{N_\phi}} \tag{4.82}$$

in which $N_\phi = \tan^2\left(45° + \frac{\phi}{2}\right)$, the well known flow value or flow number.

The analysis in terms of effective stress may be extended to include excess pore pressures and complex boundary conditions. As regards total stress analysis, Aas (1976) has given attention to the use of undrained shear strength from vane tests in an analysis.

Chapter 5

Limit equilibrium methods II – general slip surfaces and beyond critical equilibrium

5.1 INTRODUCTION AND SCOPE

This scope of this chapter includes conventional limit equilibrium methods for general slip surfaces, from the simplest to the advanced, as well as the most important developments during the last 30 years. Essential considerations in geotechnical slope analysis are outlined at different stages of this chapter. These include the choice between effective stress analysis and total stress analysis, the shape of slip surfaces and how that affects the choice of a suitable method of analysis. A procedure is presented to incorporate the effect of strain-softening and stress redistribution on the stability of a slope within the framework of a limit equilibrium analysis. There are several references to important case studies and to lessons learnt from them. Post-failure behaviour of slopes is also considered and the relevant sections include information on some exceptional landslides. However, it is outside the scope of this chapter to deal comprehensively with the subject of post-failure behaviour and landslide mobility. Therefore, introducing just the key concepts is considered appropriate. Finally, methods for the improvement of slope stability are summarized. This is also a vast subject and the coverage here is just sufficient to indicate the relevance to slope analysis.

The following discussion concerning drainage conditions and the choice of analysis related to them is also relevant to the methods of limit equilibrium already considered in Chapter 4.

5.1.1 Drainage conditions – choice between effective stress and total stress analysis

Understanding the drainage conditions in a slope is very important for correctly formulating the problem for analysis and for the choice of shear strength parameters to be used in the analysis. Analysis is often required at different stages of a project, such as 'end-of-construction' and 'long-term' stability. Additional analysis would be required for a project with multi-stage construction. Separate analyses would be required for rapid draw-down of water level where it is appropriate. For each of these stages a choice must be made between effective stress and total stress analysis.

For slopes of cohesionless soils, effective stress analysis is appropriate in all cases. However, for relatively impermeable, cohesive soils, total stress analysis is often valid for short-term (undrained) conditions while effective stress analysis is essential for stability analysis related to long-term fully drained conditions. For intermediate conditions, it is best to carry out effective stress analyses with a knowledge of pore water pressure distribution along the slip surface. This knowledge may be based on observation, testing or theoretical estimates.

For end-of-construction or short-term conditions, total stress analysis may be performed with shear strength from in-situ or undrained laboratory tests (UU or CU). For multi-stage construction of slope or for drawdown conditions, either a total stress or an effective stress analysis may be performed. For effective stress analysis, estimates of pore water pressure are required in addition to effective stress parameters of shear strength. For total stress analysis, shear strength should be obtained from undrained laboratory or field tests (e.g., field vane shear tests) carried out under loading condition which correctly represents the field conditions.

Not all soils are impermeable to the same degree as there is a wide range of soil permeabilities over several orders of magnitude. The question often arises: "Where should the line be drawn between drained and undrained conditions and what about the soils which cannot be regarded as either fully drained or fully undrained?"

According to Duncan (1992), soils with permeability greater than 10^{-4} cm/sec may be regarded as drained and those with permeability less than 10^{-7} cm/sec should be regarded as undrained. Alternatively, consider the value of the dimensionless time factor T of basic consolidation theory. A soil with a value of $T > 3$ can be regarded as drained and a soil with $T < 0.01$ may be regarded as undrained. If permeability or T values are within these extremes, then both undrained and drained analyses should be performed and a range of factor of safety values obtained for decision-making.

What pore water pressures should be used in the analyses? For all effective stress analyses, especially those for natural slopes, the pore water pressures should be estimated on the basis of observations provided that monitoring of the pressures has been carried out at the particular depths which are of interest. (See chapter 11 for case studies of urban slope stability.) Where seepage pore water pressures are applicable, a seepage analysis should be carried out for the estimation of the pore water pressures. Care should be taken to check for the presence of any artesian pore water pressures not only for natural slopes but also for man-made slopes within a hilly area. For total stress analyses, pore water pressures are assumed to be zero. Pore water pressures generated during undrained conditions are difficult to estimate and this is an important reason for adopting a total stress analysis. In all analyses, total unit weights of soils are to be used and any external water pressures acting on the face of the slope are to be included.

The reader should refer to section 5.13 for further detailed discussion concerning the choice between total stress and effective stress analysis procedures.

5.1.2   Shapes of slip surfaces

The failure of slopes in cohesive material is usually preceded by the formation and opening of tension cracks at the crest. This is followed in many cohesive soils by movement along a curved surface of sliding. According to Terzaghi and Peck (1967), the cross-section of such a surface has the least curvature at the upper end, greatest in the middle, and intermediate at the lower end; and it often resembles the arc of an ellipse. Other shapes such as the cycloid have also been mentioned in the literature. However, in stability analysis involving homogeneous soils, a slip surface is usually assumed to be circular in shape. In some cases it is assumed to be the arc of a logarithmic spiral. Taylor (1948) demonstrated that for simple homogeneous slopes the results of stability analyses based on logarithmic spiral slip surfaces are almost identical to those based on slip surfaces of circular shape. This has also been confirmed by Chen (1975) who used the limit analysis technique of plasticity (see chapter 8). The use of failure surfaces of log spiral shape in stability problems has been demonstrated by Terzaghi (1943) and Chen (1975) and the interested reader will find these books valuable.

Most observed slip surfaces are of arbitrary shape and modern slope analysis methods enable engineers to handle such slope problems with confidence. Approximations of slip surfaces by given shapes are based primarily on convenience and have proved useful in soil mechanics. Circular failure surfaces have not only proved useful for limit equilibrium studies concerning soils but have also been assumed for stability studies of slopes in soft rocks in which the mechanical properties are not dominated by structural features and discontinuities (Hoek, 1970; Hoek and Bray, 1974, 1977). In the last four decades much progress has been made in slope analysis and slip surfaces of arbitrary shape can be handled by a number of methods of analysis. With the development of specialized geotechnical software, the general use of alternative methods has also been facilitated. It is thus no longer necessary to approximate a slip surface of arbitrary shape by an arc of a circle in order to carry out a slope analysis.

For built-up slopes, distinction is made between base failure, slope failure and toe failure. In the first case the failure surface intersects the ground at some distance beyond the toe; in the second case it intersects the slope above the toe; and in the last case it passes through the toe. Base failure may indicate that the soil below the toe is unable to support the overburden pressure of the soil behind the slope. When a firm stratum is located at shallow depth, the surface for base failure is often tangent to the top of this stratum. Toe failure is most common in frictional soils and base failure may, therefore, indicate that '$\phi = 0$' conditions prevailed at the time of failure (or that weaker material was located below the toe of the slope). Possibility of slope failure arises when there is a relatively weak zone in the upper part of the slope or when the downward movement is restricted by the presence of a strong stratum at or above the level of the toe.

5.1.3 Estimating minimum factor of safety associated with a critical slip surface

This topic has been introduced briefly in chapters 3 and 4 and the following is a continuation of the discussion.

Within a slope, many potential slip surfaces, of whatever shape, can be considered for analysis of limit equilibrium. Each of these slip surfaces will have a different factor of safety. It follows that the minimum of these values is to be regarded as the relevant value of F. The slip surface with which this minimum value is associated is called a 'critical slip surface'. Thus a performance function such as the factor of safety has to be optimized in order to determine the shape and location of the critical slip surface and the associated magnitude of the minimum factor of safety. This is an important part of slope analysis and is explained further in section 5.2 dealing with short-term stability of clay slopes assuming slip surfaces of circular shape. However, the concept of critical slip surface applies to all limit equilibrium methods of slope stability considered throughout this chapter, whether the slip surfaces are of circular or arbitrary shape. Optimisation is an essential aspect of slope analysis under all conditions of construction, loading or drainage. It is unnecessary only in cases where there are one or more pre-existing slip surfaces within a slope and where analysis is to be made for potential reactivation of instability involving these pre-existing slip surfaces.

In addition to the conventional method based on repeated trials, optimization procedures include direct search methods, combination of repetitive trials and direct search methods, as well as dynamic programming.

The factor of safety is, in general, a non-linear performance function. Consequently, the nonlinear programming approach of optimization has been widely used for locating the critical slip surface by means of minimization of factor of safety. Examples of this approach include the penalty function formulation, also known as the Sequential Unconstrained Minimization Technique (SUMT), (Basudhar, 1976; Greco and Gulla, 1985; Greco, 1988; Bhattacharya, 1990; Bhattacharya and Basudhar, 2001), dynamic programming technique (Baker, 1980), alternating variable technique (Celestino and Duncan, 1981; Li and White, 1987), conjugate-gradient method (Arai and Tagyo, 1985), simplex reflection technique (Nguyen, 1985; De Natale, 1991). More recently, the Monte-Carlo method of the random walking type has also been proposed (Greco, 1996; Husein Malkawi et al., 2001a, b).

The most important merit of the penalty function methods is their flexibility; one can easily add or delete constraints, modify the objective function or constraints and interchange the roles of various parts of the problem (Fox, 1971). A critical appraisal of the application of optimization techniques to a wide variety of slope stability problems, has been presented by Bhattacharya (1990) and comprehensive reviews have also been presented by Zhang (1989) and Dawei (1994).

Optimisation may be based on the reliability index rather than the factor of safety especially if the analysis is being carried out within a probabilistic framework. It is important to note that the shape and location of the critical slip surface based on the reliability index as the performance function will, in general, be different from the shape and location based on the factor of safety. Different search and optimisation methods for slope stability problems involving slip surfaces of arbitrary shape have been developed and used by Nguyen (1985), Zhang (1989), Dawei (1994) and, Bhattacharya and Basudhar (2001) and Basudhar and Bhattacharya (2008). A number of examples have been solved considering either the factor of safety or the reliability index as a performance function (Bhattacharya et al., 2003).

5.1.4 Tension crack location and depth as part of optimisation process

It is well known that vertical or near-vertical tension cracks may occur in slopes as discussed in section 4.5.2. Sometimes such cracks are clearly visible but in other cases their presence may not be obvious. For any slope such a crack is likely to occur near the crest although the exact location may not be known for existing slopes nor predicted in advance for man-made slopes at the design stage. Tension cracks in a slope may get filled with water from precipitation, exerting an additional disturbing force which must be considered in stability analysis.

The formation of a deep crack or gap, by whatever process, can have catastrophic consequences in exceptional circumstances. An important recent example has become available after post-failure investigations of levee failures in New Orleans associated with the impact of Hurricane Katrina. Along some sections, I-walls were used along with the levees as part of the Hurricane Protection System (HPS).

Due to deflection of the I-wall under the load of the storm surge, a deep gap was formed along the I-wall on the flood side. The mechanism of failure was changed and the computed factor of safety was significantly reduced (Brandon et al., 2008; Duncan et al., 2008). The changed failure mechanism was able to explain the occurrence of those levee failures which were not due to overtopping followed by erosion. For more details refer to sections 1.2 and 1.7 and the 'important note' at the end of Example 5.3 in this chapter.

Experience has shown that the inclusion of a tension crack in slope analysis is also useful for computational reasons. Most limit equilibrium methods for slip surfaces of curved or arbitrary shape require iterative solutions. The inclusion of a water-filled tension crack facilitates convergence of such solutions. The depth of tension crack may be estimated in advance on the basis of theory [for example, Equation 4.44(a)]. Alternatively, the optimum location and depth of such crack may be determined as part of the particular limit equilibrium method of analysis. An efficient optimisation method enables the critical location and depth of a tension crack to be determined as part of the search for the critical slip surface (Zhang, 1989; Bhattacharya, 1990).

5.1.5   Back analysis of failed slopes and landslides

On the basis that occurrence of failure indicates a factor of safety value $F = 1$, an estimate of one or more shear strength parameters may be made after analysis of data from a failed slope. Firstly, however, detailed investigation must be carried out concerning the circumstances associated with the failure such as the triggering mechanism and the pore pressures at the site. It is important to learn about the type of failure and the mechanism. The shape and location of the slip surface can be inferred from surface and subsurface investigations. With a knowledge of the ground surface profile at the time of failure and the slip surface location, stability analyses may be carried out with trial values of shear strength parameters. (Some case studies of back-analysis are included in chapter 11.)

If total stress analysis is appropriate, knowledge or assumption of pore pressures along the slip surface may not be necessary. For example, this would be the case for short-term failure in a cut slope of saturated clay. Where effective stress analysis is appropriate, knowledge or assumption of pore pressures is important. One may work on the basis of the most likely piezometric surface or the most likely value of the average pore water pressure ratio. From limit equilibrium analyses, different combinations of the two shear strength parameters which all result in $F = 1$ can be estimated. It is then useful to plot one shear strength parameter against the other. This would be a plot of c versus ϕ for a specific piezometric surface or a specific average pore water pressure ratio [see Figure 5.1(b)]. If one of the shear strength parameters for the soil is known from past experience (shear strength testing, analyses of previous failures etc.), the other parameter may then be estimated with confidence.

If the pore water pressure is not known reliably, a series of c versus ϕ curves may be plotted, each associated with one pore water pressure condition. Each point on any of these curves would, of course, correspond to $F = 1$. Where one of the shear strength parameters, such as cohesion, is known reliably but the pore pressure is unknown, it would be preferable to plot ϕ against the average pore pressure ratio. For example, reactivation of a landslide along an existing slip surface is associated with residual value of angle of internal friction and zero (or near-zero) cohesion. Thus one may plot residual angle of internal friction versus the average pore pressure ratio, all points on the curve corresponding to $F = 1$ (refer case studies in chapter 11).

If two failures have occurred within a given region in the same type of soil, two c versus ϕ curves can be plotted from back-analyses, one for each failure. From the intersection of these two curves, a single pair of values (specific values of c and ϕ) can thus be determined.

Back analysis can be improved significantly if limit equilibrium analyses include optimisation to determine the critical slip surface location. A powerful and flexible limit equilibrium method is required for this type of analysis. For the same slope and for a given pore pressure condition, a particular combination of the two shear strength parameters will lead to a specific critical slip surface. As the value of the cohesion parameter increases, the depth of the critical slip surface also increases in homogeneous soil. (Accordingly the size of the potential sliding mass also increases.) The aim should be to determine a combination of c and ϕ which leads to a critical slip surface very close to the observed critical slip surface as well as a value of $F = 1$. This combination would then be the correct one for the particular case study. A suitable method and some numerical examples from the work of Zhang (1989) are presented in section 5.5.3 of this chapter.

Bhattacharya and Basudhar (1996) developed a back-analysis algorithm based on Janbu's generalised procedure of slices coupled with the Sequential Unconstrained Minimization Technique (SUMT) of optimization wherein no iteration is needed to match the predicted and the observed failure surface. In this approach, one can study the importance of imposing some side constraints defining the interval within which the parameters are most likely to lie.

Several open-pit mining failure cases were analysed by Stead (1984) using the usual approach for back analysis and later also by Zhang (1989) using a more sophisticated approach which includes the determination of critical slip surface. Guided by the shape of the observed slip surface in each case, back analyses of some of the case studies were based on the assumption of circular shape of computed slip surfaces whereas other case studies allowed the slip surfaces to be of arbitrary shape. The slope geometry for one of these cases is shown in Figure 5.1(a), along with the observed failure surface and three "predicted" critical slip surfaces of circular shape. The results of conventional back analysis are plotted as c versus ϕ curves for different pore pressure ratios r_u as shown in Figure 5.1(b). For one of the pore pressure ratios ($r_u = 0.0$), Table 5.1(a) shows the three combinations of the shear strength parameters corresponding to the three predicted critical slip surfaces. One of these surfaces is very close to the observed critical slip surface and the associated value of F is very close to 1. Therefore, this is the specific combination of c and ϕ which best explains the failure. Obviously, such a conclusion could not be reached by using conventional back analysis.

For the same case, combinations of c and ϕ were also determined for two other values of the average pore pressure ratio as shown in Table 5.1(b).

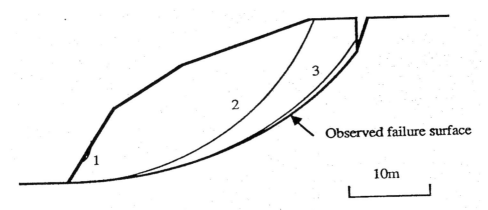

Figure 5.1(a) Back-analysis of Glyn Glas failure (after Zhang, 1989, based on Stead, 1984). With permission, see page 713, No 14.

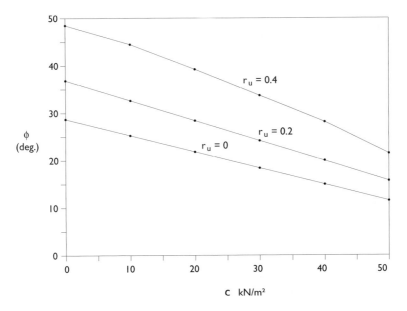

Figure 5.1(b) Results of conventional back-analysis for Glyn Glas failure (after Zhang, 1989, based on Stead, 1984). With permission, see page 713, No 14.

Table 5.1(a) Results of back analysis for Glyn Glas failure for $r_u = 0$ (Zhang, 1989). With permission, see page 713, No 14.

Slip surface	c (kN/m²)	ϕ (deg.)	F_m	F_o
1	0	29	0.25	0.97
2	25	21	0.96	1.00
3	50	12	1.05	1.06

Table 5.1(b) Back-analysis results for three values of pore pressure ratio, r_u (Zhang, 1989). With permission, see page 713, No 14.

r_u	c (kN/m²)	ϕ (deg.)	F_m	F_0
0	50	12	1.05	1.06
0.2	50	16	1.05	1.05
0.4	50	21	0.99	0.99

Note: Tables 5.1(a) and 5.1(b),
F_m: Factor of safety along predicted critical slip surfaces (1, 2, and 3).
F_0: Factor of safety along the observed failure surface.
$\gamma = 23$ kN/m³.

5.1.6   The concept of a resistance envelope

Some limit equilibrium methods were considered in chapter 4 and several others are discussed in the following sections of this chapter. In all these methods it is customary to determine minimum factors of safety by assuming trial surfaces or by adopting other optimisation procedures. A different approach can be adopted in accordance with the principle of a resistance envelope corresponding to critical or limiting equilibrium (factor of safety, $F = 1$) first explained by Casagrande (1950) and later emphasised by Janbu (1977). Several slip surfaces within a slope are assumed as usual. Using an appropriate method of analysis, the average shear strength required for critical equilibrium ($F = 1$) along each of these surfaces is determined. At the same time the average effective normal stress along each of these surfaces is also determined corresponding, in each case, to critical equilibrium or $F = 1$. The average mobilized shear strength is then plotted against the average effective normal stress. Therefore, one point on the plot represents the critical equilibrium of one assumed slip surface. When all such points are joined we get a curve called a resistance envelope. On the same diagram, the shear strength envelope of the soil is also plotted. The calculated factor of safety with respect to each slip surface or at any level of average normal stress is indicated by the vertical distance between the resistance envelope and the strength envelope (Figure 5.2). It is important to note that a resistance envelope is independent of strength parameters for given geometry of slope and given pore water pressure conditions.

An even better use of the diagram can be made as follows. By changing the relative magnitudes of c and ϕ, different strength envelopes can be drawn and the effect of variations in c and ϕ can be clearly understood from the position of the resistance envelope in relation to the strength envelopes. Resistance envelopes may be drawn in terms of both total and effective stresses and corresponding strength envelopes may also be drawn for both total and effective stresses. This concept is illustrated in Figure 5.2.

The mobilisation of strength parameters c and ϕ at different strains can be studied by plotting stress paths from the results of appropriate laboratory tests. On each stress path percentage strain is shown at different points up to failure. Then points with equal strain are joined together giving lines or curves of mobilised strength at different strains. From these curves it is easy to see how the mobilisation of c and ϕ changes with increasing strain. Often cohesion (or attraction which is the negative intercept on the normal stress axis and equals $c \cot \phi$) is fully mobilised at low strains while friction is mobilised fully only at strains close to failure. Differences in the degree of mobilisation of cohesion and friction were first shown by Schmertmann and

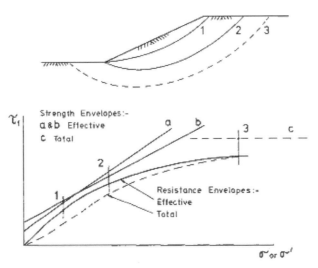

Figure 5.2 Resistance envelopes in terms of effective stress and total stress plotted along with corresponding strength envelopes. Two positions of effective stress envelope are shown. Positions 1, 2, 3 indicate levels of normal stress corresponding to trial slip surfaces shown in the upper diagram.

Osterberg (1961). In view of such differences in most cohesive soils, it is evident that resistance envelopes can be very useful since different strength lines corresponding to different mobilisation levels can be studied in relation to a resistance envelope for a given slope with known pore water pressure conditions.

5.2   SHORT-TERM STABILITY OF CLAY SLOPES

In this and several following sections, we consider methods of two-dimensional (2-D) analysis of slope stability problems, starting with the simplest methods and then covering more general methods with wider application and better accuracy. A real slip surface is idealized to be of cylindrical form. The shape of the cross-section of such a cylinder is assumed as either circular or non-circular (arbitrary shape). Three dimensional (3-D) effects and analyses are discussed mainly in section 5.12.

5.2.1   Slopes in soft clay – circular failure surfaces

5.2.1.1   Factor of safety for a given slip surface based on moment equilibrium

The factor of safety F against failure of a slope along a circular surface of sliding (Figure 5.3) is obtained as a ratio of resisting to disturbing moments taken about the centre of the slip circle. Thus,

$$F = \frac{sR^2\theta}{Wx} \tag{5.1}$$

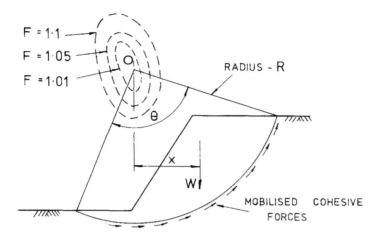

Figure 5.3 Circular failure surface in soft clay. Contours show location of centres of other trial circles and corresponding factors safety.

in which s is the average shear strength along the slip surface, R is the radius, θ is the central angle of the circular arc, and the weight W of the potential sliding mass acts at a horizontal distance x from O, the centre of the slip circle.

The analysis would be improved by including a water-filled tension crack. The moment due to this additional disturbing force would mean an additional term in the denominator of Equation (5.1), leading to more realistic modeling and a conservative solution. The estimate of factor of safety will be lower than if the water-filled crack is not included.

Modification of Equation (5.1) to include end effects is discussed in section 5.12. The shearing strength s is often assumed to be constant for a homogeneous soft clay under undrained '$\phi = 0$' conditions. Reference has already been made in chapter 2 to the '$\phi = 0$' concept for saturated soils in which failure occurs without change in volume. Under these conditions, the undrained shearing strength (or the undrained cohesion) is taken to be equal to half the unconfined compressive strength q_u i.e.,

$$s = c = \frac{1}{2}q_u \tag{5.2}$$

A better estimate of undrained shear strength results from a series of undrained triaxial tests. Correction factors may be applied to account for sample disturbance, reorientation of stresses etc. It is generally considered desirable to make use of undrained shear strength from field tests such as the shear vane tests and the cone penetration test. The results of these tests may also be used with suitable correction factors based on experience. It is useful to remember that even under '$\phi = 0$' conditions, the undrained shear strength often varies with the depth within a deposit of clay. In most soft clays, the value of undrained cohesion increases with depth and is proportional to the effective overburden pressure (See also section 8.2). Again, if there are several layers of clay, each would have a different value of undrained cohesion c (or the undrained shear strength s).

Reference has already been made to the back analysis of a failed slope in order to estimate the shear strength. Equation (5.1) may be used to estimate the average value of shear strength of soil at a site where a short-term failure has already occurred. Setting $F = 1$ (for conditions at the instant of failure) and substituting appropriate measured or estimated values for R, θ, W and x, s is easily calculated.

5.2.1.2   Locating the critical slip surface

In assessing the stability of a given slope a minimum value of F is required. This will correspond to the critical slip surface, the location of which may be found by trial and error. A number of possible slip circles are analysed and values of corresponding factors of safety noted at their centres. From contour of factors of safety thus obtained, the centre of the critical circle, the circle with the least factor of safety, is determined (Figure 5.3). The trial and error procedure for locating the critical slip surface is not efficient. As stated earlier in section 5.1.3, a variety of alternative methods have been developed for locating critical slip surfaces of both both circular and non-circular shape under a variety of drainage conditions. These alternatives are, in fact, different procedures for optimization of the performance function for slope stability which, for deterministic solutions, is the function for factor of safety, F.

5.2.1.3   Stability charts

Before the advent of the computer age, performing repetitive calculations was a tedious job. Consequently, stability charts were devised to reduce the repetitive labour to a minimum (Taylor, 1937). As mentioned in chapter 4, the concept of a stability factor N_S is useful in this regard and is defined as:

$$N_S = \frac{\gamma H}{c} \qquad (5.3)$$

in which H is the critical height of a slope, γ its unit weight and c its unit cohesion which is often replaced by the symbol for mobilised cohesion c_m. For $\phi = 0$ analyses the value of N_S depends only on the slope angle β and a depth factor n_d which is the ratio of (a) depth to a firm base (or hard layer) and (b) the slope height. For base failure (which often occurs with the critical surface tangent to a firm base located at shallow depth) it has been found that the centre of the critical circle is located on a vertical line through the midpoint of the slope.

Taylor's stability chart for '$\phi = 0$' conditions in homogeneous clay deposits is shown in Appendix II. Taylor (1937) also gave chart for locating the centre and radius of the critical circular failure surfaces in simple, homogeneous slopes. In layered deposits the critical slip surface is located predominantly in the weakest layer and fewer trials are necessary to determine the minimum factor of safety. An interesting solution for the undrained stability problem in clay whose strength increases linearly with depth is discussed in section 8.2. This solution is relevant to real deposits of normally consolidated clay. Reference is also made in that section to an alternative solution to the same problem based on the classical theory of plasticity.

5.2.2   Undrained strength of soft clay in relation to analysis (simple and advanced 'total stress' approaches)

Analyses which rely only on the undrained shear strength of clay slopes are based on a 'total stress' approach. In reality, the behaviour of all soils is determined by effective stresses which require knowledge of pore water pressures. A simple 'total stress' analysis can be carried out without knowledge of the effective normal stresses on the failure plane. Therefore it is not necessary to determine the pore water pressures which are developed during the construction of embankments or the excavation of cuts. The undrained strength is usually based on simple unconfined or triaxial compression tests or on in-situ tests such as the shear vane test and various cone tests. The current trend is to emphasise that knowledge of stress paths in terms of total and effective stresses is very useful and, therefore, it is advisable to study the 'effective stress' behaviour of a clay in addition to measuring its undrained shear strength.

It may be justified to avoid prediction of effective stresses and pore pressures for embankments since the loads imposed usually exceed the preconsolidation load of a soft clay foundation and stress paths approach the horizontal undrained shear strength line. However, there is justification for studying effective stress behaviour as far as unloading situations (excavations) are concerned since the stress paths may not approach the horizontal undrained shear strength envelope.

Improved or advanced total stress analyses have also been suggested. In these procedures, the testing program is designed to simulate different types of failure zones in a subsoil e.g., active (A), direct shear (D) and passive zone (P). This type of analysis, abbreviated as ADP analysis, was developed at the Norwegian Geotechnical Institute (Bjerrum, 1973; Aas 1976). Anisotropically consolidated undrained tests (in extension as well as in compression) are performed on clay specimens from different depths. Variations of both types of strength with depth are plotted. Similar variation is studied using direct simple shear tests. These strength relationships are used for relevant zones of the soil mass. Another advanced procedure is the SHANSEP (Ladd and Foott, 1974) developed at M.I.T. (SHANSEP stands for 'stress history and normalised soil engineering properties'). These procedures are much too complex for the ordinary practitioner who has little guidance as to the circumstances under which a simple, inexpensive, total stress analysis must be discarded. Janbu (1977) noted that there was little evidence to assess advanced procedures of total stress analysis. Even so, he cautioned that use of simple total stress analyses for excavations in clay would frequently lead to errors in calculated factors of safety and in locations of slip surfaces.

Finally it is important to note that theoretically the most accurate analysis would be one which is based on 'effective stress' approach. Unfortunately, prediction of pore water pressures during construction of embankments and excavations is difficult. The use of pore pressure parameters would enable approximate estimates to be made in advance of construction. If pore pressures are monitored during construction, analyses could then be revised at appropriate stages of a project. Effective stress analyses are, of course, expensive and there may not be sufficient justification for their use in relation to routine problems of short-term stability.

5.2.3 Stiff clays

There is no theoretical or practical justification for the use of '$\phi = 0$' concept in relation to stiff clays even when they are fully saturated. This is due to the fact that such clays are heavily overconsolidated and have a tendency to increase in volume during shear with consequent development of negative pore water pressures. As a result of negative pore pressures, these clays have a tendency to increase in water content accompanied by pore water migration. Increase in water content results in a decrease of their shear strength. Therefore, as was pointed out in chapter 2, the use of '$\phi = 0$' concept is unconservative and unsafe. Clays which are lightly overconsolidated with an overconsolidation ratio less than about 4 may be considered in the same way as normally consolidated clays. However, care must be exercised in determining the undrained shear strength parameters of heavily overconsolidated clay for use in an analysis concerned with short-term stability. In all routine problems, a total stress type of analysis may be used provided reliable values of total stress parameters, c and ϕ, for short term loading and representative of in-situ conditions, can be measured or estimated.

Measured undrained strength of stiff clays is influenced by sample disturbance, rate of loading, sample size and stress paths used for testing. Sample size is of tremendous importance in regard to fissured clays (heavily overconsolidated clays are often jointed and fissured). The operational strength of these clays is much less than their intact strength although it is somewhat higher than the strength along fissures. Reference was made in chapter 2 to a relationship between specimen size and shear strength proposed by Lo (1970). The spacing of fissures and their orientation may have a significant influence on strength. Attention should also be given to anisotropy of undrained strength which is generally attributed to pore pressure effects but may also be caused by several other factors. In general study of large scale behaviour gives a far better indication of in-situ strength than results of conventional triaxial compression tests which may be regarded as no more than an index (Morgenstern, 1977). A large range of strengths may be obtained by varying stress paths, orientation of principal stresses, sample size etc. It is also unwise to judge the strength of one clay deposit by comparing it with another deposit although the two deposits may have many similarities.

Unloading due to excavations can cause significant swelling and pore pressure changes and the only correct procedure would be to perform analyses in terms of effective stresses. Estimates of pore pressure would have to be based on calculated total stress changes and pore pressure coefficients for unloading. It is of interest to know the duration of undrained behaviour so that the limits can be defined within which a 'total stress' analysis can reasonably be applied. Long-term equilibrium pore pressures depend on seepage considerations only. With these boundary pore water pressure conditions (initial and long-term), change in pore pressure with time may be estimated by solving a two-dimensional swelling problem (Eigenbrod, 1975; Walbancke, 1975). Size effects are also important in measuring the coefficient of swelling of fissured clays. Prediction of local pore pressures in fissured clays is also complicated by the fact that infiltration of rainfall and surface water in open joints can increase the pore pressure while swelling during deformation reduces the pore pressure. In some clays discontinuities may be so well connected that assumption of undrained behaviour is invalid regardless of the magnitude of the coefficient of swelling.

5.2.4   Proportion of fissures from back analysis

Skempton and La Rochelle (1965) estimated the strength of fissured clay at Bradwell by performing back-analysis in terms of total stresses. It is useful to refer to their discussion of various factors influencing this estimated field strength. Strength along open fissures was considered to be zero, that along closed fissures to be c_j and that along intact soil equal to the peak strength c. Let L be the total length of the slip surface and $\bar{c}$ the average shear strength at failure as given by back analysis. Let L_1 be the effective slip surface length offering resistance to shear failure. This is obtained by subtracting from L a portion passing through 'burst' clay which is that portion where local bulging may occur following excavation due to relief of high horizontal stresses present in heavily overconsolidated clays. About 3 ft. on the surface of slopes at Bradwell was regarded to be in the 'burst' zone and shear strength within this zone was regarded as zero. Now for the length L_1, let f be the proportion passing through fissures, x being open fissures and $(f - x)$ closed fissures [the part $L_1 (1 - f)$ passes through intact clay]. It is assumed that a proportion r of the slip surface passes through intact soil which has been reduced by progressive failure to the residual strength c_r. Therefore peak undrained strength c applies to length $L_1 (1 - f - r)$ and residual undrained strength applies to length $L_1 r$. Equating the total strength based on average unit strength to that obtained in terms of various components:

$$\bar{c}\,L = L_1\,[c_j\,(f - x) + c_r r + c\{1 - (f + r)\}] \tag{5.4}$$

This equation is useful in computing the total proportion f of fissures in a clay mass, provided reasonable assumptions can be made concerning (a) the proportion of open to closed fissures, and (b) softening by progressive failure. As an example Skempton and La Rochelle considered $c = 1600$ lbs/sq. ft., $c_j = c_r = 900$ lbs/sq. ft., $x = 0.25\,f$, $r = 0.2\,(1 - f)$. With known values of $\bar{c} = 1120$ lbs/sq. ft., $L = 60$ ft. and $L_1 = 57$ ft., they obtained the proportion of fissures $f = 0.35$. In addition to the various factors considered above there may be softening of the clay due to its tendency under negative pore pressures (caused by excavation) to absorb water from the open fissures which have positive pore pressures due to seepage of surface and rain water. Such softening may reduce both the intact and residual undrained strengths (in terms of effective stresses the effective cohesion intercept is almost eliminated and the angle of shearing resistance somewhat reduced). After making reasonable assumptions (of a hypothetical nature nevertheless), Skempton and La Rochelle concluded that the proportion of fissures at Bradwell was between 20 and 45%. Since the fissure strength is close to the residual strength, fissure proportion is approximately equal to the residual factor R defined in chapter 2. Thus a value of R between 0.2 and 0.45 applies to the clay before long-term changes in water content and associated progressive failure effects are taken into consideration.

It is unfortunate that more case records of short-term failure in stiff clays are not available. The procedure outlined above has not been re-examined in recent years. It would be useful to have similarly documented case records enabling researchers to take a fresh look at available procedures of analysis concerning stiff fissured clays.

5.3   FRICTION CIRCLE METHOD (c, ϕ SOILS)

This method is historically very significant in the development of slope analysis. It also facilitated the first use of slope stability charts with dimensionless parameters. Although no longer widely used, it is important for facilitating an understanding of some basic concepts concerning slope analysis.

The method is useful for homogeneous soils in which the shear strength is dependent on the normal stress. In other words, it may be used when both cohesive and frictional components of shear strength have to be considered in the calculations. The method is equally suitable for total stress or effective stress types of analysis in homogeneous soils.

The resultant mobilized cohesive force C along a slip surface ab (Figure 5.4) is replaced by a force of the same magnitude C parallel to the chord ab of length L and acting at a distance x from the centre of the circle given by:

$$Cx = c_m Lx = c_m \,\overarc{ab}\, R$$

$$x = \frac{\overarc{ab}}{L} R$$

(5.5)

where, c_m is the mobilized cohesion assumed constant along the arc ab.

When there is no pore water pressure, the stability of the slope can be represented by three forces, the known weight W, the mobilized cohesive force C and the reaction P. In the triangle of forces, Figure 5.4(b), the reaction P must pass through the point of intersection of W and C. When there is seepage through the slope or pore water pressures exist due to any other reason, the resultant force U due to such pressures on the slip surface must be calculated. Then the equilibrium of forces W, P, C and U must be considered together [Figure 5.4(c)]. For equilibrium, force P must pass through the intersection of C and the resultant of W and U.

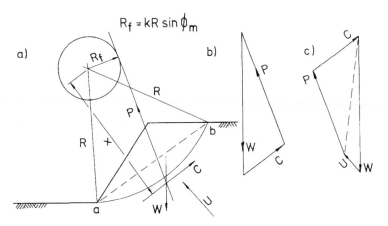

Figure 5.4 (a) Friction circle method (b) Force triangle when there is no water pressure (c) Force polygon when force corresponding to water pressure is included.

At every point the elemental frictional reaction dP act at an angle ϕ_m to the normal to the slip surface. Therefore, all elemental reactions are tangent to a circle of radius $R_f = R \sin \phi_m$ known as the friction circle. It is assumed for convenience that the resultant frictional reaction P is also tangent to this circle. The error resulting from this assumption is usually small and on the safe side. This assumption leads to a 'lower bound' to the actual factor of safety that would have been obtained with a correct position of the resultant frictional reaction. Taylor (1937, 1948) suggested that a more accurate analysis would result by taking P to be tangent to a circle of radius $R_f = KR \sin \phi_m$. The value of K is generally greater than one and the lower limit of one corresponds to a reaction P tangent to the circle of radius $R \sin \phi_m$. The value of K is statically indeterminate and depends on the distribution of intergranular (or effective) stress along the slip surface as well as on the central angle of the circular arc. Taylor determined the value of K for a uniform distribution and a sinusoidal distribution with zero values at the ends. The latter gave lower values of K for all values of the central angle of the arc. K increases in both cases as the central angle increases. The actual distribution resembles a sinusoidal one to a large extent except that it is not symmetrical. Taylor referred to the 'actual' stress distribution but did not say how this could be determined. The value of K is usually within 1.05 for circular arcs with central angles less than about 90° (see Taylor, 1948 p. 443). Thus the factor of safety for arcs with small central angles is insensitive to the distribution of normal stresses on the arc. (This conclusion refers particularly to analyses with low pore pressures.)

Lambe and Whitman (1969) found an upper bound to the factor of safety in one example by assuming the frictional reaction to be concentrated at the two ends of a slip surface. Both these end reactions are tangent to a friction circle with $K = 1$ and their resultant P is made to pass through the point of intersection of other forces (C, U and W). In the example considered the 'upper bound' to the factor of safety was $F = 1.61$ compared with a 'lower bound' of $F = 1.27$. It should be noted that the assumption (of normal stress on the slip surface) made for obtaining the upper bound is not a realistic one; hence the large difference between the two bounds. There is a narrow range of stress distributions which intuitively appear to be correct. Thus Lambe and Whitman state that, for their example a range of $F = 1.30$ to 1.36 would correspond to such acceptable normal stress distributions. The concept of upper and lower bounds to the statically admissible factor of safety is a very valuable one in both theoretical and practical slope studies. The capability to obtain these bounds is a significant advantage of the friction circle method.

Force equilibrium may be considered analytically or graphically by means of force polygons as shown in Figure 5.4. Magnitudes of forces C and P required for equilibrium are easily obtained. The factor of safety F_c may be defined as ratio of available unit cohesion c to the value of cohesion required for equilibrium c_m (c_m is given by ratio of calculated C and arc length $\overset{\frown}{ab}$). Any first trial will result in F_ϕ ($= \tan \phi / \tan \phi_m$) different from F_c. It may be required to obtain $F_c = F_\phi = F$ and this is achieved by repeated trials. It is useful to plot F_c versus F_ϕ from these trials and draw a curve connecting the various points. Then a 45° line is drawn through the origin and its intersection with the curve gives $F_c = F_\phi = F$. This value can thus be checked by direct calculation in a final trial. Such a procedure reduces the number of trials required.

Alternatively, it may be that F_ϕ is specified in the beginning and only F_c is to be obtained. In such a case trials mentioned above are not necessary. In either case, the calculations are to be repeated for a number of trial slip surfaces. The minimum factor of safety corresponding to the critical slip surface is obtained after a number of trials have been made. In order to minimise the repetitive labour involved, Taylor (1937, 1948) produced stability charts in terms of the stability factor N_S defined earlier. This chart is shown in Appendix II from which it is clear how the value of N_S varies with slope angle and friction angle. Note that the inverse of N_S is often used in charts in place of N_S itself. These curves correspond to failure which occurs along toe circles for values of ϕ greater than approximately 3°. Thus a typical base failure in a homogeneous soil is often an indication that $\phi = 0$ conditions prevailed at the time of the failure (or that the soil was not in fact homogeneous). In other words a base failure in homogeneous soil is likely to be an undrained failure involving no volume change. See Appendix II for further discussion.

It is useful to note that a consistent approach to the factor of safety is also facilitated by the use of stability charts. By using the actual available value of ϕ, a value of N_S is read from the chart for a given slope angle β. Using this value of N_S and known value of γ and H, the value of cohesion c_m required for equilibrium is obtained from $N_S = \gamma H/c_m$. Thus the factor of safety is $F = c/c_m$ in which c is the available unit cohesion. However, a value of F of 1 was used with respect to the frictional component of shearing resistance by using the available value of ϕ to read N_S from the chart. This inconsistency may be corrected by repeating the above process with a value of ϕ_m given by $\tan \phi_m = \tan \phi/F$. With values of ϕ_m and β a new value of N_S and hence c_m is obtained. This gives a new value of $F = c/c_m$. If this value is close to the value of F used in calculating ϕ_m, it is the correct value of F; otherwise further iterations are required till the same value of F applies to both c and ϕ.

Taylor (1948) discussed the use of the friction circle method comprehensively for different pore water pressure conditions such as partial or full submergence, steady seepage through a slope and rapid draw-down in the case of embankments and earth dams. However, his charts are strictly correct only for a total stress analysis and their use for arbitrary pore water pressure is not convenient. Cousins (1977) used the friction circle method with pore water pressure variations and produced charts based on effective stress parameters. For details the reader is invited to read Appendix AII.4. Effective stress stability charts have also been prepared by Spencer (1967), Bishop and Morgenstern (1960), Hoek (1970), Hoek and Bray (1974, 1977) and several others during the last three decades. Brief references to the use of stability charts are made in chapter 4 and this chapter, and their relative merits and shortcomings are also discussed in Appendix II at the end of the book.

Most stability charts have been devised for cases when the ground surface near the crest and toe of the slope is horizontal. The charts are, therefore, not directly applicable to slopes with any other geometrical configuration. Similarly the charts are not directly applicable for layered non-homogeneous deposits. Engineers with some experience may, however, use these charts profitably even for non-homogeneous and non-uniform slopes with different geometrical configurations. To do this one must use average slope inclination and weighted average of c, ϕ and γ values calculated on the basis of proportion of the length of slip surface passing through different relatively homogeneous layers. Such a procedure is useful for preliminary analyses and saves both time and expense. Detailed analyses are carried out by using more accurate methods e.g., the method of slices, different versions of which are discussed in subsequent sections of this chapter. In the age of fast computers and with the availability of specialized software packages, the use of stability charts is, of course, declining.

The approximate location of a critical surface is necessary for the use of charts in this manner for non-homogeneous soils or non-uniform slopes. When the critical surface is approximately known, weighted averages of soil parameters can be estimated. If the geological framework of the site is properly understood, the critical surface can be approximately located with confidence and an experienced person can get results within 10% of correct values. These remarks for use of charts apply to 'effective stress' charts as well as 'total stress' charts. For simple homogeneous slopes, location of critical circles can, of course, be made using charts such as those of Taylor (1937), Spencer (1967) and Cousins (1977). The latter are shown in Appendix II.

5.4 METHOD OF SLICES – FELLENIUS AND BISHOP SIMPLIFIED METHODS

The method of slices is the only general method of analysis available for dealing with irregular slopes in non-homogeneous soils and rocks in which the values of c and ϕ are not essentially constant. The method was pioneered by Fellenius (1927, 1936) and Taylor (1937, 1948) and has since been modified in different ways in order to extend its range of application and to improve its reliability and accuracy. In this section, attention is restricted to slip surfaces of circular shape. Several methods involving the procedure of slices are available to deal with slip surfaces of arbitrary shape and these methods are discussed in subsequent sections. In all methods based on the slices procedure, the potential sliding mass is subdivided, for the purpose of analysis, into a number of elements or slices. In most variations of the method of slices, the subdivision is based on vertical boundaries of slices. The vertical slices need not be equal in width. For example, slice widths may be selected in such a way that, as far as possible, the base of each slice falls within one type of soil in a layered or non-homogeneous slope. The inclination of the base of each slice, the slice weight, the material properties and pore pressures at the base of each slice are expected to be known before an analysis can be carried out. Methods with inclined slices have also been developed and used successfully. These methods are particularly good for modeling slopes with complex geology in which joints and faults may be considered as inter-slice boundaries.

5.4.1 Ordinary method of slices (Fellenius method)

Consider a trial slip circle as shown in Figure 5.5(a) and assume that the potential sliding mass has been subdivided into a number of imaginary vertical slices. Each slice is acted upon by its own weight, W, and by the boundary inter-slice or side-wall forces which have both tangential components T and normal components E. The forces acting on the base of a slice of inclination α and length l are the shear resistance S and the normal force P. A rigorous solution to the problem of stability involving the soil mass requires the following:

1   the forces on each slice must satisfy the conditions of equilibrium, and
2   the forces acting on the sliding mass as a whole must satisfy conditions of equilibrium.

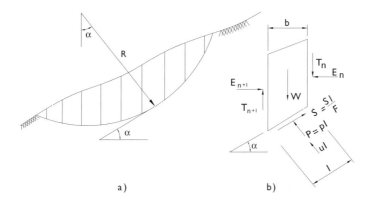

Figure 5.5 Method of slices: (a) Division of sliding mass into slices (b) Forces acting on a typical slice.

It is difficult to evaluate the forces T and E which depend on a number of factors including the stress-strain and deformation characteristics of the material of the slope. In the simplest approach, the total normal stress on the base of each slice is obtained by resolving all forces perpendicular and tangential to the base of a slice, after assuming the inter-slice forces T and E to be zero. Neglecting the inter-slice forces on each slice implies the following assumption as regards the overall equilibrium of the sliding mass consisting of n slices (Bishop, 1955):

$$\Sigma \tan \phi \left\{ (T_n - T_{n+1}) \cos \alpha - (E_n - E_{n+1}) \sin \alpha \right\} = 0 \tag{5.6}$$

where the summation is over all the slices. Such an assumption leads to an under estimate of the factor of safety [e.g., use of equation (5.7) given below]. Therefore, the results are conservative and the error is on the safe side. The inaccuracy is large for deep critical circles with large variations in α. This corresponds to arcs with large central angles. Inaccuracy also increases with increasing pore water pressures. Improved procedures are discussed subsequently.

Taking moments about the centre of the slip circle, the following equation is obtained for the factor of safety defined as a ratio of resisting and disturbing moments:

$$F = \frac{\Sigma \{cl + \tan \phi \, (W \cos \alpha - ul)\}}{\Sigma W \sin \alpha} \tag{5.7}$$

in which u is the pore water pressure at the base of any slice and the summation is over all the slices. (Note that α may have both positive and negative values.) In deriving equation (5.7) the inter-slice forces have been neglected when considering the equilibrium of each slice and the weight of each slice has been resolved tangential and normal to its base. The normal reaction at the base of the slice is thus taken equal to the component of the weight in that direction. Equation (5.7) corresponds to the Ordinary method of slices or the Fellenius method, or the Swedish method of slices.

The term ($W \cos\alpha - ul$) may become negative implying negative effective normal stress on the base of a slice which is unrealistic and unacceptable. This can happen for any slice with small W or large u or both (it is easy to check that the term is negative when u is greater than $\gamma z \cos^2\alpha$). In practice the term may be taken as zero when its value becomes negative for any slice (Whitman and Bailey, 1967). Turnbull and Hvorslev (1967) proposed a different procedure of calculating the effective normal stress directly by resolving effective forces normal to the base of a slice using an effective slice weight ($W - ub$) where b is the width of a slice. This leads to the following expression for F in which the effective normal stress is positive for all reasonable values of pore water pressure:

$$F = \frac{\Sigma\{cl + (W\cos\alpha - ul\cos^2\alpha)\tan\phi\}}{\Sigma W \sin\alpha} \tag{5.7a}$$

While the use of Equation (5.7a) is associated with acceptable normal force distribution along a slip surface, the accuracy is not necessarily improved. Inaccuracy may still be large particularly for arcs with large central angles and for problems in which pore water pressures are high.

5.4.2   Bishop simplified method

Bishop (1955) formulated the problem rigorously by including the inter-slice forces in the equations of equilibrium of a typical slice. He demonstrated the solution of the correctly formulated problem by a process of iterative calculation in which assumed values of the inter-slice or sidewall forces are improved by successive approximations. He also proposed a simplified calculation can be made which gives fairly accurate results even though the inter-slice forces are ignored. This is discussed below.

The factor of safety F is first defined as the ratio of available unit shear strength to that required or mobilised at limit equilibrium. [This is a different definition from that used in deriving equation (5.7)]. The forces acting on the base of a slice are the mobilised shear strength sl/F, the total normal force $P = pl$ and the total pore water pressure ul [Figure 5.5(b)]. Resolving these forces in the direction of the weight W (and neglecting the inter-slice forces) it is easy to get an expression for p, the local normal stress. It is seen that such an expression includes the unknown F. Now the value of p is substituted in the usual Coulomb-Terzaghi strength equation to obtain the value of s for a typical slice (again including the unknown F) as follows:

$$s = \frac{c + \left(\dfrac{W}{b} - u\right)\tan\phi}{1 + \tan\alpha \tan\phi/F} \tag{5.8}$$

in which b is the width of the slice. This equation is a consequence of calculating p by considering the vertical equilibrium of the slice, as mentioned above. The total normal force P on the slice base, the product of p and the length of the slice base, is given by the following expression:

$$P = \frac{\left\{ \dfrac{W}{b} - \dfrac{\tan\alpha}{F}(c - u\tan\phi) \right\}}{1 + \tan\alpha \tan\phi/F} \tag{5.8a}$$

Taking moments of all forces (resisting and disturbing) about the centre of the circular slip surface, equilibrium of the entire sliding mass requires that:

$$\Sigma W \sin\alpha = \Sigma \frac{sl}{F} \quad \text{or} \quad F = \frac{\Sigma sl}{\Sigma W \sin\alpha} \tag{5.9}$$

Combining Equations (5.8) and (5.9)

$$F = \frac{\Sigma\{cb + (W - ub)\tan\phi\}/m_\alpha}{\Sigma W \sin\alpha} \tag{5.10}$$

in which

$$m_\alpha = \left(1 + \frac{\tan\alpha\tan\phi}{F}\right)\cos\alpha \tag{5.10a}$$

It is important to remember for later discussion in (c) below that α may have both positive and negative values. Since F occurs in the right hand side, calculations are started with an assumed value of F and a new value of F is calculated from Equation (5.10). With this new value, calculations are repeated and such iterations are stopped when there is little difference in successive values. Convergence is usually very rapid. A simple chart for calculation of m_α facilitates the rapid determination of F. This chart is shown in Appendix II. As a first trial value, the factor of safety given by the Fellenius method (Ordinary method of slices) may be used. As a rough guide for initial calculation, F (Bishop) may be taken as 1.1 times F (Fellenius) for total stress analysis or effective stress analysis with low pore pressures and F (Bishop) may be taken as 1.2 to 1.25 times F (Fellenius) for effective stress analysis with moderate to high pore water pressures. With such initial values convergence may be obtained in 2 or 3 iterations. Occasional numerical errors are discussed in subsection 5.4.3 below.

The reason for the relative accuracy of the Bishop simplified method is that in considering only the vertical equilibrium of any slice, there is no need to account for the horizontal components of the inter-slice forces. Considering the overall equilibrium of the potential sliding mass, the assumption involved in the Bishop simplified method is (Chowdhury, 1975):

$$\Sigma(E_n - E_{n+1})\frac{\tan\phi}{m_\alpha} = 0 \tag{5.11}$$

It is thus misleading to suggest, as has sometimes been done, that this method only assumes the inter-slice forces to be horizontal.

If the factor of safety is defined as a ratio of resisting to disturbing moments, an equation for F is obtained which is identical to Equation (5.10) except that $F = 1$ on the right hand side. Equation (5.10), however, has gained wide acceptance. Development of Bishop's method for soil with anisotropic shear strength is discussed in the Appendix to this Chapter. For anisotropy with respect to cohesion alone, it is shown that no difficulties arise. However, the degree of accuracy of the Bishop simplified method for anisotropic soils has not been investigated so far.

5.4.3 Convergence problems and possible numerical errors

Convergence problems including false convergence may be encountered in applying the Bishop simplified method when the slip surface has a reverse slope near the toe of a slope (Chowdhury and Zhang, 1990). The term $(1 + \tan \alpha \tan \phi/F)$ used in Equation (5.10a) can become zero or negative near the toe of a steeply inclined slip surface when α has large negative values (reverse slope of slip surface near the toe) and ϕ is not zero. Specifically the term is zero when $\alpha = \phi_m - 90°$ where $\tan \phi_m = \tan \phi/F$. As the term approaches zero, the factor of safety is overestimated because the normal force at the base of a slice (near the steep part of a slip surface) approaches infinity. However, as the slip surface becomes steeper, the value of F is underestimated because negative values of normal force on the base of a slice introduce an incorrect direction for the shear resistance. Whitman and Bailey (1967) recommend that Simplified Bishop method should be used with caution if the term sec $\alpha/(1 + \tan \alpha \tan \phi/F)$ becomes smaller than 0.2 for any slice. Convergence problems including false convergence can be avoided (Chowdhury and Zhang, 1990) if the initial trial value of F is selected as

$$F_0 = 1 + | \tan \alpha_1 \tan \phi_1 | \tag{5.12}$$

Note that α_1 is the slope of the steepest slice near the toe and ϕ_1 is the internal friction angle for the soil through which that slice passes. The second term on the right hand side is the magnitude of the product of the two variables, $\tan \alpha_1$ and $\tan \phi_1$.

It is useful to calculate the normal stress along a slip surface using Equation (5.8a) after F has been calculated from Equation (5.10). A reasonable normal stress distribution is an indication of an acceptable solution. Although computer based solutions or specialized software are now routinely used for slope analysis, the iterative procedure involved in the Bishop Simplified Method is quite suitable for a simple calculator.

5.4.4 Pore pressures and submergence

The calculation of stability using Equation (5.7) or Equation (5.10) requires estimation of W and u for each slice in addition to the inclination of the base of each slice. The weight W of each slice should be calculated carefully based on the bulk unit weight. When the whole slice is submerged W is based on the submerged unit weight and pore pressure u is taken as the difference between pore pressure on the base of the slice and that due to the external water level from which seepage is occurring through the slope. This pore pressure may be called the 'hydrostatic excess'. When the slice is only partly submerged, use bulk unit weight (which may be saturated or partially saturated depending on the problem) above the external water level and submerged unit weight below the water level and pore pressure u again relative to the external water level. However, if there is no submergence at all, use bulk unit weight for whole slice and actual pore water pressure at the base of each slice. The determination of pore water pressure is facilitated by drawing a flow-net for the relevant seepage condition and marking the intersection of a slip surface with the equipotential lines in the flow-net.

5.4.5   Effective stress charts and average pore pressure ratio

Bishop and Morgenstern (1960) devised stability coefficients for earth slopes in terms of an average pore pressure ratio which is calculated as a weighted average of variable pore pressure ratios $r = u/\gamma h$ within an earth dam or a cut. They found a linear relationship between the factor of safety F and a given average $\bar{r}_u$ of the form:

$$F = m - n\,\bar{r}_u \tag{5.13}$$

in which m and n are stability co-efficients for the particular slope and soil properties. They performed analysis in terms of effective stress and found that the value of the factor of safety F depends only on $c/\gamma H$, ϕ and $\bar{r}_u$ for a given geometrical shape. Thus considerable simplification occurs in the number of parameters by expression of c and u in dimensionless form.

The concept of average $\bar{r}_u$ was found useful and sufficiently accurate in the examples considered. Average $\bar{r}_u$ values between 0.22 and 0.48 were obtained by Bishop and Morgenstern for typical cases of earth dams and slopes including steady seepage, end of construction and other field conditions. (The range in local values of r_u was 0 to 0. 55 at individual points of different slopes analysed).

It is well known that the condition of rapid drop in reservoir level (referred to as rapid draw-down or sudden draw-down) is often critical for water retaining embankments such as earth dams. Morgenstern (1963) prepared stability charts for rapid draw down conditions. Pore pressures after rapid draw-down are calculated in terms of the pore pressure parameters A and B discussed in chapter 2. Stability can be checked for complete or partial draw down corresponding to the actual drop in reservoir water levels. For complete draw-down the critical slip circle is tangent to the top of the assumed rigid base but for partial draw down it may be located within the slope. Therefore the factor of safety in the latter case is not found directly but by trial and error using the relevant charts. Stability charts have also been devised by Spencer (1967), Hoek (1970), Hoek and Bray (1974, 1977), and Cousins (1977) and the reader is directed to Appendix II for further discussion. Note that Spencer (1967) and Cousins (1977) have given charts for location of critical slip surfaces in simple homogeneous slopes. The reader may refer to chapter 3 for estimation of pore water pressures during rapid drawdown. For an approximate solution, the reader may refer to Appendix II.

5.4.6   Inclusion of additional external forces such as soil reinforcement

There may be disturbing forces additional to the weight of the potential sliding mass and resisting forces additional to the shear resistance along the potential slip surface. Such disturbing forces or resisting forces must be included in the stability analysis model and the equilibrium equations modified as appropriate. For instance, surcharge loads on a slope can simply be incorporated by adding to the weight of each vertical slice affected by the surcharge. On the other hand, earthquake loads are applied as pseudo-static horizontal body forces. This is explained fully in Chapter 9 and need not be considered further here. But it is useful to consider a reinforced slope in the context of a curved slip surface and a method of slices. Reinforcement force in the context of a plane surface of sliding was considered in chapter 4.

For a reinforced slope, additional term or terms corresponding to the reinforcement forces must be included in the appropriate equilibrium equation. Considering the moment equilibrium equation 5.9, there would be an extra summation term on the right hand side. In doing so, careful attention must be given to the inclination of a reinforcing force and where it intersects the slice boundaries and the base of a vertical slice. In some problems, simpler methods such as Fellenius and Bishop methods may be suitable. However, in other cases, a more rigorous method which includes interslice forces would be more appropriate and such methods are discussed in the following sections of this chapter. A couple of important points must be noted.

1   The inter-slice reinforcement forces must be considered separately from the soil and water inter-slice forces. This is because the former can be considered as known forces in contrast to the latter which are determined as part of the solution of the limit equilibrium equations.
2   If the force in the reinforcing element (soil or rock anchor) is considered as the ultimate load, a suitable 'factor of safety' ('load factor' is a more appropriate term) may be used on this force, in formulating the slope model.
3   Alternatively, the force in the anchor may be the design load (or safe load, or allowable load). In that case, a reduction factor need not be applied to the reinforcement force.
4   The factor of safety (or load factor) applied to a reinforcement force should be different from the factor of safety applied to the shear strength parameters because they are associated with quite different types and levels of uncertainty.

Note: Markedly different values of F may be obtained for a specific reinforced slope problem if the following alternative assumptions are made:

• reinforcement force factored by F while shear strength parameters considered fully mobilised.
• shear strength parameters factored by F while reinforcement force considered fully mobilised.
• shear strength parameters and reinforcement force both factored by F.

The above considerations will prove useful while using any available computer program or software developed for analysis of reinforced slopes. It will be important to establish what assumptions have been made in the program regarding the factor of safety for soil strength and the load factor for reinforcing element.

5.5 SLIP SURFACES OF ARBITRARY SHAPE

5.5.1 Janbu's generalised method

In general, a slip surface may not be even approximately circular in cross-section. It is necessary to use a generalised method of slices in which assumptions concerning the inter-slice forces do not lead to unacceptable errors. Janbu (1954a, 1957) considered the force and moment equilibrium of a typical vertical slice and the force equilibrium of the sliding mass as a whole. Using overall horizontal equilibrium as a stability criterion the following expression for the factor of safety was obtained:

$$F = \frac{\Sigma \, bs \sec^2 \alpha}{\Sigma (W + dT) \tan \alpha} \tag{5.14}$$

in which dT is the difference of tangential or shear forces on two successive slices, and

$$s = \frac{\left\{ c + \left(\dfrac{W + dT}{b} - u \right) \tan \phi \right\}}{1 + \tan \alpha \tan \phi / F} \tag{5.14a}$$

The calculations can only be made with an initial assumption about the magnitude and position of the inter-slice forces (Figure 5.6). For example one may use $dT = 0$ for initial calculations. In such a case, the value of F may be obtained by iterative calculations as in the Bishop Simplified Method so that an assumed value of F leads to

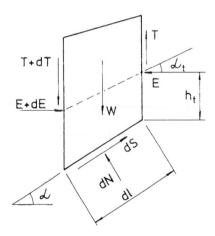

Figure 5.6 Forces on typical slice – slip surface of arbitrary shape, Janbu's method.

an improved calculated value and so on. As for the Bishop simplified method, the convergence is quite rapid. The interslice forces can then be calculated using the following equations based on considerations of equilibrium Janbu (1954a, 1957):

$$dE = (W + dT) \tan \alpha - \frac{sb}{F} \sec^2 \alpha$$

$$T = -E \tan \alpha_t + h_t \frac{dE}{b}$$

(5.15)

in which dE is the difference of normal sidewall forces on two successive slices and α_t and h_t define respectively the direction and position of the line of thrust as shown in Figure 5.6.

The calculation of interslice forces (or side forces or sidewall forces) is started from the crest of the slope, or from the top slice, on which T and E usually have zero values on one side. However, non-zero value of force E may exist for the first slice, e.g., in a problem in which there is a water pressure acting in a tension crack which forms the boundary of the first slice). Proceeding from slice to slice and using Equation (5.15) successively for each slice, the forces E and T are obtained for all the slices. The position of the line of thrust is then easily determined once α_t and h_t are known or assumed for the first slice. The resultant of E and T forces gives the line of thrust at any section.

With the computed values of inter-slice forces, the factor of safety is recalculated using Equation (5.14). Now, with this new known value of F, new values of interslice forces and a new position of the line of thrust are determined using Equation (5.15). These new forces lead to a new value of F. When successive values of F (with two successive sets of values of inter-slice forces) are nearly identical, the iterations are stopped. Convergence is usually obtained after only a few iterations.

It is useful to check whether the associated position of the line of thrust is reasonable. If the position of the line of thrust is such that tension is implied in a significant portion of the potential sliding mass, then it may not be an acceptable solution. Similarly, the failure criterion should not be violated and this can be checked by comparing forces E and T at each slice boundary. Such acceptability criteria must be satisfied in all generalised limit equilibrium procedures and are discussed further in section 5.7.

Janbu (1957) showed that preparation of charts and the study of slopes is considerably simplified by introducing a dimensionless parameter, $\lambda = \gamma H \tan \phi / c$ in addition to the parameter $\gamma H/c_m$ mentioned in chapter 4 and earlier in this chapter.

There may be boundary loads acting on the surface of the potential failure mass. To include these, the following simple modifications are required:

- In Equation (5.14a) the weight term for a slice must include any vertical load on the top of it.
- The total net external horizontal force in the direction of potential sliding must be added to the denominator in Equation (5.14). This will be outside the summation term.
- The first of equations Equation (5.15) must contain a new term dQ indicating the change in horizontal force Q across the top of any slice, and the slice weight must include the external vertical load on the slice.

- The second of equations Equation (5.15) must contain a new term $-z\,dQ/b$ where z is the depth and b the width of a slice and dQ is the change in the horizontal force Q across the top of any slice (the change is positive if it is an increase in the direction of potential movement). Details of Janbu's method have also been given in Hirschfeld and Poulos (1973).

5.5.2   Convergence problems

Convergence problems, including false convergence are encountered when applying the Janbu generalized method to individual slope stability studies especially where the curvature of part of the slip surface is large (for example, near the crest of a slope) or when the pore pressures are high. Such difficulties have been attributed to large changes in horizontal side forces in successive iterations (Wright, 1975; Zhang, 1989). Moreover, as noted in connection with the Bishop simplified method, problems may also arise if the slip surface has a reverse slope near the toe, leading to small or negative values of the term $(1 + \tan\alpha\tan\phi/F)$ for some slices. The latter difficulty can be avoided if the recommendation of Chowdhury and Zhang (1990) about the initial trial value of the factor of safety F is followed (see section 5.4.3). However, a more innovative approach is required for solution of the difficulty due to rapid changes in horizontal side force from slice to slice and from iteration to iteration. One such approach is summarized below.

5.5.3   Extended Janbu method (Zhang, 1989)

A modification of the Janbu generalized method was proposed by Zhang (1989) and implemented into an iterative computational procedure. The modeling considers the potential sliding mass in two parts, an upper part and a lower part, separated by an internal vertical surface. The upper part is relatively small in size consisting of a couple of vertical slices only and including the part of the slip surface with large curvature. The lower part is the relatively larger in size and includes the part of the slip surface with smaller curvature.

Considering the equilibrium of the smaller upper part (near the crest) yields the normal and shear forces on the internal vertical surface, separating the upper and lower parts. These forces are then applied as external forces to the larger, lower part of the potential sliding mass and the analyses are carried out right through by applying the Janbu generalized procedure. Iterative analyses are required to obtain convergence of the numerical solution. For any trial slip surface, the iterations are stopped as soon as successive changes in normal and shear forces on the internal vertical surface become negligible or insignificant. The iterative solution converges without difficulty. By comparison of solutions to problems with known alternative numerical solutions, the reliability and accuracy of the modified Janbu method was confirmed.

Combined with an optimisation procedure, the computer-based solution allows the critical slip surface of arbitrary shape to be located and the minimum factor of safety to be estimated. Moreover, if the internal vertical surface is considered as a tension crack (preferably a water-filled crack), the critical location and depth of the tension crack is determined as part of the numerical solution. Thus the modified method can be used as a powerful, flexible and versatile tool for slope stability analysis based on the limit equilibrium concept.

The modified geotechnical slope model was also found to be a good basis for analysis within a probabilistic framework.

EXAMPLE 5.1

Figure E5.1 shows slope failures in weathered rock which were analysed by Sancio and Goodman (1979) using a biplanar method of analysis [see chapter 4, section 4.5.2] and then again by Zhang (1989) using the extended Janbu method. The data are summarized in Table E5.1(a) and it may be noted that all open cracks are assumed to be dry. For impending cracks (cracks which are not yet open), the assumed tensile strength across the cracks is shown in the last column. The calculated values of the factor of safety are shown in Table E5.1(b). The values of F shown in parenthesis are those based on the extended Janbu method. It is clear that in most cases the results are in good agreement to the alternative numerical solutions based on a different method of limit equilibrium analysis used by Sancio and Goodman (1979).

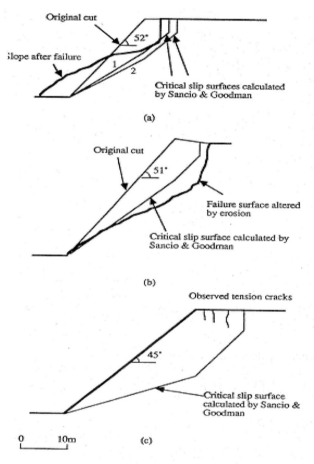

Figure E5.1 Failure of weathered rock slopes with calculated critical slip surface (after Zhang, 1989, based on Sancio and Goodman, 1979). With permission, see page 713, No 14.

Table E5.1(a) Data concerning slopes (See Figure E5.1). With permission, see page 713, No 14.

Cases	Total height of slope (m)	Unit weight (kN/m³)	φ (deg.)	c (kN/m²)	Depth of tension crack (m)	Assumed tensile strength (kN/m²)
a (1)	20.8	24.5	30	10.2	2.39	−4.8
a (2)	20.8	24.5	35	15.3	2.11	−7.1
b	30.5	24.5	35	15.0	3.00	−7.0
c	27.0	17.7	20	25.5	5.84	−7.6

Table E5.1(b) Factor of safety values calculated by Sancio and Goodman (1979), and Zhang (1989). With permission, see page 713, No 14.

Cases	Factor of safety	
	Impending crack	Open, dry crack
a (1)	0.94 (0.87)	0.94 (0.86)
a (2)	1.05 (1.10)	1.04 (1.09)
b	1.02 (1.05)	1.01 (1.04)
c	1.03 (1.06)	1.02 (1.05)

Note 1: The values in parenthesis ( ) were obtained by Zhang (1989) using his Extended Janbu method.

Note 2: Analyses with assumption of no tension crack gave values of F very close to those obtained when a dry tension crack was included.

EXAMPLE 5.2

One of the examples considered for comparison is shown in Figure E5.2: an embankment with a specified slip surface and a tension crack at the crest for which the depth may be assumed. The depth of tension crack was varied from 0 to 30% of the total embankment height. (Since the pore pressure ratio is 0.5 indicating full seepage, it is implied that the tension crack is full of water). The factor of safety in this case was found to be independent of assumed tension crack depth, a result first obtained by Spencer (1973) using a different method of slices (assumption of parallel inter-slice forces). The factor of safety range was determined to be $F = 1.44–1.45$ (Zhang, 1989), very close to Spencer's calculation, $F = 1.46$.

The conclusion that the depth of water-filled tension crack has no effect on the value of F should not be generalized. It only applies here because pore pressure ratio is 0.5 (implying full seepage within slope) and therefore water in the tension crack is simply consistent with that condition. If the pore pressure ratio was significantly smaller and a tension crack was assumed to be full of water, the depth of tension crack would certainly influence the value of F. In general, if the depth of water in tension crack is consistent with the pore water pressure condition in the slope, the tension crack will have only a marginal influence on the value of F.

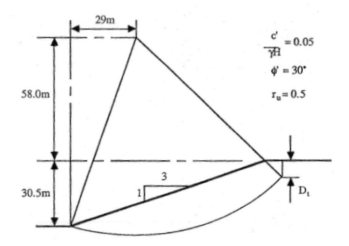

Figure E5.2 Example of an embankment with a tension crack near the crest; tension crack depth was varied for different analyses and depth of water in tension crack was assumed to be consistent with the assumed pore pressure ratio (Example 5.2). With permission, see page 713, No 14.

The situation is even more interesting where tension crack depth and location are part of the optimisation process for determining the critical slip surface and the minimum factor of safety as shown in the next example.

EXAMPLE 5.3

Another numerical example concerns the determination of the shape and location of the critical slip surface and factor of safety for a simple slope with the following parameters:

Slope Height $H = 10.67$ m
Slope Inclination $\beta = 40°$
Unit weight $\gamma = 18.87$ kN/m^3
Cohesion $c' = 19.18$ kN/m^2
Angle of internal friction, $\phi' = 28°$
Pore pressure ratio $r_u = 0.2$

Solutions based on the extended Janbu method were obtained by Zhang (1989) with several alternative assumptions. Three amongst those are summarized here.

(1) Firstly, the critical slip surface without assumption of a tension crack is shown in Figure E5.3(a) with value of factor of safety, $F = 1.38$.
(2) Secondly, tension crack is included, its location and depth being part of the optimisation process. It is assumed that depth of water in the crack is consistent with the value of pore pressure ratio. The critical slip surface is similar to

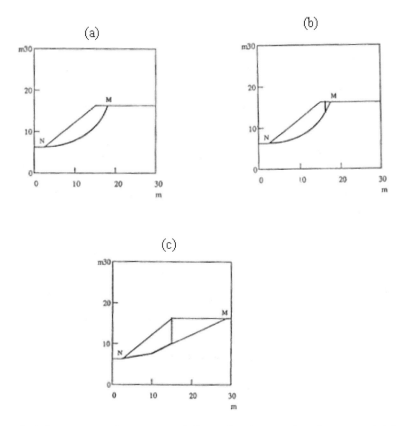

Figure E5.3 Simple slope showing critical slip surface location based on extended Janbu method assuming, from top left (a) no tension crack, (b) tension crack having depth of water consistent with pore pressure ratio, and, (c) tension crack full of water, location and depth being part of the optimisation process (Zhang,1989). With permission, see page 713, No 14.

the previous case as shown in Figure E5.3(b) and $F = 1.33$ – very close to the previous case.

(3) Thirdly, an unusual situation is considered which may or may not apply to a particular slope. In this case, a tension crack is assumed as in the second case, its depth and location being part of the optimisation process. However, the crack is assumed to be full of water although the pore pressure ratio is less than 0.5. Such a situation can arise during an intense rainstorm when tension cracks may get filled up quickly.

For this case, the critical slip surface has a very different shape as shown in Figure E5.3(c), and the factor of safety value is reduced to $F = 1.15$, significantly lower than the results for the previous two alternatives. Moreover, the critical slip surface is associated with a relatively deep tension crack. In the absence of actual case studies, it is highly questionable if such a result can be generalized although it may represent a realistic scenario for specific cases. However, see the important note below[*].

In terms of the numerical method, the important conclusion is that the shape and location of the critical slip surface and the value of the minimum factor of safety depend on the assumptions made as to the water depth in the tension crack when it is not consistent with the pore pressure ratio.

Clearly, the extended Janbu method enables the simulation of unusual, potentially dangerous situations related to the effect of intense rainstorms. However, when used with conventional assumptions, results from the extended Janbu method (Zhang, 1989) are very close to those from the original Janbu Generalised method.

EXAMPLE 5.4

This example relates to the failure of a mining spoil pile in strip coal mine (Richards et al., 1981; Richards, 1982). The geometry of the spoil pile, the observed failure surface and the water table are shown in Figure E5.4.

The basic data are:

Unit weight of spoil material, $\gamma = 17.66$ kN/m³

Shear strength parameters of unsaturated spoil material (above water table):

$c' = 130$ kN/m²
$\phi' = 36°$

Shear strength parameters of saturated spoil material along the basal slip surface:

$c' = 50$ kN/m²
$\phi' = 3°$

A back analysis was carried out by Richards (1982) using the finite element method of stress analysis. Overstressed areas and tension areas are shown in part (c) of the figure and appear to be consistent with the location of the observed slip surface.

The slip surface located by Zhang (1989) on the basis of the extended Janbu method is shown in part (a) of the figure without assumption of a tension crack and

---

[*] Important Note: Where the consequences of failure of a slope or earth structure are likely to be catastrophic, one must allow for unusual failure mechanisms. In this connection, consider the example of catastrophic levee failures in New Orleans associated with Hurricane Katrina. As pointed out in sections 1.2 and 1.7, post-failure investigations revealed unusual failure mechanisms of levees associated with I-walls. (Katrina, 2008). Due to the deflection of the I-wall under the storm surge, a gap formed along the I-wall on the flood side, right through to the bottom. This gap was observed at many locations. The observed gap can be considered as analogous to a tension crack formed in a soil or rock slope.

The failure mechanism consisted of a potential slip surface below the levee passing through the lower edge of the I-wall and ending beyond the toe of the levee. Due to existence of the gap, the lateral pressure on the I-wall was increased to hydrostatic level. Moreover, if the foundation soil was clay, the shear strength along the part of the slip surface on the flood side had to be ignored because that part of the slip surface was ineffective due to the formation of the gap. By recognizing the unusual failure mechanism and including the gap in the computation, the occurrence of failures could be explained. In one case the factor of safety reduced from 1.28 to 0.98 and in another case from 1.52 to 0.99 (Brandon et al., 2008; Duncan et al., 2008). The reduction in the factor of safety will not necessarily reduce its value below 1. Thus failure may or may not occur at a particular location, depending on the values of the relevant parameters.

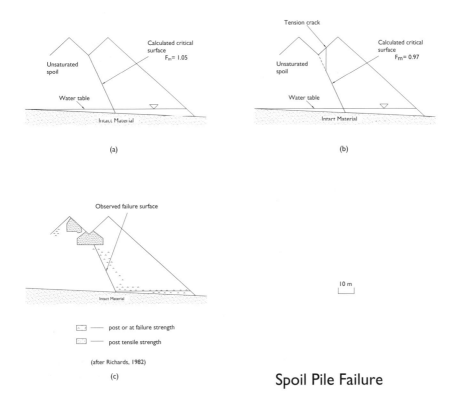

Figure E5.4 Back analysis of spoil pile failure showing slip surface predicted by extended Janbu method (a) without tension crack assumption (b) with tension crack assumption and (c) over-stressed zones and tension zones from a finite element analysis by Richards (1982) along with the observed or inferred slip surface. (after Richards, 1982, Zhang, 1989). With permission, see page 713, No 14 & 16.

in part (b) of the figure with assumption of a tension crack. In both cases the predicted critical slip surface is bilinear and its location is consistent with the observed slip surface location in part (c) of the figure and also with the stress analysis solution of Richards (1982). This can be considered a good agreement. Of course, there are some differences as would be expected between a stress-deformation analysis and a limit equilibrium analysis which is an analysis involving forces rather than stresses.

The factor of safety predictions by Zhang (1989) are $F = 1.05$ without tension crack and $F = 0.97$ with a tension crack. These results for F can be regarded as excellent for a failed slope.

5.6   OTHER METHODS FOR GENERAL SLIP SURFACES

5.6.1   *Developments before 1978*

Several methods have been developed for the stability of slopes in which the failure surface may be non-circular in shape. The methods proposed by Nonveiller (1965) and Bell (1968) are comparable in accuracy to the method proposed by Janbu (1957).

These methods do not satisfy all conditions of equilibrium. A solution developed by Morgenstern and Price (1965) was probably the first which was shown to satisfy both force and moment equilibrium. This method gained a good reputation within a short time and has retained its popularity as one of the best computer-based methods. The features of this method will be outlined in a separate section (section 5.7) and it is often referred to as the M-P method. Sarma (1973) proposed a different approach and his method is considered to be comparable to the M-P method in accuracy. The Sarma (1973) method aims at determining the critical horizontal acceleration that is required to bring the mass of soil to a state of limiting or critical equilibrium. Either (a) the critical acceleration may be taken as a measure of the factor of safety in which case no iteration is necessary or (b) the strength parameters may be reduced by a known factor of safety F and the critical acceleration computed. The value of F which gives the value of critical acceleration to be zero is the factor of safety for static conditions.

To simulate a horizontal acceleration Sarma (1973) used the conventional pseudo-static approach in which an appropriate horizontal force is applied at the centre of gravity of the sliding mass (see chapter 9). The horizontal force bears the same ratio to the weight of the soil mass as the horizontal acceleration does to the gravitational acceleration. The method involves assumptions concerning the inter-slice forces somewhat similar to those in the M-P method. The physical acceptability of the solution must be checked as in that method so that (a) failure criteria are not violated and (b) tension is not implied in the soil mass.

Spencer (1967, 1973) proposed a method which assumes the inter-slice forces to be parallel. He found the results to be fairly accurate and gave some attention to obtaining an acceptable position for the line of thrust (Spencer, 1973) in terms of effective stresses. He found that the assumption of a vertical tension crack with water pressure in it usually leads to an acceptable position of the line of thrust in terms of effective stresses. Where such an assumption is not made (or is not tenable) the position of the line of thrust may be unacceptable in some cases. He also found that the inclination of the line of thrust near the crest of a slope may have to be flatter than elsewhere.

Terzaghi and Peck (1967) outlined an approach in which the moment equilibrium of the sliding mass about an external point is considered. The factor of safety is given by:

$$F = \frac{\Sigma\{cb + (W + \Delta T_n - ub)\tan\phi\}(a/m_\alpha)}{\Sigma Wx - \Sigma\left\{W + \Delta T_n + (ub\tan\phi - cb)\dfrac{\tan\alpha}{F}\right\}(f/m_\alpha)} \qquad (5.16)$$

in which a, f and x define the position of the centre of the base of each slice with respect to the external point about which moments are taken (Figure 5.7) and m_α is given by Equation (5.10a). Iterations with successive sets of inter-slice forces are necessary as in the Janbu method.

The calculations are simplified by assuming $\Delta T_n = 0$. This approximation is considered by Terzaghi and Peck to be preferable to approximating the actual slip surface by an arc of a circle and then using a relatively accurate method for the assumed circular slip surface. For greater refinement ΔT_n must be estimated by successive approximations. Several sets of values of T_n may theoretically satisfy the conditions of equilibrium

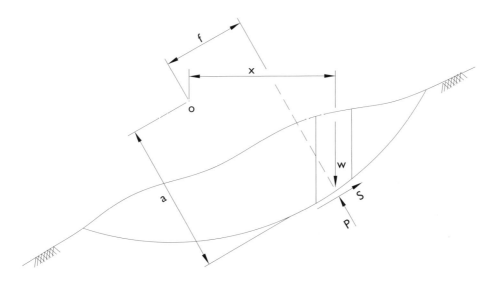

Figure 5.7 Slip surface of arbitrary shape showing dimensions *a, x, f* used in Eq.5.16 (after Terzaghi and Peck, 1967). Permission requested, see page 714, No 44.

for this statically indeterminate problems as in the Janbu method. However, there are some important restrictions on the values of T. To be acceptable, values of T must not exceed the shear strength of the soil at the particular inter-slice boundaries. Further, tensile stresses must not occur across a significant part of the inter-slice boundary. The value of F finally obtained is still not a unique one since other consistent sets of values of inter-slice forces are possible. However, the values of F obtained with different sets of values of the inter-slice forces are generally quite close to each other in their magnitude.

5.6.2   Developments over the last three decades

Almost fifty years have passed since the early methods of limit equilibrium analysis were developed for handling slip surfaces of arbitrary shapes. There is little change in the fundamental premise of the limit equilibrium approach (see, for instance, Hoek, 1987; Duncan 1992, Sharma, 2007) or in the basic assumptions and capabilities of the early methods, such as those presented by Janbu, Spencer, Sarma, and Morgenstern and Price. Details of the M-P method are presented in the following section. The early methods are still popular amongst geotechnical engineers. Although many papers have been published on proposed 'new' methods of limit equilibrium, it is not necessary to list them here because the capabilities claimed for these methods are not significantly different from the most popular early methods. Research papers on individual aspects of limit equilibrium analysis have, of course, been published in the intervening decades. For example, convergence aspects have been addressed (Chowdhury and Zhang, 1990), innovative ways have been developed for locating critical slip surfaces (Baker, 1980; Nguyen, 1985, Zhang, 1990; Bhattacharya and Basudhar, 2001), the concept of critical acceleration has been proposed as an alternative way of estimating the factor of safety, new interslice force functions have been proposed (Fan et al., 1986), non-vertical slices have successfully been considered as an alternative approach to the use of vertical slices (Sarma, 1979; Zhang and Chowdhury, 1995) and two dimensional (2-D)analyses have been extended to three-dimensional (3-D) analyses. Methods have also been proposed for combining a finite-element stress-deformation analysis, linear or non-linear, with a limit equilibrium analysis. For example, Fredlund and Scoular (1999) used the FEM stresses along a slip surface to calculate the local factors of safety and then estimated the overall factor of safety as a combination of the local factors of safety. They claimed that the basic assumptions of limit equilibrium concept were retained. Some comments on methods with non-vertical slices will be made later in this section while 3D analyses are considered in a separate sub-section.

5.6.3   Availability of geotechnical software for slopes

For using analyses in geotechnical practice, the most important development in the last decade has been the development of user-friendly slope stability software products which continue to be extended and improved in their capabilities. Nevertheless, the user of a software product must become fully aware of the assumptions and limitations associated with its use and be able to make a judicious selection amongst the alternatives and options featured in the product. Thus the user must be conversant with the fundamentals and with recent developments in geotechnical slope analysis. There may be significant differences in the capabilities of different products. One product may be suitable for rock slopes rather than soil slopes. A software product may feature numerical solutions for seepage through slopes as well as slope stability. Another product may be suited for analysis of slopes in unsaturated soil as well as saturated soil. It is important to check the range and capability of methods featured in a software product. For example, some methods may be more suited than others for investigating the actual or potential role of progressive failure at the site under consideration and other methods may be better in facilitating probabilistic modeling as a follow-up to deterministic analysis. Again, a particular method may be best suited for locating the critical slip surface or for consideration of tension cracks in a limit equilibrium analysis or both. It is also important to look for software with special capabilities such as the modeling of landslides triggered by rainfall and seismic slope analysis.

5.6.4   Non-vertical slices in limit equilibrium analysis

The use of methods with non-vertical slices deserves special comment. While such a method may be regarded as a generalised wedge method, a correct formulation requires more sophistication than a simple wedge approach. This was demonstrated by Sarma (1979) who was perhaps the first to develop a rigorous solution. Such a method can facilitate the direct and effective modeling of discontinuities in a soil or rock mass as also emphasised recently by Sitar et al. (2005). Thus, its use in slopes featuring complex geological conditions should be encouraged. To start with, both the force and moment equilibrium of the potential sliding mass must be satisfied. However, this is not sufficient for the solution to be kinematically admissible. The moment equilibrium of each individual slice should also be satisfied and this cannot be guaranteed by the fact that overall moment equilibrium is satisfied. Therefore, the moment equilibrium of each slice should be considered directly. Moreover, along each interslice boundary, the failure criterion of the material should be taken into account. Most importantly, the interslice force equation should be formulated in such a way as to be kinematically admissible (Zhang and Chowdhury, 1995). If this is done correctly, the degree of mobilisation of shear forces along an interslice boundary will differ from that along the slip surface. The former will change from one slice boundary to the next, reflecting the direction of a boundary relative to that of the slip surface. As indicated above, Sitar et al. (2005) emphasised the importance of considering the geometry of discontinuities. They also highlighted the role of kinematics in slope analysis. They referred to the full array of methods including limit equilibrium, finite-element and other methods and highlighted that, amongst all the methods, modeling the behaviour of discontinuities can be facilitated only by the distinct element method (DEM), a force-based method, and by the discontinuous deformation analysis (DDA), a displacement based method. It is interesting to note that they achieved good results for a very well known case study (the Vaiont slide) by carrying out DDA followed by static limit equilibrium analyses. Their results were comparable to those of Chowdhury (1978a) and Hendron and Patton (1985). Yet, they invoked only the deformation of blocks within the failure mass whereas the others invoked entirely different mechanisms. The Vaiont slide case study is discussed in more detail in a later section in this chapter and in chapter 7 which deals with the role of initial stresses in slopes.

Most of the methods mentioned so far are based on the assumption of vertical slices and some on the assumption of inclined slices where the boundaries may, in fact, correspond with major discontinuities. However, it is of interest to mention a proposed method based on horizontal slices (Shahgoli et al., 2001). This method is of particular value for the analysis of reinforced slopes especially where the reinforcing elements are arranged horizontally. Reinforced slopes with horizontal elements, made of steel or geosynthetics, are widely used as geotechnical structures and their design and analysis under static and seismic conditions is of considerable interest (Ling et al., 1997).

5.6.5   A variation of the method of slices and its application to the 1963 Vaiont slide

Occasionally geotechnical engineers may vary some details of the method of vertical slices procedure in a way that may or may not be consistent with basic concepts of mechanics and which may not lead to consistent results for different problems. For example, Anderson's (1985) static analysis procedure assumes the slip surface to be a series of planes and the slide is subdivided into elements with vertical interslice boundaries. In fact, this procedure may be regarded simply as a wedge method for a slip surface of multi-planar shape (refer to chapter 4). The stability of an element as a wedge is analysed and the inclination of the inter-wedge force (termed the angle of internal shearing resistance or the interslice friction angle) is assumed to be constant across all the slices or wedges, as each wedge is analysed, in turn. Iterative analyses are carried out to satisfy the force equilibrium of each slice and to match the condition of zero external force at the toe and crest. The possibility of inter-wedge movement was considered to be an inherent assumption in the use of this method. Moment equilibrium is disregarded and this is justified by referring to the nature of the landslide which is translational rather than rotational. However, from a rigorous perspective, this is a weakness in all wedge methods which rely only on force equilibrium of successive elements or wedges.

The chosen value of this inclination is presumably based on an assessment of geological and geotechnical data for a particular slope. Anderson's method was used by Hendron and Patton (1985) to carry out several two dimensional (2D) analyses of the well known 1963 Vaiont slide. The interslice friction (or angle of shearing resistance) was assumed to be 40 degrees and this value was justified on the basis of the known details, available data and other assumptions concerning the case study. However, it was found that the values of 2D factor of safety were too low. Values $F < 1$ were calculated with pore water pressure data for periods when the slide mass was observed to be stable implying $F > 1$. For periods of movement, the values of F were significantly low rather than just below 1. Consequently; 3D analyses were considered relevant and justified on the basis of the shape of the sliding surface and the configuration of the whole sliding mass.

With some modification, Andersons's static method (Andreson, 1985) was also used to develop a simple three-dimensional (3D) analysis procedure for the Vaiont slide. Shearing resistance along a vertical eastern boundary of the slide was added to the shearing resistance along the slip surface inferred from 2D analyses along three separate cross-sections. The angle of frictional shear resistance along this vertical Eastern boundary was assumed to be 36°. For both 2D and 3D analyses, the residual angle of shear resistance on basal planes was assumed to be 12°. According to Hendron and Patton (1985), this set of values of the shear strength parameters can help explain the occurrence of the four periods of movement (implying instability of the slide mass) as well as the periods of relative stability of the Vaiont slide mass. More details and some of the results are provided and discussed briefly in section 5.12.8 of this chapter and also in chapter 7 (section 7.16).

5.7   MORGENSTERN AND PRICE METHOD

A numerical solution to the limit equilibrium slope stability problem, based on the method of slices, which satisfies both force and moment equilibrium is generally called a 'rigorous' solution. The first such solution, considering slip surfaces of arbitrary shape, was developed by Morgenstern and Price (1965). The following summarises a version discussed later by Morgenstern (1968). The coordinate axes and the forces on a slice are shown in Figure 5.8. Note that the resultant forces due to pore water pressure P_W acting on the boundaries of a slice are shown separately from the total normal forces E. Resultant pore water pressure on the base of the slice is denoted by dP_b, the weight by dW, the interslice forces T and E act at y_t below the x-axis, dS is the mobilised shear strength on the slice based on factor of safety F.

This slope stability problem is statically indeterminate with high degree of indeterminacy. The following relationship is assumed between the E and T forces on a slice to make the problem statically determinate:

$$T = \lambda f(x)E \tag{5.17}$$

where λ is a parameter which must be determined from the solution and $f(x)$ is an arbitrary function which must be specified. It may be noted that Equation (5.17) corresponds to

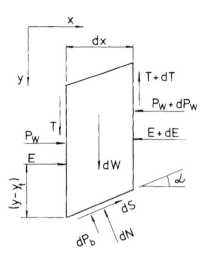

Figure 5.8 Forces on a typical slice – slip surface of arbitrary shape, Morgenstern and price method.

a total stress side force assumption. While some computer programs use this approach, others are based on a side force assumption expressed in terms of effective stresses. A user of any computer programme must find out which type of assumption has been made so that the results are processed and interpreted correctly (Starr, 1968). Regardless of how the assumption is made, results can be processed to give both effective side forces and total side forces. Considering the forces acting on a slice of width dx, moment equilibrium about the base of the slice gives the following when $dx \to 0$:

$$-T = \frac{d}{dx}\{E(y - y_t)\} - E\frac{dy}{dx} + \frac{d}{dx}\{P_W(y - h)\} - P_W\frac{dy}{dx} \tag{5.18}$$

The assumed slip surface is $y = y(x)$, the surface of the slope is $y = z(x)$, the line of action of the water pressure is $y = h(x)$ and the line of action of the effective normal force acting across the soil mass is $y = y_t(x)$.

The conditions of equilibrium in directions normal and tangential to base of slice combined with the Coulomb-Terzaghi failure criterion lead to the following equation:

$$\frac{dE}{dx}\left\{1 - \frac{\tan\phi}{F} \cdot \frac{dy}{dx}\right\} + \frac{dT}{dx}\left\{\frac{\tan\phi}{F} + \frac{dy}{dx}\right\}$$
$$= \frac{c}{F}\left\{1 + \left(\frac{dy}{dx}\right)^2\right\} + \frac{dP_W}{dx}\left\{\frac{\tan\phi}{F} \cdot \frac{dy}{dx} - 1\right\} \tag{5.19}$$
$$+ \frac{dw}{dx}\left\{\frac{\tan\phi}{F} + \frac{dy}{dx}\right\} - P_u\left\{1 + (\frac{dy}{dx})^2\right\}\frac{\tan\phi}{F}$$

In which $P_u = \cos\alpha \dfrac{dP_b}{dx}$ and $\tan\alpha = -\dfrac{dy}{dx}$ (5.20)

From Equations (5.17) and s(5.19) the following is obtained

$$\frac{dE}{dx}\left[1 - \frac{\tan\phi}{F}\frac{dy}{dx} + \lambda f\left\{\frac{\tan\phi}{F} + \frac{dy}{dx}\right\} + \lambda\frac{df}{dx}\left\{\frac{\tan\phi}{F} + \frac{dy}{dx}\right\}E\right]$$

$$= \frac{c}{p}\left\{1 + \left(\frac{dy}{dx}\right)^2\right\} + \frac{dP_W}{dx}\left\{\frac{\tan\phi}{F}\frac{dy}{dx} - 1\right\} + \frac{dW}{dx}\left\{\frac{\tan\phi}{F} + \frac{dy}{dx}\right\}$$

$$- P_u\left\{1 + \left(\frac{dy}{dx}\right)^2\right\}\frac{\tan\phi}{F}$$ (5.21)

Consider subdivision into n vertical slices with co-ordinates at boundaries x_0, x_1, x_2 .... x_n. The following linear and polynomial approximations are made within each slice.

$$y = Ax + B,\ dW/dx = px + q,\ f = kx + m$$
$$P_u = rx + s,\ P_W = U_W + V_W x = W_W x^2$$ (5.22)
$$bP_W = U_N + V_N x + W_N x^2 + Z_N x^3$$

in which x is measured from the beginning of each slice.

Now equation (5.21) may be simplified to the following from:

$$(Kx + L)\frac{dE}{dx} + KE = Nx + P$$ (5.23)

in which

$$K = \lambda k\left(\frac{\tan\phi}{F} + A\right),\ L = 1 - \frac{A\tan\phi}{F} + \lambda m\left(\frac{\tan\phi}{F} + A\right)$$

$$N = \frac{\tan\phi}{F}[2AW_W + p - r(1 + A^2)] + [-2W_w + pA],$$ (5.24)

$$P = \frac{1}{F}[(c - s\tan\phi)(1 + A^2) + V_W A\tan\phi + q\tan\phi] + [(qA - V_W)]$$

By integrating Equation (5.23) over a slice from x_i

$$E(x) = \frac{1}{L + Kx}\left[E_i L + \frac{Nx^2}{2} + Px\right]$$ (5.25)

Therefore,

$$E_{i+1} = \frac{1}{L + Kb} \left[E_i L + \frac{Nb^2}{2} + Pb \right] \tag{5.26}$$

where $b = (x_{i+1} - x_i)$ is the width of the slice.

Using Equations (5.17) and (5.18) and integrating over the range x_0 to x,

$$M(x) = E(y_t - y) = M_{eW}(x) + \int_{x_0}^{x} \left(\lambda f - \frac{dy}{dx} \right) E \, dx \tag{5.27}$$

in which $M_{eW}(x)$ is defined

$$M_{eW}(x) = \int_{x_0}^{x} \left[-P_W \frac{dy}{dx} \right] dx + \left[P_W (y - h) \right]_{x_0}^{x} \tag{5.28}$$

By substituting the assumed linear and polynomial expressions into Equation (5.19), a relation may be obtained between M_{i+1} and the width of slices. The usual boundary conditions may be specified as

$$E(X_0) = 0, \; M(x_0) = 0, \; E(x_n) = 0, \; M(x_n) = 0 \tag{5.29}$$

where n is the number of slices. Boundary conditions different from Equation (5.29) may occur e.g., with external loads on the boundary, submergence of slope, water filled tension cracks etc.

Values of λ and F may be assumed to evaluate E and M at the end of the first slice from equations (5.26) and (5.27). Then E and M are obtained for each successive slice. The last two equations of Equation (5.29) will be satisfied only when the correct values of λ and F have been assumed. The solution is obtained by iteration using a digital computer. This numerical solution is equivalent to solving a pair of non-linear simultaneous equations involving λ and F as unknowns.

Morgenstern and Price (1965) used the Newton-Raphson technique for solution. Among the early references to computer programs implementing the M-P method are those by Bailey (1966) and Hamel (1968). In the last four decades, several computer software packages have been developed which include the M-P method for slope analysis. Before working with any available M-P computer programme, a potential user must carefully check all the assumptions and numerical solution techniques in the programme, as well as the manner in which the results are processed. It is also necessary to understand any limitations and acceptability criteria that must be satisfied. It is only too easy to misuse a programme particularly when the user is inexperienced (See also Appendix III).

The factor of safety F depends on the assumed side force function $f(x)$ and thus it does not have a unique value, although the variations in F are usually very small. It is of interest to get complete information from the computer about the internal force distribution, scale factor λ, position of the line of thrust and normal and tangential forces on the base of each slice. The line of thrust in the M-P Method can be obtained in terms of effective stresses and this is helpful in assessing the acceptability of the solution. The local factor of safety is calculated as a ratio of the shear force acting at a slice boundary to the available shear resistance. The solution is theoretically not admissible if this factor of safety is less than unity. In practice, however, all the acceptability criteria are seldom satisfied over all the slices. Moreover, difference in the factor of safety between several solutions of varying degrees of admissibility is often small.

5.8   SIMPLIFIED CALCULATION AND CORRECTION FACTOR

Inspite of the widespread use of electronic computers it is frequently necessary to resort to simple solutions so that hand calculations can be made. Simple solutions are a useful check on more elaborate computer-based methods which can sometimes go wrong due to numerical difficulties or inexperience of the user or even some inherent characteristics in the methods themselves. Simple methods give a better feel of the problem and its solution and facilitate better communication not only between experts but between an expert on the one hand and a client on the other. Effective technical communication is absolutely essential for efficiency in geotechnical engineering and for this reason alone, simple methods can never be dispensed with completely.

Often simple solutions which ignore inter-slice forces are fairly accurate for long and somewhat flat slip surfaces. For other cases, correction factors may be devised. Janbu et al. (1956) gave the following version of the factor of safety which is a modification of Equation (5.14) when inter-slice forces are ignored:

$$F = \frac{f \ \Sigma bs \ \sec^2 \alpha}{\Sigma W \tan \alpha} \tag{5.14b}$$

where

$$s = \frac{c + \left(\dfrac{W}{b} - u \right) \tan \phi}{1 + \tan \alpha \tan \phi / F} \tag{5.14c}$$

and f is a correction factor which depends on the geometric ratio d/L and is plotted in Figure 5.9. As the slip surface becomes elongated and the ratio d/L decreases, the correction factor approaches unity. This correction factor f here should not be confused with the side force function $f(x)$ used as an assumed function to develop the solution known as the M-P Method.

Note that when $f = 1$, Equations (5.14b) and (5.14c) are equivalent to Equations (5.14) and (5.14a) respectively when inter-slice forces are ignored. Iterative calculation with different values of F may be done by hand and convergence is rapid. For each calculation the appropriate value of the correction factor f must be used in evaluating F from Equation (5.14b).

Sometimes the use of simplified approaches may lead to unexpected inaccuracies. This was demonstrated for circular slip surfaces by Bishop (1955). He showed that the difference between F calculated by the conventional slice approach and the

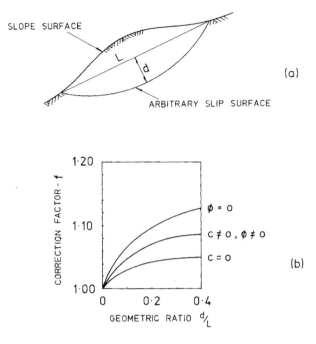

Figure 5.9 Correction factor for use in simplified calculations after Janbu et al. (1956) shown in (b) corresponding to geometric ratio d/L shown in (a).

rigorous approach increased with increase in (a) excess pore water pressure and (b) central angle of the circular arc. The errors could be as large as 50% for the analysis of stability of the upstream slope of an earth embankment after rapid draw down. However, there was a dramatic gain in accuracy if the Bishop Simplified Method was used, and the results were close to those given by a rigorous approach.

5.9 SOME EARLY APPLICATIONS

Limit equilibrium methods have been applied to a wide range of problems involving soil and rock slopes and there is little doubt of their continued popularity. It is of interest to mention some typical and unusual applications here. Hamel (1968, 1972) used the Morgenstern and Price approach to analyse a slide which was triggered by high pore water pressures developed due to the freezing of natural drainage outlets at the face of a slope. The failure surface passed through soft clay, shale and indurated clay and through an open vertical joint in overlying shale. He studied several other examples and recommended criteria for evaluating the acceptability of Morgenstern and Price solutions for (a) soil slopes and (b) rock slopes. These are given in Appendix III.

Hamel et al. (1976) used the Morgenstern and Price approach for the analysis of foundation sliding stability of concrete gravity dams and found that traditional analysis procedures gave very conservative results. The Morgenstern and Price Method which satisfies both force and moment equilibrium gave substantially higher factors of safety (25% to 30%) than conventional methods based on horizontal force equilibrium alone. It is also important to note that the factor of safety may be defined in different ways: (a) in some of the traditional methods it is the ratio of resisting to driving forces (moments) and (b) in the Morgenstern and Price method it is the ratio of available to required (or mobilised) unit shear strength. The latter definition is considered to be more appropriate.

It is interesting that sliding block or wedge analyses for typical cases appear to underestimate the factor of safety by about 20% to 30% if the inter-wedge forces are assumed to be horizontal, especially when short deep failure masses with high pore water pressures are considered and when there is a water-filled tension crack at the rear of the potential failure mass. These conditions and results correspond to the foundation-sliding stability problem considered in the above paragraph (Hamel, 1977 pers. comm.).

Janbu (1957) has shown that limit equilibrium analysis by the generalised procedure of slices can be used to solve problems of bearing capacity and earth pressure in addition to routine slope stability problems. Such solutions can be obtained quickly and efficiently. Morgenstern (1968) has also suggested that the Morgenstern and Price Method can be used for the solution of earth pressure and bearing capacity problems. The inclusion of external loads and boundary forces is possible in most methods with appropriate modifications in the relevant equations as discussed for the Janbu Method.

5.10 SPECIAL ANALYSES

5.10.1 Slope underlain by very weak soil layer such as soft clay

Often failure may involve a composite slip surface in which different sections do not merge smoothly into one another and it may be inaccurate and unsafe to approximate it by a continuous surface. Failure may involve both active and passive modes. Terzaghi and Peck (1967) referred to the example of a slope underlain by a thin layer of soft material (Figure 5.10). In such a case calculations must be made for the active pressure P_A applied by the soil on the right hand side as well as the passive resistance P_P of the left hand side wedge end. The factor of safety may be calculated by considering the force equilibrium. Assuming P_p and P_A to be horizontal and considering short-term stability, the expression for factor of safety F may be written as follows:

$$F = \frac{P_p + S}{P_A} \tag{5.30}$$

in which S is the undrained shearing resistance offered by the portion bc of the slip surface. For soft clays, S is generally independent of normal stresses and hence independent of W. Thus it is the product of undrained cohesion and length bc. Several trials may be made by selecting different positions for points c and b. The critical failure surface will correspond to the minimum factor of safety obtained in these trials. As an alternative to this approach one can use the tri-planar wedge approach discussed in chapter 4. Different tri-planar failure surfaces may be used and the minimum factor of safety determined after several trials.

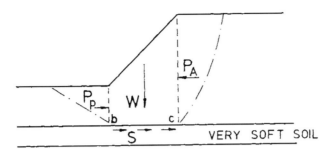

Figure 5.10 Failure of slope due to slip along layer of soft clay. (after Terzaghi and Peck, 1967). Permission requested, see page 714, No 44.

5.10.2   Considering calculated F in the context of the method of analysis

The choice of a method of analysis may have an important influence on the calculated factor of safety. Some examples have already been given earlier in this chapter. Consider now the problem of sliding on a soft layer as shown in Figure 5.10. In this situation limit equilibrium calculations may be made on the basis of the following alternative approaches.

I   Earth pressure approach [e.g., section 5.10.1 above].
II   (a) Sliding block or wedge analysis (e.g., section 4.11) or, (b) any generalised procedure of slices discussed earlier in this chapter.

It is obvious that different values of the calculated factor of safety would result in each case. In fact individual methods within group II may give different factors of safety. To a significant extent differences in *F* may be due to the different ways in which the factor of safety is defined and this aspect has been discussed in chapter 4 and earlier in this chapter. However, differences between method I and group of methods II must also arise from the fact that earth pressure theory is used in method I to calculate the net driving force. This has a fundamental significance and particular attention requires to be given to the following aspects:

1   Full mobilisation of earth pressure requires some deformation. The extent of deformation required for active failure may be different from that required for passive failure.
2   The extent of deformation required for failure in stiff soil may be quite different from that required for failure in underlying weak or soft soil.
3   The inclinations of failure planes in the field often do not correspond to those predicted on the basis of classical earth pressure theories.
4   The use of an earth pressure approach precludes consideration of inclined inter-block or inter-wedge boundaries which may be critical in some situations (e.g., Seed and Sultan, 1967, and, Sultan and Seed, 1967).

Hamel (1968) made a comparison between factors of safety based on earth pressure and Morgenstern and Price approach for one problem. The example selected from a design manual (NAVDOCKS, 1962) considers a 2:1 slope in non-homogeneous soil. The value of the factor of safety calculated in the design manual on the basis of the earth pressure approach is $F = 1.08$. Hamel found that the Morgenstern and Price method gave $F = 1.53$ (based on a constant side force distribution assumption) and $F = 1.41$ (based on a half sine wave distribution of side forces).

It is obvious from such large differences in calculated F that an acceptable value of F must depend to some extent on the method of analysis used. It is not possible to generalise and recommend that an earth pressure approach should or should not be used. In some situations, it may appear to be quite logical. In others it may present many difficulties of interpretation especially where a soil deposit has several layers with different properties. Experience is required in making a suitable choice of method of analysis in such cases. However, whatever the choice, experience may also suggest that different values of F are acceptable for different methods. For instance if the choice is an earth pressure approach (for the type of example considered above) a value of $F = 1.2$ (say) may be considered quite acceptable. On the other hand if the choice is a Morgenstern and Price approach a value of $F = 1.6$ (say) may be considered as an acceptable value. Such decisions can only be made on the basis of experience. This aspect is discussed further in section 5.14.5.

5.10.3   Clay slope underlain by water-bearing seam of fine sand

Figure 5.11 shows the forces acting on a soil slope underlain by a water bearing seam of fine sand. When the pore water pressure is low and undrained cohesion of clay controls the shear strength ('$\phi = 0$' conditions) the critical height is given from Taylor's charts for any slope less than $53°$ as:

$$H_c = 5.52 \frac{c}{\gamma} \tag{5.31}$$

The critical height is even greater if a firm base lies at shallow depth.

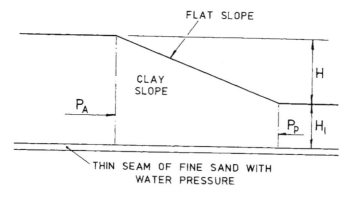

Figure 5.11 Forces in slope of clay with thin seam of water-bearing sand.

When the pore water pressure rises in the thin sand layer due to rain or melting snow, the shearing resistance of the sand layer decreases due to decrease of effective normal stress. The critical height may be estimated on the assumption that pore water pressure in the sand layer becomes equal to the total normal stress (and thus effective stress and shearing strength along the sand layer become zero). Thus, equating active and passive pressures as shown in Figure 5.11:

$$\frac{1}{2}\gamma(H+H_1)^2 - 2c(H+H_1) = \frac{1}{2}\gamma H_1^2 + 2cH_1$$

or   (5.32)

$$H = H_c = 4\frac{c}{\gamma}$$

This value of critical height is independent of the slope inclination and is close to the critical height of a vertical slope ($3.85\ c/\gamma$, according to Fellenius, 1927). This simple analysis suggested by Terzaghi and Peck (1967) explains the sudden spreading of clay slopes after wet spells, irrespective of their inclination. Such spreading may occur even when slopes are very flat. When there are several layers of permeable materials such as fine sand or silt, failure may occur by static liquefaction as soon as the porewater pressure in these layers becomes approximately equal to the overburden pressure. Such failures are very rapid in comparison to ordinary gravity slides.

5.11   AN EARLY COMPARISON OF DIFFERENT LIMIT EQUILIBRIUM METHODS

It is useful to compare different limit equilibrium methods in terms of the factors of safety obtained for specific problems. It is also useful from both practical and conceptual aspects to study the differences in assumptions in various methods. Comparison of the type and extent of information that can be obtained is also valuable.

Differences in accuracy (in the determination of the value of F) depend mainly on the type of problem. In some problems the results of simple methods may not differ significantly from those of more accurate methods while in others the differences may be unacceptable (Bishop 1955; Whitman & Bailey, 1967; Wright, 1975; Chowdhury, 1975). Table 5.2 shows a comparison of three methods for four different types of problem made by Whitman & Bailey (1967). It is clear that the ordinary method of slices underestimates the factor of safety and is therefore conservative and safe. However, the extent of underestimate may be so large that the solution would prove to be uneconomical. Again, it should be noted that different methods will in general lead to different positions of the critical slip surface. This is not a matter of much concern if the critical slip surface is largely controlled by geological aspects, which can be identified before analysis. Table 5.3 gives a summary of the significant features of several methods to which reference has been made so far.

Table 5.2 Comparison of factors of safety *F* obtained by different methods of slices (Whitman and Bailey, 1967). With permission from ASCE, see page 713, No 15.

	Value of F		
Example case	*O. M. S.*	*B. S. M.*	*M. P. M.*
(1) Homogenenous soil and no pore pressure	1.49	1.61	1.58–1.62
(2) Long term stability of embankment on organic silt. Three different soils	1.09	1.33	1.24–1.26
(3) Immediate stability of the same embankment as in 2	0.66	0.7–0.82	0.73–0.78
(4) Submerged slope of	1.14	2.00	2.01–2.03
Rockfill resting on inclined core of cohesive soil	1.84*		

O. M. S. = Ordinary method of slices (also called Fellenius Method).
B. S. M. = Bishop Simplified Method.
M. P. M. = Morgenstern and Price Method.
*The first value corresponds to use of total unit weight and pore pressure and the second to use of submerged unit weight. This points to a special difficulty of the Ordinary method of slices in exceptional cases.
Note: The range of results in M. P. M. is based on choice of assumption concerning interslice forces. The two values for case 3 by B. S. M. were due to some difficulty in determining the shear force at the base of a slice near the toe as discussed by Whitman and Bailey (1967).

Table 5.3 Features of different slope stability methods suitable for curved or composite slip surfaces and for non-homogeneous soils.

Method	*Features*
Fellenius	Underestimates factor of safety. Errors large for deep failure masses with high pore pressures. Calculation very simple, no iteration required. Strictly applicable to circular failure surfaces only. Adequate for total stress analyses of circular failure surfaces but not always suitable for effective stress analyses.
Bishop simplified	Normal force on slice base obtained by resolving forces on a slice in a vertical direction. Results are fairly accurate. The method is strictly restricted to slip surfaces of circular shape. Iterative procedure required for solution but convergence rapid. Errors possible where portion of slip surface has steep negative slope near toe. Suitable for both total and effective stress analyses of circular failure surfaces in soil and soft rock.
Janbu	Requires assumption regarding position of line of thrust. Iterations made with successive sets of inter-slice forces till convergence reached. Suitable for slip surfaces of arbitrary shape. Convergence generally rapid. Necessary to check acceptability of solution in terms of any implied tension or violation of failure criterion. Suitable for total and effective stress analyses of soil and rock slopes.
Janbu simplified	Use of correction factors necessary. Suitable for slip surfaces of arbitrary shape in soil and rock mostly for preliminary work.

(Continued)

Table 5.3 (Continued).

Morgenstern and Price	Versatile method which satisfies both force and moment equilibrium and accounts for inter slice forces. A side force function must be assumed. The method is applicable to failure surfaces of arbitrary shape and arbitrary boundary conditions. Acceptability of solution must be checked-as in Janbu method. Considerable experience and judgment required to use the method reliably, to assume side force functions which lead to acceptable results and to interpret the results. Useful for both effective and total stress analyses of soil and rock slopes.
Spencer	Originally devised for circular failure surfaces, but adapted for non-circular failure surfaces (Spencer, 1973; Wright, 1975). Assumes inter-slice forces to be parallel. Accuracy acceptable. Satisfies both force and moment equilibrium. Use of computer desirable. Specially devised in relation to embankment stability problems, but may be used for all types of problems.
Sliding Block or Wedge (See Chap. 4)	Can be used for typical non-circular failure surface (bi-planar and tri-planar) which have been observed in practice. Very well suited to many rock slope problems and some soil slope problems. Care should be exercised in selecting inclination of inter-wedge forces. Inclination of inter-wedge forces especially important for short deep failure masses with high pore pressures. In special cases it may be more appropriate to base the calculation on active and passive pressures (section 5.10).

Note: (a) In all the methods considered above, except the Fellenius method, the factor of safety F is defined as the ratio of unit shear strength available at a point to unit shear strength mobilised or required at the same point. F is assumed constant along slip surface. (b) Friction circle method is not included because it is suitable only for homogeneous deposits. For such cases it has the advantage that upper and lower bounds to F may be found.

5.12   THREE-DIMENSIONAL EFFECTS

Idealisation of real three-dimensional (3D) slope problems as two dimensional (2D) problems is often valid However, in some cases three-dimensional effects may be significant and, therefore, 3-D analyses are justified. Generally the value of the factor of safety F will be underestimated by using a 2D analysis where a 3D analysis is appropriate. It is also important to consider back-analysis of a failure which may be carried out to understand the failure as well as to estimate the shear strength. A slope failure is like a full scale test with the factor of safety at the time of failure having the value $F = 1$. A 2D back analysis of a 3D slope failure would overestimate the shear strength if F(3D) is greater than F(2D), which is the general case.

5.12.1   Developments over the last four decades

Several methods of 3D limit equilibrium analysis ranging from the relatively simple to the sophisticated have been developed and many comparisons of 2D and 3D analyses have been made. In a review of methods developed over the period 1969–1992, Duncan (1992) noted that most researchers reported the 3D values of F (F_3) to be greater than the corresponding 2D values (F_2). In one case F_3 was as high as 1.5 F_2. However, some investigators reported instances or example cases with $F_3 < F_2$. Such results appeared unrealistic to other researchers and the reliability of the particular methods or comparisons was questioned. Cavounidis (1987) concluded that, in cases where F_3 was found to be less than F_2, either inappropriate factors of safety were compared or the methods were based on simplifying assumptions, or important aspects of the problem were neglected. In terms of the reliability of some of the 3D methods, it is interesting to note that Chen and Chameau (1982) found that results from an extended Spencer-type 3D limit equilibrium analysis compare well with a finite-element analysis.

An interesting 3-D approach for saturated slopes in discontinuous rock has been described by Hatzor and Goodman (1997). The approach is based on block theory combining limit equilibrium and kinematic methods using stereographic projection and vector analysis. Two historic block failures on the left abutment of Pacoima Dam, California, were back-analysed. Water pressures within the boundary joints were introduced by parametric addition of vectors. The effect on water pressure on the factor of safety F was, of course, significant. More importantly, the rate of change of F with joint water pressure in the base joints was higher for double plane sliding and lowers for single plane sliding. The stability of the right abutment was also analysed by block theory and, in contrast to the left abutment, it was found to be safe by virtue of kinematics alone. This result about the right abutment has been validated by field experience since it has survived several episodes of strong ground motion.

Some aspects of different approaches and methods for 3-D analyses are presented in the following sub-sections. Here the emphasis is on relatively simple approaches. Detailed discussion of relatively rigorous 3D approaches is outside the scope of this book. Specialized computer software is now commercially available not only for 2D analyses but also for 3D analyses. Such software may include methods ranging from relatively simple to rigorous or sophisticated.

5.12.2   Weighted average procedure

Slides in cohesive materials are often three-dimensional in character. In some cases three-dimensional effects may not appear to be important while in others it may be necessary to account for such effects. Two-dimensional analyses may be carried out for several cross-sections within a sliding mass, each taken perpendicular to the length direction of the mass. Approximate calculation of the three-dimensional factor of safety may be made as follows:

Consider several parallel cross-sections through the slope. For these let A_1, A_2, A_3, etc. be the areas and F_1, F_2, F_3 ..., the limit equilibrium factors of safety (2D), calculated for each cross-section respectively. The overall factor of safety (3D) may be defined as follows (see e.g., Sherrard et al., 1963; Lambe and Whitman, 1969):

$$F = \frac{F_1 A_1 + F_2 A_2 + F_3 A_3 + \cdots\cdots}{A_1 + A_2 + A_3 + \cdots\cdots} \tag{5.33}$$

5.12.3   Inclusion of end effects

Where the failure mass is long and the cross-sectional area of the potential failure mass is nearly uniform at various sections along its axis, end effects may be directly included in an analysis. Consider for example '$\phi = 0$' type of analysis discussed in section 5.2.1.

Let the failure length be l. Shear failure is resisted (a) along the cylindrical surface of sliding of length l and radius R giving a resisting moment of $sR^2 \theta l$ and (b) at the two ends, giving a combined resisting moment of $2M_0$. Considering a small elemental area dA within the cross section at a distance r from the centre of the circle, M_0 is given by the summation $M_0 = \Sigma\Sigma c \, dA \, r$ where c is the undrained cohesion for the small elemental area dA. Therefore, the increased factor of safety is given by:

$$F = \frac{sR^2 \theta l + 2\Sigma\Sigma c \, dA \, r}{Wxl} \tag{5.1a}$$

Where l is very long in comparison to M_0, Equation (5.1a) reduces to the two-dimensional form [Equation (5.1)] discussed in section 5.2.1. In a similar manner, end effects can be provided for in other problems where both c and ϕ are included in analysis. Similarly, the analysis may be extended to cases where the cross-section of the slip surface is wedge shaped or of arbitrary shape.

Baligh and Azzouz (1975) studied three-dimensional effects on the stability of cohesive slopes using a computer program in which the failure mass was considered to be a surface of revolution extending along the ground surface for a finite length. (The two-dimensional case corresponds to an infinitely long cylinder). Different geometries and shapes were considered to analyse the "end effects" by attaching either an ellipsoid or a cone at each end of a finite cylinder. The Ordinary method of slices was adopted for analysis, the aim being only to compare factors of safety F for different shapes. It was found that F increased generally from its two-dimensional value. For long shallow failures (in which the ratio of length along axis of slope to depth of failure is greater than eight) the increase is of the order of 5% and can be disregarded. For short deep slope failures in which this ratio is less than 2 to 4, the increase in factor of safety may be greater than 25% and three-dimensional effects must therefore be considered. They also found that the prediction of length of failure is difficult since it is very sensitive to slope and material parameters.

5.12.4 A general three-dimensional approach

Hovland (1977) proposed a general but simplified (approximate) approach for three-dimensional (3D) slope stability analyses aimed at finding a factor of safety F defined as the ratio of the total available resistance along a failure surface and the total mobilised resistance along it. From the simple definition adopted above, the 2D factor of safety F_2 for a slope of height h may be expressed as follows:

$$F_2 = \frac{c}{\gamma h} A_2 + \tan\phi \, B_2 \tag{5.34}$$

where

$$A_2 = \frac{\Sigma \sec\alpha}{\Sigma \dfrac{z}{h}\sin\alpha} \quad \text{and} \quad B_2 = \frac{\Sigma \, z \cos\alpha}{\Sigma \, z \sin\alpha} \tag{5.35}$$

in which α is the inclination of the base of any slice and z its height and the slice width is considered constant. A_2 and B_2 are functions only of geometry and determine how cohesion and friction components of resistance respectively are influenced by geometry.

The 3D factor of safety F_3 may be presented in a similar form considering the soil mass above the failure surface to be divided into a number of vertical soil columns. Assume the xy plane to be horizontal and z axis to be vertical and y axis to be in the direction of downslope movement. Let Δx and Δy define the cross sectional area of a vertical soil column on the xy plane and assume that both Δx and Δy are constant for all slices. Then we have the expression:

$$F_3 = \frac{c}{\gamma h} A_3 + \tan \phi \, B_3 \qquad (5.36)$$

in which

$$A_3 = \frac{\Sigma_x \Sigma_y \sec \alpha_{xz} \sec \alpha_{yz} \sin \theta}{\Sigma_x \Sigma_y \frac{z}{h} \sin \alpha_{yz}}$$

$$B_3 = \frac{\Sigma_x \Sigma_y \, z \cos (\mathrm{DIP})}{\Sigma_x \Sigma_y \, z \sin \alpha_{yz}} \qquad (5.37)$$

in which α_{xz} and α_{yz} are the dip angles in the xz and yz planes respectively and DIP and θ are given by: (DIP follows usual geological definition).

$$\cos (\mathrm{DIP}) = \left(1 + \tan^2 \alpha_{xz} + \tan^2 \alpha_{yz}\right)^{-\frac{1}{2}} \qquad (5.38)$$
$$\cos \theta = (\sin \alpha_{xz} \, \sin \alpha_{yz})$$

The factors A_3 and B_3 represent the influence of the problem geometry including the shape of the 3D failure surface.

Hovland (1977) made a number of 2D and 3D studies by the simple method outlined above and found that 3D factors of safety are usually higher than 2D factors of safety. However, it is interesting that in some situations 3D factors of safety were lower than 2D factors of safety. His studies also showed that landslides in cohesive soils may follow a wide shear surface geometry approaching a 2D case. On the other hand, slides in cohesionless soil may follow a 3D wedge type surface. In general the ratio F_3/F_2 is quite sensitive to the values of c and ϕ and also the shape of the 3D surface. The difference between F_3 and F_2 is not a consequence of end effects alone but also of the different extent to which resisting and driving forces are altered in going from a 2D to a 3D situation. Hovland defended the use of a simple approach which ignores inter-slice forces on two grounds: (1) Assumption of inter-slice forces in conventional 2D analyses does not necessarily make them realistic since 3D effects are ignored; (2) the proposed method can be used in combination with finite element analyses which enable computation of stresses and deformations throughout a continuum.

5.12.5   Lateral curvature (curvature in plan) of a slope

The lateral curvature of a slope may have a significant influence on its stability. The usual assumption in two-dimensional analyses is that a slope is very long and straight in its lateral direction. This assumption may not be justified in some natural slopes where effects of curvature may be important. Similarly these effects may be significant in mining excavations. Reference is made in chapter 8 (section 8.2) to an interesting study for axisymmetric slopes (vertical wells). This study was made with mining situations in mind and showed the beneficial effects of curvature on slope stability (Jenike and Yen, 1963). However, care should be exercised in making qualitative judgements concerning the effects of curvature which may be either concave or convex. The influence of pit geometry on the stability of excavated slopes in open cast mines was discussed by Hoek (1970). He pointed out that there was a tendency for convex slopes to suffer instability in comparison to concave slopes. This difference in behaviour was attributed to the difference in stress conditions. Concave shapes tend to introduce compressive stresses and to increase stability by arching action. Convex shapes on the other hand tend to assist relaxation of normal stresses with consequent decrease of shear strength and opening of joints and fissures in some cases. However, improved drainage conditions in convex slopes may compensate for this reduction in stability. Clearly there are a number of complex factors to be considered in any particular problem and any conclusions must be reached after comprehensive evaluation of all influencing factors.

Based on their experience with rock slopes, Hoek and Bray (1977) recommend that the slope angle of a concave slope can be $10°$ steeper than that required by conventional limit equilibrium methods if the radius of curvature of the slope is less than the height of the slope. On the other hand if a convex slope has a radius of curvature less than the slope height, the slope angle should be $10°$ flatter than the angle required by two-dimensional analysis. Once again these recommendations should be treated only as a guide. In addition to rock slopes these recommendations were considered to be applicable to the design of waste tips which may have undesirable convex curvature due to dumping procedures.

5.12.6   Shape or curvature of slope profile or slope face

As the height of a soil or rock slope increases, the critical stable angle or inclination of slope decreases. This conclusion is generally valid when the material of any slope has some cohesion. Therefore for high slopes the slope angle must decrease with depth below the surface. In other words relatively steep angles can be tolerated towards the crest of a slope but the slope must be made flatter with increase in the depth. An important exception is the case where a weathered zone exists at the surface. Such a zone would have a low shear strength in comparison to unweathered material. Thus steepening such a slope near the crest may not be feasible. The concept of increasing slope inclination towards the top of a homogeneous slope is of tremendous practical importance in very high rock slopes particularly in open cut mining operations.

Beneficial effects may also be obtained by making a slope face concave. As concavity of a slope face increases the factor of safety F increases and as the face is made convex, the value of F decreases (Rana and Bullock, 1969; Hoek and Bray, 1977).

5.12.7   An example of 3D factor of safety calculations – analysis of the 1963 Vaiont slide

The reader may first refer to section 5.6.5 where mention was made of a variation of the method of slices used by Hendron and Patton (1985) for an analysis of the 1963 Vaiont slide. The chair-shaped configuration of the Vaiont slide in cross-section is well known. Most investigators and commentators have considered the lower or basal part of the slip surface to be near-horizontal. However, Hendron and Patton (1985) drew attention to the 1960 unpublished geological maps developed by Giudici and Semenza, before and after the landslide which indicate that the lower part of the slide surface dips upstream (to the east) in the range 9–22 degrees.

They argued that as a consequence of these geological conditions, the three-dimensional aspect of the slide mass must be considered in an assessment of its stability and performance during the period of reservoir filling and the subsequent catastrophic failure of the landslide mass. They proposed the inclusion, in the stability analysis, of the additional shearing resistance along a vertical boundary at the eastern end of the slide. They speculated that this eastern boundary of the slide was associated with the location of one or more faults. Either the eastern boundary of the slide was formed during the occurrence of the old, undated slide which is presumed to have occurred at this site, or it may have been formed during subsequent geological processes. They pointed out that a lateral fault was shown on the unpublished 1964 and 1965 geological maps of Rossi and Semenza. Moreover, field evidence was claimed to have been found by Hendron and Patton (1985) which confirmed the spatial transition or connection between the fault surface and the slide surface close to the eastern boundary.

Two-dimensional analyses by the modified method of slices were carried out on three separate cross sections. For each cross-section, F (2D) was computed considering the following six cases of pore water pressure distribution along the slip surface:

Case (a) assumed high artesian pore water pressures on the rear part of the slip surface associated with high rainfall and a high reservoir level of 710 m.

Case (b) assumed relatively lower artesian pore water pressures on the rear part of the slip surface associated with relatively low rainfall, and a reservoir level of 710 m.

Case (c) assumed high artesian pore water pressures on the rear part of the slip surface associated with high rainfall and a lower reservoir level of 650 m.

Case (d) assumed relatively lower pore water pressures on the rear part of the slip surface associated with relatively low rainfall, and a reservoir level of 650 m.

Case (e) assumed high artesian pore water pressures on the rear part of the slip surface associated with high rainfall and no reservoir.

Case (f) assumed relatively lower pore water pressures on the rear part of the slip surface associated with relatively low rainfall, and no reservoir.

Most of the calculations gave values of F (2D) less than 1. Taken as a whole, the calculated 2D values of factor of safety were too low for landslide mass to have been stable over its history even before the construction of the dam and the filling of the reservoir. For example, based on a residual friction angle of 12° along the slip surface, which was considered reasonable after comprehensive investigations, and considering no pore water pressure along the slip surface (dry case), values of $F = 0.8$

Table 5.4 Comparison 2D and 3D factor of safety for various cases of analysis of the 1963 Vaiont Slide (after Hendron and Patton (1985).

Case	F (3D)	F (2D)		
		Section 1	Section 2	Section 3
(a)	1.00	0.52	0.90	0.45
(b)	1.10	0.62	1.06	0.51
(c)	1.08	0.60	0.99	0.50
(d)	1.18	0.70	1.10	0.56
(e)	1.12	0.63	1.0	0.51
(f)	1.21	0.73	1.20	0.57

Comments: The approach summarized above is one element in a complex explanation for the occurrence of the Vaiont slide, an explanation proposed by Hendron and Patton (1985). However, there have been many investigations and analyses of this landslide and thus there are several alternative explanations. This has been a controversial subject and remains so today (see also chapter 7 for alternative explanations).

For most explanations of the landslide, there is an important point to be noted, an apparent paradox related to stability analysis concerning catastrophic landslides such as this one. On the one hand, very low shear strength and high pore water pressure along the slip surface are necessary to explain the decrease of stability to critical equilibrium and an even lower strength and/or higher pore water pressures are necessary to explain the catastrophic landslide which followed. On the other hand, a much higher strength alone can explain why the landslide mass was stable before the Vaiont dam was constructed and the reservoir filling process started.

and $F = 0.66$ were obtained for two of the three cross-sections analysed; $F > 1$ was, however, obtained for the third cross-section.

After careful examination of all the results, it was concluded that the missing element was the three-dimensional aspect of stability of the potential landslide mass. In order to calculate the 3D factor of safety, the shearing resistance over the whole section at the Eastern end was calculated and added to the shearing resistance over the whole of the 2D slip surface. The total was then divided by the disturbing force over the whole of the slip surface.

For each of the cases listed above (combinations of each reservoir level (710 m, 650 m and 0) with the artesian pore pressure related to rainfall cases (high and low), the results for $F(3D)$ are shown in Table 5.4 along with $F(2D)$ for the three cross-sections of the slide mass.

5.13 'TOTAL STRESS' VERSUS 'EFFECTIVE STRESS' ANALYSES

This section follows on from the introduction to this subject in section 5.1.1. Having described a number of limit equilibrium methods, it is desirable to consider again the choice between 'total stress' and 'effective stress' approaches in the actual application of a method of analysis. In the 'total stress' approach shear strength parameters based on undrained tests are used and pore water pressures are ignored. In the 'effective stress' approach effective shear strength parameters based on drained tests (or undrained tests with pore pressure measurements) are used. In addition, a knowledge of pore pressures in the field is necessary. The estimation of these pore water pressures in the field in advance of construction is often difficult. Skempton's well known pore pressure equation in terms of coefficients A and B can be used but reliable values of these coefficients must be estimated based on testing and experience.

One advantage of the 'effective stress' approach is that, when actual pore pressures from piezometers installed in the field become available, the analyses can be updated. In principle, both methods of analysis should lead to the same factor of safety, whether short-term (end-of-construction) or long-term stability of a slope is being analysed. However, experience has shown that each method has advantages in particular situations.

Usually total stress analysis requires less work than effective stress analysis. However, the latter approach is more logical and straightforward because, in reality, strength is controlled by effective stresses. While a total stress analysis is simple in itself, shear strength parameters have to be measured and selected with great care. The test conditions must correspond to the conditions of consolidation (isotropic or anisotropic) that exist in the field followed by shear under conditions of drainage that may be applicable. These conditions are not always easy to select and set up. Consideration must also be given to the requirement of undisturbed samples for testing especially in natural soils. Undrained strength required for use in a total stress analysis is usually far more sensitive to sample disturbance than are drained strength parameters. On the other hand, tests to determine effective stress parameters from drained tests are often time consuming. Also the accuracy of estimated field pore pressures required for effective stress analyses is often in doubt.

A comparison of the two approaches is presented in Table 5.5, for the following conditions:

1 End of construction conditions (or conditions during construction) in saturated cohesive soils of low permeability, e.g., excavation in saturated soil where period of construction is short in comparison to time required for pore pressure equilibrium.

2 End of construction condition in partially saturated soils of low permeability, e.g., earth dam in which period of construction is short in comparison to time required for consolidation.

3 (a) Steady seepage condition for earth dam; (b) Long-term condition for natural or excavated slope.

4 Rapid draw-down condition for earth dam or for natural slope forming the sides of a reservoir (assuming material of low permeability).

5 Conditions intermediate between construction and long-term in excavated slopes.

6 Earthquake loading of earth or rockfill dams, embankments etc. (a) Material of low permeability, e.g., earth fill; (b) Material of high permeability, e.g., free-draining rockfill.

Table 5.5 Effective stress versus total stress analysis.

Condition	Comments on type of analysis
1	(i) Total stress analysis with strength from UU tests generally satisfactory. Advanced total stress analyses use more elaborate test procedures for cuts in soft clay. Total stress analyses for stiff clays require great care (especially if the clays are fissured) in the determination of in-situ undrained strengths. Laboratory undrained strengths are always too high and $\phi = 0$ assumption leads to error on the unsafe side. (ii) Effective stress analyses are more justified in theory and more logical for cuts but require estimation of pore pressures in advance of construction. However, actual pore pressures can be measured during construction and new analyses made to check earlier analyses. For construction pore pressures, see Appendix II.
2	(i) Total stress analysis with strength from UU tests generally satisfactory (use of parameters c, ϕ). (ii) Effective stress analyses are based on estimated pore pressures based on pore pressure parameters measured in laboratory tests which simulate the field loading condition. Analyses can be checked where pore pressures are monitored during construction.
3	(i) Effective stress analyses should be made using pore pressures corresponding to full reservoir. Appropriate flow net facilitates pore pressure determination. (ii) Effective stress analyses should be carried out using pore pressures corresponding to equilibrium ground water condition. Appropriate flow net facilitates pore pressure determination.
4	(i) Total stress analyses are generally based on the assumption that effective normal stress on the failure surface after drawdown is the same as the effective normal stress prior to drawdown. Thus effect of change in pore pressure (due to load reduction) on strength is disregarded. Such a procedure is conservative (Bishop, 1952; Johnson, 1975). Strength is generally determined from CU tests. Johnson (1975) recommends that combined CD-CU strength envelope be used, the changeover point being that normal stress at which the two envelopes intersect. In the low normal stress range CU envelope gives high strength which implies reliance on shear strength associated with negative pore pressure. Therefore it is better to use CD strengths in this low stress range so that no reliance is placed on negative pore pressures. In reality dissipation of pore pressure may occur. Ignoring this leads to conservative results. Terzaghi and Peck (1967) recommend that consideration should be given to the rate of drawdown, permeability and dimensions of mass affected by drawdown to examine the appropriate values of strength between the upper and lower limits given by CD and CU tests. CAU tests are considered preferable to CIU tests. (ii) Effective stress analyses must be based on estimated pore pressures. Pore pressure parameters are to be determined from appropriate tests which simulate undrained load reduction due to drawdown. The procedure is explained by Bishop (1954). Once again attention should be given to actual drainage conditions i.e., rate of drawdown should be compared to permeability and size of soil mass to determine if undrained or relatively drained conditions prevail during drawdown. (See also Appendix II).
5	Effective stress analyses may be used with estimated pore pressures or pore pressures measured in the field. Estimation of pore pressures may be made on the basis of empirical data or analysis of a two-dimensional swelling problem. Some references are given later in this chapter (section 5.17).

(Continued)

Table 5.5 (Continued).

6	(i) Total stress analysis with shear strengwth parameters from anisotropically consolidated, cyclic loading undrained tests for slopes which allow little dissipation of pore pressure during earthquakes. Estimation of pore pressures for effective stress analysis is difficult in such cases. (ii) Effective stress analyses are suitable for free draining material. Again, strength parameters should be from cyclic tests as in (i) above.
	Note: Seismic response (dynamic) analyses are increasingly being used for such problems in addition to pseudo-static analyses (see chapter 9).

5.14   CHOICE AND USE OF LIMIT EQUILIBRIUM METHODS – GUIDELINES

5.14.1   Essential first steps

1   Visualise the probable shape of slip surface or slip surfaces. Understanding the geological framework of site is of paramount importance in this regard. Special attention must be given to the existence of major discontinuities, existing slip surfaces, stratification, non-homogeneity, tension cracks and open joints. Once the likely shape of slip surface is approximately known, its critical location can be determined rapidly and reliably using an appropriate method of analysis. In homogeneous soil or soft rock slopes without discontinuities, assume slip surface of circular shape unless local experience dictates otherwise. In earth dams and embankments give consideration to method of construction, zones of different materials, and nature of foundation in order to visualise probable shapes of slip surfaces.

2   Distinguish clearly between first-time slides and possible renewed movements along existing slip surfaces. Rely only on the residual strength along parts of assumed slip surfaces which correspond to existing shear zones or old slip surfaces.

3   Make decisions on relative factors of safety with respect to cohesion and friction. It may not be justified to have $F_c = F_\phi$. Whenever possible compare strength parameters from back analyses of case records with those from laboratory and field tests. Examine the reliability of data concerning strength parameters and pore, water pressures. Consider possibility of artesian pore pressures and perched water tables by examining significant geological details. Give consideration to seepage and submergence and draw down conditions where appropriate.

4   Make decisions concerning use of effective stress or total stress type of analysis on the basis of section 5.13. In particular, consider type of material, whether analysis is for short-term or long-term conditions, whether reliable estimate of pore pressure can be made in advance and whether pore pressures are to be monitored in the field.

5.14.2   Choice of method of analysis

1   For long uniform natural slopes where failure surface is parallel to ground surface, simple infinite slope equations given in chapter 4 are fairly accurate.

2   For shallow, very long planar failure surfaces which are not parallel to the ground surface, Fellenius approach will give fairly accurate results. (A planar failure surface may be regarded as a circular one with infinite radius).

3   For bi-planar and tri-planar failure surfaces, Fellenius approach may be used only for rough preliminary analysis. Large inaccuracies can be expected particularly if the slip surface is not a shallow one and if pore pressures are high. Janbu's simplified equation with correction factors will give better preliminary results. Wedge or sliding block analyses must be used for greater accuracy in determining factor of safety and critical failure surface location. In some cases discussed in previous sections, a solution based on balance of active and passive pressures may be more logical. Accurate results should be obtained using a generalised procedure of slices.

4   For surfaces which can be approximated by arcs of circles, preliminary studies are facilitated by the use of stability charts. In the age of computers, the use of charts is declining. Yet, there is some merit in using charts for preliminary analysis. Charts for total stress analysis must be distinguished from those for effective stress analysis. Examine carefully the geometry for which charts are applicable. For slopes in non-homogeneous soil make decisions on average slope inclination. Also calculate weighted averages of soil properties based on proportion of slip surface which passes through different types of material. The approximate location of slip surface must be known for adopting this procedure. Preliminary analyses may also be made using Fellenius approach but high inaccuracies can be expected particularly for deep circles and where pore pressures are high. For more accurate studies, use Bishop simplified method.

5   For slip surfaces of arbitrary shape use a generalised procedure of slices. Preliminary studies may be made using Janbu's simplified procedure (without inter-slice forces) and correction factors. For more accurate studies, Janbu's generalised procedure, Spencer's procedure, M-P method or Sarma method may be used. Several software packages are available. However, the user must check the performance of the software and the accuracy of the results. Reliability of analyses can be checked by plotting normal force distributions on failure surface and by examining acceptability criteria, e.g., violation of failure criterion, tension in parts of failure mass etc.

6   For failure along single planes in rock, use the simple procedure explained in chapter 4. When there is no single dominant discontinuity but planar or approximately planar failure surface is expected, critical failure plane inclination must be obtained by trial and error minimisation process with respect to F. Care must be exercised in the choice of software packages and in checking their performance. In all rock slope problems, attention must be given to continuity of jointing, relative strength of intact rock and joints, filling of discontinuities, open joints etc.

5.14.3   Sensitivity of calculated F

The sensitivity of the factor of safety to strength parameters has been emphasised in chapter 4. Particular attention was also given to the need for proper interpretation of strength data especially when a strength envelope is curved (section 4.8). The selection of strength parameters appropriate to the stress level in a given problem is most essential. Regardless of stress level, however, there may be considerable scatter in shear strength parameters of the same soil tested in different laboratories. According to Johnston (1969), Lee and Singh (1968) and Singh (1970), the scatter may easily be $\pm 25\%$ for ϕ values, $\pm 50\%$ for c values and the variation in shear strength of a soil at a given normal pressure may be of the order of $\pm 30\%$. Therefore, sensitivity analyses are often necessary to study the variation of F with variations in c and ϕ values corresponding to different estimates or to different field conditions. The use of the concept of a resistance envelope for sensitivity studies has been explained earlier in this chapter (section 5.1). An alternative approach would be to draw curves of equal factors of safety on plots of $c/\gamma H$ against F for a given slope geometry and pore pressure conditions. The charts prepared by Singh (1970) on these lines are based on analysis without pore water pressure (total stress approach) and are, therefore, of limited use. However, the approach may be explained simply by writing F in the form suggested by equation (5.34):

$$F = Ac + B \tan \phi \tag{5.34a}$$

in which A and B are functions only of geometry of sliding mass and assumed failure plane and given pore pressure conditions. Assuming a given value of F a curve representing this value can be drawn on a plot of c or $c/\gamma H$ on y axis versus $\tan \phi$ on the x axis. Now a new value of F may be assumed and a different curve representing this new value drawn. Thus a series of curves are drawn corresponding to given slope and failure surface geometry and pore pressure conditions. On such a chart different points may then be plotted, each point representing one combination of c and ϕ which is considered to be feasible from soil testing, past experience or field conditions. The location of different points corresponding to different combinations of c and ϕ enables a study of the range of possible F values for a given slope.

5.14.4 Sensitivity of F to tension cracks

Let us now consider the sensitivity of factor of safety to tension cracks. The importance of tension cracks and open joints in both soil and rock slopes has already been mentioned in chapter 4, and, earlier in this chapter, results of several slope stability problems with tension cracks have been cited (Zhang, 1989, see also Chapter 7). In geotechnical practice related to slope engineering (and, in particular, preventive and remedial measures against slope failures) due emphasis is given to drainage of surface water away from tension cracks and to covering cracks with plastic sheets etc. Yet it is somewhat surprising that water-filled tension cracks have not received adequate emphasis in soil mechanics where slope analysis has been discussed. It is possible that water-filled tension cracks may have a negligible influence in the case of embankments (e.g., Spencer, 1967; 1968; 1973) since the assumed tension crack depth is small. However, in problems concerning excavations and disturbed natural slopes, deep cracks may develop and the effect of water in these cracks may be to lower the factor of safety significantly. Note also that in the studies made by Spencer only homogeneous slopes with circular slip surfaces were considered. In practice soils may be non-homogeneous and failure surface shapes may be complex. The effect of water pressure in tension cracks may be much greater in translational slides than in slides of a rotational character.

It is useful to study for both rock and soil slopes the influence of (1) distance of tension crack from slope crest b, (2) depth of tension crack Z_c and (3) depth of water in crack Z_w on the factor of safety F. As an example consider a study of block sliding on clay layers made by Hoek and Bray (1977). The value of F dropped from about 2.2

at $Z_u/H = 0.25$ to about 0.5 at $Z_w/H = 0.5$ for a value of $b/H = 0.25$ (a crack depth equal to slope height H was assumed i.e., $Z_c/H = 1$). As the value of b/H increased the factor of safety also increased for the same values of Z_w/H. For a value of $Z_w/H = 0.5$, approximate values were $F = 0.5$ for $b/H = 0.25$ and $F = 1.2$ for $b/H = 0.5$. For similar studies, concerning the effect on factor of safety, of the location and depth of tension cracks, the reader may refer to Zhang and Chowdhury (1989).

Robertson (1971) suggested a new method for accounting for cracks in slope stability analysis. He proposed that a vertical crack divides the potential failure mass into a lower failing segment and an upper hanging segment. A force P is assumed to develop between the two segments along the assumed failure surface. The force P may be defined as follows:

$$RF = DF + P \tag{5.39}$$

in which RF and DF are respectively the total resisting force and driving force along the failure surface. Since the factor of safety F may be defined as $F = RF/DF$, we have from Equation (5.39),

$$F = \frac{RF}{DF} = \frac{DF + P}{DF} = 1 + \frac{P}{DF} \tag{5.40}$$

If P is positive, $F > 1$ and the failing segment will not slide; while, if P is negative, $F < 1$ and the slope has failed. If an equal and opposite force P is applied to the failing segment, then $RF = DF$ and $F = 1$. Therefore P may be considered as a force which must be applied to bring the failure mass to critical equilibrium. By assuming different positions of the crack, the range in which negative values of P are implied can be studied by plotting F and P against position of crack in the slope. For this range F has a value below unity. Again, for a low value of slope height H, no position of the assumed crack may give a negative value of P (or $F < 1$). The slope height may then be increased step by step and the height at which cracking will occur may then be determined by plotting minimum F against slope height. On such a plot the slope height corresponding to $F = 1$ gives the height at which cracking can be considered to develop. In practice slip surfaces of different geometry must be tried to determine minimum F values for each slope height. The crack position is defined by the point at which $P = 0$ and $dP/ds = 0$ simultaneously where s denotes the distance along the failure surface. Robertson's approach must be used only after careful attention to relevant information about theoretical or observed depth of cracks, observed position of cracks etc. It assumes that the slope material has no tensile strength and this assumption is usually considered to be acceptable. However, assumption of crack from the surface right down to the failure surface may not always be justified.

Reference was made earlier in this chapter to the extended Janbu method proposed by Zhang (1989) which also considers the potential sliding mass in two parts separated by an imaginary vertical boundary or by a tension crack. The upper part is chosen to be relatively small and, bounded by the steeper part of the slip surface, and, the larger lower part is bounded by the rest of the slip surface. This is similar to the procedure of Robertson (1971) mentioned above.

5.14.5   The factor of safety in practice

In chapter 3, (section 3.2.5), reference was made to the acceptable values of the factor of safety for natural slopes and landslide management on the one hand (Cornforth, 2005) and for constructed slopes on the other (Duncan 1992). In each case, a minimum or threshold value of F will depend on a number of factors including the type of project, the consequences of potential failure and the way in which the values from analysis are estimated. Here we continue the discussion concerning the meaning or interpretation of estimated values of factor of safety and related aspects.

The precise meaning of the factor of safety in geotechnical practice is difficult to establish. There is a wide range of acceptable values of calculated F and opinions may differ not only from one country to another but from one organisation to another. In fact there may be important differences of opinion between recognised experts. It is relevant to quote the following (De Mello, 1977, p. 333): "Although limit analysis must continue to be used (to tie in with the past and for convenience) it should be definitely dissociated from any implication that $F = 1.0$ signifies incipient real failure. This point is important on several counts ... that various methods of analysis give nearly identical results (e.g., Wright et al., 1973), the respective certainty is only of equivalence of various computations within a presumed model, and not of equivalence of model to reality". The reader may compare these remarks with the introductory remarks made in chapter 8 about agreement between limit equilibrium solutions and solutions based on the limit analysis technique of plasticity. The reader may also recall the introductory remarks made in chapter 4.

An interesting example of how practising engineers may interpret computed F values on the basis of experience was given at the 1977 Penrose Conference in Vail, Colorado, U.S.A. It was stated that two leading geotechnical engineers had come to the following agreement while testifying on opposite sides of litigation concerning failures (J.V. Hamel, pers. comm. 1977).

$F = 0.8$: 100% probability of failure
$F = 1.0$: 50% probability of failure
$F = 1.2$: about 10% probability of failure.

These examples illustrate the futility of specifying an acceptable value of F for all situations. Presumably the nominal failure probabilities quoted above relate to a specific method of slope analysis based on limit equilibrium concepts. The same geotechnical engineers would probably have arrived at quite different conclusions if the method of analysis was different, since F values may differ by as much as 30% depending on the particular limit equilibrium method of analysis used [an example was given in section 5.10.2]. Similarly, if F is calculated on the basis of stress analysis, it may have a different meaning in relation to the nominal probability of failure.

Quite clearly, analyses are often (if not always) necessary as a basis for design and decision-making and to quote again De Mello (1977, p. 330): "Although it has been emphasised that the root problem in design might be to obviate the very need for a stability computation, understandably one must not forego some conventional computation of F. The first obvious hope is that the F value should be developed to reflect a real estimate of the probability of failure ...". In practice, it is, therefore, necessary to develop, on the basis of experience, the range of acceptable F values for specific problems on the basis of specific methods of analysis. The range of acceptable F values for deep excavations may be different from the range which is acceptable for earth dams. Again, for the same problem, an acceptable range of F on the basis of limit equilibrium may be different from an acceptable range of F on the basis of stress analysis. Secondly, it is essential to obtain lower and upper bounds to the value of F (on the basis of any method of analysis which happens to be the choice) considering pessimistic and optimistic forecasts with regard to geological details, strength parameters, pore water pressures, gravitational and other forces as well as initial or in situ stresses. Thirdly, acceptable values of F to be used in design must be related to the consequences of failure. Minor slope failures along highway cuts may be more acceptable in economic terms than adoption of high F values with a view to preventing failure completely.

Fourthly, one must recognise the fact that different parameters of strength, weights, forces and pore water pressures may be known with different degrees of confidence. As such, it would be useful to have different acceptable F values for cohesive component of strength, frictional component of strengths, weights etc. For example Londe suggested the following on the basis of his experience for rock slopes (Hoek and Bray, 1977):

$F_c = 1.5$ for cohesive component of strength or c parameter
$F_\phi = 1.2$ for frictional component of strength or ϕ parameter
$F_u = 2.0$ for pore water pressures
$F_w = 1.0$ for weights and forces.

Lastly, it is necessary to emphasise once again that calculated F values may have little significance if sufficient attention has not been given to site conditions and geology before developing idealised cross-sections for analysis. There are specific areas in which geologists and engineers make the best contribution to slope problems; and Peck (1977) made the following comments in this regard.

"Geologists are good at recognition of landslides and landslide topography and at understanding geological structure and stratigraphy, slide processes and slide features, ground water and hydrogeology. Geologists are poor at quantifying properties of earth materials, seepage pressures and pore pressures and in performing equilibrium calculations. They are overzealous in classifying slides with little regard to fundamental causes. On the other hand, engineers tend to look at a landslide as just another structure but are good at equilibrium calculations and at estimating seepage pressures and pore pressures and at carrying out quantitative studies of remedial measures. Engineers are, however, poor at visualising the anatomy of slides and tend to over-idealise slide masses. They are also poor at picking most probable slide surface which is often governed by geological details. They are usually poor at picking out differences from one site to another and at interpretations of subsurface conditions. They tend to interpret slides on mechanistic rather than geological basis." Peck concluded that there are very few people with complete background in geology and engineering and, therefore, there is need for teamwork and communication.

5.14.6   Important considerations in all types of analysis

1   Inclusion of tension cracks and open joints in analysis must not be forgotten. Where appropriate, assume water in these cracks. The pressure of water in tension

cracks may have an important influence on stability. Estimate tension crack depth carefully as explained in chapter 4.

2   Sensitivity analyses may be made by varying one parameter at a time, e.g., depth of tension crack, location of tension crack, cohesion parameter, friction parameter. Plot each parameter against F. Use concept of resistance envelopes to study influence of c and ϕ on F in cohesive slopes.

3   Where strength envelopes are curved, exercise great care in selecting c and ϕ values. Selected values must correspond to stress level appropriate to problem. For shallow slip surfaces c and ϕ are selected from portion of strength envelope in the low normal stress range, for deep slip surface values of c and ϕ are selected from portion of strength envelope in the high normal stress range.

4   Consider three-dimensional effects carefully. For rock-wedge problems use appropriate procedures referred to in chapter 4. For general use, weighted averages procedure discussed in this chapter is usually appropriate. In some cases, direct provision may be made for end effects. Curvature of slope in plan can have either a beneficial or an adverse effect on stability. Curvature of slope face can be important especially in high slopes.

5   For slopes with high initial lateral stresses, or for high embankments and earth dams in which deformations are important, consider concepts presented in chapters 6 and 7 and shear band concepts presented in chapter 8. For understanding landslides of exceptional character and propagation of slip surfaces in slopes, these concepts are particularly useful.

6   Consider progressive failure possibilities and especially the role of slope disturbance, tension cracks, geological details, strain-softening, non-uniform stress and strain distribution in initiating or accelerating progressive failure.

7   Examine possibilities of delayed failure due to decrease in shear strength parameters with time, increase of pore pressure with time, and any other factors.

5.15 VARIATIONAL CALCULUS AND SLOPE STABILITY

The determination of the critical surface of sliding in a homogeneous slope without discontinuities is usually a trial and error (or iterative) process in which the value of the factor of safety from each trial is compared with values obtained from previous trials. Not only is the process cumbersome but the final result often corresponds to a specific shape of slip surface assumed in advance, e.g., circular or log spiral. The calculus of variations may be used to study maxima and minima of functionals which are applications of a set of functions. It aims at finding those functions in a prescribed class called admissible functions for which a given functional has extreme values. In the case of the stability of slopes the function $y(x)$ to be considered is the one which describes the surface of sliding. The factor of safety F associated with any surface is the functional to be minimised. If the function $y(x)$ is such that it extremises the functional F, then F satisfies the corresponding Euler equation of variational calculus (Berg, 1962).

Let the factor of safety F (or the functional) be given by:

$$F = \int \frac{f(x,y,y')\,dx}{g(x,y,\,y')\,dx} \tag{5.41}$$

This is a common form of expression for F being the ratio of integrals for disturbing and resisting forces along a slip surface. However, it cannot represent a ratio of the resisting and disturbing moments as well because neither the shape of the slip surface nor the stress distribution along it is known in advance. The Euler equation to be satisfied so that F as defined above is a minimum is given by Revilla and Castillo (1977) as follows:

$$\int \frac{f(x,y,y')\,dx}{g(x,y,y')\,dx} = \frac{\dfrac{\partial f}{\partial y} - \dfrac{d}{dx}\left(\dfrac{\partial f}{\partial y'}\right)}{\dfrac{\partial G}{\partial y} - \dfrac{d}{dx}\left(\dfrac{\partial G}{\partial y'}\right)} \tag{5.42}$$

The function $y(x)$ which gives the minimum factor of safety (and hence describes the critical slip surface curve) must satisfy Equation (5.42). Both end points to the curve may or may not be specified. A slope may be uniform or defined by broken lines. Several conditions such as transversality, continuity and boundary conditions are required to enable a unique solution to be found.

Revilla and Castillo (1977) gave solutions for a slope in cohesive material ($\phi = 0$) and used Janbu's (1954b) equations as a basis for defining the functional. They found that the critical slip surface is located deeper and is longer in extent as the steepness of the slope decreases. Comparison with results obtained on the basis of conventional limit equilibrium methods showed that the factors of safety are smaller when variational calculus is used. For example, important differences from Taylor's (1948) results were found for a wide range of slope angles. These results are shown in Figure 5.12. The critical slip surfaces are markedly non-circular in shape and do not pass through the toe as would have been expected from conventional solutions for some range of slope angles. Studies in which slip

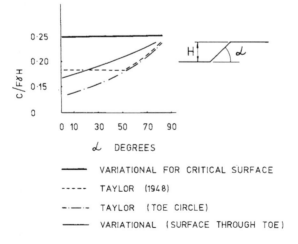

Figure 5.12 Comparison of stability factor $c/F\gamma H$ for $\phi = 0$ analysis using variational calculus with conventional slip circle results (after Revilla and Castillo, 1977). With permission, see page 713, No 19.

surfaces were selected to pass through the toe showed somewhat better agreement with Taylor's results.

It has always been suggested on the basis of approaches such as plasticity and limit-analysis (chapter 8) that conventional limit equilibrium methods give conservative results. In other words it is believed that the factors of safety are underestimated and correspond to 'upper bound' solutions as defined in limit-analysis technique of plasticity discussed in chapter 8. (Upper bound 'solution' should not be confused with an upper bound to factor of safety which would be unconservative. Upper bound solution gives an upper limit to the load required for failure or an upper limit to the disturbing forces. Therefore it gives a lower limit or a lower bound to the factor of safety). This is now contradicted by results discussed above which indicate that much lower factors of safety are possible. Further, the shape and location of a critical slip surface may itself be different from the one predicted by a conventional approach. Morgenstern (1977) commented on some difficulties in the application of variational calculus to slope stability problems and cautioned against ignoring these difficulties. He found that many studies [e.g., Baker and Garber (1977), Ramamurthy et al., (1977)] appeared to ignore shear forces between slices as well as the requirement of moment equilibrium. This may explain the difference in results referred to above since the condition of moment equilibrium is not automatically satisfied on the critical surface of arbitrary shape obtained from the calculus of variations while it is automatically satisfied for circular failure surfaces assumed in Taylor's solution (for the $\phi = 0$ case considered). However, the contribution of this factor may not be as important as the contribution of other obvious factors. In the $\phi = 0$ case, the differences in shape and location of the slip surface must be responsible for a major part of the disagreement between the two solutions.

In comparing factors of safety F (especially when $\phi > 0$), attention must be given to the way in which F itself is defined. For example Equation (5.41) is based on the ratio of resisting to disturbing forces. This is different from the definition (ratio of available to mobilised unit shear strength) which has gained acceptance e.g., Bishop Simplified Method, ϕ-circle Method, Morgenstern and Price Method.

Another important point deserves comment. It has been shown in connection with studies based on plasticity and limit analysis that a logarithmic spiral represents the critical shape of slip surface for a frictional material. Such a surface is of the form $r = r_0 \exp(\theta \tan \phi)$ which reduces to a circle $r = r_0$ when $\phi = 0$. Chen (1975) proved the validity of a log-spiral surface on the basis of variational calculus and also showed that it gave the minimum weight of a sliding mass. Yet, Revilla and Castillo (1977) found non-circular surfaces for their '$\phi = 0$' analyses although they also used variational calculus in a different way. Therefore the manner in which the problem is defined has a significant influence on the solution.

In view of all the factors discussed above, reconciling different approaches is neither always necessary nor always useful. Yet, the role and power of the method based on calculus of variations is evident and more research is certainly warranted. A lot more research and development has been carried out over the last three decades and a literature review should be useful to the student scholar.

5.16 SIMULATING PROGRESSIVE FAILURE WITHIN THE FRAMEWORK OF LIMIT EQUILIBRIUM – THE EFFECT OF STRESS REDISTRIBUTION IN SLOPES OF STRAIN-SOFTENING SOIL

Conventional methods of limit equilibrium are based on the assumption that the factor of safety is constant along the assumed slip surface. Consequently, if the computed value of F is greater than 1, it is implied that there is no local overstressing or local failure anywhere along the slip surface. Therefore, strain-softening, stress-redistribution and progressive failure cannot be taken into consideration. However, if local factor of safety can be distinguished from the overall factor of safety, the limit equilibrium approach can be extended to simulate stress redistribution and progressive failure in a slope comprising strain-softening material. After defining local factor of safety, overstressed segments of the slip surface can be identified and then a number of steps follow logically in the simulation process. Consider, as usual, the subdivision of a potential sliding mass into a number of vertical slices. Thus there will be the same number of segments of the potential slip surface forming the bases of these slices. Consider a vertical slice of weight W with base length L and inclination α. The local factor of safety may be defined as the ratio of shear strength to shear stress as follows:

$$F_\ell = \frac{\tau_f L}{W \sin \alpha} \tag{5.43}$$

where,

$$\tau_f L = c'L + (W \cos \alpha - uL) \tan \phi' \tag{5.44}$$

in which c' and ϕ' are the shear strength parameters and u is the pore water pressure. Local failure of the slice will occur if,

$$W \sin \alpha > c'L + (W \cos \alpha - uL) \tan \phi' \tag{5.45}$$

Applying this inequality to all the segments of the slip surface, overstressed or failed segments of the slip surface can be identified.

Assuming that the soil is perfectly brittle strain-softening, the shear strength parameters of overstressed slices will reduce to residual values c_r and ϕ_r, whereas the remaining segments of the slip surface will still be at the peak shear strength c' and ϕ'. The following steps are involved:

i   Using any limit equilibrium method, calculate first the overall factor of safety based on peak shear strength all along the slip surface. Designate this value as F_0.

ii Secondly, using the same method, calculate the overall factor of safety after the shear strength parameters of overstressed segments of the slip surface have been reduced to residual values. Designate this value as F_1.

Unless there is a situation in which none of the segments is overstressed, it is clear that $F_1 < F_0$.

iii Consider now an unfailed segment of the slip surface (segment not yet over-stressed). Initially the shear stress was τ_0 corresponding to overall factor of safety F_0, and, on the first iteration, the shear stress is τ_1 corresponding to overall factor of safety F_1, where

$$F_0 = \frac{\tau_f}{\tau_0} \quad \text{and} \quad F_1 = \frac{\tau_f}{\tau_1} \tag{5.46}$$

Thus the excess shear stress on the particular segment is given by

$$\tau_e = \tau_1 - \tau_0 = \tau_f \left[\frac{F_0 - F_1}{F_0 \, F_1} \right] \tag{5.47}$$

iv Adding this excess shear stress to the initial shear stress on the segment, one can calculate the total shear stress. Then one can check if this total shear stress exceeds the shear strength of the segment, i.e., whether

$$(W \sin \alpha + \tau_e L) > \tau_f L \tag{5.48}$$

If this inequality applies, this segment has been overstressed and its shear strength parameters must be reduced to residual values.

This procedure can be applied to all the unfailed segments to identify which ones are now overstressed.

v Once all such segments have been identified and their shear strength parameters reduced accordingly, the next limit equilibrium analysis can be carried out yielding a new overall factor of safety. Designate this as F_2, where F_2 will be less than F_1 unless none of the unfailed segments was shown to be overstressed.

vi Now start the next iteration. For each of the still unfailed segments, calculate the excess shear stress from the following

$$\tau_e = \tau_2 - \tau_1 = \tau_f \left(\frac{F_1 - F_2}{F_1 \, F_2} \right)$$

vii Adding this to the initial shear stress for each unfailed slice, calculate the total shear stress and check if this exceeds the shear strength.

If no new segment is found to be overstressed, the analysis is complete and F_2 is the final factor of safety. Otherwise make the next limit equilibrium analysis and calculate F_3. Usually convergence is achieved in three or four iterations.

5.16.1   Applications of the above procedure

1   The procedure outlined above is illustrated by an example below (Example 5.5).
2   The student will find it very useful to carry out a re-analysis of the Bradwell Slip (Skempton and La Rochelle, 1965) using the above procedure. The student should

study the original paper thoroughly to understand the nature of the failures and to finalise the input parameters. The results can be very sensitive to the geometry of the slope and the slip surface.

Preliminary analyses carried out by Matthews (1983) and Heins (1986) were successful in simulating progressive failure but to different degrees.

i   For example, for Bradwell Slip 1 Mathews (1983) obtained the following results:
Slip circle 1 analysed with only 11 vertical slices
$F = 1.35$ (using peak undrained shear strength), $F = 0.67$ (using undrained residual strength), and
$F = 0.90$ (after iterations for stress redistribution).
Slip Circle 2 analysed with 10 vertical slices
$F = 1.37$ (using peak undrained strength), $F = 0.73$ (using undrained residual strength), and $F = 0.99$ (after iterations for stress redistribution).

ii Heins (1986) analysed only slip circle 2 but his result after redistribution was $F = 1.27$ for 10 slices. He then increased the number of slices up to 120 but the lowest value after redistribution was $F = 1.17$. (The value of F for peak and residual strength were close to those obtained by Matthews). It seems that the differences in the result for the final value of F, after stress redistributions, is probably due to differences in approximating the shape of slope and slip surface.

3 Another very useful exercise for the student will be to re-analyse the 1984 failure of Carsington Dam (Skempton and Vaughan, 1993). The upstream slope failed when the embankment was at full height of 37 m and post-failure investigations revealed that the upper shear failure occurred through the rolled clay which contained shear surfaces due to rutting. The lower part of the slip surface was located in a layer of yellow clay, which contained solifluction shears. Investigations further confirmed both these materials to be brittle. Using the finite element method, the role of progressive failure was confirmed by Potts et al. (1990). Using the above procedure, the author carried out a very preliminary analysis and obtained a factor of safety close to 1 after just a couple of iterations of stress redistribution (Chowdhury, unpublished notes, 1994).

EXAMPLE 5.5

The slope geometry is shown in Figure E5.5 along with a slip surface of circular shape. The data are

Height, $H = 25$ m
Inclination, $\beta = 22°$
Central angle, $\theta = 68.7°$
Unit weight of soil, $\gamma = 18.8$ kN/m³
Peak shear strength parameters: $c' = 30$ kN/m², $\phi' = 20°$
Residual shear strength parameters: $c'_r = 10$ kN/m², $\phi'_r = 12°$

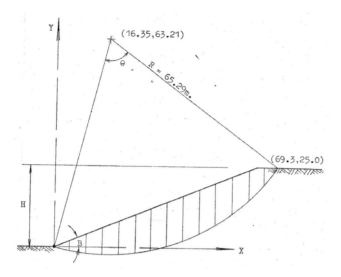

Figure E5.5 Slope Section for Example 5.5.

Table E5.2 Results of analysis of Example 5.5.

F value for	Ordinary method of slices	Bishop simplified method	Remarks
Peak Shear Strength Parameters for all the segments, i.e., $F = F_0$	1.57	1.65	–
Residual Shear Strength Parameters for all the segments, i.e., $F = F_r$	0.77	0.82	–
$F = F_1$	1.27	1.33	–
$F = F_2$	1.21	1.26	–
$F = F_3$	1.21	1.26	convergence

Summary of results

One solution was based on the Bishop simplified method and another on the Fellenius method (Ordinary method of slices). For both solutions, the potential sliding mass was subdivided into 14 vertical slices with a slice width of 5 m. The results are shown in the Table E5.2.

Concluding comments

Table E5.2 clearly demonstrates the effect of local overstress and the consequent stress re-distribution in strain-softening soils such as in the slope section in Example 5.5.

When such effect is considered, convergence was achieved in 3 iterations. While the final value of F ($=F_3$ or F_2) is found to be approximately 23 to 24% less than $F = F_0$ based on peak strength parameters for all the segments, it is found to be approximately 54 to 57% more than $F = F_r$ based on residual strength parameters for all the segments.

In other words, assuming peak strength for all the segments overestimates the factor of safety by nearly 30%, while assuming residual shear strength for all the segments underestimates the factor of safety by nearly 35%.

5.17   LESSONS FROM CASE STUDIES OF CLAY SLOPES

This section summarises the results of analyses, field observations and laboratory tests carried out before 1978 and also the interpretations based on such research. Several decades later, the conclusions are still considered valid and many of the associated uncertainties are still considered to be important.

5.17.1   End-of-construction failures in clay

Study of slope failures is often useful in investigating the causes of failure. The extent to which such studies can be used to establish the reliability of a method of analysis depends on a number of factors such as (1) the accuracy of data concerning slope geometry, strength parameters, pore water pressures, and soil profile; and (2) the accuracy with which the mechanism of failure has been understood. In general, back-analyses have limited aims. The investigator is often concerned with the determination of the factor of safety applicable to the potential failure mass at the instant of failure. The actual factor of safety at that instant is considered to be unity. Therefore the success of a method of analysis is measured by the extent to which the computed factor of safety approaches unity. Limit equilibrium methods are generally used in such studies either exclusively or in combination with other procedures such as stress analysis by the finite-element method. Widespread use of limit equilibrium methods does not mean that they have been completely successful in explaining failures. On the contrary, it reflects lack of sufficient progress in the development and application of other techniques.

The results of a number of case histories concerning failures of excavations in saturated clay as well as the failures of fills on saturated clay were given by Bishop and Bjerrum (1960). '$\phi = 0$' conditions were considered appropriate to these end-of-construction failures which were assumed to have occurred under undrained conditions. Consequently undrained shear strengths applicable in each case were used in total stress limit equilibrium calculations. The values of factors of safety are shown in Table 5.6.

These results can be interpreted to confirm the validity of '$\phi = 0$' analyses for failures at end-of construction in intact clays since the computed values of F are reasonably close to one in all cases except Bradwell. The failure at Bradwell was in stiff-fissured clay and it is widely recognised that '$\phi = 0$' analysis is not suitable for such materials. Terzaghi and Peck (1967) pointed out that a '$\phi = 0$' concept is not applicable to heavily overconsolidated clays because of their dilatant behaviour. In dilatant materials it would be unconservative to use a '$\phi = 0$' approach.

In fissured materials, there is an additional difficulty since the intact strength is much higher than the bulk strength of the soil mass including fissures (see chapter 2).

Table 5.6 $\phi = 0$ analyses of short-term failure giving values of factor of safety F (after Bishop and Bjerrum, 1960).

	Location	Computed F
Excavations in saturated clay	Huntspill	0.90
	Congress St.	1.10
	Bradwell	1.70
	Skattsmanso	1.06
	Skattsmanso	1.03
Fills on soft saturated clay	Chingford	1.05
	Gosport	0.93
	Panama 2	0.93
	Panama 3	0.98
	Newport	1.08
	Bromma II	1.03
	Bocksjon	1.10
	Huntington	0.98

(Attention to fissured clays and in particular to undrained failures at Bradwell has also been given earlier in this chapter in section 5.2). Therefore, the factor of safety is significantly overestimated if the strength from usual laboratory specimens is used. Secondly, the operational strength of fissured clays (to which reference has already been made in chapter 2 and earlier in this chapter) is considerably reduced due to the weakening effect of fissures. Thirdly, the presence of fissures may result in a significant increase in bulk permeability of the clay mass with consequent possibility of volume change and pore water migration during failure. If deformation is accompanied by volume change, the '$\phi = 0$' concept is invalid. It should be noted, however, that the bulk permeability does not necessarily increase in fissured clays and in support of this contention reference to earlier work on Brown London clay is made in section 5.17.4.

Returning now to intact clays, the closeness of the computed factor of safety F to unity may be interpreted in other different ways as well. The results may indicate that failure is not progressive and that orientation of stresses and decrease of shearing resistance by strain-softening do not influence the factor of safety. Alternatively, however, the influence of different unknowns (progressive failure, strain-softening etc.) may be self-compensating. The reader would naturally be keen to know the performance of 'total stress' or undrained analyses since 1960 (the date of publication of data in Table 5.6). By and large analyses based on 'total stress' approach are still considered reliable for short-term stability of cohesive soils. However, the success of this approach depends largely on the reliability with which in-situ undrained shear strengths can be determined. The factors which influence this strength for heavily over-consolidated fissured clays are many and complex and great care is necessary in the interpretation of the results of any analysis. Even in respect of normally or lightly overconsolidated clays Janbu (1977) expressed some reservations about the adequacy of a 'total stress' approach particularly for short-term stability of excavations. He referred to six case histories including three short-term failures in which resistance envelopes in terms of effective stresses corresponded well with effective stress envelopes of shear strength. Steady seepage conditions were assumed to have developed during the period of excavation. According to Janbu, such an assumption is logical because swelling moduli of clay are 5 to 10 times the compression moduli and the time to reach steady pore pressure or groundwater conditions is measured in weeks or months at the most (comparable to period of construction). This view is in sharp contrast to the observation that pore pressure equilibration takes considerable time even in fissured clays (Vaughan and Walbancke, 1973; Skempton, 1977). It would, therefore, be unwise to generalise from Janbu's experience and assume that steady seepage conditions are relevant to the investigation of short-term stability of all normally or lightly overconsolidated clays. (For design purposes such an assumption may be conservative and safe for excavations provided parameters of strength for effective stress analysis are chosen with care. In zones of swelling considerable loss of cohesion intercept may occur).

While for excavations Janbu did not give results of alternative 'total stress' calculations, he did make comparative studies for some natural slopes. For the latter he found a 'total stress' approach totally unreliable with minimum factors of safety as low as 0.5 corresponding to the condition of failure. On the other hand effective stress analyses gave minimum factors of safety close to unity. Total stress analyses gave ridiculously low factors of safety (0.25–0.5) even for stable (unfailed) slopes. These findings of Janbu are not surprising since it is well known that, for natural slopes (in contrast to cut or fill slopes), effective stress analyses with appropriate seepage pore pressures alone are relevant.

5.17.2   Long-term failures in intact clays, progressive failure and renewed movement

Effective stress analyses have been found to be very useful for the study of long-term stability of clay slopes. Delayed failures are a distinctive feature of slopes in overconsolidated clays although such failures do occur in other types of soil as well. These failures correspond to drained conditions and it is logical to use effective shear strength parameters preferably those from drained tests. Analyses must, of course, be made considering actual pore water pressures at the time of failure. Table 5.7 shows computed values of F, for slopes at failure, in different types of intact clay. It is significant that the computed factor of safety is reasonably close to one in most of these cases.

These examples appear to support the use of effective-stress limit equilibrium analyses to study drained failures in intact clays. The selection of strength parameters

Table 5.7 Factors of safety for long-term slope failures in intact clays (after Lambe and Whitman, 1969). With permission, see page 713, No 4.

Location and references	Soil type	F
Lodalen, Norway, Sevaldson (1956)	Lightly overconsolidated	1.05
Drammen, Norway, Bjerrum and Kjaernsli (1957)	Normally consolidated	1.15
Selset, England, Skempton and Brown (1961)	Overconsolidated	1.03
Breckenridge, Canada, Crawford and Eden (1967)	Lightly overconsolidated	1.12
Siburua, Venezuela, Wolfskill and Lambe (1967)	Compacted plastic clay	1.02

and pore water pressures is crucial in these analyses and even minor errors in these will cast serious doubt on computed factors of safety. Even when all the data concerning strength parameters and pore water pressures are reliable, an important uncertainty concerning the role of progressive failure remains. The question arises: "Do failures occur at the peak strength or at strength lower than the peak?"

According to Skempton (1970), first-time slides in slopes in intact (non-fissured) clays generally correspond to strengths only slightly less than the peak strength. Bjerrum (1967) suggested that progressive failure would result in a decrease of the shear strength below the peak. He cited examples of first time failures in which shear strengths mobilised at failure were closer to the residual than to the peak strength. (There have been suggestions that some of Bjerrum's examples were in reality not first-time slides (Palladino and Peck, 1972). He did not differentiate between intact and fissured clays since he felt that other criteria were significant in relation to the possibility of progressive failure in overconsolidated clays and clay-shales. In fact Skempton (1970) agreed that it would be unsafe to generalise from his experience that peak strength was mobilised at failure in all intact overconsolidated clays. According to Bishop et al. (1971) overconsolidated clays with a high value of the brittleness index (defined in chapter 2) often exhibit a tendency for progressive failure while clays with a low value of brittleness index do not show a significant tendency for progressive failure. Brittleness index depends on the stress level and its value decreases consistently with increasing effective normal stress even when the shear strength envelope is linear. A failure occurring at low stress levels may be progressive since the brittleness index is high while a failure occurring at high stress level may involve very little decrease of strength by a mechanism of progressive failure before a slide occurs. In some soils (particularly those with low plasticity) the brittleness index is low even at low stress levels and progressive decrease of strength is very unlikely.

From a fundamental point of view, the brittleness of a soil may be considered in terms of the following factors: (a) dilatancy accompanying failure as in the case of dense sands and overconsolidated clays. Although the former have lower brittleness index than the latter, only small strains are required for decrease of strength to the residual, and progressive failure is important, (b) reorientation of clay particles in the zone of failure which requires large displacements and is, therefore, an unlikely mechanism for progressive failure in first-time slides, (c) cementation bonds which may be the factor contributing to a high cohesion intercept in undisturbed clays. At low stress levels (typically 0.4 kg/cm^2) there is a significant loss in drained strength due to dilatancy and destruction of cohesive bonds. At high stress levels (typically 3.5 kg/cm^2) the loss due to these factors is small and particle re-orientation is required for further loss. Bishop et al. (1971) pointed out that majority of examples of progressive failure were to be found in the low stress range.

To summarise, there are three somewhat differing views about the strengths operative at failure in first-time slides in intact overconsolidated clays. According to one view (Skempton, 1970) peak strengths are mobilised at failure. According to a second view progressive decrease in strength occurs before a slide if three criteria concerning recoverable strain energy are satisfied (Bjerrum, 1967). According to a third view (Bishop et al., 1971) progressive decrease of strength may occur if the brittleness index is high. Since this index depends on the level of effective normal stress, the size of the slide is important in determining the potential for progressive failure. There is some similarity between the last view and one of the three criteria in the second view (see chapter 2 for Bjerrum's criteria). Finally it must be remembered that the normal effective stress along a slip surface may vary significantly depending on the geometry and inclination of the slope and the shape of the slip surface. This variation in stress level may contribute to variation in the brittleness index which in turn would lead to variation in mobilised strength at failure. Therefore the strength could vary in an arbitrary manner from peak to residual along a given slip surface (Bishop, 1971). Peck (1967) discussed other important aspects concerning the variation of mobilised shear strength along a slip surface. He presented experimental results of R.J. Conlon which show that the horizontal displacement required to reach peak and residual shear strengths increases significantly with increasing normal stress on the failure plane upto a limit. Beyond this normal stress the horizontal deformation required to reach peak strength decreases slightly. Based on these results and typical normal stress distribution along failure surfaces, he reached the important conclusion that failure is likely to progress from the crest of a slope. Combined with the usual appearance of tension cracks at the crest before complete failure, these interesting results strongly lead to the view that simultaneous failure in slopes is rarely possible. (Peck was cautious to point out that there may be other factors to consider and, therefore, failure need not necessarily start at the head of a slide).

Recent literature concerning first-time slides is lacking in examples which support progressive failure as it is usually understood i.e., mobilisation of average shear strength less than the peak strength along the failure surface at the time of failure. Some failures in Seattle which Bjerrum (1967) considered to be first-time slides are regarded by Palladino and Peck (1972) as failures along existing discontinuities at shear strengths equal to the residual value. Failure conditions for initial East and West Culebra slides along the Panama Canal were reconstructed and analysed (Lutton and Banks, 1970) and showed average mobilised strengths close to the peak ($c' = 0$, $\phi = 19°$) for the fractured, highly slickensided, Montmorillonite rich clay-shale, the Curracha shale. Extensive movements occurred in 1914 and 1915 with consequent reduction of strength to values nearing the residual. Pore pressure observations revealed that swelling continued to occur for several decades. This would, of course, contribute to reduction of strength with time. Similar observations were made by Peterson (1954) for shales in river valleys excavated by natural erosion processes and analysis of such processes has been made by Koppula (1970). Lutton (1975) and Banks (1975) studied the entire Galliard cut along the Panama Canal and found that structural features (bedding plane, in particular) were very important for sliding to occur. In some cases, three-dimensional wedge analysis, normally used for hard rock slopes, may be appropriate. Even with displacements of 1.2 ft. at the surface, strengths close to the peak were mobilised and high resistance was offered by the shales when failures occurred across bedding.

James (1971a) analysed re-activated slides to determine the decreased friction angle after initial movement. Comparing this to initial ϕ computed from analysis of first-time slides, he estimated the decrease of ϕ. He then plotted this decrease against field strain, defined as the ratio of slip movement to length of slip plane. A useful curve showing increase in drop of ϕ with increasing field strain was obtained for London, Oxford and Lias clays. It was found that a field strain of 0.1 was needed to reduce ϕ by a few degrees. Large movements which are required to cause a decrease of shear strength below the peak may explain why back-analyses generally show that first-time slides occurred at strength close to the peak. It seems that deformations required to reduce the strength need not be so large for failure along bedding as for failure across bedding (James, 1971b; Matheson, 1972). Morgenstern (1977) suggests that compatibility of such deformations as well as discontinuous development of shear zones should be considered in future analytical studies of progressive failure. Discontinuous shearing has been emphasised by Skempton (1966a) and by Morgenstern and Tchalenko (1967a,b).

Despite the fact that many case histories suggest that, in intact overconsolidated clays (or for that matter other clays as well), first-time long-term failures occur at average strengths close to the peak, the following points should be noted.

- There are usually many uncertainties about pore pressures and geological conditions pertaining to slope failures.
- Peak strengths measured in the laboratory are not always truly representative of peak strengths operative in the field.

Besides these points, it is important to remember that a failure occurring at an average strength close to the peak strength may still be 'progressive' in the sense that it did not occur simultaneously over the whole failure mass. Apart from long-term pore pressure effects or rheological decrease of shear strength, it is logical to expect that failure will occur first in areas which are overstressed in relation to the shear strength. In this respect, it is unfortunate that progressive failure is usually taken to signify only the fact that failure occurred at an average strength less than the peak.

In contrast to first-time slides, re-activation of movements along old slip surfaces or shear planes is usually associated with mobilised shear strength close to the residual strength value. Back-analyses have shown shear strengths close to the residual in many cases involving different types of soils (e.g., Early and Skempton, 1972; Hamel and Flint, 1972; Hamel, 1973a,b). However, there may be some differences between values of inferred field residual shear strength and residual strength measured in the laboratory. This aspect has also been discussed in chapter 2.

Renewed movements along old shear zones or slip surfaces are not always easy to recognise. Detailed local geological investigations and careful geotechnical studies are equally important to establish whether or not the whole or part of a slip surface has been involved in previous movements. The existence of shear zones on which strength has fallen close to a residual value can be attributed to several phenomena other than landsliding e.g., tectonic folding, valley rebound, periglacial phenomena and non-uniform swelling. (See Morgenstern, 1977 for detailed discussion and many references.)

5.17.3   Long-term failures in fissured clays

Case records concerning failures in London clay are the most significant in respect of fissured clays. Long-term failures in this material have been summarised at various times by Skempton (1964, 1970, 1977). Once again limit equilibrium methods alone have been extensively used. Such analyses can generally explain most of the failures if the values of shear strength parameters chosen for analysis are those corresponding to the fully softened condition when the cohesion parameter c is zero or very small (of the order of 1 kN/m² for brown London clay). The values of pore water pressure corresponding to equilibrium values are applicable for the long-term stability of overconsolidated fissured clays. Analyses are very sensitive to the values of cohesion parameter c and the pore pressure parameter $\bar{r}_u$. Skempton (1977) found from several case histories that a range in $\bar{r}_u$ of 0.25 to 0.35 gave estimates of average shear strength at failure in the range $c' = 1$ kN/m², $\phi = 20°$ to $c' = 0$, $\phi = 20°$ in brown London clay. The values from back calculations in respect of actual failures agree closely with drained softened strength parameters obtained in the laboratory for this soil. In laboratory tests, specimens were normally consolidated from a slurry and showed nearly the same drained strength as was measured for fissures and joints in the clay. The mechanism of progressive decrease in strength from a high peak value ($c' = 14$ kN/m², $\phi = 20°$ for 38 mm triaxial samples to $c' = 7$ kN/m², $\phi = 20°$ for 250 mm samples) to the fully softened value is not fully understood. Softening as a mechanism of progressive failure was first postulated by Terzaghi (1936) as a consequence of stress release due to excavation followed by entry of rain water in the fissures, non-uniform swelling and consequent further cracking and weakening of the soil mass. Skempton (1948) gave some attention to the rate of softening of stiff-fissured clays in terms of undrained strength, applicable for 'total stress' analysis. Even in the nineteenth century, Rankine (1862) considered the possibility that clays may lose their cohesion and Baker (1881) noted from experience that slopes steeper than 3:1 in London clay were generally not stable in the long-term. (Skempton, 1977)

Data from Patton (1966), Marsland (1967) and Mitchell (1976) suggest that softening reduces the dilatant characteristics of a fissured clay at low effective stress levels. Chandler (1974) found that failures in weathered Lias clay occurred at strengths close to the fully softened strength particularly when the clay was also brecciated. His results gave some support to the view that softening is time-dependent. Loss of cohesion appeared to be greater with increasing age of slope failure. Clay which was both weathered and brecciated could lose the whole of cohesion intercept in 80 to 100 years while clay which was only weathered retained some cohesion.

Eigenbrod and Morgenstern (1972) studied a first-time slide in fissured, heavily overconsolidated upper Edmonton formation. Part of the slip surface passes through a bentonitic formation which was found to be pre-sheared. If residual strength was assumed for this part of the failure surface and allowance made for perched water tables, analysis showed that peak softened strengths were mobilised along the rest of the slip surface. According to Morgenstern (1977), this case history supports softening mechanism, indicating a softening clay shale across bedding planes and a pre-sheared clay along bedding.

Non-uniform mobilisation of shear strength (usually designated as progressive failure) may also have some role to play in first-time failures of slopes in fissured clays. However, most of the evidence supports softening (gradual loss of cohesion) as the mechanism of failure. Yet failure may not be simultaneous throughout a potential sliding mass. In that sense, failure of a progressive nature can never be ruled out.

Finally, it is again important to note that the residual strength of fissured overconsolidated clays is often much lower than the fully softened strength (e.g., residual $c' = 0$, $\phi = 13°$ for brown London clay). This strength is generally mobilised only after a slip has occurred requiring minimum displacements of the order of 1 or 2 m. As in the case of intact clays reactivation of movements along old slip surfaces may correspond to this much reduced shear strength. There are many examples of renewed movements at shear strengths close to the residual in fissured clays (e.g., London clay) and in clay shale (e.g., the famous slides along the Panama Canal). However, it is perhaps important to consider the stress level of a new slide in comparison to the stress level of an old slide on the same slip surface. As Bishop et al. (1971) pointed out the stress level may have an important influence on the mobilised shear strength even in relation to renewed movements. It is also important to consider the direction of renewed movements relative to direction of original slide.

5.17.4   Time to failure

It is well known that first-time slope failures in clays, and notably those in fissured clays, occur many years after a cutting has been made. Often the delay is of the order of decades. The problem of delayed failure is, of course, a complex one and the reasons for delay have not been fully understood except in isolated cases. Delays are of interest in short-term, intermediate and long-term failures. Vaughan and Chandler (1974) found that some short-time slope failures occurred during excavation while others occurred after a delay extending upto about 50 days. In their survey slope heights ranged from 4.5 to 15 metres and slope angles from 45° to 85°, higher slopes being generally less steep. A consistent relationship between calculated strength at failure and depth of cut was noted. Skempton (1977) noted delays in failure between 3 and 35 years for London clay slopes ranging in inclination from 1½:1 to 2¾:1 and in height from 6 to 17 metres. In the same soil he found the delay in long-term failures to range from 46 to 65 years in slopes ranging from 3:1 to $3\frac{2}{3}$: 1 and in height from 6 to 12.2 metres.

There are many instances in which failures appear to occur without any apparent cause. Peck (1967) described an interesting case record in which failure could have been triggered by exceptional rainfall or a seismic tremor. However, the slope survived both events and there was significant delay before the failure actually occurred. In a similar manner it is sometimes difficult to establish even an approximate relationship between the time to failure on the one hand, and material parameters and external influencing factors on the other.

Significant progress has, however, been made in explaining the delay in long-term failures of slopes in brown London clay. Originally it was believed that progressive decrease of the strength from a peak value to a lower value was a phenomenon which involved a delay similar to that characteristic of the long-term failures. Since the clay is fissured, it was thought that the increase of pore water pressures to equilibrium values would occur relatively fast. The bulk permeability was believed to be high due to the fissures and consequently it was assumed that pore water pressure equilibrium would be rapidly established. However, based on long-term field observations of pore water pressure in stable and failed cut slopes, this view was shown to be incorrect for brown London clay.

The relationship between age of cutting and the value of pore pressure parameter $\bar{r}_u$ is shown in Figure 5.13. The delay in failure was found to be of the same order as the delay in rise of pore water pressure to equilibrium values (Vaughan and Walbancke, 1973; Skempton, 1977). Calculations by Eigenbrod (1975) also show that the time scale of pore pressure equalisation can be many tens of years. Some delay may, however, be associated with decrease of strength from a peak value to a fully

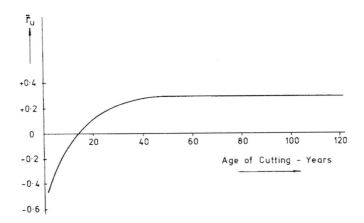

Figure 5.13 Relationship between age of cutting and average pore pressure ratio for Brown London
clay (depth of cutting more than 6 metres). Eight points corresponding to back analysis of slope failures ($\bar{r}_u$ for $F = 1$) lie close to this curve. Also, four points corresponding to
field observations at different sites lie very close to this curve (after Skempton, 1977).
Permission requested, see page 714, No 43.

Table 5.8 Comparison of delay in failures in first-time slides in London clay (after Lo and Lee, 1973).
With permission, see page 713, No 18.

| | Time to failure | | |
Location of slide and reference	Actual years	Predicted years	Remarks
Northolt, Skempton (1964)	19	14	Based on 6% decrease of
Sudbury Hill, Skempton and Hutchinson (1969)	49	42	drained strength per log cycle of time. No
Upper Holloway, DeLory (1957)	81	55	delay assumed in pore pressure equilibrium.

softened value although the evidence available suggests that this is not significant for
brown London clay.

For clays in general, many factors may be responsible for delay in failure e.g. (1)
decrease of strength from a peak value to that mobilised at failure may take time in
some materials, (2) creep movements often precede failure and a significant magnitude
of pre-failure displacement due to creep may take considerable time, (3) rheological
decrease of strength with time may be important. The role of these factors is at best
understood only qualitatively. Moreover, there may be other factors such as reorientation of stresses and non-uniform soil strains which also influence the delay in failures.

The manner in which a finite-element analysis may prove useful in studies of time
to failure was demonstrated by Lo and Lee (1973), who provided an explanation
for the magnitude of delay in three slides in London clay assuming a 6% rheological
decrease of strength per log cycle of time. Their results are of interest in spite of the
fact that the delay in these failures is now considered to be due to the delay associated
with attainment of pore pressure equilibrium as discussed in the previous paragraphs.
Their results are summarized in Table 5.8.

The following are the Steps in the analysis of Lo and Lee (1973) mentioned above:

1   Assume that a cutting is made in strain-softening or brittle soil. A finite element analysis which takes into consideration the relevant failure criterion and the brittle nature of the soil is used to accurately identify zones of failure at any stage provided (a) the initial stress field is known so that tractions to simulate excavation can be calculated. (This means a knowledge of K_0 for the soil), (b) the excavation is simulated in incremental steps and, (c) changes in pore water pressure are taken into consideration. Suppose that pore pressure equilibrium is rapid and final equilibrium values are obtained shortly after excavation. Calculate the factor of safety at end of construction for the relevant critical slip surface. (Such a surface is generally known for any case history but is found by trial and error if slip has not occurred). The factor of safety is based on peak strength along that part of the slip surface which is outside the failed region and reduced strength for the remaining part. This is the factor of safety at end of construction or at time $t = 0$ and may be designated as F_0.

2   Now it is desired to find the decrease in F based on a rheological decrease of peak strength at the rate of x per cent per log cycle of time. Repeat the above analysis with strengths reduced by x_1, x_2, x_3, etc. per cent corresponding to time intervals $t_1, t_2, t_3, \ldots$ etc. The corresponding factors of safety are F_1, F_2, F_3, etc. Plot F as a function of time t. The value of t at which $F = 1$ can be found from such a graph. This represents the time required for failure on the basis of the assumptions made.

The question now arises as to the use of a similar approach when delay in failure is due to some other causes e.g., due to delay in pore pressure equilibration. This may be done by performing the following steps:

1   Establish F_0 for the end-of-excavation condition assuming that the pore pressures are the sum of initial values and negative excess pore pressures due to unloading obtained in terms of Skempton's pore pressure parameters.

2   Assuming the relationship between pore pressure parameter r_u and time t in the field to be known as in the case of brown London clay (Figure 5.13), find F_1, F_2, F_3 etc. corresponding to r_{u1}, r_{u2}, r_{u3} associated respectively with times t_1, t_2, t_3.

3   Plot F versus t and read value of t for $F = 1$. This is the time to failure. Similarly, consideration can be given to the combined effects of rheological decrease in strength and delay in pore pressure equilibration.

5.18 POST-FAILURE BEHAVIOUR OF LANDSLIDES WITH PARTICULAR REFERENCE TO EXCEPTIONAL ROCKSLIDES

Due to a number of reasons, the stability of an initially stable slope may decrease to a state of critical equilibrium so that a slope failure or a landslide occurs. The concept of limit equilibrium does not facilitate the prediction of the speed with which failure would occur. The failure event may be gradual or fast or very fast and catastrophic. Understanding and analysis of the post-failure phase is also beyond the scope of the limit equilibrium concept. Yet, it is often important, and sometimes essential, to consider the transition from stability to failure as well as to estimate the velocity and travel distance of a landslide. In particular, exceptional landslides occur from time to time and the speed of post-failure movements as well as the magnitude of travel distances may be baffling.

Based on the uncertainties in understanding and analysis of landslides, broad categories of landslides are suggested below. Some examples of exceptional historical rockslides are given followed by a summary of suggested mechanisms for their post-failure travel. Alternative calculations concerning the speed of travel of one historical rockslide are also given.

5.18.1   Broad categories of landslides

Scholars and researchers have realized that the occurrence, associated mechanisms and post-failure behaviour of landslides can be explained well in some instances but not in others. Besides, there is a vast range in the size (volume), geology, environmental conditions, earth materials, velocity and travel distance of landslides. Moreover, there can be several basic causes and main triggering agents.

Chowdhury (1980) suggested three broad categories of landslides to differentiate the degree to which the cause and occurrence of landslides can be understood within the limits of current knowledge. The suggested categories are:

I   Landslides resulting from exceptional causes such as:

   i   earthquakes of relatively large magnitude
   ii   exceptional precipitation and
   iii liquefaction of extra-sensitive clays, poorly compacted fill or loose sand masses.

In terms of size, velocity and impact, such landslides have a large range and can include catastrophic events. While most landslides in this category may be explained within the framework of widely accepted concepts, a complete understanding of some events may still be difficult. Exceptional events may not always lead to expected outcomes. An extension of known methods of analysis is often necessary to understand exceptional landslides. There are numerous examples of exceptional landslides in the literature. For example, Seed (1968) attributed the occurrence of some exceptional landslides to the liquefaction of isolated sand or silt lenses in a mass of cohesive soil followed by a mechanism of progressive failure.

II Ordinary Landslides or landslides resulting from known or usual causes which can be understood fairly well on the basis of widely accepted concepts and theories.

In this category one may include failures of natural slopes, embankments and excavated slopes due to factors such as external disturbance, erosion, wave action, change of shear strength with time or increase of pore water pressures following rainfall. Over many decades, hundreds of cases of slope investigation and analysis have been reported and discussed in the literature. In many cases, slope behaviour has been interpreted reasonably well on the basis of conventional theory. This does not always imply success either (i) in the prediction of slope failure, or (b) in obtaining reliable results from quantitative back-analysis.

III Landslides which occur without any apparent cause or with unusual aspects including unusual post-failure behaviour. Often these are very large and rapid landslides. Consider the following examples:

1 The Mayunmarca rockslide Peru, 1974

This rockslide and debris flow occurred in the Andes of Peru in 1974 (Kojan and Hutchinson, 1978) and had a volume of a thousand million cubic meters (10^9 m^3) and velocities approaching 130 km/hour. There was no immediate or obvious triggering agent. To explain a condition of critical or limiting equilibrium ($F = 1$) on the flat lower slopes, high pore water pressures would be required. However, all the evidence pointed to the absence of pore pressures and, in fact, dry or moist (low water content) conditions prevailed. To explain velocities approaching 130 km/h, pore pressure would have to be artesian since, even for $F = 1$, pore pressures required would have to be equivalent to $r_u > 0.5$.

2 The Frank Slide (Canada), 1903

This rockslide occurred in the Turtle Mountains near the Crowsnest Pass area of Southwestern Alberta, Canada in 1903 with an approx. rockmass volume of 30.5×10^6 m^3 (approx. weight 90×10^6 tonnes). The slide moved very rapidly after detachment. The average thickness of debris over an area of 2.67 km^2 has been estimated at 13.7 m with a maximum of up to 150 m.

The Frank slide is considered to be an example of a classical natural rockslide However, it has also been suggested that mining activity at the foot of the slide area might have provided a trigger for the catastrophic landslide. Several months prior to the event, some movements had been observed by miners and, in the final stages, coal began to mine itself. While the observations could be interpreted as a period of creep preceding the occurrence of the main event, qualitative or quantitative analysis has not been able to simulate the effect of mining at the toe of the potential sliding mass. The analyses of Krahn and Morgenstern (1976) show that the effect of mining excavation was small and they conclude, among other things, as follows:

"It is difficult to ascertain what finally triggered the slide. Factors which have been cited as possible causes are ice wedging in cracks at the top of the mountain, earthquake tremors, water pressure effects and mining at the base of the mountain. Although small, none of these effects can be ruled out. Procedures for rock slope stability are not sufficiently sensitive to discriminate between them".

The rockmass moved very rapidly after the occurrence of the slide. Estimates of duration of the event vary from 20 to 120 seconds. During this period the debris moved down from the east face of the Turtle Mountain across the entrance of the Frank mine, across the Crowsnest river, the southern end of the town of Frank, the main road from the east and the Canadian Pacific mainline through the Crowsnest Pass and then traveled upslope on the opposite side of the valley coming to rest 120 m above the valley floor. Even if transformation of a stable mass to a condition of critical equilibrium $(F = 1)$ is accepted, the extremely rapid motion characterizing the unusual post-failure behaviour cannot be explained at all.

3   The Vaiont Rockslide (Italy), 1963

Aspects of this catastrophic landslide are mentioned at several places in this book, including chapters 1, 2, 4, 5 (this chapter) and chapter 7. In particular, two alternative interpretations of this slide are discussed in this chapter and chapter 7 (See 7.15).

4   The Elm Rockslide (Switzerland), 1881

This catastrophic landslide occurred near the village of Elm in Switzerland on September 11, 1881. Like the Frank slide it is often characterized as a natural event and yet its occurrence appears to have been a direct consequence of an excavation more than 50 m deep into a slate seam at the base of the hill from which the potential sliding mass was to detach itself. A large crack developed and, well before the main event, millions of cubic metres of the rock mass were creeping slowly downwards. When this huge mass was detached, the hamlet of Untertal was buried, a part of Elm village was destroyed and 115 people died. Pioneering work concerning the understanding of this landslide was done by Heim (1932) whose observations have been cited in all subsequent studies. He noted that the travel distance of the rock mass was far in excess of that predicted on the basis of a reasonable coefficient of friction within a frictional sliding model. He called the event a 'sturzstrom' which may be described as 'an exceedingly rapid debris flow generated by a rockfall or rockslide'. Heim concluded that the rockfall at Elm did not slide; it crashed and its debris flowed.

He also noted that other, very large rockslides exhibited similar behaviour. The larger the volume of a sliding mass, the greater is the discrepancy between observed and estimated travel distance. Thus a back analysis based on actual (observed) travel distance shows a discrepancy between actual and estimated coefficients of sliding friction. This discrepancy increases as the size (volume) of sliding mass increases.

No stress analysis has been performed to study the effect of mining at the toe. Just as in the case of Frank slide, such analyses may prove to be inconclusive as to the full significance of mining activity for the occurrence and post failure velocity and travel of the slide.

5.18.2   Suggested mechanisms for exceptional landslides

The following mechanisms have been suggested for the unusual post-failure behaviour of exceptional landslides. All of these are controversial and not widely accepted within the geotechnical engineering profession. There are also significant differences of opinion amongst geoscientists, researchers and scholars as to the applicability of one or more of these mechanisms to individual catastrophic landslide events. Detailed presentation and discussion of the following suggested mechanisms is considered to be outside the scope of this book.

I Air-layer lubrication and postulating that movement of landslide debris occurs on a cushion of compressed air (Shreve, 1966, 1968).

II Pore fluid vaporization as a consequence of heat generated during very rapid movement. It is postulated that the developed gaseous pore pressure reduces the shear strength of the moving debris Habib (1976).

III Fluidisation by air or other gas. It is postulated that friction between individual particles within the debris is reduced to zero and thus they become highly mobile (Thrush, 1969).

IV Turbulent grain flow: It is postulated that turbulent flow of a dispersed particulate mass occurs with an interstitial fluid which may be air or dry dust (Bagnold 1954, 1956). The concept of grain flow recognizes that a static granular mass cannot flow without some degree of dilation and dispersion. The dispersive stress originates from grain collisons in a suspension of high concentration. According to Hsu (1978), the postulate of Sturzsstrom motion suggested by Heim (1932) for the Elm rockslide is similar to what Bagnold postulated later for a turbulent grain flow.

5.18.3 Travel angle of landslides based on completed motion after detachment

The travel distance of landslides is often characterized in terms of a travel angle (or shadow angle) α defined as follows:

$$\tan \alpha = \frac{H}{L} \tag{5.49}$$

in which H is the vertical drop (vertical projection of the travel distance) of the debris (soil or rock mass) and L is the horizontal projection of the travel distance. The travel distance may be along a single plane or multi planar (Figure 5.14). Heim (1932) called α the Fahrboschung angle.

Based on sliding friction, for many rock materials, a typical value of tan $\alpha = 0.6$ ($\alpha = 31°$) should be expected. However, values based on observations at the sites of many large rockslides are considerably smaller than 0.6. According to Heim (1932), the travel distance of a sturzstrom depends on the size of the traveling mass, the height of fall and the regularity of the path of motion. He suggested that tan α may be regarded as the equivalent coefficient of friction associated with the motion of a landslide mass. He defined this angle (α) as the inclination of the line joining the uppermost point where the rock mass broke away to the terminus of the debris. (A better measure may be the inclination of the line joining the centres of gravity of a mass before and after the travel associated with the event). (At Elm the values of alpha based on the alternative definitions are 16° and 23° respectively.)

He listed 7 rockfalls in increasing order of volume (ranging from 0.5 million cubic metre to 12000 million cubic metre. The observed angle α (apparent friction angle) decreased from 33° (tan $\alpha = 0.65$) for the smallest landslide to 8° (tan $\alpha = 0.14$) for the largest. The relationship between size and apparent friction angle showed a consistent decrease in the latter with an increase in the former, although it is not a simple relationship. This is sometimes referred to as the scale effect in large rockslides.

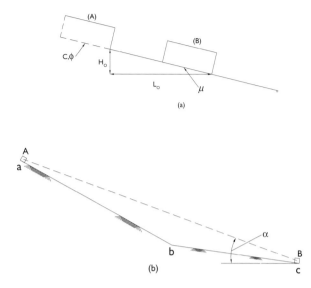

Figure 5.14 Potential movement of rock mass: (a) along single plane surface, (b) along bi-planer path; the travel angle is the angle between the line AB and the horizontal, as shown.

Cruden (1976) listed 7 prehistoric rockslides in the Canadian Rocky mountains with volume ranging from 4.13 million cubic metres to 498 million cubic metres. The value of tan α decreased from 0.32 to 0.21 but the relationship between size and apparent friction coefficient was not consistent.

EXAMPLE 5.6

This example relates to the 1881 Elm landslide event (Heim, 1932). In its simplified version, the travel path for the Elm slide consists of 2 parts. The first part may be regarded as a plane inclined at 45° to the horizontal with a length of 719 m and the second part a plane inclined at 4° to the horizontal with a length of 1513 m (Figure E5.6).

According to the interpretation and estimate of Heim based on observations of eye witnesses, the total time of travel was 45 seconds. The time of travel and the total distance traveled are to be reconciled based on suitable assumptions concerning the coefficient of sliding friction.

Solution

A comparison of travel times based on different assumptions has been made by Chowdhury (1980) and the following is a summary of that contribution.

Note: In addition to calculation of travel distances and velocities, Chowdhury (1980) has provided a comprehensive discussion concerning the concept of stored elastic energy which may be released at the time of occurrence of a very large rockslides. Such a phenomenon would imply a non-zero initial velocity at the time of detachment of the landslide mass. It is postulated that the released energy would be converted into kinetic energy. Consequently, such a phenomenon could explain travel distances being

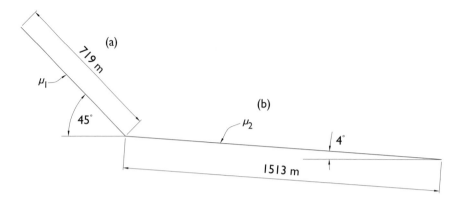

Figure E5.6 Bi-planar travel path of ELM slide.

larger than those estimated on the basis of a reasonable coefficient of sliding friction as the landslide mass travels. Thus such a postulate could explain the significant scale effect observed in these large rockslides as far as travel distance is concerned. For details of the concept of released energy associated with large rockslides, the reader may refer directly to Chowdhury (1980).

The following is limited to the calculations of time of travel and velocities based on a sliding block model.

Consider a rigid block traveling along an inclined plane of inclination β. Assume the coefficient of sliding friction is μ where $\mu = \tan\phi$, and ϕ is the angle of sliding friction. The acceleration of the block is related to the inclination of the inclined plane, the coefficient of friction and gravitational acceleration g, as follows:

$$a = g \, (\sin \beta - \mu \cos \beta) \qquad\qquad\qquad (E5.1)$$

Alternative 1. Assuming $\mu = 0.3$ ($\phi = 16° \, 42'$) on both the steep (upper) and flat (lower) parts of the travel path.

Denote acceleration along the steep part of the travel path as a_1 and along the flat part as a_2.

From the above equation, $a_1 = 4.86$ m/sec^2 and $a_2 = -2.25$ m/sec^2.

The maximum velocity of motion is attained at the end of the steep travel path and is calculated as 82.54 m/sec.

Considering the travel distances, the corresponding travel times based on simple equations of motion are: $t_1 = 17.2$ seconds, $t_2 = 36.2$ seconds. Thus total estimated time is 53.4 seconds (in comparison to 45 seconds interpreted on the basis of observations).

Conclusion: While the calculated travel time is reasonable, the assumption of a low value of friction angle would be regarded as unrealistic unless the mechanisms involved during motion is very different from that based on a conventional sliding block model.

Alternative 2. Assuming a more realistic value of $\mu = 0.6$ ($\phi = 31°$) along both the upper and lower parts of the travel path.

The calculated travel distance is much smaller than that observed and the calculated travel time is also much smaller than that interpreted on the basis of observation. As an exercise, the reader may perform the detailed calculations in the same way as for the above alternative (Answers: travel distance along the flat part = 672 m, time along flat part of the travel path = 16.1 seconds, total time of travel = 26.4 seconds).

Conclusion: The assumed coefficient of friction is reasonable but calculated travel distance and calculated travel time do not match the corresponding observed values.

Alternative 3. Assuming a coefficient of friction of 0.6 along the steep upper part of the travel path and 0.3 along the flat lower part.

The motion on the upper part would be regarded as sliding since the mass was not yet fully broken up nor had it attained the maximum velocity. On the other hand, a reduced coefficient of friction of 0.3 may be adopted for the flat lower part of the travel path. This can be justified since the second stage of motion was characterised as a sturzstrom by Heim, and turbulent grain flow by Hsu (1978). According to the latter, based on interpretation of Heim "the kinematic treatment of the Elm sturzstrom, based on an assumption of frictional sliding, was applicable even if the sturzstrom did not slide but moved like a fluid on account of grain collisions."

The calculated accelerations are: $a_1 = 2.77$ m/sec^2 and $a_2 = -2.25$ m/sec^2.

The travel times are: $t_1 = 10.3$ seconds and, $t_2 = 36.2$ seconds, and total time $t = 46.5$ seconds. This is closer to the observed value of 45 seconds than the estimate made for alternative 1. However, this solution implies a non-zero initial velocity for the detached mass. The portion of released energy converted to kinetic energy must be sufficient to impart an initial velocity of 53.2 m/sec to the slide mass which would increase to a maximum velocity of 82.54 m/sec at the end of the steep part of travel path and then decrease to zero after traveling a further 1513 m along the flat part of travel path.

Alternative 4. Assuming a coefficient of fiction of 0.6 on the steep part of the path and 0.2 along the flat part of the path: Assuming no released energy at the start of motion, the maximum velocity is calculated to be 63.11 m/sec. Accelerations are: $a_1 = 2.77$ m/sec, $a_2 = -1.27$ m/sec. Travel times are: $t_1 = 22.78$ sec, $t_2 = 49.58$ sec and total time of travel, $t = 72.36$ sec (compared to observed value of 45 sec).

Also, distance along the flat part of the path, $s_2 = 1564.36$ m (compared to observed value of 1513 m). The time is significantly overpredicted although distance traveled is approximately equal to that observed.

(To get the travel distance nearly equal to 1513 m, it is necessary to have friction coefficient of the upper part of travel path as $\mu_1 = 0.61$ rather than 0.6).

By varying the two friction coefficients, a number of results which fit within the observed travel distance have been obtained and are presented in Figure E5.7 as plots of distance traveled versus velocity.

Final comment on alternative 4
Assuming no released energy, a very low friction coefficient for the flat part of the travel path is required in order to get the travel distance close to the observed. While a very low friction coefficient for the flat part of the travel path could be explained in

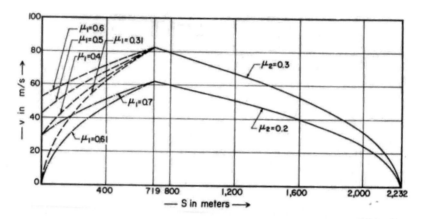

Figure E5.7 Relationship of travel distance and velocity with different assumptions of sliding function coefficients for the ELM slide. (after Chowdhury, 1980). With permission, see page 713, No 17.

terms of the postulate of turbulent grain flow etc., the assumption significantly over-predicts the total time of travel.

Conclusion

Among the four alternatives considered above, the third alternative offers the explanation that best fits with the observed data on total travel distance and total time of travel. There seems to be merit in postulate of released energy and in the postulate of turbulent grain flow for the second part of travel path.

5.19   UNDERSTANDING ORDINARY SLOPE FAILURES BEYOND CRITICAL EQUILIBRIUM

5.19.1   Stability to critical equilibrium and failure

A limit equilibrium method applied to a slope enables an analysis of its safety under a set of conditions that control the stability. If the slope is stable under the prevailing conditions, it has a real factor of safety $F > 1$. Depending on how accurately the parameters controlling stability are estimated and how good the mechanistic model and the method of analysis are, the calculated factor of safety will be close enough to the real factor of safety. However, to be realistic, one must expect some degree of uncertainty associated with the estimated value of F.

A change in the conditions controlling stability of the slope may occur due to different reasons such as increase in pore water pressure associated with rainfall infiltration or, alternatively, the action of cyclic forces associated with the occurrence of an earthquake. Thus the stability of a slope will decrease and it may reach a state of critical equilibrium ($F = 1$). As the stability decreases further ($F < 1$), an overall failure of the slope will occur. Such a failure may take any of several possible forms, the most familiar being a 'slip' or a 'slide' in which the sliding mass moves along a slip surface in an outward and downward direction. The slip surface may be an existing one from an earlier sliding movement or it may be a new one formed during the process of failure in homogeneous soil. Often the conditions are non-homogeneous and whole or part of the slip surface may follow a discontinuity such as a joint or a fault or a weak soil layer.

As we consider this transition to failure, several questions arise, such as:

How much deformation of the failure mass will occur and how fast? Will the failure mass be detached from the slope and, if so, how far and how fast will the detached mass travel below the slope? Will the detached mass stay intact or will it suffer fragmentation and to what extent? Under what conditions will the movement become a debris flow or a flow slide?

These questions are beyond the scope of the concept of limit equilibrium or methods of analysis based on that concept. However, a limit equilibrium analysis method can be used to simulate the transition from stability to critical equilibrium. More importantly, it may facilitate an understanding of the initiation of rainfall-induced debris flows. Therefore, it has provided a useful tool for understanding certain phenomena observed in the field.

However, going beyond critical equilibrium and incipient failure, the simulation of post-failure behaviour requires modelling and analysis based on the principles of dynamics or viscous fluid flow or both, taking into consideration site specific factors such as the topography of the terrain below the slope over which the travel slope debris has to occur.

Relatively simple analyses may be made if the failure mass is detached as an intact mass or if such an assumption is justified for the purpose of analysis. A simple approach may prove to be quite reliable, if in addition to the mass remaining relatively intact during motion, the ground topography and path of motion are both relatively simple. As shown in the previous section, the velocities and total travel distances can be estimated based on realistic assumptions concerning the coefficient of sliding friction during movement. For an observed case, the results can be validated by comparing the observed distance with the estimated distance. Moreover, if the observed travel time is known, the estimated travel time must be compared with the observed time.

5.19.2   The importance of very small movements of a failed but undetached mass

The movement of a failed sliding mass may have a magnitude within a very wide range from very small (millimetres deformation of the undetached failure mass) to very large (hundreds of metres travel of the detached debris) and velocity may take a magnitude within a wide range from extremely slow to very rapid. It is also important to note that the landslide volume can also vary from very small to very large, whatever the speed of movement.

Without local experience and expertise, recognition of extremely slow movements from visual observation alone is difficult. Instrumentation such as inclinometers are generally used for monitoring very small landslide movements (see chapter 11). Often very small landslide movements are of stick-slip type, occurring intermittently during or after significant rainfall and ceasing as the rainfall ceases. Such small movements deceptively give the impression of being harmless. However, experience has shown that the long-term, cumulative effect of such movements is often potentially destructive to houses and infrastructures in urban areas. This cumulative effect increases as landslide magnitude (volume) increases.

5.19.3   Estimating deformations

Using a limit equilibrium analysis in combination with a basic dynamic analysis, it is possible to estimate the deformation of a slope under a change of conditions controlling stability. This has been demonstrated most effectively for the estimation of earthquake induced slope displacements by the 'sliding block method' proposed by Newmark in 1965. This well known and popular method will be discussed further in the separate chapter on earthquake slope stability (Chapter 9). Some researchers have suggested the use of a similar approach for displacement caused by increase of pore water pressure. However, stress-deformation analysis such as FEM is a more versatile approach (see chapter 6).

On the other hand, the sliding block model for earthquake slope or embankment analysis remains very popular although it is recognised that, in projects where detailed studies can be justified or where complex behaviour needs to be investigated, FEM dynamic analyses can provide very valuable insights.

5.19.4   Rainfall-induced debris flow initiation

Rainfall-induced debris-flows occur in many regions of the world and can be very destructive. There is often significant uncertainty associated with the occurrence of debris-flows and it is difficult to predict which potential slope failures will be just slides and which will become debris flows.

One must, however, distinguish between debris flows and flowslides. Flowslides are also triggered by rainfall but involve cohesionless soils and often occur on steep slopes such as sand or pyroclastic deposits. Flowslides travel faster and have a longer run-out distance than debris flows. The mechanism of initiation of flowslides has both similarities and differences with that of the initiation of debris flows and a lot more research is needed to explore these mechanisms in detail. Based on published research, the following summary refers specifically to debris flows.

There is general agreement amongst researchers and experts that increase in pore water pressure is the most important factor in the initiation of debris-flows. This can occur in various ways. Firstly, rapid infiltration of rainfall through permeable slope materials in the source area may initiate a debris flow. Secondly, a perched water table may develop at the interface between a permeable soil layer and a relatively impermeable boundary such as rock or clay. Thirdly, in partially saturated slopes of residual soil, negative pore water pressures (suctions) may be eliminated during rainfall infiltration causing rapid reduction of the shear strength and slope stability. The effect on stability will be more marked if positive pore water pressures develop within the soil mass.

As pore water pressure increases sufficiently, a stable mass will transform from stability $(F > 1)$ to critical equilibrium $(F = 1)$ and initial failure $(F < 1)$. This failure may be associated with a limited initial movement. So how does the failure mass transform into a debris-flow? Two mechanisms have been postulated, one for contractive soil behaviour and the other for dilatant soil behaviour.

If the soil behaviour is contractive, the initial movement leads to increase in pore water pressure and total loss of shear strength. The soil mass suffers what might be called static liquefaction and is transformed into a viscous liquid which moves rapidly as a debris-flow.

If the soil behaviour is dilatant, pore water pressure will fall after the initial movement and thus the movement should stop. However, if rapid rainfall inflow occurs to counteract the fall in pore water pressure, the soil may still be transformed into a debris-flow.

Research has shown that the initial movement occurs under drained conditions and the second phase of static liquefaction occurs under undrained conditions (Sitar et al., 1992). Shear strength parameters from drained strength tests give factors of safety significantly greater than those calculated on the basis of undrained tests. Research has also led to the conclusion that the undrained shear strength parameters should be estimated from stress-path controlled tests on anisotropically consolidated undisturbed soil specimens (ACU tests). The relevant field stress path is one in which the total normal and shear stresses on the failure plane remain constant; only the pore water pressure changes. Thus the effective-stress Mohr circle of stress has a constant diameter as it moves left towards the strength envelope until the latter becomes tangent to that Mohr circle.

It is important to note that there may be other causes and mechanisms specific to particular soil types, geology and location. Progressive failure phenomena may play an important part in some cases. For example, a small debris flow may become a much larger one by a process of failure progression and extension.

Observed debris-flows in different parts of the world have occurred under a wide variety of conditions and there are significant differences in the causes, the patterns of occurrence and in volume, velocity and impact. In addition to rainfall patterns, the history of previous landsliding in the region and also at particular sites can prove helpful in understanding previous failures and also in assessing the hazards of new failures. For example,the case of Otari debris flow disaster (Kawakami, et al., 1999) is very interesting in this regard and demonstrates the difficulties in predicting or mitigating such disasters.

5.19.5   Methodology for analysing a rock avalanche

There is a wide variety of landslide phenomena which involve significant volumes of soil or rock or both travelling vast distances which can be very large and at velocities which can be very rapid. These include soil and rock flows and avalanches, wet or dry, with or without known triggering agents. It is beyond the scope of this book to discuss all such phenomena. A brief reference to a proposed methodology for the analysis of a rock avalanche is made here for completeness since the post-failure movement of rock mass was not included in the discussion so far. Three zones are identified in such problems: the detachment zone, the transition zone and the deposition zone. Couture et al. (1999) proposed a comprehensive methodology and applied it to the La Madeleine Rock Avalanche (Savoie, France).

The methodology comprises the following:-

- The gathering of information and its documentation: This includes recorded historical events, geological information, geomorphology, previous investigation reports, topographic and geological maps, air photos, climate data (failure may be related to climate factors) etc. A digital terrain model (DTM) helps the representation of morphology.
- Field work including field testing including physical and mechanical properties of rocks and rock joints.
- Laboratory testing and interpretation, including shear strength and other mechanical properties of rock mass, intact rock and rock joints.
- Analyses related to stability, energy balance with emphasis on the fragmentation process, mobility and post-failure behaviour.

Among other things such as the causes and mechanisms of failure, the proposed methodology aims at an evaluation of the block size distribution in the detachment zone as well as in the deposition zone. It also aims at an understanding of the boundary conditions along the travel path.

5.20 IMPROVING SLOPE STABILITY

5.20.1   Introduction

There are a number of methods which can be used for improving slope stability or slope stabilisation. The objective is to increase the factor of safety or the reliability index to a desired level under the operating conditions over the design life of a slope. Alternatively, the objective may be to decrease the probability of failure (or, more precisely, the annual probability of failure) to a desired level. Probability concepts have been introduced in Chapter 3 and the reader will find a comprehensive discussion of probabilistic slope analysis in chapter 10.

An increase in safety or reliability of a slope or a decrease in the probability of slope failure may be achieved through an increase in the forces that resist potential sliding or a decrease in the disturbing forces, or both.

Widely used methods of slope stabilisation include (a) slope drainage (surface and subsurface), (b) modification of the slope geometry by cut and fill operations, (c) use of restraining structures (such as retaining walls, anchors and piles) and reconstruction of a slope after removal of the landslide mass or loose debris. The choice of method will depend on the type of slope, its location, potential failure mechanisms, observed performance, consequences of future failure, and the performance required after improvement.

5.20.2   Preliminary steps for slope improvement

Ideally, slope improvement or stabilisation in urban areas should be considered as a preventive strategy which includes a systematic observational approach. In general, slope improvement should not be considered as a set of actions to be taken following a complete or catastrophic slope failure. Early signs of slope movement or distress should alert the responsible authority to the need for slope improvement. This is particularly important in urban areas where the economic consequences of complete collapse of a slope are often significant. In many cases, the consequences for human safety and environmental damage are also significant. Once a slope of marginal stability has been identified, it is necessary to carry out detailed field studies, determine the shear strength parameters and pore water pressures, establish the causes of slope distress and observed movement, and consider potential failure mechanisms. The next step would be to carry out analyses and determine the existing factor of safety F under the relevant conditions. Further analyses can then be carried out to quantify the improvements required to achieve the desired increase in the value of F.

Thus one can quantify the required decrease in disturbing forces (e.g., gravity loads), or the required decrease in pore water pressure (to increase shear strength) or the required anchor force.

For an existing landslide, first-time or reactivated, the causes of failure must be fully understood before selecting a method for stabilising it. Back analysis of slope failures or landslides, to which many references have been made throughout this chapter, can provide very useful insights into the causes and mechanisms of failure. Moreover, one can determine the average shear strength parameters operative over an observed slip surface. Consequently, case studies which include comprehensive back-analyses, are the best source of knowledge about the performance of slopes and landslides. Some well-documented case studies may include the performance of slopes or landslides after remediation or stabilisation has been carried out. Monitoring of a slope or landslide site after remediation is important to assess the long-term performance and reliability.

5.20.3   Brief outline of some stabilisation methods

5.20.3.1   Drainage

Drainage can include surface drainage and subsurface drainage systems. The latter include horizontal or inclined drains, trench drains, drainage wells and galleries. Drainage is one of the best methods for improving the stability of slopes and hillsides subject to infiltration from rainfall and snow melt. Rainfall induced slope failures occur frequently in many regions of the world. Following a significant rainfall event, many new or first-time landslides may occur within urban areas, along hill roads and near railway lines. Moreover, existing landslides in urban areas and along transportation routes may be reactivated.

5.20.3.1.1   Slopes of saturated soil

As the increased distribution of rainfall-induced pore water pressure over a potential slip surface within a slope reaches a critical value, a slide will occur. Thus the aim of drainage is to decrease infiltration and hence the positive pore water pressure so that shear strength and stability are not reduced to critical levels.

5.20.3.1.2   Slopes of unsaturated soil

Positive pore water pressures are generally not responsible for failures of unsaturated slopes, as discussed in chapter 2 and elsewhere in this chapter. Therefore, it is important to ask 'can drainage also be effective in improving the stability of unsaturated slopes?' Since rainfall infiltration eliminates suction (negative pore water pressure) in unsaturated soil, a component of shear strength related to suction is reduced and thus the factor of safety can decrease below the threshold value of 1 as infiltration proceeds. Therefore, the aim of drainage in such soils should be to prevent infiltration reaching the unsaturated soil zones. If this is done, drainage can be effective for improving the stability of slopes of unsaturated soil.

SURFACE DRAINAGE

The aim of surface drainage is to direct water away from the slope or landslide area, prevent ponding near and above the head of the slope. This can be achieved by improving the slope surface to remove irregularities and establishing surface drains with lining and making sure the water is directed to existing streams or established drainage channels. Infiltration may also be reduced by the use of vegetation which improves the evapo-transpiration and thus reduces runoff and infiltration.

HORIZONTAL DRAINAGE SYSTEM

Slopes with potentially deep slip surfaces require subsurface drainage because the high pore water pressure is due to water flow from a large catchment. One of the methods is to drill holes laterally into the face of slope at a small inclination (few degrees) to the horizontal. Perforated pipes are inserted into these holes. These inclined drains are generally referred to as horizontal drains. Usually it is a system of drains rather than just one or two drains. Several locations for installation are selected on the basis of access for the equipment and ability to reach the whole of the area to be drained. A number of drains are drilled in different directions from each of these locations and appear, in plan, arranged like a fan. The lengths of drains must be sufficient to tap the aquifer. Water flows by gravity through the drains and is conveyed to a collection point well away from the slope. The quantity of flow will depend on soil mass permeability and local geological details. Thus some horizontal drains may be more effective than others. The reduction of pore water pressure with time may be monitored by piezometers installed in the slope.

TRENCH DRAINS

These are trenches filled with clean, permeable granular materials such as rock and gravel. The depth should be enough to reduce the pore pressure significantly and if possible, greater than the depth to the potential slip surface. The achievable depth would depend on the stability of the sides of the trench. The fill materials are deposited in the trench according to size in accordance with filter criteria.

Excavating a long trench parallel to the slope has the potential to destabilise a slope. Therefore, trench drains are generally oriented perpendicular to the slope so that the process of excavation causes the least adverse effect on the stability. Several of these drains may feed into a connecting drain parallel to the slope. Such a drain should be completed in short sections in order to minimise adverse effect on stability. The connecting drain should have some inclination in order to facilitate flow under gravity.

DRAINAGE WELLS

For a relatively deep soil mass, which consists of several layers of different permeability, vertical drainage wells are more effective than horizontal drains in collecting the water. Of course, the wells must be connected to horizontal drains or pipes to convey the collected water outside the slopes. A system of wells will reduce the water table below the original level, the extent of lowering depending on the spacing between the wells. As the spacing increases, the effectiveness in lowering the water table reduces. The drawdown of the water table is maximum at each well itself and minimum at the midway point between two wells. It is important to plan an optimum spacing in accordance with the objectives of a project and based on well flow theory. During construction, the effectiveness of the spacing can be monitored.

DRAINAGE GALLERIES

These are tunnels drilled into a deep slope or landslide. Smaller diameter drains are then drilled into the soil mass from within the gallery. Such a system is required for relatively large soil masses where deep drainage is required, and also for sites where other methods cannot be used due to local site constraints.

5.20.3.2   Retaining structures

These may include gravity retaining walls, soil nailed walls and mechanically stabilised earth walls. The objective is to provide an additional restraining force or resisting force to the slope in order to achieve a desired value of the factor of safety F. Thus analyses are first performed to estimate the required additional force. Once this is determined, the wall can be designed using conventional geotechnical design procedures.

This method provides restraint at the boundary of a potential sliding mass and, therefore, it may be unsuitable for a large landslide mass or where the main slip surface is quite deep or where there are several potential failure modes and where more slip surfaces can develop within the mass.

Another point to note is that movement must occur to a certain extent before the additional force can be mobilised by the restraining structure.

5.20.3.3   Prestressed anchor system

Prestressed anchors may be used, each with a bearing pad to transfer the loads to the slope surface. Alternatively, such anchors may be used in combination with a retaining wall. The advantage over a gravity wall is that the required additional force can be transferred to the slope without allowing any movement. Again, slope analysis is carried out to determine the additional force required in each anchor. A factor of safety or load factor should be used on the ultimate anchor capacity to estimate the working load. This value of the factor of safety depends on considerations which are different from those which govern the factor of safety of the slope. The latter depends on uncertainties in soil shear strength and other geotechnical parameters while the former will depend on the uncertainties in evaluating the anchor capacity and the consequences of the failure of an anchor.

5.20.3.4   Reinforcing piles

Pile groups may be installed within a potential sliding mass and into more stable soil. The installation may be either as drilled shafts or as driven piles. The former process would minimise the disturbing effect on the stability of a slope. The piles are oriented along one or more lines, parallel to the slope, and thus provide additional resistance to potential failure or sliding movement. Such piles are subjected to shear and moment and must be analysed accordingly. The extra lateral resisting force required from each pile may be obtained by carrying out a slope stability analysis. The spacing of piles within each row must be optimised based on past experience, analysis and judgement. Analytical studies for the use of piles in slope stabilisation and the design of such piles has been considered by a number of researchers including Poulos (1995, 1999), Yamagami et al. (2000).

5.20.3.5   Modification of slope geometry

The method involves a reduction of slope inclination or of slope height or both. Thus the net gravitational disturbing force and moment are reduced and the stability is improved. In general, an improved balance of forces is achieved by cutting and removal of material from the upper part of a slide, or installing a fill at the toe of a slide or both. The optimum location of cutting and fill can be decided on the basis of analyses. Another aim may be to increase the shear strength along part of the potential slip surface. This may be achieved by excavating landslide material from the lower part of the slide to a depth well below the slip surface and replacing it with a buttress formed of well compacted earth material of adequate strength and provided with good drainage at its base.

5.20.3.6   Other methods

There are other methods of slope stabilisation which have been successfully used from time to time. These include drainage by well points, use of cement grout, use of lime piles, use of stone columns, use of lime slurry piles, thermal treatment of soil and, of course, the use of vegetation.

5.20.3.7   Concluding remarks

More than one of the available slope improvement methods may have to be used together to stabilise a complex site or for achieving a high reliability even in less complex situations. Methods of limit equilibrium analysis described in chapter 4 and this chapter are quite well suited for assessing what changes are required to achieve a given level of safety or reliability. For instance, one may use one of the suitable methods to determine the decrease in pore water pressure required or the additional force required in an anchor. For existing landslides detailed back analyses are most important for gaining an insight into the influence of different parameters on stability.

To asses the improvement in slope reliability within a probabilistic framework, it is necessary to use concepts and methods of analysis outlined in chapter 10.

APPENDIX TO CHAPTER 5

C5.1   Slope analysis including anisotropy

To analyse the stability of a slope in anisotropic soil, it would be necessary in most cases to use an appropriate method of slices for circular or non-circular slip surfaces as the case may be. In certain simple problems, exact integration may be possible. However, in general, a simple numerical approach based on the method of slices will prove to be useful.

C5.2   For '$\phi = 0$' conditions

Equation (2.53) is valid and thus undrained cohesion varies along a slip surface, depending on the direction θ.

   The factor of safety for a circular sliding surface is easily obtained by putting $\phi = 0$ in the general expression for Bishop simplified method and using Equation (2.53) for c, as:

$$F = \frac{\Sigma(c_h \cos^2 \theta + c_v \sin^2 \theta)\, b \sec \alpha}{\Sigma W \sin \alpha} \tag{C5.1}$$

in which θ is given by either Equation (2.54) or Equation (2.55) as the case may be.

   Similarly, Equation (2.53) may be substituted in the relevant equations for factor of safety F, considering a sliding surface of arbitrary shape discussed in the main body of this chapter (Chapter 5).

C5.3   For $\phi > 0$ cases

Next it is of interest to consider a problem in which ϕ has a non-zero value. It is now useful to return to Equation (2.52). The second term in brackets is in fact the normal stress on the plane of inclination θ. Therefore Equation (2.52) may be written as follows:

$$s = (c_h \cos^2 \theta + c_v \sin^2 \theta) + \sigma \tan \phi \tag{C5.2}$$

in which σ is the normal effective stress on the plane of inclination θ. Using this equation, Bishop simplified approach gives the following equation for the factor of safety:

$$F = \frac{\{(c_h \cos^2 \theta + c_v \sin^2 \theta)\, b + (W - ub) \tan \phi\}/m_\alpha}{\Sigma W \sin \alpha} \tag{C5.3}$$

where m_α has been defined in chapter 5 (Equation 5.10a). Again, a choice has to be made between Equation (2.54) and Equation (2.55) for the variable angle θ. Similar modification of equations for factors of safety in relation to slip surfaces of arbitrary inclination may be made as long as ϕ is considered to be independent of direction. If ϕ is also anisotropic with direction and the general form of strength equation [Equation (2.51)], is to be obeyed, then it is necessary to know the stresses completely at each point along the assumed slip surfaces. Considering soil mass with isotropic strength a limit equilibrium approach will yield only the normal and shear stresses on the slip surface. In order to estimate the principal stresses an assumption will have to be made that the slip surface represents the theoretical failure plane. With this assumption Mohr circle construction will enable the determination of principal stresses for the isotropic case. However, this approach is not possible in an anisotropic situation. At the outset a limit equilibrium solution cannot be obtained because the shear strength is dependent on the stresses at each point which are unknown. Again, Mohr circle construction for the anisotropic case presents problems because the relevant Coulomb line cannot be drawn.

The problem could be solved by performing stress analysis using the finite element method as discussed in chapter 6. The shear strength at each point could then be estimated from known stresses and anisotropic strength parameters in horizontal and vertical directions (alternatively defined as shearing strengths obtained when major principal stress is inclined at zero and 90 degrees respectively with the horizontal). The factor of safety could then be obtained on the basis of known strengths and shear stresses from the stress analysis solution.

Chapter 6

Stress-deformation analyses and their role in slope analysis

6.1 INTRODUCTION

6.1.1 Range of advanced numerical methods for stress-deformation analysis

Often assessments of slope stability based on limit equilibrium methods of analysis are sufficient for geotechnical purposes. Advanced numerical methods can provide the means for improving these assessments and supplementing them. Moreover, there are cases when it is necessary to have reliable and accurate assessments of stresses, strains and deformations within slopes, embankments and systems of which they are components. For such assessments, advanced numerical methods of analysis are not just desirable but necessary. As numerical methods have advanced rapidly in range and scope over the last few decades, it is useful to know what is available today. Here we make a brief survey before proceeding to the need for stress-deformation analysis in the next sub-section.

The most widely used method of advanced numerical analysis, and arguably the most important, is the Finite Element Method (FEM) and the basics of this method are presented briefly in this chapter. Solutions can be based on the assumption of linear-elastic, multi-linear elastic, hyperbolic elastic, elastoplastic or general non-linear behaviour. Among other attributes, FEM is able to analyse slopes and earth structures with arbitrary geometry, irregular boundaries as well as non-homogeneous and aniso-tropic zones. A variety of numerical analysis software packages include FEM as one of the methods However, only some of these are specially suited to geotechnical analysis. For example ABAQUS is a general purpose software package while the software from GEO-SLOPE has been developed specifically for slope analysis, and includes limit equilibrium, seepage and stress-deformation modules.

For geotechnical applications, it is important to distinguish between short-term behaviour requiring undrained analyses involving slopes and embankments of satu-rated cohesive soil and long-term behaviour requiring drained analyses of slopes and embankments in saturated cohesive soils. More sophisticated, coupled analyses are required for simulating the complete, time-dependent behaviour involving slopes or earth structures.

The other advanced numerical methods include the Boundary Element Method (BEM), the Explicit Finite Difference Method (EFDM), Discrete Element Methods such as the Distinct Element Method (DEM) and Discontinuous Deformation Analysis (DDA). The well known software package FLAC, based on finite-difference approach, is used for analyses based on EFDM. Based on the same approach, the well known software packages UDEC and 3-DEC are used for DEM analyses.

Methods based on the principles of continuum mechanics include FEM, BEM and EFDM. However, there are problems and situations in which the behaviour of a soil or rock mass or medium is largely governed by discontinuities because of finite deformations and rotations of individual blocks which can occur in a discontinuous or jointed medium. Individual blocks may even separate or develop new contacts during such behaviour. Methods which simulate or analyse such behaviour include DEM and DDA. The former (DEM) is a force-based method while the latter (DDA) is a displacement-based method. These methods have the ability to simulate the kinematics and dynamics of a large number of individual blocks without assuming failure modes in advance. DDA may be used as a tool to illustrate how kinematics influences the mode of failure and the mobility of blocks in discontinuous rock masses and enables the computation of displacements along the discontinuities as demonstrated by Sitar et al. (2005).

The capabilities, advantages and limitations of different methods have been discussed in many papers and reviews such as Sitar et al. (2005) and Carter et al. (2000). A focused geotechnical perspective, considering mainly the role of FEM, has been provided by Potts (2003). Geotechnical engineers now recognize, in particular, the role of stress-deformation analyses for understanding important aspects of slope behaviour such as progressive failure (Potts et al., 1990; Dounias et al., 1996; Potts et al., 1997; Leroueil, 2001; Charles and Bromhead, 2008).

Specialists in numerical methods are fond of pointing out, with considerable justification, that advanced numerical methods are superior to limit equilibrium, plasticity and limit analysis methods in terms of satisfying equilibrium, compatibility and boundary conditions and in their ability to incorporate elastoplastic and elasto-viscoplastic constitutive models. Although closed-form elastoplastic solutions also satisfy equilibrium, compatibility and boundary conditions, such solutions are very few and, therefore, cannot be applied to most real situations. Closed-form solutions based on the assumption of linear elastic soil behaviour are more numerous but applicable to only a limited range of geotechnical problems. Analysis of real cases of slopes and earth structures on the basis of either elastic or elastoplastic closed form solutions may lead to inaccurate or misleading conclusions. However, such solutions have been immensely useful in the development of geotechnical analysis and enable a student to gain an enhanced understanding of concepts related to analysis.

Limit equilibrium methods satisfy overall equilibrium but not compatibility and they satisfy only the failure criterion of the material and not any other constitutive law. Lower Bound limit analysis theorem satisfies equilibrium but not compatibility whereas the Upper Bound theorem satisfies compatibility but not equilibrium. The Bound Theorems are based on the assumption of perfectly rigid plasticity. Limit analysis methods, which are briefly considered in the next chapter, have a useful but very limited role with regard to slope analysis. In contrast, limit equilibrium methods are useful in solving a wide range of practical problems despite the theoretical shortcomings mentioned above. However, numerical stress-deformation analyses are very useful in many cases and are essential in some situations as discussed below. Moreover, some investigators have made a case for including the stresses from FEM analyses to improve the accuracy of limit equilibrium solutions (Krahn, 2001). A simple summation of strength over an appropriate slip surface is often used for such a stability analysis. Alternatively, strength reduction methods can be used for deformation analyses up to overall collapse (Zienkiewicz et al., 1975; Donald and Giam, 1988; Matsui and San, 1992; Ugai and Leshchinsky, 1995; Griffith and Lane, 1999). To implement such an approach, elastoplastic analyses are carried out successively, after decreasing the magnitude of the shear strength parameters in small incremental steps until the solution no longer converges indicating that a state of critical equilibrium and collapse has been reached.

6.1.2   Need for stress-deformation analysis

Conventional methods of slope analysis are based on the concept of limit equilibrium and enable only the calculation of the critical height or the minimum factor of safety of a slope. These methods are not usually concerned with the stress distribution within a slope either above or below assumed surfaces of failure. Similarly strains and deformations within a potential sliding mass cannot be determined from the results of limit equilibrium studies. Often it is important to learn about expected deformations or to compare observed deformations with calculated values. In such cases stress-deformation analyses are thus desirable, if not necessary.

It is possible to determine an approximate stress distribution on an assumed slip surface corresponding to a limit equilibrium solution. However, each method is based on a different set of assumptions and the stress distribution on a surface corresponding to one method may differ considerably from that corresponding to another method.

Often the limit equilibrium slope problem is statically indeterminate and, even with the same method of analysis, different stress distributions on the failure surface may be found which are statically admissible. Consequently, values of factor of safety which are significantly different may result from different assumed stress distributions on a given assumed slip surface. In this connection reference was made in chapter 5 to an example by Lambe and Whitman (1969, pp. 360–63) which they solved by the friction circle method. Thus the value of F actually obtained depends not only on the method of analysis but also on the assumed or implied stress distribution on the assumed failure surface.

From the previous paragraph it is obvious that the stresses on an assumed failure surface which correspond to a limit equilibrium approach may bear little or no relationship to the actual stress distribution on that surface. For this reason alone, a stress analysis approach would appear to be most desirable. The simplicity of limit equilibrium methods is their main appeal. However, they require little or no consideration to be given to the type of slope (natural, excavation or embankment) or the history of slope formation. A geotechnical expert may exercise his judgment in regard to these matters by selecting appropriate values of safety factor and using one limit equilibrium method in preference to another but this does not necessarily result in a marked improvement in understanding slope behaviour. Similarly there is no requirement for consideration of initial stresses and their possible influence on slope stability where limit equilibrium methods are used for analysis. In view of these limitations the need for stress-deformation studies to supplement conventional stability analyses has been felt for decades.

The determination of stresses on an assumed slip surface appears to be important in the context of limit equilibrium approaches. However, from a realistic geotechnical engineering viewpoint it is the overall stress distribution within a slope which is of interest and not that on isolated or imaginary slip surfaces. The overall stress distribution controls deformations, movements and the development of failure zones within a slope depending on its material properties. Stress concentrations may have a significant influence on the initiation and growth of slip surfaces especially in homogeneous slopes. Geological factors and in particular discontinuities certainly have a dominant influence on many slope problems. Yet knowledge of stress distributions resulting from different conditions is crucial in understanding slope behaviour and analysing slope performance. The main reasons for adopting an approach based on stress analyses are summarised below.

6.1.3   Specific advantages of stress-deformation analyses

1   It is useful to know the state of stress within a soil mass both before and after the formation of a slope. The magnitude and orientation of principal stresses often vary from point to point and study of this variation enables accurate analyses of slope behaviour to be made.

2   Knowledge of the stress field is necessary in order that the existence of zones of active or passive failure can be checked by applying the relevant failure criterion (usually the Coulomb-Terzaghi criterion). Zones of overstress or failure may exist in a soil or rock slope even if the overall stability is adequate. These overstressed zones may be significant in relation to the possibility of progressive failure. Also knowledge of these zones is extremely useful in making decisions on further slope alterations, and in planning preventive or remedial measures against possible slides.

   Conventional limit equilibrium methods give little or no information concerning localised failure zones. The stresses on an assumed failure surface are based on an assumed state of incipient failure but do not in general correspond to critical equilibrium or $F = 1$. Even when an actual failure is being studied (after the event) limit equilibrium calculations do not give a complete or true picture of the conditions leading to the failure.

3   Results of stress distribution studies enable choice to be made in relation to the stress conditions under which laboratory tests for material parameters should be made. These conditions may relate to stress level, stress path and principal stress orientation. For example, active conditions underneath an embankment are adequately represented by a triaxial compression test, passive conditions away from the toe of an embankment by a triaxial extension test, and conditions in the intermediate zone by a simple shear test.

4   An adequate technique of stress analysis enables the determination of strains and deformations within a soil mass. It is of great interest to locate zones in which excessive deformations have occurred or can occur. Moreover, non-uniform stress and strain distribution may, in some cases, lead to progressive failure due to the strain-softening behaviour of many soils and rocks.

5   Often the extent of deformation is a far better indication of stability and performance than the conventional factor of safety which cannot be related to expected movements. Information on deformations is particularly important in the case of embankments, earth dams, and rockfill dams in which it may be necessary to limit

the extent of movement and distortion (within the structure or its foundation or both).

Data about expected deformations can be very useful in planning and developing the software of field instrumentation and performance monitoring. The application of stress analysis to study movements of articulated conduits under earth dams on compressible foundations has been discussed by Rutledge and Gould (1973).

6   It is well known that incremental nature of construction processes such as excavation and filling has a significant influence on the final stresses and deformations. Thus the influence of history and method of construction on the behaviour of a slope requires careful analysis. This can only be achieved by 'incremental' as different from 'single lift' stress analyses as discussed in subsequent sections of this chapter. (Incremental analyses are also called 'stage analyses' or 'sequential analyses').

7   Excavation and embankment construction result in the development of excess pore water pressures which may be either positive or negative (as explained in chapter 2). The determination of these increments to existing pore water pressures is always desirable and often necessary. Excess pore water pressures have a direct influence on the short-term and long-term stability of fills and excavations. Dissipation of excess pore pressures in materials of low permeability requires a great deal of time. A slope may fail either as a consequence of increases in positive pore pressures or due to the dissipation of negative pore water pressures. As explained in chapter 2, estimation of excess pore pressure requires a knowledge of increments in total principal stresses caused by imposed loads or removal of slope material. Therefore stress analysis is essential for accurate estimation of pore pressures.

Data about expected pore pressures can be useful in planning and developing software for monitoring pore pressure. Comparison of estimated and observed pore pressures enables progress to be made in procedures used for investigation, analysis and instrumentation.

8   The advantages of stress analysis in relation to full scale tests on trial embankments are quite obvious from the preceding paragraphs. However, stress analyses also have an important role in relation to centrifugal model tests for slopes. The manner in which loads on a model slope in a centrifuge increase or decrease can be simulated by appropriate alteration in slope dimensions to be used in successive analyses corresponding to different centrifuge speeds.

9   Slopes may fail due to causes other than shear failure. Reference was made in chapter 1 to the possibility of embankment and slope failures due to sinking, spreading, piping etc. The possibility of such failures must be assessed by considering a number of relevant factors including changes in stress distribution and expected deformations. Reference was made in chapter 1 to the failure of Teton Dam and it may be recalled that stress analyses were useful in understanding the possible causes for the initiation of failure by piping.

6.1.4   Beginnings of a numerical approach for embankment stress analysis

Few closed-form or analytical solutions for stresses and deformations in embankments or excavations have been developed. A couple of decades before the powerful and versatile finite element method was developed and successfully used, Bishop (1952) carried out a numerical study of embankment stresses. He considered an isotropic elastic triangular dam (embankment) and foundation system and studied the stresses by developing a finite-difference formulation of the elasticity problem and using a relaxation technique for its solution. Known stress conditions were assumed on finite boundaries located a reasonable distance away from the dam. The selection of stress boundary conditions was facilitated by invoking St. Venant's principle. The solution approximates to that for an infinite extent of the foundation and is independent of elastic parameters. On the basis of a comprehensive study Bishop concluded that limit equilibrium methods of analysis offer no reliable information about the actual stresses. In order to justify the assumption of elastic behaviour, he argued that, at the usual factor of safety used in design (of the order of 1.5), plastic failure would be limited to relatively small zones.

In real problems the foundation has a finite extent and the stresses depend on the Poisson's ratio of the material. However, the general trend of results showing non-uniform distribution of normal and shear stresses is similar to that found by Bishop (1952). Only the vertical normal stress within an embankment may be estimated approximately as the vertical head of soil at any point (i.e., the unit weight multiplied by the depth). This will usually give an overestimate of the vertical stress which may be as high as 15% in some locations. Often a dam (embankment) has deformation properties different from its foundation and this non-homogeneity may have significant influence on the stresses. The foundation may also have significant 'elastic' (as opposed to strength) anisotropy, deformation moduli being different in horizontal and vertical directions. Studies in which these factors are taken into consideration are facilitated by an application of the finite element method which is discussed below. The finite element method also enables the determination of stress changes due to excavations and boundary loads with any arbitrary distribution. There is usually little or no difficulty in handling displacement boundary conditions which may have to be imposed to obtain realistic solutions. Non-linear material behaviour and dependence of deformation parameters on stress level can be taken into consideration. It is possible to study the development of plastic failure by invoking an appropriate yield criterion.

6.2   THE FINITE ELEMENT METHOD

6.2.1   Basis of the method

Over the last four decades, the finite element method (FEM) for numerical solution of a wide range of problems in continuum mechanics has been very successful. Consequently, the use of FEM has gained wide acceptance amongst geotechnical engineering researchers and practitioners. The use of a computer is essential, and the phenomenal growth in computing power has indeed contributed to the development and use of numerical solutions based on FEM.

Many computer software packages have been developed and it is, therefore, necessary to understand the basic philosophy, structure and operational details pertaining to a software package before it is used. Several different finite element methods have been developed. One feature common to all these methods is that a continuum is divided into discrete parts called 'elements'. The elements are separated from each other by imaginary lines or surfaces and are assumed to be interconnected only at a finite number of nodal points situated on their boundaries (Figure 6.1). In geotechnical applications the most convenient and popular formulation is the one for a compatible model in which nodal point displacements are assumed to be the only unknowns. This is generally known as a displacement formulation. When displacements have been determined, the computer software proceeds to calculate respectively the element strains and the element stresses. Simple procedures can be devised to compute the nodal point stresses from the element stresses.

In the formulation itself, a choice has to be made concerning the element shapes. Triangular elements have often been used in geotechnical applications although rectangular, quadrilateral and isoparametric elements are sometimes used as well. The popularity of triangular elements is due to convenience in formulation and due to the ease with which irregular boundaries can be approximated. The element subdivision need not be uniform and smaller elements are, in fact, necessary in regions where stresses are expected to vary rapidly. For example, in slope problems, it would be necessary to have a finer mesh in the toe region and close to the slope surface. The size of elements can be increased in regions well away from the slope surface and in regions with low stress gradients.

The second most important choice in the displacement formulation concerns the assumed variation of displacements within each element. In general, it is not easy to ensure that the chosen displacement function will satisfy the requirement of compatibility between adjacent elements. Fortunately, continuity of displacements between adjacent elements of triangular shape is ensured if the displacement variation within these elements is assumed to be linear. Any distributed loads and boundary stresses are approximated by a system of forces concentrated at the nodes such that overall equilibrium is satisfied. Often there may be violation of local equilibrium within

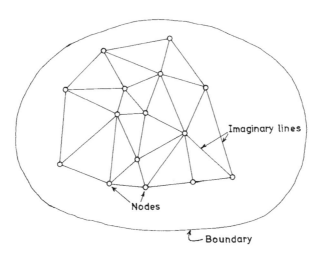

Figure 6.1 Finite elements of a continuum. Triangular elements connected only at nodal points located at the corners of elements.

elements or on their boundaries due to the approximation involved. When this occurs to a significant degree, the solution can be improved by the adoption of a finer mesh, by the choice of alternative element shapes and by increasing the number of nodal points on the element boundaries.

It has been shown that finite element idealisation is equivalent to the minimisation of the total potential energy of a system in a prescribed displacement field. Convergence to the correct result is dependent on the appropriateness of the chosen displacement field. Zienkiewicz (1971) has referred to three convergence criteria: (1) the chosen displacement function should not permit the straining of an element when the displacements of the nodes are due to rigid body displacement only. (2) when the nodal displacements are compatible with a constant strain condition, the displacement function must be such that constant strain can be obtained and (3) the strains at element interfaces must be finite even though they are indeterminate. The criteria are necessarily satisfied in the limit when element sizes tend to zero. However, their imposition on a 'finite' element is desirable in practice.

6.2.2   Two-dimensional displacement formulation

Consider a two-dimensional problem when a continuum has been divided into a number of finite elements of triangular shape. The relationship between generalised displacements $\{f\}$ and nodal point displacements $\{\delta\}$ may be expressed thus:

$$\{f\} = [N]\{\delta\} \tag{6.1}$$

in which the matrix $[N]$ depends only on the shapes and sizes of elements and is obtained from the assumed linear displacement field simply in terms of the nodal point co-ordinates of an element. The strains $\{\varepsilon\}$ are related to the displacements as follows, assuming deformations to be small:

$$\{\varepsilon\} = [B]\{\delta\} \tag{6.2}$$

in which the matrix $[B]$ depends only on the nodal point co-ordinates.

Next the relationship between stress and strain components is required and this is expressed through another matrix, called $[D]$ matrix. The elements of this matrix should represent the assumption concerning the stress-strain behaviour of the material (soil or rock) being modeled. Assuming a linearly elastic response during an increment of loading or unloading, the stresses are related to the strains by an appropriate elasticity matrix $[D]$ thus:

$$\{\sigma\} = [D]\{\varepsilon\} \tag{6.3}$$

On the assumption of elastic behaviour, the elements of Matrix $[D]$ are easily obtained from Hooke's law. For isotropic elastic materials it depends only on the modulus of elasticity, E and the Poisson's ratio, v. In problems of soil mechanics, it is often considered desirable to express $[D]$ in terms of shear modulus G and bulk modulus K which are simply related to E and v (see chapter 2). It is usual to make the assumption of plane strain applicable to long embankments, earth dams, excavations and retaining walls. Therefore, in that case, the elasticity matrix [D] would be different from that corresponding to that for plane stress problems. It may be of interest to consider soil or rock as anisotropic materials. A transversely-isotropic model of behaviour is often assumed since natural formations and man-made fills are deposited in layers suggesting differences in properties parallel and perpendicular to strata respectively. From generalised Hooke's law, it is found that assumption of a plane of isotropy (parallel to the plane of bedding, deposition or strata) reduces the number of elastic parameters considerably. However, five parameters are required in comparison to only two for an isotropic material. The basis for determination of these parameters has been discussed elsewhere (Chowdhury, 1972; Bowles, 1977).

In general, soil behaviour cannot be described as linearly elastic although, in specific situations, anlalyses on the assumption of linear elastic behaviour may lead to reasonable outcomes. In a subsequent sub-section, more detailed reference is made to the advantages and limitations of both the simpler and the more sophisticated methods of FEM analysis.

A whole range of constitutive models have been developed by researchers and successfully incorporated into stress-deformation analyses (Duncan, 1992, Carter et al., 2000). These include assumption of linear and non-linear elasticity and assumption of plasticity. Some models are based on idealized theories of soil behaviour such as the critical state concept (Potts, 2003). Researchers have also tried different methods for simulating strain-softening behaviour or degradation of material shear strength with increasing strain (Potts et al., 1990, 1997; Dounias et al., 1996)

Thus the [D] matrix should correspond to the particular stress-strain model being adopted for analysis. While evaluating finite element software for use in individual applications, a geotechnical engineer should learn about the standard or well known constitutive models that are available. Also the user should learn about the non-linear solution strategy adopted in the software.

As stated earlier, particular attention should be given to appropriate drainage conditions to be assumed in the analysis. If short-term stresses and deformations of a saturated earth structure are to be evaluated, undrained FEM analyses are appropriate and thus the input data should be chosen accordingly. For example, undrained values of the elastic modulus would be appropriate. If the long-term stresses and deformations are also required for the same structure, the corresponding FEM analyses would be drained effective stress analyses and the input data would be chosen accordingly. For example drained value of the elastic parameters would be used. For simulating the complete, time-dependent response, including both short-term and long-term performance, a coupled, effective stress analysis would be required. The input data would include the full range of soil parameters including compression and expansion (contraction and dilation) rather than just the shear strength parameters and the elasic modulii.

While evaluating finite element software for use in individual applications, a geotechnical engineer should learn fully about the assumptions on which the software code is based and about the capabilities of the software. For example, the user should be able to know the answer to questions such as the following: Can the software handle only linear elasticity or also non-linear elasticity? Can solutions based on well known plasticity models be obtained? What particular non-linear solution strategy has been adopted in the software? If the software includes a special constitutive model, what type of soil does that model represent? As has been pointed out by Potts (2003) there is no standard non-linear strategy and the results achieved are influenced by the choices made. Therefore, much depends on the judgment of the geotechnical expert and the reliability of the software used.

Considering the applied nodal forces and distributed loads, the total potential energy of the system comprising the assemblage of elements and the external loads must be a minimum. This requirement leads to a relationship between the nodal forces and nodal displacements for each element. Since each node may be common to several elements, these relationships require assembly in an appropriate manner and the complete system of equations may be written as follows:

$$[S]\{\delta\} = \{F\} \tag{6.4}$$

in which $\{\delta\}$ are the nodal displacements, $\{F\}$ the resultant nodal forces and $[S]$ is the combined stiffness matrix for the assemblage of elements which approximate the continuum. It is assembled from individual element stiffness matrices $[S_e]$ which depend on matrices $[B]$ and $[D]$ as follows:

$$[S_e] = \int B^T DB \, dxdy \tag{6.5}$$

in which the integration is over the area of each element in an x, y co-ordinate system.

For two-dimensional problems with simple triangular elements, Equation (6.4) represents a system of 2 m equations where m is the number of nodes and matrix $[S]$ is square and symmetrical. Assembly and solution of this system of equations is conveniently handled by computer using appropriate matrix and numerical procedures.

Once both displacements at each nodal point are known from the solution of the linear simultaneous equations, the computer software is designed to calculate the strains and stresses. The details of formulation, assembly and solution are discussed in many papers and books and reference may be made, for instance, to Zienkiewicz and Cheung (1967), Zienkiewicz (1971), Desai (1972), Desai and Abel (1972) and Desai (1976). Over the last 30 years many advances have been made in the range and sophistication of stress-deformation methods in general and of the finite element method in particular as outlined by Sitar et al. (2005), Potts (2003) and Carter et al. (2000).

These publications describe a variety of geotechnical applications and refer to specific computer techniques and softwares. As stated earlier, finite element computer softwares are now widely available and some softwares are specifically designed for application to soil and rock mechanics problems. Before a software product is adopted for use it is essential to study all its features such as its capacity (the maximum number of nodal points and elements it can handle), types of boundary conditions that can be specified, element shapes, assumed displacement functions etc. Some software products may be suitable only for linear-elastic analysis only while others may be suitable for problems in which non-linear material behaviour and appropriate failure criteria are considered. Similarly some softwares may be suitable for stage or incremental analysis which are theoretically necessary and practically desirable for embankments and excavations while other softwares may be suitable only for single stage analyses. The latter softwares might, of course, be quite suitable for some geotechnical applications such as retaining walls, footings under certain conditions Special softwares may be required to analyse an incompressible material. For example, short-term behaviour of saturated soft clays is considered to be like that of an incompressible material. (See section 6.5.5).

6.2.3   Review of linear, non-linear and sophisticated models for FEM Solutions

FEM analyses of slopes, embankments, earth dams and landslides have been carried out by geotechnical engineers and researchers for about 40 years. Relatively simple analyses based on assumption of linear-elastic stress-strain behaviour continue to be performed, as also analyses based on more realistic assumptions. At the other extreme, increasingly sophisticated constitutive models have been developed and analyses carried out using such models. There is still a lot of mystique about the need and value of sophisticated elastoplastic and elasto-viscoplastic models. However, each type of analysis has advantages and limitations and this was clear from the findings of a 25-year review carried out by Duncan (1992).

In that comprehensive review of published papers spanning the period 1967–1992, the purpose and scope of many FEM analyses was summarized and the success in capturing slope and embankment behaviour assessed. One table listed 20 different cases in which linear-elastic FEM analyses were carried out. A second table listed 19 cases in which multi-linear elastic FEM analyses were carried out. A third table listed 21 cases in which FEM analyses were carried out on the assumption of hyperbolic elastic stress-strain relationships as suggested by Duncan and Chang (1970). In a fourth table, 17 cases were listed in which FEM analyses were carried out based on elastoplastic and elasto-viscoplastic models. It was concluded that each of the models has a legitimate role although it is important that both merits and limitations are recognized.

In each and every case, the input data should be obtained carefully and evaluated for accuracy. Quite clearly, for instance, deformations computed on the basis of a linear elastic analysis would be very sensitive to the values of elastic modulus and Poisson's ratio or, alternatively, the bulk modulus and the shear modulus.

6.2.4   Features of the simpler models: linear elastic, multi-linear elastic, hyperbolic elastic

The most attractive feature of linear-elastic analyses is their simplicity and the most important limitation is that the results are good only at low stress levels when the strains are small enough to justify assumption of linear elastic behaviour. The attractive feature of multilinear elastic analyses is that non-linear behaviour can be captured. However, the drawback is that the details of the model have to be adjusted for each individual case since each case has a different non-linear response. Hyperbolic elastic analyses can model non-linear behaviour in a more organized way but they still cannot model real behaviour logically. For example, it is not possible to distinguish between elastic and plastic deformations.

6.2.5   Features of elastoplastic and viscoplastic models

Elastoplastic and elasto-viscoplastic analyses reflect real soil behaviour more closely than simplistic idealizations of stress-strain curves. Such models aim at capturing the response of slopes and earth structures over the full range from initial deformation to failure and beyond. However, these models are complex and may not be well suited for general use by geotechnical engineers. Moreover, the more sophisticated the model, the greater the difficulties of obtaining the right parameters accurately. Moreover, a sophisticated model may be limited in its application to particular types of soil or soils for which it was developed.

6.2.6   General comments about all models

There is no doubt about the flexibility and versatility of the finite element method. FEM analyses can be used to simulate a wide range of conditions governing geotechnical performance of slopes and embankments. As Duncan (1992) pointed out from his comprehensive review, results from FEM analyses were in reasonable agreement with other evidence (such as measured deformations) in most cases. However, the tendency for calculated values to be higher than measured values was noted. Reasons suggested for this included the fact that soil stiffness in the field is usually greater than that estimated from laboratory tests on soil specimens, that sample disturbance is unavoidable in any case, that soil samples are tested under axi-symmetric conditions while the field deformations occur under plane strain conditions, and that, in some cases, 2D analyses are not good enough to represent 3D behaviour such as that of an earth dam located within a deep gorge or within a V-shaped valley with steep sides.

Like all geotechnical analyses, the results are influenced by uncertainties including soil variability. Attention should therefore be given to all sources of uncertainty including the input data on soil properties and also on the sequence of construction and operations that would be followed in the field.

6.2.7   Range and complexity of data and parameters required
for some sophisticated models

Let us now consider some FEM analyses based on sophisticated models and try to get an awareness of the type of input parameters that are involved in such analyses. The performance of an excavation in overconsolidated London clay was simulated on the basis of a strain softening soil model (Potts et al., 1997). The values of shear strength parameters were: peak effective cohesion = 7 kPa, peak effective angle of internal friction = 20°, the devatoric plastic strain at which a shear strength starts to fall from peak to the residual = 5%, the deviatoric plastic strain at which shear strength falls to the residual value = 20%, residual effective cohesion = 2 kPa and the residual angle of internal friction = 13°.

The analyses were carried out for a 3:1 slope, 10 m high with coefficient of earth pressure at rest $K = 1.5$ and surface suction = 10 kPa. Analyses showed the propagation of an almost horizontal shear band from just below the toe of the excavation. Nine years after the excavation, the failure surface is still just below the excavation but 14.5 years after the excavation, just before actual collapse, the failure surface is almost completely defined.

Let us consider next the use of an elastic-viscoplastic model to analyse the deformation pattern of five landslides sites in Japan (Hiroaki et al., 1999). The landslides varied in length from 70 m to 600 m, in width from 30 m to 320 m and in velocity from 5 mm/year to 3300 mm/year. Shear strength parameters also varied: effective cohesion from 0 to 19.6 kPa and internal friction angle from 17.4 to 33.4 degrees. The soil elastic modulus was taken as 17,640 kPa and for the bedrock 4,900,000 kPa. The Poisson's ratio varied from 0.31 to 0.25. Appropriate phreatic surface was chosen for the analyses. The changes in pore water pressure with changes in rainfall (rise and fall of the phreatic surface) were not considered in these analyses and that was recognized as a source of uncertainty.

Field measurements of deformation at surface and at depth up to the sliding surface were carried out with inclinometers and extensometers. Calculated horizontal displacements at the ground surface and along the sliding surface were compared with the measured displacements.

In the development of the model for FEM analysis, the total strain rate was considered as the sum of elastic and viscoplastic components. The viscoplastic strain rate was a product of three terms: a fluidity parameter γ which governs the displacement velocity, a flow function based on the Mohr-Coulomb yield function F, and the derivative of the yield function. By matching the measured and calculated values of deformation at different times from the start of measurements, values of the fluidity parameter γ were back-calculated. After that, a fitting value of γ was chosen for the rest of the analyses.

The modeling was considered to be successful in capturing the time-dependent behaviour of these landslides over a number of years. The effect of dewatering at one of the landslide sites was also investigated. The calculated stabilizing effect on displacements was found to correspond well with reduced values of deformation measured after the completion of dewatering.

6.3 MATERIAL PARAMETERS FOR STRESS ANALYSIS

In order to perform finite element analyses for soil or rock masses it is necessary to use appropriate values for material parameters. In general the medium cannot be regarded as elastic although a linear relationship between stresses and strains may be assumed for small incremental steps of loading. Therefore, the deformation parameters may be regarded as pseudo-elastic parameters. It is always necessary to distinguish between stress increment and stress level. While giving further attention to the relationship between components of stress and components of strain expressed in matrix form by Equation (6.3) we will consider only small incremental changes in the components because it is only then that use can be made of elastic theory in geotechnical problems. Here attention is restricted to two-dimensional problems involving plane-strain deformation (zero strains in the direction z are considered here; the z direction would thus correspond to the longitudinal axis of long slopes, embankments, dams, etc.).

The following should be regarded only as a basic introduction to the determination of parameters for linear elastic analyses based on laboratory tests. Elastic parameters may, however, be estimated in ways other than based on laboratory samples. For example, appropriate data may be available from field tests. Alternatively, where field deformations have been measured, elastic modulii may be calculated from back-analyses. Because of such possibilities and other reasons, alternative expression of stress-strain relations in terms of bulk modulus K and shear modulus G should be considered. This approach is preferable to using the relationships on the basis of elastic modulus E and Poisson's ratio μ. It seems more logical to consider volumetric and shear strains separately. Moreover, precise value of Poisson's ratio is not required.

6.3.1 Isotropic parameters

The use of triaxial compression tests for determination of strength and deformation properties of soils and rocks is common. Thus if plots of deviator stress versus principal strains were made from such tests, it would be useful to obtain elastic parameters E and v as follows:

$$\frac{d(\sigma_y - \sigma_x)}{d\,\varepsilon_y} = E, \quad \frac{d(\sigma_y - \sigma_x)}{d\,\varepsilon_x} = \frac{-E}{v} \tag{6.6}$$

Plane strain compression tests would be more useful than triaxial compression tests for two reasons. Firstly these tests are more suitable for use in problems involving plane strain deformation than are triaxial compression tests. Secondly it is possible to determine anisotropic parameters from such tests and this is shown below. Although plane strain compression tests are not common, they have been used successfully by research workers for a number of years.

Equation (6.6) shows that pseudo-elastic parameters at a given level of deviator stress may be obtained on the basis of the slopes of deviator stress-strain curves. Usually a set of such curves would be available corresponding to different cell pressures (stress levels) used in triaxial testing. These curves would enable non-linear and stress-dependent material behaviour to be taken into consideration.

6.3.2 Anisotropic parameters

Consider a transversely-isotropic medium having five independent elastic parameters. Assume xz to be the plane of isotropy. Let E_1 and v_1 represent the modulus of elasticity and Poisson's ratio in the planes parallel to the plane of isotropy, xz; let E_2 and v_2 be the modulus of elasticity and Poisson's ratio perpendicular to the plane of isotropy (i.e., in the y direction) and G_2 be the shear modulus in the y direction. [The shear modulus G_1 in xz plane is not an independent parameter and is obtained from E_1 and v_1 i.e., $G_1 = E_1/2(1 + v_1)$].

From Equation (6.3) we have for plane strain conditions from generalised Hooke's Law (Lekhnitskii, 1963):

$$\varepsilon_x = A\,\sigma_x + B\,\sigma_y$$
$$\varepsilon_y = B\,\sigma_x + C\,\sigma_y \tag{6.7}$$
$$\gamma_{xy} = \tau_{xy}/G_2$$

in which

$$A = \frac{1-v_1^2}{E_1}, B = \frac{-v_2(1+v_1)}{E_2} \quad \text{and} \quad C = \frac{1-nv_2^2}{E_2}, \quad \text{where } n = \frac{E_1}{E_2} \tag{6.8}$$

For isotropic medium $E_1 = E_2 = E$, $v_1 = v_2 = v$, $n = 1$ and $G_2 = G_1$. Therefore, there are only two independent parameters.

Consider a constant cell pressure plane strain compression test on a sample with its plane of isotropy horizontal and assume curves of deviator stress versus axial and lateral strain are available. Differentiating the first and second of Equation (6.7) with respect to normal strains in x and y directions respectively (where y is the vertical or axial stress direction), we have

$$\frac{d\sigma_y}{d\varepsilon_y} = \frac{d(\sigma_y - \sigma_x)}{d\varepsilon_y} = \frac{1}{C}$$

$$\frac{d\sigma_y}{d\varepsilon_x} = \frac{d(\sigma_y - \sigma_x)}{d\varepsilon_x} = \frac{1}{B} \tag{6.9}$$

Thus, from the slopes of appropriate curve, B and C may be obtained for a particular stress level corresponding to the constant cell pressure. Consider now an identical sample of soil oriented with its plane of isotropy along the $y - z$ plane in a similar compression test as before and at the same constant cell pressure. For this case Equation (6.7) may now be rewritten as:

$$\varepsilon_x = C\sigma_x + B\sigma_y$$

$$\varepsilon_y = B\sigma_x + A\sigma_y \tag{6.7a}$$

Differentiation gives:

$$\frac{d\sigma_y}{d\varepsilon_x} = \frac{d(\sigma_y - \sigma_x)}{d\varepsilon_x} = \frac{1}{B}$$

$$\frac{d\sigma_y}{d\varepsilon_y} = \frac{d(\sigma_y - \sigma_x)}{d\varepsilon_y} = \frac{1}{A} \tag{6.9a}$$

From available curves of deviator stress versus axial strain B and A may be obtained for a particular stress level.

In plane strain only the four parameters A, B, C and G_2 are required for deformation studies. The parameter G_2 may now be obtained by considering the curve of another identical specimen with its plane of isotropy inclined at $45°$ to its base. It has been shown (Chowdhury, 1972) that the following equation is obtained for such a sample:

$$\frac{d\sigma_y}{d\varepsilon_y} = \frac{d(\sigma_y - \sigma_x)}{d\varepsilon_y} = \frac{4}{A + C + 2B + 1/G_2} \tag{6.10}$$

Knowing A, C and B from equations relating to the first two orientations for any stress level, G_2 may be obtained for the same stress level from Equation (6.10). Since real materials may not exhibit ideal anisotropy, it is obvious that there may be differences between values of B obtained from Equations (6.9) or (6.9a).

Isotropy is a special case as explained above and testing in only one orientation is necessary for a truly isotropic material. Plane strain equations for isotropy are of course somewhat different from Equation (6.6) which is based on the simple cylindrical compression test.

The above equations are valid only for a total stress approach if applied to results of undrained compression tests. In such a situation the parameters would be regarded as total stress deformation parameters. Where the equations are applied to the curves from drained tests, the parameters are of course suitable for use in effective stress analyses. Further attention to the distinction is given by Chowdhury (1972).

6.3.3   Influence of deformation parameters on stresses and deformations

Even a simple linear elastic model of soil or rock behaviour can be useful for studying the influence of deformation parameters on stresses and displacements. Figure 6.2 shows the significant influence of Poisson's ratio on shear stresses, vertical displacements and horizontal displacements along the base of symmetrical embankment of height H and 3:1 side slopes which has an elastic foundation. Here embankment and foundation are assumed to have the same properties and only single stage embankment construction is considered. The results are presented in a normalised form so as to make them independent of height H. The base of the foundation is assumed as rigid and rough and vertical sides as rigid and smooth.

Figure 6.3 shows the influence of anisotropy with respect to elastic moduli on stresses due to excavation. Only a single stage excavation is considered here and all other elastic parameters are maintained constant. It is obvious that while the vertical normal stress is insensitive to the ratio E_2/E_1, horizontal normal stress is very sensitive to this ratio. The results are valid only for excavation in the assumed soil with initial stresses represented by a value of $K = 1.6$. (K is the ratio of initial horizontal to initial vertical normal stress). The importance of K is fully explained in the next two sections.

Figure 6.4 represents the results of a very interesting study. An isotropic embankment of height H with side slopes of 2:1 and 3:1 is built on an isotropic foundation such that $E_1 = E_2 = E$ and $v_1 = v_2 = v$ for both embankment and foundation, but the embankment has $G_1 = G_2$ because it is isotropic while the foundation has a given G_2/E_2 ratio different from isotopic. This ratio is kept constant and only the orientation of the plane of isotropy is varied. The influence of relatively small variation in this orientation on horizontal shear stresses and horizontal displacements along the base of the embankment are shown. (Orientation $\beta = 0°$ corresponds to planes of isotropy parallel to horizontal base of foundation or embankment). It can be seen that at any point horizontal displacements increase in the direction in which the plane of isotropy dips downwards. When the planes of isotropy dip in

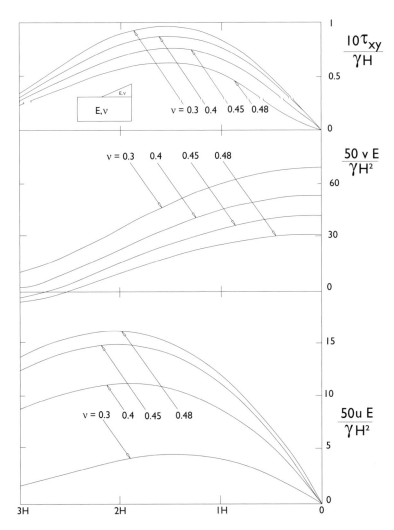

Figure 6.2 Influence of Poisson's ratio on shear stresses and on displacements (vertical *v* and horizontal *u*) along the base of a dam on an elastic foundation with elastic modulus *E*. The dam is symmetrical with 3:1 side slopes and height *H*. Results are presented in a normalised form. Horizontal axis shows distance from centre-line; the centre line is indicated by zero distance (after Chowdhury, 1970a).

the opposite direction, horizontal displacements at the same point decrease. These results appear perfectly reasonable but could hardly have been predicted before stress analysis. The power of the finite element technique in analysing different geological situations is quite evident from this example. In both Figures 6.3 and 6.4 the bottom horizontal boundary is assumed rigid and rough and vertical side boundary as rigid and smooth.

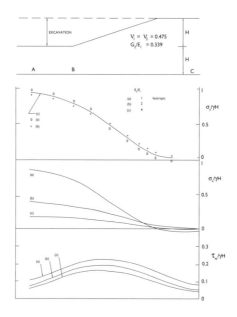

Figure 6.3 Stress increments along horizontal line ABC at depth 2H due to excavation in initially horizontal ground with $K = 1.6$ and assuming linear anisotropic soil behaviour: Influence of E_2/E_1 with other parameters constant. Normal stress increments plotted above the horizontal axis are negative or tensile, indicating that initial normal stresses are reduced by the excavation (after Chowdhury, 1972).

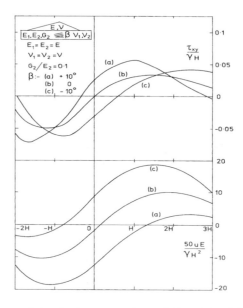

Figure 6.4 Isotropic, unsymmetrical embankment on anisotropic foundation: Influence of variation in inclination of plane of isotropy of foundation on horizontal shear stresses and horizontal displacement u along base of embankment with side slopes 2:1 and 3:1, (after Chowdhury, 1972).

6.4   INCREMENTAL BODY FORCE STRESSES

6.4.1   Embankment analysis in stages

The most significant forces in many problems involving soils and rocks are body forces.

Traditionally soil masses were analysed in their final form as if the weight was applied simultaneously to the completed shape of such a mass or structure. For built up bodies like embankments it was shown by Brown and Goodman (1963) that an analysis which takes into consideration the incremental processes of construction may yield values of stresses and displacements which differ significantly from those obtained by a 'single-stage' analysis. A closed form solution for the plane strain problem of stresses within an incrementally built wedge with infinite sides was given by Goodman and Brown (1963). At each stage of construction one side of the wedge was considered to be horizontal. These studies led to an interest in incremental studies of real embankments and excavated slopes. Fortunately finite element techniques were already available and made studies of realistic problems possible. Clough and Woodward (1967) analysed an embankment on a rough rigid base and found significant differences in the deformations and shear stresses calculated by single-stage and incremental analyses. (Differences in vertical normal stresses calculated by single-lift or incremental analyses are not significant). For instance, incremental analyses show that maximum vertical displacements during construction occur close to the mid-height of an embankment. Single stage analyses on the other hand show that the maximum vertical displacements occur at the crest which is unrealistic because the top layers are not subjected to any loading. Figure 6.5 shows contours of horizontal and vertical displacements obtained by both single-lift and incremental analyses for a 100 ft. high isotropic embankment on a rough rigid base analysed by Clough and Woodward (1967). For an embankment with same geometry and boundary conditions

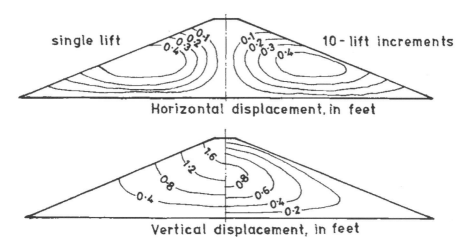

Figure 6.5 Comparison of single-lift and incremental (10 lifts of 10 ft. each) analyses for a 100 ft. high embankment on rough, rigid base: (a) horizontal and (b) vertical displacements assuming values of $E = 2000 \times 10^3$ lb/ft^2, $v = 0.4$ (after Clough and Woodward, 1967).

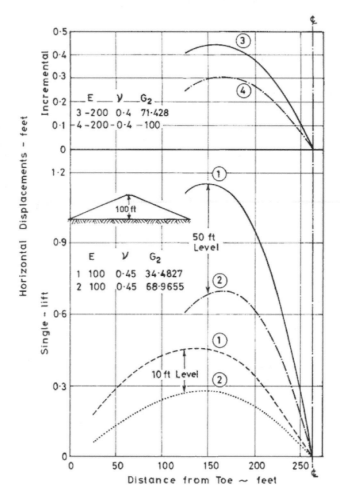

Figure 6.6 Embankment displacements (horizontal) assuming anisotropic shear modulus G_2 in vertical direction but isotropic elastic modulus and Poisson's ratio. Values from both incremental and single-lift analyses are shown. E and G are in units of 10^3 lbs/ft^2. 10 lifts of 10 ft. each are considered in incremental studies shown by curves (3) and (4) (after Chowdhury, 1970a).

but anisotropic properties, Figure 6.6 shows the results of both single-lift and incremental analyses.

A relatively small increase in the value of G_2 from the isotropic value of 71.428 units to 100 units results in a significant decrease of horizontal displacements in incremental or stage analyses. (See curves (3) and (4) for displacements along horizontal plane at 50 ft. level; the lower curves (1) and (2) for 10 and 50 ft. levels correspond to different soil parameters and to single stage analyses only).

The simulation of embankment construction in a multi-stage analysis does not present any difficulties. The construction of an individual embankment layer is equivalent to the application of gravitational loads equal to the weight of the layer. The layer is divided into small elements interconnected at nodal points and the body forces acting on elements are distributed to the nodal points in an appropriate manner. With these nodal forces as external loads a particular stage of analysis is completed and the software then proceeds to consider the next layer and execute the next stage of an incremental analysis.

It has already been mentioned that for embankments incremental analyses may give results markedly different from those given by single stage analyses even when material behaviour is assumed to be linearly elastic. In general soil masses show marked departure from linear elasticity. Therefore, it would be desirable to take into consideration the real stress-dependent, stress-strain behaviour of soils. Similarly realistic incremental analyses must take appropriate failure criteria into consideration.

6.4.2   Multi-stage excavation in linear and non-linear material

When an excavation is analysed on the basis of linearly elastic, isotropic response of the ground to the unloading process, the results of an incremental analysis do not differ from those of a single stage analysis, assuming no failure has occurred anywhere. Some difference in results close to the final excavated surface may appear in numerical solutions due to the manner in which the slope is idealised into an assemblage of small elements. These errors are usually small and can be ignored. However, when the material in which the excavation is made departs from linear elastic behaviour, incremental analyses which simulate the real process of excavation give results which are different from those obtained from single-stage analyses. The same conclusion applies to an excavation in which the material is assumed to obey some yield criterion or failure law even though the behaviour before yield is considered to be linearly elastic. Failure at a given point may occur during any stage of an incremental analysis and change the nature of the continuum (or assemblage of elements) in subsequent stages. This could not be simulated in a single stage analysis.

6.4.3   Simulation of excavation

There is a basic difference between how an excavation is simulated and how an embankment load is applied in a finite element analysis. When a layer of soil or rock is excavated from existing ground, it is not merely a case of removing the weight of the overburden. Consideration must be given to the stresses existing in the original ground before an excavation is made.

In Figure 6.7a which shows one symmetrical half of an excavation let abc represent the first layer of excavation and bde the next. Before any excavation is made there are stresses acting at points such as g and f. These stresses have both shear and normal components and the direction and magnitude of principal stresses depends not only on the depth of overlying material but also on the geological and stress history of the deposit. After the excavation the stresses at both points are zero. Therefore the simulation of an excavation such as abc requires the application on the surface abc of surface tractions (normal and shear stresses) equal and opposite to the existing normal and shear stresses. From these tractions, loads on the nodal points located on the surface abc may be calculated. It is these loads which are then used as the external loads in a finite-element analysis of the soil mass below abc. The analysis gives the stress changes or increments at each point below the surface. These are added to the initial stresses at corresponding points in Figure 6.7b.

Thus 'new' normal and shear stresses at points such as h and k along the surface bde can be calculated. Let this surface represent the next stage of excavation. To simulate this excavation, tractions equal and opposite to the 'new' stresses must be applied to simulate the excavation. From calculated tractions, applied loads on the nodes located on the surface bde are easily computed.

With these loads analysis is carried out of the soil mass located beneath bde. The area to be analysed is reduced with each incremental stage and this must be considered carefully in any computer software. Sometimes this is achieved by assigning very small values of the elastic modulus for elements which are redundant at any stage.

If the boundaries of the area to be analysed are not well defined, these are chosen to be as far from the final excavated surface as possible. The boundary conditions need to be defined by specifying displacements on all nodal points located on the boundary. For example, assumption of a rigid rough base would mean that all displacement along $\overline{23}$ are zero. Assumption of a rigid but smooth vertical boundary

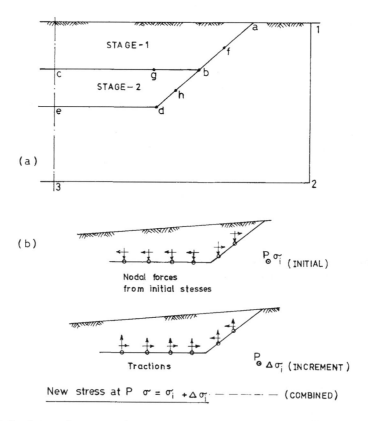

Figure 6.7 Simulation of incremental or stage excavation in stress analysis: (a) stages 1 and 2, (b) application of tractions in any stage. [Ground surface may be horizontal as in (a) or sloping as in (b)].

would mean that all horizontal displacements along $\overline{12}$ are zero but vertical displacements are unspecified and can take any value.

Embankments and excavations may be analysed on the basis of plasticity theory using the finite element method (chapter 8). However, the incremental nature of the problem has not yet been solved on the basis of plasticity or limit analysis.

6.5 NON-LINEAR MATERIAL BEHAVIOUR AND SPECIAL PROBLEMS

6.5.1 Introduction

In general soil masses show a marked departure from linear elasticity. Therefore it is desirable to take into consideration the real stress-dependent, stress-strain behaviour of soils. There are no stress-strain theories which have a general application to soil masses. Consequently the elastic model of soil behaviour is used and adjustments to obey real non-linear curves made in a step-by-step manner. Provided loading can be simulated in small increments, it is reasonable to assume proportionality between stress and strain increments within each stage. Iterative procedures are necessary for each stage of analysis and with suitable adjustments during iterations piecewise approximations are accomplished successfully by using the finite element method. Nonlinear stress analyses have become attractive to geotechnical engineers ever since Clough and Woodward (1967) demonstrated the application of a finite element approach for a real embankment-foundation system. They used a variable elasticity procedure which is one of the three techniques that can be used as discussed below in (b). In general it is necessary to consider an appropriate failure criterion in terms of effective stresses, even though stress analysis is carried out using a total stress approach. It is also necessary to distinguish between soil parameters for loading from soil parameters for unloading. Also it may be desirable to check during the analysis if computed stresses imply 'loading' or 'unloading' of a particular element, whatever the nature of external loads.

In multi-stage analyses of embankments and excavations little extra effort is required to account for non-linear behaviour since the loading is already applied in incremental steps. In solutions based on the variable elasticity technique, incremental pseudo-elastic parameters may be selected on the basis of (1) tangent moduli measured directly from sets of stress-strain curves (e.g., Clough and Woodward, 1967) or (2) secant-moduli derived from octahedral normal and shear components of stress and strain (e.g., Girijivallabhan and Reese, 1968) or (3) idealisation of real soil behaviour as bilinear or hyperbolic response (e.g., Dunlop and Duncan, 1970; Duncan and Chang, 1970; Chang and Duncan, 1970) or (4) idealisation by mathematical functions (Desai, 1971; Desai and Wu, 1976). Non-linear problems have also been solved on the basis of elastic-plastic idealisation (e.g., Ozawa and Duncan, 1976) or on the basis of idealised theories for sand and clay dealing with stress dilatancy and critical state concepts respectively (e.g., Smith, 1970; Smith and Kay, 1971).

Detailed comments on alternative ways of performing nonlinear analyses have been provided, among several others, by Duncan (1992), Carter et al. (2000) and Potts (2003). There is no unique way of dealing with non-linearity and what is presented below should be regarded as just an introduction. The requirements and capabilities of software to be used will often determine the strategy to be adopted for non-linear analyses. The knowledge and experience of the user will help greatly in selecting input parameters on the right basis and with a good degree of reliability and accuracy.

6.5.2   *Alternative approaches for non-linear problems*

Three alternative techniques are possible for carrying out adjustments in order to satisfy non-linear stress-strain behaviour. To understand the basis of these techniques, let us assume that at the outset of an incremental stage of loading initial stresses and strains exist in the elements of a continuum. Let the initial stresses be denoted by $\{\sigma_0\}$ and initial strains by $\{\varepsilon_0\}$. The relationship Equation (6.3) may now be written in the following general form:

$$\{\sigma\} = [D]\,(\{\varepsilon\} - \{\varepsilon_0\}) + \{\sigma_0\} \tag{6.3a}$$

The use of this general form does not necessitate any major change in the formulation or in the corresponding computer software. Iterations for non-linear problems may now be made by successive adjustment of either the basic elasticity matrix $[D]$ or the initial stress matrix $\{\sigma_0\}$ or the initial strain matrix $\{\varepsilon_0\}$. The first approach is called 'variable elasticity' or 'variable stiffness' approach, the second is called an initial stress approach and the last an 'initial strain' approach. Once again it is necessary to remember that we are dealing with incremental stresses and strains and not with stress levels. Therefore initial stresses and initial strains mentioned here may be considered only as a computational device which enables adjustments to be made in stress and strain increments in a particular stage of loading. Real initial stresses and strains may exist in a continuum to start with and the stress levels after each loading increment is obtained by adding to these real initial stresses the computed stress increments which have been adjusted for non-linear behaviour.

In the variable elasticity technique the matrix $[D]$ is considered to be a function of the strains or strain level reached by the corresponding elements. This matrix is adjusted for all elements in each iteration so that stresses and strains obey the given non-linear stress-strain relationship. The stiffness of each element and the overall stiffness matrix for the continuum, therefore, change with each iteration. Although a standard linear elasticity software can be used, the stiffnesses have to be reformulated and new equations solved in every iteration. It is easy to understand the variable matrix $[D]$ in terms of tangent moduli or secant moduli of non-linear stress-strain curves for soils.

In an initial stress approach, the value of $\{\sigma_0\}$ is adjusted after each iteration so that the given non-linear equation can be satisfied. This is achieved by determining the difference between the true stresses (corresponding to computed strains) and the stresses computed in the elastic solution. This stress difference is redistributed so that equilibrium is maintained. The process may be likened to one of stress transfer. The same stiffness matrices are used at every iteration and the process is therefore economical in terms of computer time. The elastic constants used need not necessarily be those used in the first iteration and may be altered to ensure rapid convergence.

Initial strain approaches are based on adjustment of the initial strain matrix $\{\varepsilon_0\}$. These methods are useful when stress level cannot be uniquely specified in terms of strains which is the basis of 'initial stress' procedures. Instead it may be possible to specify increments of strain or strain level in terms of stresses. The strains correspond-ing to the actual stress-strain relationship are compared to the elastic strains and the difference is adjusted in a suitable way to maintain equilibrium. Like the initial stress approach the method is economical in terms of computer time.

Despite some advantages of the last two approaches, the variable elasticity approach has been widely used in geotechnical applications with a great deal of suc-cess. Its continued popularity is due to the fact that it is easier to visualise the physical picture of a material which changes moduli in accordance with the given stress-strain curve. The initial strain approach is useful in problems such as those of creep while the initial stress approach can prove useful in usual stability problems particularly those involving strain softening. The difference between the two approaches is shown in Figure 6.8.

For plasticity problems involving irreversible straining beyond the stresses at yield (defined by an appropriate yield criterion), it may be useful to formulate a modified elastic plastic matrix $[D]_{ep}$ in place of the usual $[D]$ matrix. This is done in accordance with the flow rule defining plastic strain increments in relation to the yield surface. Both ideal and strain-hardening plasticity can be handled in this way but the iterative process must be followed using loads in small increments. This is necessitated by the incremental formulation of the basic plasticity relationships. 'Initial strain' and 'initial

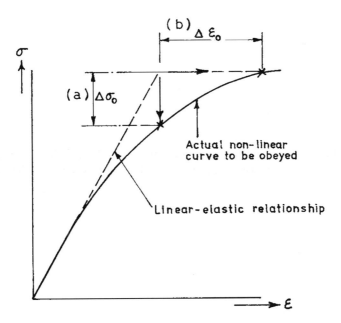

Figure 6.8 Adjustments from linear solution to given non-linear curve using (a) initial stress (b) initial strain approach.

stress' procedures have been used successfully in the application of finite element techniques to plasticity problems. According to Zienkiewicz (1971) the initial stress process is advantageous because any unloading proceeds on an elastic basis. He recommends that for elements which have yielded the stresses should be reduced to the yield condition after each iteration since departure from the yield surface occurs after every finite step of loading. The incremental stress-strain relations of plasticity are valid only after yield and where yield has not taken place, only an elastic stress-strain relationship should be used.

6.5.3   Equations based on hyperbolic response

In a large number of successful applications of the finite element method for non-linear problems, stress-strain curves have been idealised by a hyperbolic relationship relating deviator stress to axial strain of the form:

$$(\sigma_1 - \sigma_3) = \frac{\varepsilon}{a + b\varepsilon} \tag{6.11}$$

The original evidence for the validity of such a relationship for sand was given by Kondner and Zelasko (1963) and for clay by Kondner (1963). If Equation (6.11) is rearranged and ratio of axial strain to deviator stress is plotted against axial strain, we get a straight line plot from which a and b are easily obtained. The initial tangent modulus E_i is related to lateral stress (e.g., in a triaxial test).

$$E_i = KP_a \left(\frac{\sigma_3}{P_a} \right)^n \tag{6.12}$$

in which P_a is the atmospheric pressure in the same units as the lateral stress σ_3 and, K and n are experimental parameters. Unloading and reloading modulus is different from the initial tangent modulus for loading and may be written as:

$$E_{ur} = K_{ur} P_a \left(\frac{\sigma_3}{P_a} \right)^n \tag{6.12a}$$

in which K_{ur} and n are determined experimentally. Differentiating Equation (6.11) to obtain an expression for tangent modulus E_t at any levels of deviator stress and lateral stress, expressing the failure deviator stress in terms of c and ϕ by Coulomb's equation in terms of principal stresses, using R_f as a ratio of ultimate failure strength to peak failure strength and using Equation (6.12), we have (Duncan and Chang, 1970):

$$E_t = KP_a \left(\frac{\sigma_3}{P_a} \right)^n \left[1 - \frac{R_f (1 - \sin\phi) (\sigma_1 - \sigma_3)}{2c \cos\phi + 2 \sigma_3 \sin\phi} \right]^2 \tag{6.13}$$

It is usually assumed that the unloading and reloading modulus depends only on the lateral or confining stress and not on the deviator stress as shown by Equation (6.12a) whereas tangent modulus for loading depends on both lateral stress and deviator stress Equation (6.13). Incremental Poisson's ratio may be calculated from axial and volumetric strain increments as follows:

$$v = \frac{d\varepsilon_1 - d\varepsilon_v}{2d\varepsilon_1} \tag{6.14}$$

Duncan and Chang (1970) reported that for one particular sand, K was 295 for very loose state and 2000 for very dense state (corresponding values of K_{ur} were 1090 and 2120 and those of n were 0.65 and 0.54). Typical values of R_f range from 0.75 to 1. For a clay, values used by Duncan and Chang were $K = 47$, $n = 0$, $R_f = 0.9$. Chang and Duncan (1970) also used simple procedures for clay relating tangent moduli for loading and reloading to stress increment and void ratio changes in one-dimensional compression. They also studied the influence of consolidation pressure on the initial tangent modulus and found that the value of n in Equation (6.12) would usually be close to one. The continued popularity of hyperbolic stress-strain idealisation for use in finite element studies is shown by many recent applications to embankments, earth dams etc. reported in Desai (1976, Vol. II, pp. 611–23, 650–62, and 662–86).

Alternative formulation in terms of determining incremental values of K and G rather than those of E and μ should also be considered. It may prove to be more suitable as mentioned earlier.

6.5.4   Joints and discontinuities and interface elements

1   A special application of the 'initial stress' technique concerns problems in which it is necessary to ensure that no tension is developed within a continuum. This concept is often useful in problems of soil and rock mechanics. Zienkiewicz et al. (1968) developed the 'no tension' solution specifically for materials such as randomly jointed rock. An elastic analysis is carried out and wherever tension exists, it is eliminated by reducing the tensile principal stresses to zero. The removal of stress is compensated for by appropriate nodal forces to maintain equilibrium and these forces are the applied loads in the subsequent iteration. In a realistic 'no-tension' solution it is necessary to consider the possibility of closing of fissures on re-application of loads. Also a limited capacity to carry tensile stresses may be specified in preference to 'no tension'.

2   The existence of individual faults and joints in rock mechanics problems may have to be considered in an analysis. Zienkiewicz (1968) gave some examples of how faults may be considered even in an ordinary linear elastic analysis. A wide fault was treated as a no stress boundary and no restraint on displacement was assumed along the fault. A narrow fault filled with mylonytes may be able to transfer normal compressive stresses but may show little resistance to shear. Either it may be represented as an anisotropic layer in which shear modulus and elastic modulus parallel to the layer are given small values or bar type elements may be assumed to connect the main elements on either side of the fault so that the bar elements offer no restraint to motion along the fault surface. In both techniques tension should be avoided. On the other hand joints may exhibit friction

and non-linear stress-strain behaviour. Therefore non-linear analysis techniques may be necessary for handling jointed materials.

3　Special procedures for handling joints and in particular the use of joint elements have been devised. The joints may be classified according to their stiffness in normal direction K_n and shear direction K_s (where K_n is the ratio of increments in normal stress and normal displacement and K_s the ratio of increments in shear stress and shear displacement,) and by their strength. Failure in tension or shear, rotation of blocks, development of arching etc. can be represented in this manner (Goodman et al., 1968; Duncan and Goodman, 1968). The use of hyperbolic equations for interface or joint elements was demonstrated by Clough and Duncan (1971). These equations are similar to Equations (6.11)–(6.13) of this section. For other applications the reader may refer to Goodman and Dubois (1972), Goodman (1976) and Sharma et al. (1976). The last reference concerns use of interface elements in non-linear sequential analysis of a rockfill dam.

An alternative technique called the discrete element technique has also been proposed to deal with discontinuities. In this technique (Wang and Voight, 1969; Ko, 1972) dual nodes are used along discontinuities but special joint elements are not adopted. This method allows local inelastic displacement (slip and separation) along the discontinuity according to prescribed criteria. The application of this technique to open pit jointed slopes has been discussed by Ko (1972) who found that it had some distinct advantages over other techniques. Ko felt that the technique was simpler and gave realistic results. In particular he found studies of mode of unloading to be useful for a specific slope problem.

The application of finite element analysis to a study of rock slopes with high tectonic stresses has been demonstrated by Dodd and Anderson (1972). In plane strain analysis the stress in the direction of zero strain is dependent only on the Poisson's ratio and other principal stresses. However, the actual stress in that direction may be a tectonic stress many times the gravitational stress. Dodd and Anderson showed that this stress had a significant influence on the results from stress analysis. Their technique was a modified two-dimensional one because a truly three-dimensional technique was not found to be applicable.

As stated at the very beginning of this chapter, for discontinua like jointed and fractured rock masses, more logical and effective alternatives to the FEM are now available. These include the Distinct Element Method (DEM) and the Discontinous Deformation Analysis (DDA). For DEM, appropriate and powerful software tools such as FLAC, UDEC and 3-DEC have been available for more than two decades. Until recently, little was known about the application of DDA. Recently Sitar et al. (2005) have used this approach successfully and tackled the well known problem of the Vaiont slide.

6.5.5　Incompressibility

Undrained deformation of saturated soft clay is accompanied by no change in volume. Such a condition can be obeyed only when the finite element analysis is made with a value of Poisson's ratio v equal to 0.5 (for isotropic materials). A value of 0.5 for this ratio creates numerical difficulties in the solution (all terms in the elasticity matrix become infinite). The use of values very close to 0.5 is also not effective in all situations. However, special formulations have been developed to handle incompressible materials and corresponding special computer softwares, although more expensive (because of increased computer time required in relation to conventional computer softwares) are available. These may be used for studying slopes of saturated clay undergoing undrained deformation. Special numerical methods for dealing with incompressibility have been proposed by Herrman (1965), Christian (1968), Chowdhury and King (1972) etc.

6.5.6   Analysis of mining spoil pile stability (Richards et al., 1981; Richards, 1982)

A good example of the application of both limit equilibrium (LE) and finite element (FEM) analyses to a built-up structure has been provided by Richards et al. (1981) and Richards (1982). These analyses were part of the research and investigations for spoil piles associated with Goonyella mine in Queensland, Australia. The observed failures revealed a two-wedge failure mechanism involving tensile failure at the top and shearing of strain-softening material along the basal shear plane of very low inclination. The rear shear surface was typically very steep and is associated with a tension crack at the top.

Both types of analyses (LE and FEM) validated the observed failure mechanism. Two-wedge LE back-analyses gave peak strength values for the rear or escarpment plane and residual strength values for the basal plane. Large strains were observed at the toe of the piles and thus progressive failure initiates at the toe.

The initial FEM analyses were carried out using pre-existing joint elements located along the observed failure planes. This type of analysis works well only if near-zero tensile strength is assumed in the upper part the escarpment zone.

However, a non-linear analysis incorporating detailed data from shear tests on the spoil was also performed. Such an analysis was carried out without assuming the failure planes in advance. The location of the failure zones (shear and tensile at top and base respectively) was identified by the analysis and hence the observed mechanism was validated. Some details of the non-linear analysis procedure are summarized below.

Simple constant-strain, 3-node triangular elements were adopted although there was an option of 6-node triangles as well. Non-linear elasticity was incorporated in the analysis by using incremental construction sequences with 4 iterations per increment. Tangential moduli were used. New stresses were calculated after iteration for the recalculation of the tangential moduli.

After every second iteration,the redistribution of stresses from yielded elements was carried out. Non-linear material properties of the continuum elements were characterised by hyperbolic stress-dependent relationships for incremental loading.

An element which reaches the yield criterion for shear has its shear modulus reduced to the failure value (zero) and the element is converted into a slip element with a finite thickness. The slip direction for non-dilatant yield was calculated to be that of the maximum shear strain corresponding to the incremental nodal displacements at yield. This is not related to geometry as in the case with joint elements. The geometry of the mesh had no significant effect on the results.

After yield the excess shear stress was redistributed to adjacent elements using the initial stress method originally proposed by Zienkiewicz (1968). The analysis simulates the stress-softening characteristics of the spoil materials with residual stress operative in the elements which have undergone significant strain.

According to Richards (1982) the results were no better than those sustained by using alternative approaches based on plasticity and viscoplasticity (Zienkiewicz et al., 1975). However, the use of a non-linear approach (with recourse to slip elements after yield) proved more effective for directly incorporating constitutive stress-strain relationships from the test results carried out with conventional equipment (direct shear and triaxial tests).

Typical hyperbolic equations used were of the following form:

$$K = K_1 \sigma_0^n + K_0 \tag{6.15}$$

$$G = G_1 \sigma_0^m \left[1 - \left(\frac{\tau}{\tau_f} \right)^p \right] + G_0 \tag{6.16}$$

in which

$$\sigma_0 = \frac{1}{3}(\sigma_1 + \sigma_2 + \sigma_3) \tag{6.17}$$

$$\tau = \frac{1}{2}(\sigma_1 - \sigma_3) \tag{6.18}$$

$$\tau_f = c_p \cos \phi_p + \frac{1}{2}(\sigma_1 + \sigma_3) \sin \phi_p \tag{6.19}$$

More details of the non-linear approach summarized above as well as the numerical values of different parameters for the spoil pile are given in Richards, et al. (1981) and Richards (1982).

6.6   POST EXCAVATION STRESSES

Consider a horizontal ground surface and a point in the ground located at a depth z. The following initial total stresses (vertical and horizontal normal (principal) stresses respectively) act at the point:

$$\sigma_v = \gamma z, \quad \sigma_h = K \gamma z \tag{6.20}$$

in which γ is the bulk unit weight of the material and K is the co-efficient of earth pressure at rest. Now consider that the pore water pressure at the same point is u; then the effective principal stresses are given by:

$$\sigma_v' = (\gamma z - u) \quad \text{and} \quad \sigma_h' = K_0 \sigma_v' = K_0(\gamma z - u) \tag{6.21}$$

in which K_0 is the co-efficient of earth pressure at rest in terms of effective stresses. From Equations (6.20) and (6.21) we have:

$$K = K_0 + r_u (1 - K_0) \qquad (6.22)$$

in which $r_u = u/\gamma z$ is the pore pressure ratio which for a saturated soil with water table at the ground surface has a value γ_w/γ in which γ_w is the unit weight of water. When $u = 0 = r_u$, $K = K_0$.

Values of horizontal stresses greater than vertical stresses have been reported for many soil and rock deposits. In overconsolidated clays values of K_0 as high as 3 were reported for London clay by Skempton (1961). These high values of K_0 have since been confirmed by many workers on the basis of laboratory and in-situ measurements. [See, for instance, Windle and Wroth (1977)].

The extent of stress release during excavation depends on the initial stress field and it is obvious that the value of K_0 has a primary significance in these problems. Finite element studies of excavations have shown (Duncan and Dunlop, 1969; Chowdhury, 1970a) that initial stresses have a considerable influence on the magnitude of shear stresses after excavation, even when linear elastic behaviour is considered. Shear stresses around excavated slopes of all inclinations are much higher for overconsolidated clays with high values of K_0 than in corresponding slopes in soils with low values of K_0. This is not surprising since initial shear stresses before excavation are already high when K_0 is high. When the ground surface is horizontal shear stresses are zero only on horizontal and vertical planes. On all other planes shear stresses exist and the maximum shear stress on 45° planes is half the difference of the principal stresses:

$$\tau_{max} = \frac{1}{2}(\sigma_h - \sigma_v) = \frac{1}{2}(K - 1)\ \gamma z \qquad (6.23)$$

or,

$$\tau_{max} = \frac{1}{2}(\sigma_h' - \sigma_v') = \frac{1}{2}(K_0 - 1)(1 - r_u)\gamma z \qquad (6.23a)$$

The ground is free of shear stress only when the parameter K_0 has a value exactly equal to one, which is rarely the case. While the initial maximum shear stresses have uniform inclination at all points, excavation results in a reorientation of the maximum shear stress directions from point to point. The magnitudes of the maximum shear stresses increase depending on the initial shear stresses and the inclination of the excavated slope. Due to these increases in magnitude and changes in orientation, failure may develop at various locations within the soil mass even when the limit equilibrium factor of safety is high for end of construction conditions. Table 6.1 shows a comparison of percentage increase in the largest maximum shear stresses over the initial maximum shear stresses while Table 6.2 shows a comparison of undrained shear strengths required to prevent failure on the basis of (a) largest maximum shear stress being exceeded and (b) $\phi = 0$ limit equilibrium analyses.

These tables show that (a) the post excavation factor of safety against local failure decreases with increase in the magnitude of $(K-1)$ which gives a measure of the initial shear stresses of uniform orientation. Thus even when K is less than one, initial shear stresses are high and consequently post excavation shear stresses are high, and (b) the post excavation factor of safety against local failure becomes a smaller proportion of the corresponding limit equilibrium factor of safety as the value of K or the inclination of the slope increases.

Dunlop and Duncan (1970) used a bilinear stress strain curve to study failure around excavated slopes. In the elastic range a modulus value dependent on stress level was selected and after failure the element modulus was assigned a very small value. Typical moduli were 100 times the shear strength of the clay before failure and 10^{-4} of this value after failure. Undrained shear strength was either assumed to be constant or to increase with depth as in normally consolidated clays. Dunlop and Duncan found that (1) For clays with values of K greater than one local failure develops near the toe and

Table 6.1 Percentage increase due to excavation in the greatest maximum shear stress as a proportion of γH in which H is height of slope (i.e., in $\tau_{max}/\gamma H$) (after Chowdhury, 1970b, Duncan and Dunlop, 1969). With permission from ASCE, see page 713, No 20 & 21.

Slope inclination	K = 0.81	K = 1.6	Location
3:1	63	16.6	base
1.5:1	89.5	30	base
Vertical	500	237	toe
Vertical cut to rigid base	710	340	toe

Note: Largest values of $\tau_{max}/\gamma H$ were higher for $K = 1.6$ due to initially high shear stresses e.g., (a) in a 3:1 slope the value was 0.70 for $K = 1.6$ and 0.31 for $K = 0.81$ and (b) in a vertical slope it was 1.01 for $K = 1.6$ and 0.57 for $K = 0.81$.

Table 6.2 Comparison of shear strengths required to prevent failure (after Duncan and Dunlop, 1969). With permission from ASCE, see page 713, No 21.

Slope inclination Hor. to ver	K	(a) Largest max. shear stress	$s_u/\gamma H$ based on (b) Conventional value	Ratio $\dfrac{(a)}{(b)}$
3H:1V	0.81	0.31	0.16	1.94
	1.60	0.7	0.16	4.37
1.5H:1V	0.81	0.36	0.175	2.06
	1.60	0.78	0.175	4.45
Vertical	0.81	0.57	0.26	2.19
	1.60	1.01	0.26	3.89
Vertical cut to rigid base	0.81	0.77	0.26	2.96
	1.60	1.32	0.26	5.07

Note: The conventional value determined by a $\phi = 0$ limit equilibrium analysis was referred to as the 'average stress' in the original table.

progresses inwards but for clays with low values of K local failure develops at the crest and progresses downwards. (2) When strength increases with depth failure begins at the crest and progresses downwards but when strength is constant with depth failure begins at the base and progresses upwards. (3) When excavation reaches a stage so that failure zone encompasses a large part of the region adjacent to the slope of a normally consolidated clay, the limit equilibrium factor of safety is close to one. This is not so for analyses in which initial stresses and strength profiles are assumed to represent over-consolidated clays. The factors of safety using conventional methods are of the order of 2 even at the terminating stages of the analyses. The failure zones do not indicate the possibility of curved surfaces of sliding of the type assumed in limit equilibrium analyses.

6.7 COMPUTED STRESSES AND SAFETY FACTOR

Definitions have been proposed from time to time for 'local factors of safety' and 'overall factors of safety' based on known or calculated stresses (e.g., Brown and King, 1966; Duncan and Dunlop, 1969; Wright et al., 1973; Resendiz, 1974). However, geotechnical engineers and researchers who have grown accustomed to limit equilibrium calculations are often reluctant to adopt a definition of F on the basis of known or calculated stresses, even though this approach is entirely logical. It is, therefore, interesting to note encouraging signs of a possible change in attitude as reflected in current literature.

It is important to note here that limit equilibrium factors of safety may not be widely different from stress analysis factors of safety for embankments (e.g., Wright et al., 1973) although reservations have been expressed by Resendiz (1974). However, there may be considerable differences between limit equilibrium and stress analysis factors of safety for natural and excavated slopes depending on the level and type of initial or in situ stresses and other factors.

Consider an excavated slope and an arbitrary surface ab along which the likelihood of failure is to be assessed (Figure 6.9). The principal stresses at points along the surface are known from stress analysis. Therefore the normal stresses σ and shear stresses τ along the surface can be calculated. The factor of safety F may be defined as a ratio of the total shear strength to the total shear stress as follows:

$$F = \frac{\int (c + (\sigma - u) \tan \phi) \, dL}{\int \tau \, dL} \tag{6.24}$$

in which the integration is over the whole length of the failure surface. It is worth noting that limit equilibrium is not assumed and the factor of safety assumes a more realistic meaning particularly when $F > 1$ (i.e., when considering a safe slope). There are two other ways in which the factor of safety may be defined when the stresses everywhere are known.

The factor of safety may be defined as the ratio of available shear strength to that required for equilibrium (or mobilised strength). Equating total mobilised strength to the shear stress, we have:

$$\int \left(\frac{c + (\sigma - u) \tan \phi}{F} \right) dL = \int \tau \, dL \tag{6.25}$$

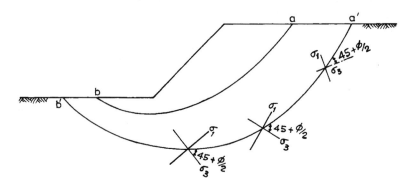

Figure 6.9 Trial slip surfaces: Surface *ab* is an arbitrary one but surface *a′ b′* is drawn so that minor principal stress has a constant inclination with the surface at every point as shown.

Equation (6.25) will reduce to equation (6.24) only when F is considered constant along the whole of the slip surface. The assumption of a constant F is usual in limit equilibrium methods but the two definitions do not give the same expression for F in those methods even on the base of constant F. For example the Bishop simplified method gives an expression for factor of safety which contains the unknown F. However, if the first definition above is used, the expression for F remains unchanged except that right hand side does not contain F which is replaced by one in the term m_α (see chapter 5).

A third approach is to consider the overall factor of safety as an average of local factors of safety along the slope which gives:

$$F = \frac{1}{L} \int_0^L \left(\frac{c + (\sigma - u)\tan\phi}{\tau} \right) dL \tag{6.26}$$

It is obvious that there are large variations in local factors of safety and for this reason averaging local factors of safety will not lead to the same overall factor of safety as is obtained by taking the ratio of resisting to disturbing forces over the whole surface.

Brown and King (1966) made some interesting studies based on stress analysis by finite elements in which trial surfaces were selected in a consistent manner in accordance with the angle of obliquity of the failure plane (Figure 6.9). The assumed failure plane makes an angle $\theta = (45° + \phi/2)$ with the direction of minor principal stress at every point and this is in accordance with the Mohr-Coulomb failure theory. Its use in connection with active and passive states of failure is well known. The orientation of principal stresses was already known from finite element analysis and varied from point to point. Therefore an irregular surface was obtained by drawing lines from one finite element to another at constant inclination θ to the variable direction of the minor principal stress. Each irregular surface was a close approximation to a reasonably shaped curved surface. Brown and King (1966) commented that the shapes of the surfaces were somewhat similar to those observed in actual failures.

A starting point was chosen at the bottom of a slope and in most cases an end point was located at the top. The shapes of these trajectories were found to depend on the initial stress ratio K. Studies were then made for slope stability for $\phi = 0$ conditions in order that the results for these surfaces could be compared to those from a conventional limit equilibrium solution. The stability factor $(c/\gamma h)$ was found to be dependent on the value of K (the initial stress ratio or the co-efficient of earth pressure at rest) for (a) excavation cases and (b) embankment cases in which the failure surface passed through the original ground. The results are summarised in table 6.3. Note that, in table 6.3, h was taken as the distance of the slip line propagation point from the embankment top.

It is worth noting that factors of safety are higher than those from the corresponding solution by any limit equilibrium method for this $\phi = 0$ study. The limit equilibrium value is independent of K but values from stress analysis are dependent on this value. It can be concluded on the basis of these limited studies that the limit equilibrium approach is conservative and this view is generally accepted in soil mechanics. For further discussion on this point refer to chapter 8. Brown and Goodman (1963) also reached this conclusion on the basis of their closed-form solution to the problem of an incrementally-built wedge.

Wright et al. (1973) also compared finite element solutions and corresponding stability results of a number of built-up slopes with the results of conventional stability analyses made by the Bishop Simplified Method. They decided to include a wide range of slope heights and strength parameter c and ϕ. In order to achieve this, the value of the dimensionless parameter $\lambda = \gamma H \tan \phi / c$ first introduced by Janbu (1957) was varied from 0 to 50. As would have been expected linear elastic finite element studies showed that the factor of safety F varied significantly along the length of the slip surface (assumed to be circular). This is in sharp contrast with the assumption of a constant factor of safety made in limit equilibrium calculations. (The local factor of safety at each point was calculated in their study as the ratio of available strength to shear stress at that point, the stresses being those from a finite element analysis). It is interesting to see from Table 6.4 that the factor of safety required to prevent local overstress is generally not more than 1.5 to 2. [(Bishop, 1952) also referred to plastic failure being restricted to small areas with this order of factor of safety]. As regards the average factor of safety from a stress analysis, this was somewhat higher

Table 6.3 Comparison of stability factors for '$\phi = 0$' studies (after Brown and King, 1966). With permission, see page 713, No 22.

Slope	Range of $c/\gamma h$	Conventional value
Excavation $K = 1$	0.0935 to 0.1405	
Embankment $K = 1$	0.149 to 0.156	$c/\gamma H$ for critical toe circle
Embankment $K = 0.25$	0.1435 to 0.152	0.170

Note: Results for embankment cases are included only for the cases where they were different for the two K values.

Table 6.4 Values of factor of safety required to prevent local overstress for c, ϕ soil (after Wright et al., 1973). With permission from ASCE, see page 713, No 23.

Value of λ	Slope ratio		
	1.5:1	*2.5:1*	*3.5:1*
0	1.46	1.44	1.49
2	1.32	1.23	1.23
5	1.34	1.18	1.14
20	2.27	1.21	1.10
50	4.36	1.737	1.12

than the value from Bishop Simplified Method but never greater than about 8%. The normal stress distribution on the failure surface agreed reasonably well in the two types of analysis. Results from some non-linear analyses were also reported to have shown similar agreement. While embankment stresses are not dependent on the initial ground stresses, the general agreement is still somewhat surprising in view of the completely different assumptions made in the two approaches. Therefore, it is useful to recall that averaging a variable factor of safety is a different definition for the overall factor of safety than is adopted in the Bishop Simplified approach. Perhaps differences would have been more evident in the two types of solutions if the same definition could be used for the factor of safety or if the stress analysis factor of safety were defined in one of the other alternative ways discussed earlier in this section. Without alternative calculations it is difficult to assess how meaningful it may be to average local factors of safety.

Variation of factor of safety and overstressing of some areas indicates that conditions for progressive failure may develop in slopes of a wide range of inclinations even when the average factor of safety is greater than one. Therefore finite-element analyses are useful in indicating the likelihood of progressive failure even when limit equilibrium methods have predicted that simultaneous failure will not occur.

Resendiz (1974) commented on the results of Wright et al. (1973). The former found differences as large as 30% between stability values from non-linear finite-element analyses and limit equilibrium stability values. The stress analysis factors of safety were always higher as expected. He suggested that the potential failure surface be drawn as a locus of maximum major principal strain and found that such a surface approximated to a circular arc. The procedure suggested by Brown and King (1966), on the other hand, does not produce slip surfaces which approximate to circular arcs.

Hovland (1977) proposed that in his method of slope analysis for three-dimensional problems it would be useful to define F on the basis of stresses calculated by using the finite element method. If this were done there would be no need to develop a rigorous three-dimensional method of slices in which inter-slice forces are accounted for. For a problem with three-dimensional slices or columns such an extension would be a formidable task. Even if a rigorous extension was achieved the results obtained by using the extended method may not necessarily reflect the correct results. On the other hand if F is based on a realistic stress distribution (three-dimensional finite element programs have been developed and used successfully), the results are likely to represent a significant step closer towards reality. A value of F based on stress analysis would certainly be an improvement on Hovland's (1977) approach which is simply an extension of the Fellenius method to three-dimensional problems.

The second example concerns the definition of local and overall factors of safety for earthquake stability of Hawkins dams (see chapter 9). Lee and Roth (1977) found it useful to define local factors of safety on the basis of stresses calculated by dynamic analyses corresponding to the selected ground motions. They also found it worthwhile to calculate overall factors of safety (on different assumed failures) considering both static and dynamic stresses calculated by corresponding analyses. Static analyses were made for pre-earthquake stresses due to soil weight; seepage forces etc. and dynamic (earthquake) stresses were superimposed on these static stresses. From the combined stress field normal and shear stresses were obtained along any assumed slip surface enabling the calculation of an overall factor of safety as a ratio of total shear strength to total shear force along that surface.

6.8 MODELLING PROGRESSIVE FAILURE IN SLOPES OF STRAIN-SOFTENING SOIL

6.8.1 Brief overview of available methods

Attention has already been drawn in this chapter to recent advances for tracking failure zones within a soil mass on the basis of the failure criterion and these include the methods surveyed by Carter et al. (2000), the strain-softening model used for slopes in stiff clays by Potts et al. (1997) and the "strength reduction techniques" mentioned earlier (e.g., Zienkiewicz et al., 1975; Matsui and San, 1992).

Advanced FEM models are required for the study of progressive failure involving strain-softening materials. Such models have been used to study both embankments and cut slopes in order to gain an improved understanding of failure mechanisms. Reference is made to a few relevant examples below:

The 1984 failure of Carsington dam occurred through two strain-softening materials, a brittle core and a brittle foundation clay (Skempton and Vaughan, 1993). Using an advanced FEM model, the important role of progressive failure was confirmed by Potts et al. (1990). The role of progressive failure and cracking in old British dams was studied by Dounias et al. (1996) and the delayed collapse of cut slopes in stiff clay was studied by Potts et al. (1997). Further reference is made to some of these analyses in chapter 8 of this book.

In sharp contrast to these sophisticated methods, an extended limit equilibrium approach can also be used successfully to model progressive failure. This has already been discussed in section 5.16 and illustrated by Example 5.5. Such methods have significant practical value but are also subject to important limitations. For example, strains and deformations within the slope cannot be estimated. Thus further research is required to extend the scope and versatility of the simpler methods.

6.8.2   Overstressed elements in a slope and calculating excess shear stress

In the light of recent advances related to the modeling of progressive failure in slopes, the following treatment of brittle strain-softening behaviour is just a basic introduction to the subject. Details of advanced finite element models are outside the scope of this book.

Let the effective principal stresses at a point be σ_1 and σ_3. The principal stress difference at failure may be designated by $(\sigma_1 - \sigma_3)_f$ and is given by (2.15) in accordance with Coulomb-Terzaghi criterion as follows:

$$(\sigma_1 - \sigma_3)_f = 2c \cos\phi + (\sigma_1 + \sigma_3) \sin\phi \tag{2.15a}$$

Substituting the values of σ_1 and σ_3 on the right hand side, the left hand side may be calculated. Failure is considered to have occurred in terms of the Mohr Coulomb criterion if $(\sigma_1 - \sigma_3)$ equals or exceeds $(\sigma_1 - \sigma_3)_f$. In order to simulate the failure conditions the stresses must be adjusted so that excess given as follows is reduced to zero:

$$\text{Excess} = \Delta = (\sigma_1 - \sigma_3) - (\sigma_1 - \sigma_3)_f \tag{6.27}$$

This excess is transferred from the point under consideration to the surrounding continuum. In finite-element analysis this means that the excess must be distributed to the remaining elements in an appropriate manner. To do this appropriate nodal forces are generated from the element stiffness matrix as explained by Zienkiewicz et al. (1968) in connection with their attempt to simulate rock as a no-tension material. Thus the stress changes in the x, y plane are given by:

$$\{\Delta\sigma\} = \begin{Bmatrix} \Delta_x \\ \Delta_y \\ \Delta_{xy} \end{Bmatrix} = \frac{1}{2} \begin{Bmatrix} -\Delta\cos 2\theta \\ \Delta\cos 2\theta \\ -\Delta\sin 2\theta \end{Bmatrix} \tag{6.28}$$

where θ is the inclination of σ_1 to σ_x.

By applying equal and opposite stress increments the nodal forces are given as follows:

$$\{F\} = \int [B]^T \{-\Delta\sigma\} dv \tag{6.29}$$

where integration is over the volume of the element. In the next iteration of stress analysis these nodal forces influence the rest of the elements and are thus distributed throughout the continuum.

The overstressed element is to be brought to the failure condition by removing the excess shown above. However, it is essential to consider any change that may occur in the mean normal stress while excess shear stress is being adjusted. Chowdhury and Gray (1976) proposed that the mean normal stress should be maintained constant

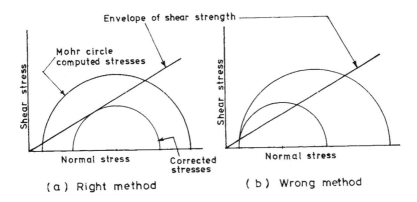

Figure 6.10 Modification of shear stress in an overstressed element (a) right method (b) wrong method, (after Chowdhury and Gray, 1976).

while the stress difference is appropriately adjusted as shown in Figure 6.10(a). This appears logical since the shear strength is maintained while removing the excess shear stress. The alternative shown in Figure 6.10(b) would be the wrong approach because the failure criterion is violated

While this simple approach for simulating strain-softening behaviour provides a good insight into the stress adjustment process, it is neither a formal approach nor rigorous. In a solution based on the theory of plasticity, an appropriate flow rule would be used and the adjustment of stresses would accordingly follow from the adopted failure criterion and the adopted the flow rule.

6.8.3 Iterative FEM analyses in strain-softening soil

Next it is of interest to consider a strain-softening material and this may be handled by considering the stress strain curve as bilinearly elastic (Figure 6.11a). A step-by-step procedure for removing the excess shear stress from overstressed elements in the manner discussed above has been suggested by Lo and Lee (1973). To conform to the post-peak stress strain relationship, a positive modulus E_2 is used for the corresponding elements rather than a negative one. After several iterations the excess shear stress in overstressed elements becomes negligible. Elements which have in the meantime attained the residual failure condition are assigned very small values of the elastic modulus to correspond to the last (horizontal) part of the stress-strain curve.

The experimental determination of the post-peak stress-strain or load deformation relationship is not easy and it is sometimes appropriate to consider a strain-softening material as a brittle one with an abrupt drop from the peak to residual strength (Figure 6.11b). The excess principal stress difference on overstressed elements is now given as in Equation (6.27a).

$$\text{Excess} = \Delta = (\sigma_1 - \sigma_3) - (\sigma_1 - \sigma_3)_r \tag{6.27a}$$

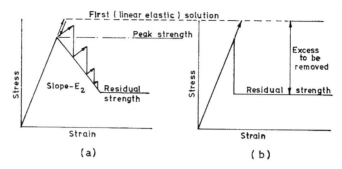

Figure 6.11 Idealised stress-strain relationships for strain-softening material: (a) Removal of excess shear stress by iterative process using positive elastic modulus for branch with negative slope; (b) Brittle material in which excess from residual is removed directly (after Lo and Lee, 1973). With permission, see page 713, No 24.

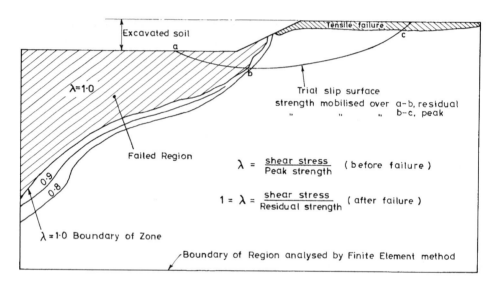

Figure 6.12 Location of failure zone due to excavation in ground with $K_0 = 2$: Plots of λ in brittle strain-softening material (after Chowdhury and Gray, 1976).

in which

$$(\sigma_1 - \sigma_3)_r = 2c_r \cos \phi_r + (\sigma_1 + \sigma_3) \sin \phi_r \tag{2.15b}$$

in which c_r and ϕ_r are the residual shear strength parameters of the strain-softening material.

Once again the excess shear stress is converted into nodal forces and then put back into the continuum during the next iteration. A very small value of the elastic modulus is assigned to the failed elements which are at the residual state after excess shear stress has been removed from them. The results can be plotted as contours of λ which is defined as follows:

$\lambda = (\tau/s_p)$, if s_p is not exceeded in the element
$\lambda = 1 = (\tau/s_r)$, if the element has failed
$\lambda = 1$ shows the failed zone as shown in Figure 6.12.

With given slope angle, the size of the failure zone increases not only with increase in the height of the slope but also with increase in the value of initial stress ratio K for overconsolidated soils. The higher the initial stress ratio for overconsolidated soils the greater the size of the failure zone. Finite element solutions using plasticity theory are mentioned in chapter 8. (See also Palmer, 1973b.)

6.9   CHANGES IN WATER TABLE AND PORE PRESSURES

In many problems concerned with long-term stability of excavated slopes, considerations must be given to the drop in water table from an initial position (before excavation) to the final one after pore pressure equilibrium has been reached. Knowing these pore pressures initial and final effective stresses may be calculated. Therefore, if the excavation is to be simulated in a one-stage finite-element analysis, it is easy to calculate the tractions to be applied to the final excavated surface. Thus the nodal loads can be determined as those based on effective stress tractions.

However, a multi-stage analysis is essential if the material is non-linear or if failure criteria have to be obeyed. Consider the first stage of such an analysis. Unloading leads to negative excess pore water pressures (pore pressure relief) which depend on changes in 'total' stress and pore pressure coefficients A and B. In an 'effective stress' analysis, these changes are not known. Therefore pore pressure increments cannot be calculated and, in turn, surface tractions to simulate an excavation stage cannot be calculated. The problem can be solved by using a careful combination of 'total stress' and 'effective stress' approaches. Stress analysis may be performed using a 'total stress' approach. During each stage, pore water pressure increments can then be calculated from total stress increments knowing the values of pore pressure parameters A and B. The total pore water pressure at each point may then be obtained, enabling a determination of current effective stresses at that point. The failure criterion can then be checked in terms of these effective stresses and thus failed elements identified. Excess shear stress can, therefore, be redistributed as explained in the previous section and the next stage of excavation can then be simulated.

After all the excavation stages have been considered, the failure zone at-the-end-of-excavation can be identified. This relates to immediate or short-term failure conditions. The final stage of analysis would consist of simulating the change to equilibrium pore water pressure conditions. This corresponds to a rise in pore water pressure for most elements and may cause the failure zone to increase considerably. This final situation after the adjustment of water level to the equilibrium position would indicate conditions in the long-term. Further details of trialing such an approach can be found in Chowdhury and Gray (1976).

6.10   LIMIT EQUILIBRIUM ANALYSIS WITH KNOWN FAILURE ZONE

A stress-analysis procedure which takes into consideration an appropriate failure criterion is very useful especially when a drop in strength to the residual is considered. Thus a slip surface may be chosen in the ordinary manner (Figure 6.12) and a limit equilibrium analysis performed. For that part of the slip surface which passes through the failed zone, residual shear strength parameters are appropriate whereas for the remaining part, peak strength parameters are used. Lo and Lee (1973) performed such analyses and found an approximately linear relationship between the residual factor R (see chapter 2) and the factor of safety F_c which takes into consideration the drop in strength along that part of the slip surface which passes through the failed zone.

It is useful to remember that the stresses throughout the slope are already known from an FEM analysis and the factor of safety could have been determined from these stresses as discussed before rather than by resorting to a limit equilibrium approach. Thus, combining a stress analysis solution with a conventional limit equilibrium approach in this way is hardly necessary. While Lo and Lee (1973) presented a simple and user-friendly stress-analysis approach, the evaluation of overall factor of safety is somewhat inconsistent with that approach. Furthermore, one may question about the modeling of pore water pressure changes during the incremental process of excavation. In discussing some case histories concerning long-term stability of slopes in London clay, Lo and Lee (1973) appear to have simulated the change in water table to the final equilibrium value in the very first stage of excavation. This may not be realistic because the establishment of pore water pressure equilibrium may take considerable time, even in fissured clays (Skempton, 1977), a fact not widely known at the time of the publication of Lo and Lee's paper.

Chapter 7

Natural slope analysis considering initial stresses

7.1 INTRODUCTION

7.1.1 *Importance of in-situ stresses*

The importance of geological and topographical setting in relation to natural slopes has been emphasised at appropriate places in the previous chapters. Simple infinite slope analyses with and without pore water pressure were considered in chapter 4. The influence of pore water pressure on the stability of layered natural deposits was also considered in the same chapter. However, little attention was given to the in situ state of stress apart from considering stresses due to overburden pressure.

Knowledge of in situ or initial stresses has been of interest to geotechnical engineers and engineering geologists for a long time. In a qualitative way it has been recognised for many decades that in situ stresses are important for analysis and design of strutted excavations, tunnels and underground openings. Awareness of the fundamental and practical importance of lateral ground stresses to slope stability has also increased, beginning perhaps with the work of Skempton (1961). However, popular methods of analysis based on the concept of limit equilibrium, which continue to dominate professional practice, still do not include consideration of the in situ stress field.

The mechanical behaviour of soils is dependent on stress paths and this fact is important for a proper understanding of the role of in situ stresses in geotechnical problems (see, for instance, Henkel, 1970). Increasing use of stress deformation studies and the availability of a powerful and versatile numerical technique (the finite element technique discussed in the previous chapter) for performing such studies has led to a better appreciation of the importance of initial ground stresses. It would be true to say that the relevance of in situ stresses to stability studies concerning slopes and excavations was not widely recognised until the finite element method became available as a valuable tool for stress analysis. During the last fiftty years or so, a number of slope stability investigations and analyses have been made in which the role of in-situ stresses has been considered. Studies of excavations were discussed in chapter 6. These were based on the assumption of in-situ horizontal and vertical principal stresses which is usually made when the initial ground surface is horizontal. Further consideration to the concept of an in situ stress field considering sloping ground is given in section 7.4.

7.1.2   Magnitude and measurement of in-situ stresses

In the previous chapter an initial state of stress was defined in terms of the parameter K for total stresses and the parameter K_0 for effective stresses. Consistent with
accepted practice two important assumptions were made, namely: (1) The vertical
and the horizontal, normal stresses at any point are the principal stresses when the
ground surface is horizontal, and (2) the vertical normal stress at any point is equal
to the corresponding overburden pressure at the same point. It is necessary to point
out that this simple description of in situ stresses may not always be sufficiently accurate, even when a mass of soil has a horizontal surface. Due to tectonic stresses (and
perhaps other unknown factors) the principal stress orientation may be different from
horizontal and vertical. Again it may sometimes be inaccurate to assume the vertical
normal stress to be equal to the overburden pressure particularly in rock masses.

Where the ground surface is sloping with a given uniform inclination to the horizontal, the description of an in situ or initial state of stress is based on the concept
of conjugate stresses (Taylor, 1948) which is considered in some detail in section 7.4.
For the present, let us consider the magnitude of initial stresses based on assumptions
considered above.

Jaky (1944) proposed a semi-empirical expression for the determination of K_0:

$$K_0 = 1 - \sin \phi \tag{7.1}$$

in which ϕ is the effective angle of shearing resistance. Laboratory tests on soil samples under conditions of no lateral strain have shown that Equation (7.1) is generally
valid for normally consolidated clays. Terzaghi (1925) and Bishop (1958) reported
that, from laboratory measurements, K_0 lies between 0.3 and 0.8 for such clays. On
the basis of a detailed experimental study, Brooker and Ireland (1965) proposed the
following relationship for normally consolidated clays which is almost identical to
Equation (7.1) for practical purposes:

$$K_0 = 0.95 - \sin \phi \tag{7.2}$$

Again for sands the results of Brooker and Ireland (1965) support Jaky's equation. There is insufficient evidence to establish the accuracy of Equation (7.1) or
Equation (7.2) for field values of K_0 in normally consolidated clays.

Laboratory measurements are valuable in understanding the development of lateral stresses during loading, unloading and reloading of a specimen of soil under
conditions of no lateral strain. However, such measurements cannot simulate other
varied natural factors which influence in situ stresses e.g., soil structure, cementation
between particles, weathering and secondary time effects associated with loading and
unloading. In the case of rocks, the type of laboratory testing used for measurement
of K_0 is not suitable at all. Therefore, in situ measurements are always desirable for
soils and essential for rocks.

As long ago as 1936, it was found that values of K_0 greater than one may apply to
overconsolidated soils. On the basis of oedometer tests it was suggested that the value
of K_0 was 2.2 in Devonian clay shales at Svir 3 power station in Russia (Samsioe,
1936). Kjellman (1936) conducted laboratory tests on sand and concluded that the

value of K_0 increased with increasing overconsolidation ratio and stress history in addition to the drained angle of shearing resistance. They measured values of K_0 as high as 3 for remoulded clays with high values of overconsolidation ratio.

Qualitative and quantitative field evidence of high K_0 values has been found in many parts of the world (e.g., Langer, 1936; Smith and Redlinger, 1953; Peterson, 1954; Skempton, 1961; Bjerrum, 1967; Windle and Wroth, 1977). It is now well known that the value of K_0 for overconsolidated clays may approach the value of the coefficient of passive pressure and that the soil may be close to a state of passive pressure at failure at locations where the overconsolidation ratio is sufficiently high. There is also a growing body of evidence of high in situ lateral stresses in rock masses based either on geological investigations or on field measurements, (e.g., Hast, 1958, 1967; Hooker and Johnson, 1969; Durney, 1972; Dodd and Anderson, 1972; Blackwood et al., 1976).

The value of K_0 at any location may be inferred from in situ measurements. The determination of true in situ stresses in undistrubed soil or rock is almost impossible in the sense that local disturbance of soil or rock will result from the insertion of a measurement device. Such disturbance is bound to alter the local stresses. However, different techniques for in situ measurements are constantly being improved and it is becoming possible to make reliable estimates of true in situ stresses. In situ measurements in rock may be made by pressure cells directly installed in boreholes (e.g., Hult et al., 1966). Similar direct measurement techniques have been used in soils. For example, piles instrumented with load cells were used by Kenney (1967a). Techniques based on stress relief (e.g., the overcoring technique) have been used with success in rocks (Hast, 1958; Obert, 1967). Improvements in overcoring technique were reported by Blackwood et al. (1976). Hydraulic fracturing is another technique which has been used in both soils and rocks (e.g. Kehle, 1964; Fairhurst, 1964; Haimson, 1968; Bjerrum and Anderson, 1972; Bjerrum et al., 1972). Pressuremeter tests, using different kinds of instrument, have also been used to measure in situ stresses (e.g., Menard, 1957; Baguelin et al., 1972; Windle and Wroth, 1977).

As stated earlier, in situ stresses in soil may also be inferred from laboratory tests on undisturbed samples (Skempton, 1961; Bishop et al., 1965; Knight and Blight, 1965; Blight, 1967; Davis and Poulos, 1963; Poulos and Davis, 1972; Abdelhamid and Krizek, 1976; Menzies et al., 1977). In situ stresses may also be inferred from field observations and back analyses of failure (Skempton, 1961) or measurements during underground operations such as tunnelling (Endersbee, 1969) or a study of fractures of rock cores (Obert and Stephenson, 1965) etc. In some cases, it may also be possible to infer the initial state of stress by comparing observed deformations in actual excavations with results of finite element studies in which the value of K_0 is varied. In the next section, attention is given to the relationship between K_0 shear strength parameters and changes in pore pressure in a soil sample during loading or unloading.

7.2   RELATIONSHIP BETWEEN K_0, SHEAR STRENGTH AND PORE PRESSURE COEFFICIENTS

It is useful to refer to a key paper for understanding the role of initial stresses and for estimating the value of K_0 in London clay (Skempton, 1961). This paper was published at the time of investigations concerning the failure of an excavation at Bradwell (see also Skempton and La Rochelle, 1965). The procedures suggested by Skempton are summarized in this section. It is interesting that his predictions concerning the value of K_0 have since been confirmed by laboratory and field measurements. Among those were measurements made with a self-boring type of pressuremeter developed at Cambridge University (Windle and Wroth, 1977).

Firstly a relationship can be established between capillary pressure p_k which exists in a saturated soil specimen after it has been extracted from the ground, the effective overburden pressure p which acted on the specimen before it was extracted, and K_0.

The total stress on the specimen is zero when it has been extracted, and the pore water pressure is negative (suction). Therefore, based on the principle of effective stress for a saturated soil, the effective stress (capillary pressure) must be equal and opposite to the negative pore water pressure u. The simple expression for the capillary pressure is:

$$p_k = 0 - u \tag{7.3}$$

The suction u is the algebraic sum of the initial pore water pressure u_0 (which may simply be due to a particular height of water above the point under consideration) and the change in pore water pressure Δu due to removal of load on the specimen. The changes in total principal stresses on the specimen are:

$$\Delta\sigma_1 = 0 - \sigma_v = -(p + u_0), \quad \Delta\sigma_3 = 0 - \sigma_h = -(K_0 p + u_0) \tag{7.4}$$

To estimate the excess pore pressure Δu due to this unloading, we use Skempton's (1954) pore pressure equation, [noting that, for saturated soil, pore pressure coefficient B in Equation (2.47) is 1]:

$$\Delta u = \Delta\sigma_3 + A|\Delta\sigma_1 - \Delta\sigma_3| \tag{7.5}$$

It is extremely important to note that $\Delta\sigma_3$ here is the lateral principal stress (it acts in both the horizontal directions). It is the major principal stress in this case if we are considering an overconsolidated clay with $K_0 > 1$. Also the second term of Equation (7.5) involves the magnitude of the deviator stress. These matters are important and are further clarified by examining the original form of Equation (7.5):

$$\Delta u = \frac{1}{3}(\Delta\sigma_1 + 2\Delta\sigma_3) + \left(A - \frac{1}{3}\right)|\Delta\sigma_1 - \Delta\sigma_3| \tag{7.5a}$$

Substituting the values of the principal stress changes from Equation (7.4) in either of Equations (7.5) or (7.5a):

$$u = u_0 + \Delta u = -p\{K_0 - A_s(K_0 - 1)\} \tag{7.6}$$

in which A_s is the value of A for swelling under removal of load. From Equation (7.3) we have:

$$p_k = p\{K_0 - A_s(K_0 - 1)\} \tag{7.7}$$

Next we need to know the relationship between the capillary pressure p_k and other conventional parameters such as undrained shear strength and effective stress parameters. Let the undrained shear strength of a soil specimen be c. Consider an unconfined compression test to failure. Before the specimen is tested it has an effective stress p_k and total stresses are zero (both lateral and axial). At failure, it still has a zero total lateral stress, but the axial total stress is equal the unconfined compressive strength. Under the undrained conditions, excess pore pressure Δu_f will develop. Therefore, the new lateral effective stress is given as follows:

$$\sigma_3' = p_k - \Delta u_f \tag{7.8}$$

In an unconfined undrained test the principal stress changes usually are:

$$\Delta \sigma_3 = 0 \quad \text{and} \quad (\Delta \sigma_1 - \Delta \sigma_3)_f = 2c \tag{7.9}$$

in which the subscript f refers to deviator stress change at failure. Note that the difference of total principal stresses and effective principal stresses remains the same. Here undrained strength or cohesion c is the radius of the Mohr-circle for either type of stress. It is also useful to note that when there is no reorientation of principal stresses (as in conventional tests) the deviator of the principal stress difference is the same as the difference of the changes in principal stress i.e.,

$$\Delta(\sigma_1 - \sigma_3)_f = (\Delta \sigma_1 - \Delta \sigma_3)_f \tag{7.10}$$

From Equations (7.5) and (7.9) it is now easy to estimate the pore pressure change Δu_f giving

$$\Delta u_f = A_f \left| \Delta \sigma_1 - \Delta \sigma_3 \right|_f = A_f \cdot 2c \tag{7.11}$$

in which A_f is the pore pressure parameter at failure. From Equations (7.8) and (7.11):

$$p_k = \sigma_3' + A_f \cdot 2c \tag{7.12}$$

To estimate σ_3' it is easy to see from the geometry of the effective stress Mohr-circle in Figure (7.1) that:

$$c = \frac{1}{2}(\sigma_1' - \sigma_3')_f = c' \frac{\cos \phi'}{1 - \sin \phi'} + \sigma_3' \frac{\sin \phi'}{1 - \sin \phi'} \tag{7.13}$$

Therefore, knowing c, c' and ϕ', σ_3' can be estimated. With knowledge of this stress and A_f, the capillary pressure p_k may be estimated from Equation (7.12). Knowing the capillary pressure and A_s, K_0 may be estimated from Equation (7.7) for the particular depth to which the effective overburden pressure p corresponds. Thus K_0 is dependent only on the ratio p_k/p and A_s.

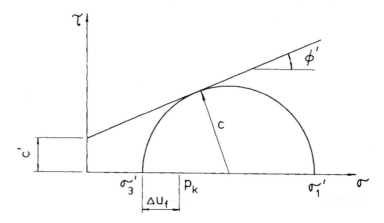

Figure 7.1 Effective stress Mohr circle at failure corresponding to an undrained test on a sample in a triaxial test.

Skempton also estimated p_k in the following alternative ways:

1   Measure volume changes in the consolidation stage of drained tests. Plot volume changes against effective pressure. Pressure corresponding to zero volume change is the capillary pressure. This is called the swelling pressure test.
2   The swelling pressure is given approximately as the pressure which just prevents a volume change when a specimen in the oedometer is immersed in water. Both procedures (1) and (2) are based on the assumption that swelling pressure is equal to the capillary pressure, but the following procedure (3) is based on direct measurement of pore water pressure suction.
3   Subject a specimen to a cell pressure x and measure pore pressure under no volume change conditions and let it be y. Then the effective stress in the specimen was $(x-y)$ since the pore pressure suction was $(y-x)$.

Reasonable agreement was found among estimates made by all these methods and that based on Equation (7.12). Using a value of $A_f = 0.25$, $c' = 380$ lb/ft^2 and $\phi' = 20°$, and using values of c at different depths (c increased consistently with depth), values of p_k/p at different depths could be calculated. To calculate K_0, the value of A_s was determined from a special triaxial test in which a specimen was consolidated and then all stresses reduced to the same value. A_s was found to be 0.3. K_0 was found to vary with depth, with a maximum value of 2.8 at a depth of about 20 ft. Note that the value of $A_f = 0.25$ was only relevant to these quick tests in which no pore pressure migration could take place. The value was 0.55 for slow undrained tests in which equalisation of pore pressure was possible.

7.3   ESTIMATING K_0 FROM THE BACK ANALYSIS OF A FAILED SLOPE

The short-term failure of a 37 ft. deep excavated slope gave Skempton the opportunity to obtain an independent estimate of the value of K_0 in London clay. He found reasonable support for estimates based on the method explained in the previous section. Therefore, it is of great interest to outline the procedure that may be followed for estimating K_0 on the basis of data concerning the stability analysis of a failed slope.

Failure corresponds to a factor of safety of unity. Therefore, from a 'back analysis', an estimate can be made of the shear stress at failure on the slip surface (mobilized shear strength). The total stress can be estimated in the usual way, from the soil unit weight and depth of any vertical slice. Knowing the total stress and shear stress, and using the Coulomb-Terzaghi equation, the pore pressure at failure at any point is given by:

$$u_f = \sigma - \frac{\tau - c'}{\tan \phi'} \tag{7.14}$$

in which σ is the total normal stress and τ the shear stress as well as the shearing resistance at the time of failure at the particular point.

Now the final pore pressure at failure u_f is the sum of the known initial pressure u_0 and the change in pore pressure Δu during excavation up to failure.

Therefore, change in pore pressure is given by

$$\Delta u = u_f - u_0 \tag{7.15}$$

The change in pore pressure during excavation may be estimated from an equation for excess pore water pressure such as Equation (7.5) or Equation (7.5a). In his calculations Skempton considered a generalised form of his equation in which the increment of intermediate principal stress $\Delta \sigma_2$ was taken as half the sum of $\Delta \sigma_1$ and $\Delta \sigma_3$. (Although no reasoning was given in his paper, this could be justified by assuming that the slope failure occurred under plane strain conditions. For plane strain, $\Delta \sigma_2 = v (\Delta \sigma_1 + \Delta \sigma_3)$ and $v = 0.5$ for deformation under no volume change which is a reasonable assumption for the short-term failure). The generalised form of Equation (7.5) and Equation (7.5a) which Skempton used contains increments in all the three principal stresses and is written as follows:

$$\Delta u = \frac{1}{3}(\Delta \sigma_1 + \Delta \sigma_2 + \Delta \sigma_3) + \alpha \sqrt{(\Delta \sigma_1 - \Delta \sigma_2)^2 + (\Delta \sigma_2 - \Delta \sigma_3)^2 + (\Delta \sigma_3 - \Delta \sigma_1)^2} \tag{7.16}$$

in which, for plane strain deformation under undrained conditions, one may substitute the following:

$$\Delta \sigma_2 = \frac{1}{2}(\Delta \sigma_1 + \Delta \sigma_3) \tag{7.16a}$$

Note that for triaxial test conditions

$$\Delta \sigma_2 = \Delta \sigma_3 \tag{7.16b}$$

and

$$\left(A - \frac{1}{3}\right) = \alpha \sqrt{2} \tag{7.16c}$$

Table 7.1 Typical values of pore pressure parameter A (after Lambe and Whitman, 1969). With permission, see page 713, No 4.

Material (fully saturated)	A at failure i.e. A_f	A for foundation settlement
Very loose fine sand	2 to 3	–
Sensitive clay	1.5 to 2.5	>1
Normally consolidated clay	0.7 to 1.3	0.5 to 1
Lightly overconsolidated clay	0.3 to 0.7	0.25 to 0.5
Heavily overconsolidated clay	−0.5 to 0	0 to 0.25

for which Equation (7.16) becomes identical to Equation (7.5) or Equation (7.5a). When applying the pore pressure equation for failure conditions, the coefficient A_f will replace A in Equation (7.16c). Similarly, α_f will replace α in Equation (7.16).

From Equation (7.16) we get an equation relating unknowns $\Delta\sigma_1$ and $\Delta\sigma_3$ since Δu is known from Equation (7.15). Now these increments in principal stresses may also be obtained by subtracting the total principal stresses before excavation from the total principal stresses after excavation. The latter are known because the stability analysis gives the normal and shear stress on the failure plane at failure. Therefore, a Mohr-Coulomb plot can be made to get σ_{1f} and σ_{3f}. The initial principal stresses are known to be equal to γz and $K\gamma z$ respectively. Therefore, ignoring the reorientation of principal stresses, which is a necessary, though questionable, approximation, we have

$$\Delta\sigma_1 = \sigma_{1f} - \gamma z, \quad \Delta\sigma_3 = \sigma_{3f} - K\gamma z \tag{7.17}$$

Thus $\Delta\sigma_1$ is known from Equation (7.17) and $\Delta\sigma_3$ contains the unknown K and hence K_0. [Note that K and K_0 are related by Equation (6.22).]

Substituting Equation (7.17) and Equation (7.16a) or Equation (7.16b) in Equation (7.16) which contains $\Delta\sigma_1$ and $\Delta\sigma_3$ as the only unknowns, K_0 is obtained provided A (and hence α) is known. It may be noted that Skempton (1961) did not explain the procedure precisely in the manner outlined above although he gave the reasoning on which it is based. His approach was summarised as a relationship between A_f and K_0 which he plotted for two different values of c. The value of A_f measured in slow laboratory tests was 0.55. However, as Skempton pointed out, there would be greater pore pressure migration in the field and that the probable value would be about 0.65. Increase of A_f from 0.55 to 0.65 increased K_0 from 2 to 2.5 in his calculations. The tremendous importance of A_f is obvious.

Typical values of A for different types of soil are given in Table 7.1 for failure as well as for conditions before failure (under working loads).The latter values would be suitable for analysis of foundation settlement.

7.4 INITIAL STRESSES IN SLOPING GROUND

The concept of conjugate stresses for uniform natural slopes is well known in soil mechanics and a formal proof for the validity of such a stress field was given by

Taylor (1948). Consider a very small element at depth z below the surface of a slope of uniform inclination β (Figure 7.2a). The total stress on a vertical plane acts parallel to the slope and is designated σ_β and the total stress on planes parallel to the slope acts in a vertical direction and is called σ_v. The latter stress is expressed in terms of the weight of the overburden above the element and the second in terms of conjugate stress ratio K as follows:

$$\sigma_v = \gamma z \cos \beta, \quad \sigma_\beta = K \gamma z \cos \beta \tag{7.18}$$

The representation of the two-dimensional state of stress by Equation (7.18) has gained wide acceptance not only in soil mechanics but generally in the whole field of geotechnical engineering. These stresses are not 'normal' stresses but have both shear and normal components. Therefore, consideration of an effective stress ratio (such as K_0) requires care. However, where $\beta = 0$, Equation (7.18) is identical to Equation (6.20) which gives the initial stress ratio in terms of total stresses when the ground is horizontal. Therefore, the description of K as a conjugate stress ratio which becomes a total principal stress ratio for $\beta = 0$ is quite adequate. Further, when pore water pressure is zero K becomes the effective principal stress ratio K_0 when $\beta = 0$.

Now considering the stress components in the x–z plane we have from Equation (7.18) two normal stresses and a shear stress (Figure 7.2b):

$$\sigma_z = \gamma z \left(1 + K \sin^2 \beta\right)$$
$$\sigma_x = K \gamma z \cos^2 \beta \tag{7.19}$$
$$\tau_{xz} = K \gamma z \sin \beta \cos \beta$$

Let the pore water pressure at depth z be u; then, assuming saturated conditions we have (from the principle of effective stress) the following equation for K_0 which

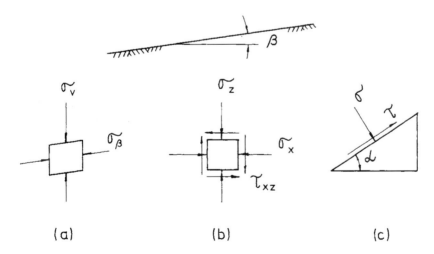

Figure 7.2 Stresses within a long uniform natural slope: (a) conjugate stresses (b) normal and shear stresses on an element (c) stresses on a plane at any arbitrary inclination.

may be defined as the ratio of effective normal stresses on horizontal and vertical planes respectively.

$$K_0 = \frac{\sigma_x - u}{\sigma_z - u} \tag{7.20}$$

When $\beta = 0$, K_0 becomes the ratio of effective principal stresses in horizontal and vertical directions. Therefore the general definition of K_0 is adequate. Note that the effective stress principle cannot be applied to σ_v and σ_β which have both shear and normal components and, therefore, there is no such thing as an 'effective' conjugate stress ratio. A conjugate stress ratio has to be defined in terms of 'total' stresses.

From Equation (7.19) and Equation (7.20) the relationship between K and K_0 is easily shown to be the following:

$$K_0 = \frac{K \cos^2\beta - r_u}{1 + K \sin^2\beta - r_u} \tag{7.21a}$$

or, rearranging the above,

$$K = \frac{K_0 + r_u(1 - K_0)}{\cos^2\beta - K_0 \sin^2\beta} \tag{7.21b}$$

in which $r_u = u/\gamma z$ is the dimensionless pore pressure ratio. With these relationships it is possible to interpret measured data, concerning K_0, in terms of the conjugate stress ratio K. When $\beta = 0$, Equation (7.21b) reduces to Equation (6.22) as expected. Figure 7.3 shows curves relating K and K_0 for different values of r_u considering a slope inclination of 15°. From Equation (7.19) the total principal stresses σ_1 and σ_3 are given as follows:

$$\sigma_{1,3} = \gamma z \left\{ \left(\frac{1+K}{2} \right) \pm \frac{1}{2} \sqrt{K^2 + 2K(\sin^2\beta - \cos^2\beta) + 1} \right\} \tag{7.22}$$

When $\beta = 0$, it is easily seen that $\sigma_1 = \gamma z$ and $\sigma_3 = K\gamma z$, as expected. The principal stresses are inclined at an angle θ to the x-axis given by:

$$\tan 2\theta = \frac{2K \sin\beta \cos\beta}{K \cos^2\beta - 1 - K \sin^2\beta} \tag{7.23}$$

Two values of 2θ differing by 180° are obtained; therefore two values of θ differing by 90° correspond to minor and major principal stresses.

Denote the term in brackets in Equation (7.22) by K_1 when plus sign is taken and K_3 when minus sign is taken, we have:

$$\sigma_1 = K_1\gamma z, \quad \sigma_3 = K_3\gamma z \tag{7.22a}$$

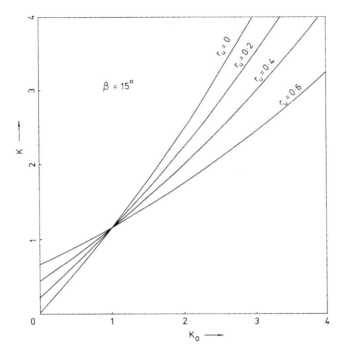

Figure 7.3 Relationship between K and K_0 for a slope of given inclination $\beta = 15°$ and for different values of pore pressure ratio r_u.

The intermediate principal stress acts in a direction perpendicular to xz plane. If the slope surface has no inclination in the y direction, this principal stress may be taken as K_2 times the overburden stress, in which K_2 depends on the stress history etc. Assuming $K_2 = K$ for simplicity:

$$\sigma_2 = K\gamma z \tag{7.24}$$

In general, K_2 may be different from K and it is difficult to establish any relationship between the two. However, on the above assumption it would be possible to determine the relationship between capillary pressure and K for a specimen extracted from ground beneath a slope (following the same procedure as explained in section 7.2), noting that:

$$\Delta\sigma_1 = -K_1\gamma z, \quad \Delta\sigma_3 = -K_3\gamma z, \quad \Delta\sigma_2 = -K\gamma z \tag{7.25}$$

The usual equations Equation (7.5) and Equation (7.5a) cannot be used since in these equations the intermediate principal stress is assumed equal to one of the other principal stresses. Therefore, Equation (7.16) may be used instead. From Equation (7.16) and Equation (7.25) an equation similar to Equation (7.7) may be obtained. Knowing capillary pressure from Equation (7.12) and Equation (7.13), the value of K can be obtained. Once K is obtained, the value of K_0 can be obtained from Equation (7.21). From Equation (7.22) and Equation (7.22a), the influence of the slope angle β on the relationship between K and p_k is obvious.

Generalisation of the procedure for determining K or K_0 for sloping areas suggested above has not been applied to any practical problems. It would be of great interest to study the influence of slope angle on estimated values of K_0.

7.5   LIMITING VALUES OF K

It is now useful to consider the initial state of stress in terms of classical soil mechanics and in particular the Mohr-Coulomb (or Terzaghi-Coulomb) failure criterion. A natural slope can only exist in its stable form if plastic failure has not occurred throughout the soil mass. Therefore, the initial state of stress should be such that the relevant failure criterion is not violated. This means that there are limits to the value of K. If its value decreases beyond a certain limit, the soil mass will fail in the active mode corresponding to an active Rankine state. On the other hand, if the value of K exceeds an upper limit, the soil mass may fail in the passive mode corresponding to the passive Rankine state. For example, it is well known that for a cohesionless soil mass with a horizontal surface the value of K must lie between K_a and K_p as follows:

$$K_a < K < K_p \tag{7.26}$$

where

$$K_a = \tan^2(45° - \phi/2), \quad K_p = \tan^2(45° + \phi/2) \tag{7.26a}$$

If a cohesionless soil mass has a sloping surface with an inclination β we have again:

$$K_a < K < K_p$$

where

$$K_a = \frac{\cos\beta - \sqrt{\cos^2\beta - \cos^2\phi}}{\cos\beta + \sqrt{\cos^2\beta - \cos^2\phi}}, \quad K_p = \frac{1}{K_a} \tag{7.26b}$$

For a soil with both c and ϕ (in effective stress terms) the values of K_a and K_p are dependent on the slope inclination β, the unit weight γ and the pore pressure u. Using the Coulomb-Terzaghi equation in terms of principal stresses and substituting the value of the existing principal stresses from Equation (7.22), the limiting values of K are given by the following (assuming $u = 0$):

$$\sqrt{K^2 + 2K(\sin^2\beta - \cos^2\beta) + 1} = \frac{2c}{\gamma z}\cos\phi + (1 + K)\sin\phi \tag{7.27}$$

When u is not zero, the extra term $(-2u \sin\phi/\gamma z)$ appears on the right hand side. When $\beta = 0$, Equation (7.27) gives the following limiting values for K:

$$K > K_a = \frac{1 - \sin\phi}{1 + \sin\phi} - \frac{2c}{\gamma z}\frac{\cos\phi}{1 + \sin\phi}$$

$$K < K_p = \frac{1 + \sin\phi}{1 - \sin\phi} + \frac{2c}{\gamma z}\frac{\cos\phi}{1 - \sin\phi}$$

(7.27a)

Most slopes fail in the active mode. However, conditions may arise in which part of the soil mass fails in the passive mode during slope failure. This was discussed briefly in section 5.10. High local values of K indicating local passive failure do not necessarily indicate that a full scale slide involving the whole slope must develop. Skempton (1961) found that at shallow depths soil at the Bradwell site was in a state of passive failure. Yet slides did not develop until the excavation had reached a 37 ft. depth.

The fact that high values of K can be applicable to soil or rock at shallow depths is extremely important. This means that the concepts presented in this chapter may be valid for shallow slides as well as deep-seated ones. The value of K is always important except perhaps for very superficial slope movements, erosion etc. In overconsolidated soil, the value of K may decrease with depth since the overconsolidation ratio often decreases with depth. Considering rock slopes, it may be noted that Jaeger (1971), in his Rankine lecture, referred to the possibility of high lateral stresses in the surface layers of rock slopes. He considered the effect of an assumed lateral force directly in a limit equilibrium analysis of a rock wedge.

There are, of course, several qualifications to be made. In many real situations, in situ soil or rock may be covered with talus or colluvial material. The existence of such material may be of primary significance to the stability of many slopes. The initial stress field, and hence the value of K, for the upper layer of colluvium may be quite different from that of the intact material. In particular consideration must be given to previous deformations and movements of an extensive nature affecting the upper layers of colluvium or residual soil. Such deformations may have relieved the upper layers of high lateral stresses. Geological details, discontinuities and weathering profiles are often very important and this should never be forgotten. In this chapter, attention is concentrated on the significance of an initial stress field and an effort is made to show how knowledge of initial stresses may help to quantify stability. Such calculations as are proposed should help the experienced slope engineer to verify his judgment based on considerations of geology and on conventional calculations. To the student and researcher, this chapter should serve as a reminder of the need for consistency and clarity in regard to analytical procedures.

Like many other analytical procedures an engineer must have a reasonable overall knowledge of conventional methods, their merits and shortcomings, before he tries the application of new procedures. Indiscriminate replacement of guidelines based on experience by new approaches, however logical, is not likely to prove helpful. An intelligent practitioner must carefully weigh all data, conventional calculations as well as results based on new approaches.

7.6   STRESSES ON ANY PLANE

It is now of interest to consider the stresses on a plane inclined at an arbitrary inclination α to the horizontal. By analysing an element such as the one shown in Figure 7.2c for equilibrium, the following equations are obtained for normal stress σ and shear stress τ on the plane of inclination α:

$$\sigma = \gamma z \ \{\cos^2 \alpha (1 + K \sin^2 \beta) + K \sin^2 \alpha \cos^2 \beta - K \sin^2 \alpha \sin \beta \cos \beta\}$$
$$\tau = \gamma z \ \{\sin \alpha \cos \alpha (1 + K \sin^2 \beta - K \cos^2 \beta) + (\sin^2 \alpha - \cos^2 \alpha) \ K \sin \beta \cos \beta\}$$

$$(7.28)$$

Knowing the initial stress parameter K, the existing normal and shear stresses within any slope of uniform inclination may be calculated. It is of interest to consider some special cases:

- For planes parallel to the slope, the angle α is equal to the angle β and the stresses are:

$$\sigma = \gamma z \cos^2 \beta$$
$$\tau = \gamma z \cos \beta \sin \beta$$

$$(7.29)$$

These are the well known equations which have been widely used in soil mechanics in connection with 'infinite' slope analysis. Examples are given in Chapter 4 and Chapter 9. It is interesting that these stresses are independent of K, a fact which explains why this parameter, and hence lateral stresses, have been ignored in conventional treatment of long natural slopes. For any plane which is not parallel to the surface of a slope, the normal and shear stresses are dependent on the value of K. Therefore, realistic stability calculations must take this fact into consideration.

- Consider the hypothetical condition $K = 0$. The stresses are given from Equation (7.28) as follows:

$$\sigma = \gamma z \cos^2 \alpha$$
$$\tau = \gamma z \cos \alpha \sin \alpha$$

$$(7.30)$$

These equations are independent of the slope inclination β and may easily be recognised as those which are used in connection with planar failure surfaces in limit equilibrium methods as well as in connection with curved surfaces when the ordinary method of slices (which ignores inter-slice forces) is used. Once again it is obvious that these equations are unrealistic since the value of K is assumed to be zero.

7.7   THE CONCEPT OF INHERENT STABILITY

It is useful to differentiate between a 'stable' slope and an 'unstable' slope although no slope is stable for an unlimited time or in an absolute sense. The concept of a stable slope may be considered valid for a set of known conditions at any given instant. The question arises: "How can the stability of a slope be quantified?". As Wilson (1970) observed in his Terzaghi lecture, it is always possible to balance driving forces and resisting forces in some way to explain a failure which has already occurred but it is far more difficult to predict the performance of an embankment or an excavation which is stable. Again he commented that while observational data about slope movements may help understand slope behaviour, it does not help to quantify the safety of a stable slope or explain the reasons for such safety or stability. The problem is much more difficult when we are concerned with natural slopes rather than excavations or embankments. Geological factors and stress history are usually of prime significance. It would be desirable to consider such slopes in terms of initial or in situ stresses in addition to shear strength parameters, slope inclination and pore water pressure which are already recognised to be important.

The stability of a natural slope may be quantified, as is done in limit equilibrium methods by defining a factor of safety in terms of shear strength and shear stresses. However, these must be related to the realities of the initial stress field which exists in the slope in its stable condition. Such a factor of safety is a function of the conjugate stress ratio (or initial stress parameter) K. In the following sections it will be shown that the value of K has a significant influence on the magnitude of the safety factor for a stable slope.

The value of K for a slope could also be interpreted in another way by considering the possibility of the development of zones of active or passive failure. The factor of safety against failure by plastic flow could be taken as a ratio K_a/K or K_p/K. If the ratio K/K_a exceeds one, the material of a slope is safe from active failure. The higher the value of K/K_a, the higher the factor a of safety against active failure. Similarly if the ratio K_p/K exceeds one, the slope is safe against passive failure. As the ratio increases, the factor of safety against passive failure increases. However, this approach is not sufficient in slope stability analysis. It is more useful to consider a mass bounded by a potential slip surface. Therefore, we return to the well known concept of a factor of safety against sliding on a given surface.

7.8 PLANAR FAILURE

Consider the possibility of slip along planar surfaces which may or may not be parallel to the surface of a slope. In this connection it is convenient to define a local or directional factor of safety F_α at any point within a slope. Such a factor of safety is dependent on the inclination α of the plane under consideration. It may be defined as the ratio of shear strength to shear stress on the relevant plane giving:

$$F_\alpha = \frac{c}{\tau} + \left(\frac{\sigma - u}{\tau}\right) \tan \phi \tag{7.31}$$

in which the normal stress σ and shear stress τ are given by Equation (7.28) and depend on the value of the conjugate stress ratio K. When $c = 0$, it is useful to consider the ratio $F_\alpha/\tan \phi$. Assuming $u = 0$, plots of $F_\alpha/\tan \phi$ are shown in Figure 7.4 for different values of β. The results are independent of depth z and soil unit

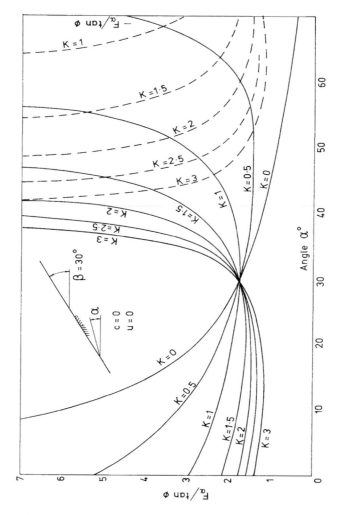

Figure 7.4 Curves showing the relationship between directional (or local) safety factor and inclination of corresponding plane for different values of K when $\beta = 30°$ and $r_u = 0$. Dotted curves correspond to negative values of $F_\alpha/\tan \phi$.

weight γ. It is interesting to find that inherent factors of safety are dependent on K except when $\alpha = \beta$. Figure 7.5 shows such plots when both positive and negative values of α are considered. Figure 7.6 applies to the case when unit cohesion $c \neq 0$. Here the dimensionless parameter $c_m/\gamma z$ is plotted against ϕ_m where $c_m = c/F_\alpha$ and $\tan \phi_m = \tan\phi/F_\alpha$. Once again the influence of K on the inherent factor of safely F_α and can be seen.

It is interesting to note that the factor of safety is not necessarily a minimum for planes parallel to the slope (i.e., $\alpha = \beta$). Considering the case with $c = 0$, $u = 0$, it can be shown that only when $K = 1$ is the value of F a minimum for $\alpha = \beta$.

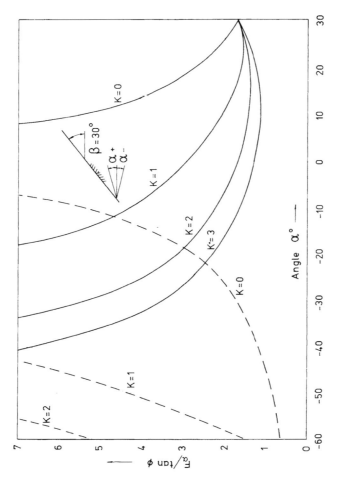

Figure 7.5 Curves showing the relationship between directional (or local) safety factor and inclination of corresponding plane for different values of K when both positive and negative values of α are considered. Dotted curves correspond to negative values of $F_\alpha/\tan \phi$.

From plots of F_α against α, it is seen that there are ranges of values for which F is close to the minimum and that outside these ranges F rises sharply. This indicates that basal failure surfaces of flat inclination and rear failure surfaces of steep inclination are most likely in natural slopes. Such surfaces have often been observed in actual failures (see, for example, Bjerrum, 1967) and are considered in section 7.10. It is necessary to point out that there may be other factors which are of obvious importance in the development of flat basal slip surfaces (and steep rear failure surfaces). These factors are usually related to geological details e.g., weak beds or strata, adverse inclination or dip of a key layer, tectonic activity and valley stress relief. The concept of an initial stress field enables the problem to be considered in a more complete or comprehensive manner.

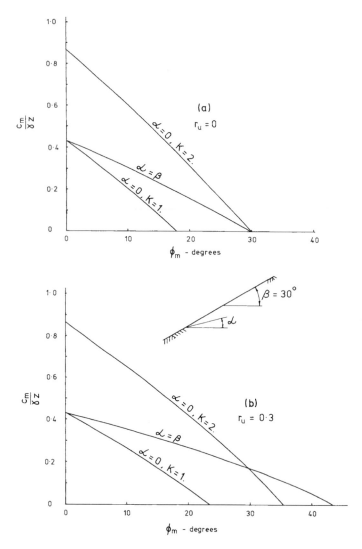

Figure 7.6 Relationship between c_m and ϕ_m for different values of α and K for a 30° slope (where $c_m = c/F_\alpha$ and $\tan \phi_m = \tan \phi/F_\alpha$) assuming (a) $r_u = 0$ and (b) $r_u = 0.3$.

7.9 ULTIMATE STABLE ANGLE OF NATURAL SLOPES

It is of interest to reconsider the question of the ultimate stable angle of natural slopes which was discussed briefly in section 4.4. Consider the slope material to be cohesive but at the residual state as regards its shearing resistance such that $c = c_r = 0$, $\phi = \phi_r$. Assume a horizontal failure surface within a slope of inclination β. Table 7.2 shows, for specific values of β, ϕ_r and r_u, and considering the potential slip surface to be horizontal, the values of factor of safety F for two values of K.

Table 7.2 Factor of safety on a horizontal surface
within a slope (after Chowdhury, 1976).

$r_u = 0.5$	K	F
$\beta = 10°$	1.00	1.13
$\phi_r = 20°$	1.50	0.77
$r_u = 0$	0.45	1.00
$\beta = 30°$		
$\phi_r = 10°$	1.00	0.50

Table 7.3 Value of K which all give $F_\alpha = 1$ for different conditions
(after Chowdhury, 1976).

ϕ_r^0	$\beta°$	r_u	K
10	5	0.5	1.03
20	10	0.5	1.14
30	15	0.5	1.37
40	20	0.5	1.89

Table 7.3 shows different values of K which all give a factor of safety of one on a horizontal surface when ϕ_r and β are varied but their ratio (ϕ_r/β) and r_u are kept constant. The tables 7.2 and 7.3 clearly demonstrate the influence of K on factors of safety considered on a plane with a given inclination.

Discussion in geotechnical engineering of the 'ultimate stable angle' of natural slopes has concentrated merely on the value of ϕ_r. Thus in every case the factor of safety is assumed to be nearly one when β is half of ϕ_r, assuming r_u to be approximately half (see chapter 4). It is well known that current hypotheses cannot always explain observed slope performance data from both unstable and stable slopes. Usually this is attributed to lack of accurate information about geological details and pore water pressures. However, in part at least, this may also be due to the fact that the value of K is ignored. Consideration of this value together with potential failure surfaces at different inclinations to the surface will provide useful information concerning the inherent stability of natural slopes. Consequently a better understanding of the conditions for long-term stability can be expected. As discussed in chapter 4, there are other factors which may exert considerable influence on the ultimate stable slope angle. Geological environment, climate and erosion patterns are some of the obvious factors which influence slope form in the long term.

7.10 BI-PLANAR SURFACES OF SLIDING

Reference was made earlier to the fact that many actual failures take place along slip surfaces which can be approximated by two planes. These may be called bi-planar failure surfaces and the most striking example is that of the Vaiont slide (Muller, 1964) which had a 'chair-shaped' sliding surface. Other examples have been given by Hamel and Flint (1972), Broscoe and Thompson (1967), Bjerrum (1967) etc.

Figure 7.7a shows a bi-planar surface with one plane segment of inclination θ_1 and the other of inclination θ_2. H is the depth of their point of intersection below the surface. The overall factor of safety F against sliding along this potential surface of sliding may be defined as the ratio of available total shear strength to the total shear force along the surface. This may be obtained by simple integration and is given by

$$F = \frac{2c(A+B) + H \tan \phi \,(AM_1 + BM_2)}{H(AN_1 + BN_2)} \tag{7.32}$$

in which $A = \operatorname{cosec}\,(\beta - \theta_1)$, and, $B = \operatorname{cosec}\,(\theta_2 - \beta)$.

$M_1 = \sigma/\gamma z$, $N_1 = \tau/\gamma z$, are obtained from Equation (7.28) after replacing α with θ_1; similarly M_2 and N_2 are obtained after replacing α with θ_2 in Equation (7.28).

When $c = 0$, Equation (7.32) simplifies to:

$$F = \frac{AM_1 + BM_2}{AN_1 + BN_2} \tan \phi \tag{7.33}$$

Therefore, F is independent of H and γ when $c = 0$ irrespective of the value of K, θ_1 and θ_2. This equation, Equation (7.33) would, for instance, be useful when $c = 0 = c_r$ and $\phi = \phi_r$. Such an assumption is considered reasonable for old slip surfaces when assessing the potential for renewal of instability in the case of an existing landslide.

Consider a simple example in which $\theta_1 = 0°$ and $\theta_2 = 90°$ as shown in Figure 7.7b. Conventional methods ignore the lateral stresses with the result that the calculated factor of safety would be infinity in this case since the shear stress on the horizontal surface is considered to be zero. In alternative conventional terminology it may be stated that the weight of wedge has no component in the potential direction of

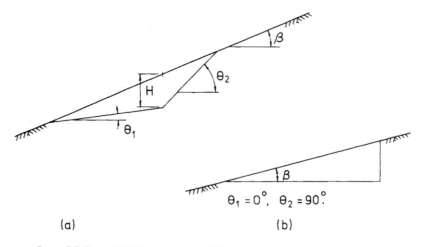

(a)   (b)

Figure 7.7 Potential failure surfaces of bi-planar shape within natural slopes.

Table 7.4 Variation of factor of safety F with K for bi-planar surface in Figure 7.7b (after Chowdhury, 1976).

K	0	0.5	1	1.5	2	3	5
$\dfrac{F}{\tan\phi}$	Infinity*	6.2	3.9	3.1	2.7	2.3	2

Note: An infinite value of F for K = 0 corresponds to a limit equilibrium solution. Normal and shear stresses are calculated from the components of the weight of an element or slice. Thus the shear stress on a horizontal plane is zero.

movement or along the surface of sliding. However, the actual factor of safety is finite and is given by the following (for $c = 0$):

$$F = \frac{(M_1 + M_2 \tan\beta)}{(N_1 + N_2 \tan\beta)} \tan\phi \tag{7.34}$$

Note that Equation (7.32) to Equation (7.34) have been derived on the assumption that pore water pressure $u = 0$. However, the inclusion of pore water pressures in the analysis presents no difficulty.

From Equation (7.34) the variation of ($F/\tan\phi$) with K for a slope with $\beta = 30°$ is shown in Table 7.4.

In Table 7.4 the shear stresses and shear strengths on the vertical segment of the failure surface have been included. An open crack coinciding with the vertical segment of the failure surface (e.g., a tension crack) would justify ignoring shear stress and strength on this segment. The resulting factors of safety are consistently lower. For example, $F/\tan\phi = 2.9$ for $K = 1$ and $F/\tan\phi = 1.04$ for $K = 5$. These results are explained in terms of the change in the sign of the shear stresses for steep inclinations of any failure surface. This is clear from Figure 7.4 which shows a change in the sign of F_α when α is greater than a certain value depending on K and β. These negative shear stresses thus contribute to the 'apparent' stability while it is assumed that failure or sliding has not occurred. However, when a tension crack develops, the contributions to shear stress and shear strength from the relevant part of slip surface have to be ignored.

7.11 POTENTIAL SLIP SURFACE OF ARBITRARY SHAPE

For a potential slip surface of arbitrary shape the inclination α may vary from point to point and it is necessary to include this variation in the calculation of the overall inherent stability in terms of the factor of safety F. This may be achieved by numerical integration after dividing the soil mass into a number of vertical slices. Let the width of a slice be b and base inclination (along the surface of sliding) be α. The following equation may be written for F:

$$F = \frac{\sum\{b\,c\sec\alpha + b(\sigma - u)\tan\phi\sec\alpha\}}{\sum b\,\tau\sec\alpha} \tag{7.35}$$

in which σ and τ depend on the value of K as shown by Equation (7.28) and u is the pore water pressure, the value of which may be variable. The equation may be simplified if the slice width b is assumed to be constant.

Equation (7.35) is based on the definition of a factor of safety as the ratio of resisting to disturbing forces. As has been shown in chapters 5 and 6, there are alternative definitions and F may be taken as the ratio of available to mobilised shearing resistance. This ratio (the local factor of safety) varies from point to point. In limit equilibrium methods the factor of safety is assumed to be constant all along a potential failure surface. However, in the present case the stresses are assumed to be known and the variation of local factor of safety cannot be ignored. Averaging the local factors of safety leads to the following:

$$F = \frac{1}{L}\int F_\alpha dL = \frac{1}{L}\sum\left\{\frac{c+(\sigma-u)\tan\phi}{\tau}\right\} b \sec\alpha \tag{7.36}$$

in which L is the total length of the potential failure surface. Obviously Equation (7.35) and Equation (7.36) will not lead to the same result.

In the case of a failure surface of circular shape, Equation (7.35) also gives the ratio of resisting to disturbing moments. Note that the stresses are known everywhere within the soil mass and there is no need to account for the inter-slice forces. In limit equilibrium calculations, the stresses on the potential failure surface are unknown and their determination on a rigorous basis requires a consideration of the inter-slice forces for the condition of limit equilibrium. In connection with the initial stress approach it seems more logical to accept the first definition of overall factor of safety leading to Equation (7.35). However, application of Equation (7.36) would also be of significant interest in order to compare the results with those obtained on the basis of Equation (7.35).

7.12   EXAMPLE – CIRCULAR FAILURE SURFACE

Figure 7.8 shows a potential failure surface of circular shape in a natural slope. For simplicity it is assumed that $c = 0$ and $u = 0$. The overall factor of safety was

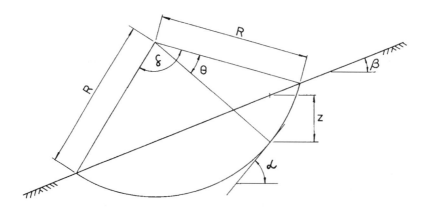

Figure 7.8 Potential slip surface of circular shape within a natural slope.

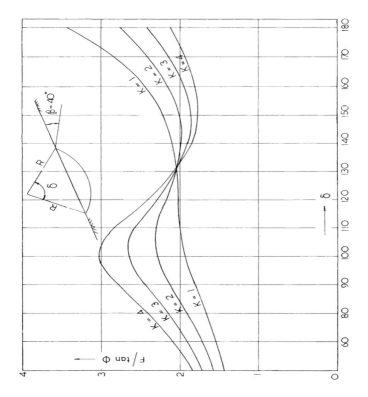

Figure 7.9 Variation of inherent factor of safety with central angle of circular slip surfaces with constant radius (for different values of K).

computed for different values of the central angle and for different slope inclinations using Equation (7.35). The results for different values of K are shown in Figures 7.9 and 7.10. At first glance the results are somewhat surprising since the inherent factor of safety appears to increase with increase in K. Once again these results must be considered in relation to the variation in the local or directional factor of safety with change in the orientation of the failure plane from point to point. The overall factor of safety calculated on the basis of initial stresses cannot be regarded absolute in any sense. In fact it may be interpreted in quite the opposite way and represents the potential for progressive failure as will be seen in the subsequent section.

7.13   SIMULATING PROGRESSIVE CHANGE IN STABILITY

7.13.1   The simulation process

In order to explore the potential for progressive failure, it may be worthwhile to consider the gradual transformation of the stress state within a sloping soil or rock mass from an initial stress field to a simple gravitational stress field that one might consider within the framework of limit equilibrium. The implicit assumption of a

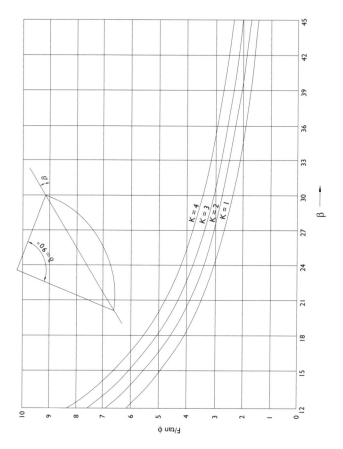

Figure 7.10 Variation of inherent factor of safety with slope inclination for different values of K assuming constant central angle.

conventional limit equilibrium solution is that such a transformation occurs simultaneously throughout a potential sliding mass. In this case, for simulation of the potential for progressive failure, one would have to consider particular modes of progression which are considered relevant and feasible. For the sake of simplicity and continuity with general limit equilibrium methods, the concept of a potential slip surface may, however, be retained in such a simulation.

One of the aims of such a simulation would be to study the change in the factor of safety of the slope during the process of transformation of the stress field from the initial stress field to a simple gravitational one. Consequently, it would be possible to determine the stage of progression at which the factor of safety is a minimum. One can also determine if the factor of safety falls below unity and, if so, the stage of progression at which this occurs for the given or assumed mode of progression.

Progressive change from an initial stress might be simulated in a number of ways depending on the conditions and processes which are considered relevant. Here we will restrict our attention to spatial progression from one end of the slip surface to the other. First we may consider a small element of the slip surface and assume that the stresses in the sloping mass above that portion have been transformed to gravitational stresses. The adjacent element of the slip surface is then included in the simulation and thus a larger part of the sloping mass is considered to be transformed from initial stress field to simple gravitational stress field. As the simulation process continues, an increasingly larger part of the slip surface is included until the whole of the sloping mass is considered to be transformed from an initial stress field to a simple gravitational stress field.

7.13.2 Defining an overall factor of safety at any stage

Consider that, at a given stage in the process of progression and associated stress transformation, a part A of the soil mass has its stress field transformed to a simple gravitational one. Let this part be bounded by portion L_1 of the slip surface. Let the factor of safety of this mass of soil from limit equilibrium considerations be F_1. The remaining part B of the soil mass is still at the initial state of stress and the factor of safety along the part L_2 of the failure surface which bounds B may be obtained in the manner discussed in the previous section. Let this be F_2.

F_1 and F_2 may be expressed in terms of disturbing and resisting forces thus:

$$F_1 = \frac{R_1}{D_1}, \quad F_2 = \frac{R_2}{D_2} \tag{7.37}$$

The overall factor of safety F is given by:

$$F = \frac{(R_1 + R_2)}{(D_1 + D_2)} = \frac{(F_1 D_1 + F_2 D_2)}{(D_1 + D_2)} \tag{7.38}$$

7.13.3 Change in stability considering two alternative modes of progression

Part A is small in the beginning and L_1 is small. Progressively part A becomes larger, L_1 increases and part B as well as L_2 become smaller. When and if the whole sloping mass is transformed into a simple gravitational stress state, the final value of F will not depend on the initial stress field. It will depend on the gravitational stress field and thus may be estimated from the weight and geometry of the sliding mass. Thus the value of the factor of safety F changes from the inherent value based on initial stresses to the conventional limit equilibrium value as the progressive transformation of stress field is simulated.

Chowdhury (1977b) has shown that, for a potential sliding surface of circular shape, the factor of safety F changes in different ways, depending on whether when spatial progression is assumed to develop (a) from the toe of the slope, or (b) from the crest of the slope.

In the former case, the value of F first increases to a maximum before reaching the limit equilibrium value and in the latter case the value of F first decreases to a minimum before reaching the limit equilibrium value. This minimum value decreases as the value of K increases. This shows that the higher the value of K, the greater the

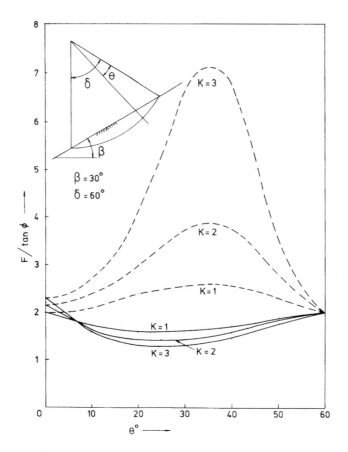

Figure 7.11 Variation of overall factor of safety with extent of progress to limit equilibrium in natural slope assuming progressive transformation from (a) crest: full lines (b) toe: dotted lines.

potential for progressive failure. The results showing maxima and minima are evident in Figure 7.11 for a circular failure surface.

These results concerning progressive change in the stress field have a far reaching significance in relation to the stability of natural and man-made slopes and have been discussed in some detail by Chowdhury (1977a, b; 1978a). The application of these concepts to the catastrophic Vaiont slide is discussed later in this chapter (see section 7.15).

7.13.4   An alternative method for simulation of progressive change in the stability of an idealized embankment

Here it is of significant interest to invite attention to the simulation of the change in factor of safety of an idealized embankment (top of Figure 7.12). The development of a slip surface was simulated as the propagation of a crack (Romani et al., 1972). The stresses due to the construction of the embankment were assumed to be the initial stresses and crack propagation was assumed to occur in two alternative ways: (a) from the toe upwards, and (b) from the crest downwards The results are shown in bottom part of

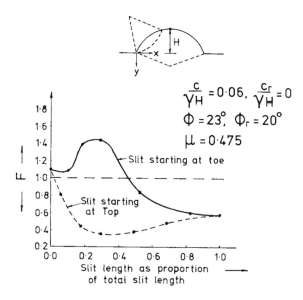

Figure 7.12 Variation of factor of safety F as a slit propagates in an idealised embankment from crest or toe. Horizontal axis shows length of slit as a proportion of the final slit length which is equal to the length of the circular are shown dotted, (after Romani et al., 1972). With permission from ASCE, see page 713, No 26.

Figure 7.12. While the problem is very different from that of natural slope stability considered above, and a different approach was used for the simulation and estimation of factor of safety curves, the shapes of the curves are very similar to the corresponding curves for the natural slope stability problem of Figure 7.11.

This striking similarity implies that the initial stress approach can be applied to general slope stability problems and need not be restricted to natural slopes. However, the methodology and the details of a simulation process must be suited to the significant aspects of any specific slope problem. The results of simulation and analysis must be interpreted and assessed on the basis of engineering judgment and experience.

7.14   APPLICATION TO ALTERED SLOPES

In practice it is often necessary to analyse the stability of altered natural slopes including cuts and embankments. In such cases inherent stability may be considered in terms of the altered stresses which are a sum of the initial stresses and the stress changes caused by excavation or embankment loading. The determination of stress changes will usually require a numerical solution based on the finite-element technique. The principles to be considered in stress analysis involving slopes have been considered in detail in chapter 6.

Having established the stress state after slope formation or slope disturbance, the inherent factor of safety may be considered simply by integrating the shear strength and shear stresses over a potential slip surface and taking their ratio. The next step would be to simulate the transformation of the slope from this state to one of limit equilibrium in the manner discussed above. In this process the minimum factor of safety with a particular slip surface and a specific mode of failure progression can be estimated.

A realistic analysis must take into consideration all relevant factors such as pore water pressures, tension cracks, water pressure in the tension cracks etc. The movement of the potential sliding mass theoretically begins when F, the overall factor of safety during the transformation process, falls just below unity. This point may be identified on the curve in which F is plotted against the extent of transformation to limit equilibrium. The approximate calculation of velocities and displacements after this point is facilitated by the rest of the curve. The exact solution of the dynamic problem is difficult since the results obtained concerning F are not strictly valid once the motion of the sliding mass begins. An estimate of accelerations, velocities and displacements may be made by assuming that the statical calculations of factor of safety are approximately valid even when F falls below one.

In conventional slope stability studies, only the static factor of safety is considered and little attention is given to the dynamics of slides. This is precisely because conventional studies are based on an over-simplification of the mechanics of slope failure. The factor of safety is calculated by assuming that conditions for limit equilibrium develop suddenly and simultaneously. Furthermore only one single value of F is obtained and on the basis of such a value, it is simplistic to attempt calculations concerning the dynamics of any slide.

In the method proposed here it would be easy to include strain-softening behaviour as an additional feature of a simulation. For example, it may be suggested that as soon as a soil mass is transformed into limit equilibrium the shear strength falls to an ultimate or even a residual value. The relevant part of the slip surface could then be assumed to have corresponding reduced shear strength when further progress of limit equilibrium is simulated. As a greater proportion of the soil mass is transformed to limit equilibrium, a greater proportion of the potential failure surface may be assigned the reduced strength. The overall factors of safety at any stage are then influenced by (a) the reorientation of stresses depending on the initial stress field and (b) the strain-softening behaviour of the slope material.

Effective stress analyses are usually relevant in an analysis of a natural slope which has not been recently altered. However, either a total-stress analysis or an effective-stress analysis may be relevant to an altered slope such as an excavation. Total stress analysis would be a choice for studying the short-term stability of a built-up or excavated slope of saturated clay. The concepts presented in this chapter may, therefore, be useful in both types of analysis depending upon the nature of the problem.

7.15   ROCK-SLIDE AT THE SITE OF THE VAIONT DAM AND A SUMMARY OF SOME ANALYSES CARRIED OUT AFTER ITS OCCURRENCE

7.15.1   Unusual nature of the catastrophic landslide

The slide which occurred on the upstream side of the Vaiont dam in Italy in 1964 has been studied by many investigators. It is probably the most famous and unique case history among a number of known catastrophic landslide events which have occurred in different parts of the world. Many such events have not been fully explained on the basis of the widely accepted methods of analysis. However, there is often agreement among aspects about the explanations of some of these landslides after the event. In the case of the Vaiont landslide there is general agreement only on the fact that the landslide could not have been predicted and that, even decades after its occurrence, key aspects cannot be explained to the satisfaction of experts around the world.

There are other unique aspects. For example, several catastrophic landslides have occurred at sites about which little information concerning geotechnical and geological aspects was known before the event. On the other hand, a lot was known about the location of this landslide, being the site for the Vaiont dam for which comprehensive investigations were undertaken. The behaviour of the site was observed during the construction of the dam, during reservoir filling and during stages when the reservoir water was lowered. Slope movements were noted and the potential for instability became obvious to the engineers, especially after a small landslide occurred. However, when the final event occurred, it was enormous beyond any expectation in its magnitude, velocity and impact.

The slide involved a volume of approximately 250 million cubic meters and generated a wave about 90 m above the crest of the dam. Because of the wave, adverse impacts occurred both upstream and downstream of the dam. The slide occurred with extreme violence and estimates of velocity based on external observations range from 18 m/s to 50 m/s (Banks and Strohm, 1974).

The failure was of a progressive nature and intermittent movements had been observed at the site for a number of years. In fact, a small slide occurred in November, 1960. The main failure appeared to have progressed from the top of the slope downwards.

Many investigators have used limit equilibrium methods to understand the occurrence of the landslide, but with only limited success. The occurrence, magnitude and velocity of exceptional landslides are notoriously difficult to predict. However, after the event, it is often possible to provide one or more alternative explanations on the basis of investigation and analysis. But the Vaiont slide is one of those catastrophic events which has defied any consistent explanation within the bounds of geotechnical knowledge and consistent with the basic concepts and observations.

In the case of the Vaiont slide, limit equilibrium methods appear to suggest that the strength was extremely low at the time of failure and reduced dramatically from its original value. Investigations and analyses were made by Muller (1964), Kenney (1967c), Broili (1967), Hendron and Patton (1985), among many others.

7.15.2   Back-calculated shear strength based on critical equilibrium

The high velocities attained by the slide would suggest an internal frictional angle as low as 7 degrees with zero cohesion. However, such a low value of shear strength before the occurrence of the slide would not be acceptable because of the stability of the site before and during the construction of the Vaiont dam. As stated in the next

Table 7.5 Back-calculated values of ϕ required for critical equilibrium ($F = 1$) with $c = 0$ for Vaiont slide (after Jaeger, 1972). With permission, see page 713, No 25.

Water level above sea level	Lowest values		Highest values	
	ϕ	Author	ϕ	Author
600	18.8	Muller	22.1	Nonveiller
650	20.1	Kenney	22.1	Nonveiller
700	17.5	Mencl	28.5	Nonveiller

sub-section, such a low value would also not be consistent with the assessment of the geological and geotechnical information at the site.

Considering just the state of critical equilibrium, significantly higher values were estimated. By 1972, a review of back-analyses based on limit equilibrium approaches suggested that ϕ values for critical equilibrium ($F = 1$) ranged from 17.5° to a maximum of 28.5° assuming cohesion c was zero in each case. Some calculated values are shown in Table 7.5.

A decade and half later, Hendron and Patton (1985) carried out a comprehensive investigation and came to the conclusion that the value of the internal friction angle along the slip surface must have been much lower. For their analyses, they adopted a value of just 12 degrees for the internal friction angle. They acknowledged that 2D factors of safety on this basis are too low to explain the long period of relative stability before and during the construction of the dam especially given their additional assumption of high artesian pore water pressures. Therefore, they had to make a number of other assumptions which would be considered questionable under widely accepted concepts. Because of the nature and extent of their assumptions concerning key parameters and the explanations offered, a summary of their approach and findings have been included in this book including the final section of this chapter (refer to sections 2.3.2, 5.6.5, 5.12.7 and 7.15). Any final judgment about their explanation for the landslide and the assumptions on which it is based would require a consensus amongst other experts.

7.15.3   Shear strength of rock materials

Failure occurred mainly in the limestone for which ϕ values are generally much higher than those predicted. Even if it is accepted that the ϕ values had reached a residual state due to tectonic shearing or large pre-failure deformations (Skempton, 1966b), the calculated values are still quite low. Lo et al. (1972) surveyed the literature and found that residual ϕ values below 28° had not been measured for limestones. No evidence of any significant clay layers was found in any of the detailed investigations. The presence of extensive clay layers could have reduced the mobilised shear strength considerably. Further, even if ϕ values of the order of 20°–28° were accepted at the instant of failure ($F = 1$), the enormous velocities of the slide cannot be explained on this basis. In fact it has been suggested that the value of ϕ would have to be smaller than 7° over the entire slip surface to explain velocities of the order of 25 m/sec. (Jaeger, 1972). Until the investigation of Hendron and Patton (1985), there was no evidence cited in relevant publications concerning the existence of clay layers even along parts of the slip surface. However, they came to the view that extensive clay layers did exist along the slip surface and postulated that the field residual shear strength must have been very low. They adopted a value of 12° for the angle of shearing resistance. As stated earlier, a consensus from other experts would be required before their conclusion about the shear strength is judged to be realistic.

7.15.4 Pore water pressure assumptions

The possibility that high artesian pore water pressures might have existed at the site at the time of the slide had also been investigated well before the investigation of Hendron and Patton (1985)*. However, available evidence had not supported such a suggestion. Even with assumed artesian pressures, limit equilibrium analyses give realistic values of ϕ only for static calculations (Lo et al., 1972). Once again the high velocities could not be explained at all. It was generally agreed that actual pore water pressures correspond to the reservoir level at the time of the slide. Even for a material with $c = 0$, submergence can reduces the factor of safety to some extent when the slope surface and the slip plane are not of uniform inclination. Therefore, reservoir filling could have been the final trigger mechanism for the slide. With these facts, reconciling the failure and observed movements to the actual shear strength of the material requires consideration of a neglected factor such as the initial stress field. This is discussed below.

7.16 SIMULATION OF PROGRESSIVE FAILURE BASED ON INITIAL STRESS APPROACH (CHOWDHURY, 1978a)

7.16.1 Assumption of a reasonable initial stress field

Chowdhury (1978a) used the approach outlined earlier in this chapter for analysis of the Vaiont slide in order to simulate the transformation of the slope from stability to critical equilibrium and consequent failure. No information concerning initial stresses was found in the literature and two values of the conjugate stress ratio ($K = 1$ and 2) were assumed. From published accounts and discussions of the geology of the site, it is obvious that there has been considerable valley stress relief by removal of material at the site. In view of this factor and tectonic activity, the order of K assumed appears to be quite reasonable. It is generally agreed now that high in-situ stresses existed at the site of the Vaiont landslide (L. Muller, Salzburg, 1977 pers, comm.).

7.16.2 Estimation of factors of safety

Analyses of stability were made considering (a) no pore pressure and (b) pore pressure corresponding to reservoir level at the time of the slide. Altogether three cross-sections were analysed. (Figures 7.13 and 7.14). The results are shown in Table 7.6 in which

---

* Hendron and Patton based their analysis and explanation of the Vaiont slide on several assumptions, including the assumption of very high artesian pore pressures along the rear part of the slip surface. Their results are considered separately in the next section.

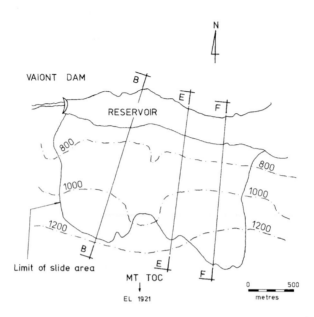

Figure 7.13 Plan of slide area at the Vaiont dam in Italy showing location of sections considered in analysis.

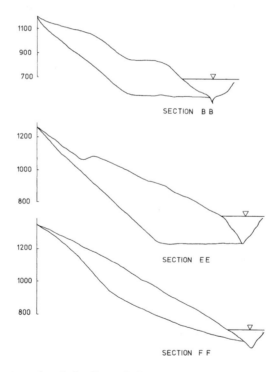

Figure 7.14 Cross sections identified in Figure 7.13 and adopted for analyses by Chowdhury (1978a). The levels are in metres, and the reservoir level at the time of slide is also shown.

Table 7.6 Minimum overall factors of safety during failure progression – Vaiont slide
(after Chowdhury, 1978a). With permission, see page 713, No 27.

Section	Value of K	PWP condition	Minimum F/tan ϕ
BB	1	No PWP	2.1
		Reservoir	1.6
	2	No PWP	1.78
		Reservoir	1.36
EE	1	No PWP	1.98
		Reservoir	1.63
	2	No PWP	1.83
		Reservoir	1.51
FF	1	No PWP	1.72
		Reservoir	1.63
	2	No PWP	1.46
		Reservoir	1.42

Note: PWP = Pore Water Pressure.

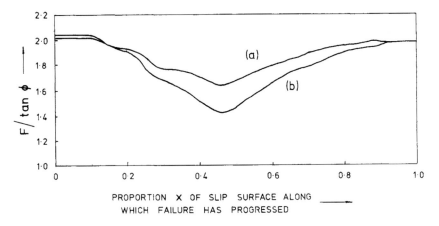

Figure 7.15 Plot of ratio of factor of safety and tan ϕ against x, the extent of failure progression
when (a) $K = 1$ and (b) $K = 2$ (after Chowdhury, 1978a). With permission, see page
713, No 27.

values of the minimum factor of safety are shown as a ratio of tan ϕ, assuming $c = 0$.
The change in the factor of safety with extent of failure progression from the top of
the slide is shown for one cross-section in Figure 7.15.

7.16.3   Approximate estimation of accelerations

In order to calculate accelerations and velocities, the following procedure was adopted.
For each progressive stage of failure the values of acceleration were calculated after
the factor of safety had reached a value equal to unity. The value of ϕ was assumed

Table 7.7 Maximum and average calculated accelerations – Vaiont slide (after Chowdhury, 1978a). With permission, see page 713, No 27.

Section	Value of K	Max. a/g	Average a/g
BB	1	0.70	0.17
			0.29*
	2	1.58	0.52
EE	1	0.68	0.33
	2	1.16	0.63
FF	1	0.76	0.19
			0.34*
	2	1.68	0.58

Note: The value marked * is obtained if negative acceleration towards the end of failure progression is neglected.

to be 28°, the lowest residual value mentioned earlier for limestones. Acceleration a_x relevant to distance of progression x was approximately calculated as follows:

$$a_x = \frac{\text{Driving forces} - \text{Resisting forces}}{\text{Mass of slide}}$$

The approximation involved concerns the assumption of constant mass after the motion has begun and the assumption of resisting forces over the whole of the slip surface. From curves of acceleration versus extent of failure progression x, values of average and maximum acceleration were calculated and these are given in tabular form in Table 7.7 as proportions of the gravitational acceleration g.

7.16.4   Approximate estimation of velocities

The distance travelled by the sliding mass at Vaiont is estimated to be 400 m. Using values of average acceleration given in Table 7.7 average velocities can be calculated. For $K = 1$, and reservoir conditions, the predicted velocities are of the order of 19 m/s to 26 m/s and for $K = 2$, the predicted velocities are of the order of 32 to 34 m/s. The time of travel predicted is in the range of 11–22 seconds. Jaeger (1972) refers to calculations based on external observations which gave a time of travel of 20 seconds. The predicted velocities are also in excellent agreement with the range 18 m/s to 50 m/s which has been suggested on the basis of external observations (including wave height in the reservoir) at the time of the slide. Further, there is remarkable agreement between predicted velocities for different cross-sections for $K = 2$ (and also for $K = 1$ if negative accelerations in the last stages of failure progression are ignored).

7.16.5   Supporting comments

In the opening paper to the 25th Geomechanic Colloquy held at Salzburg in October, 1976, Muller (1977) stated the following after giving a number of examples about the influence of an initial stress field in the earth's crust: "Today I am convinced that the catastrophic slide at Vaiont would have been considered and judged in a different manner after the event, if already then we could imagine that this sliding mass was lying on a rock body under high stresses and that this mass was jerked off like an arrow from a bow".

In a broader presentation the same remark had been discussed one year before by Muller at the conference of the Sonderforschungsbereich 77 Felsmechanik Karlsruhe and a similar note was made in the publication Vol. 2 of the International Symposium "Interprevent 1975" at Innsbruck (L. Muller, pers. comm., 1977). It is useful here to recall that Muller made several detailed studies of the Vaiont slide from the time of its occurrence (e.g., Muller, 1964, 1968) and his remarks give tremendous support to the initial stress approach adopted by Chowdhury (1978a).

7.16.6   Conclusion

Progressive failure calculations presented here take into consideration an initial stress field in the rock mass and its subsequent reorientation during the progress of the rock mass from relative stability to critical equilibrium and then to catastrophic failure. This approach appears to provide a reasonable explanation for the Vaiont slide. No other explanation has been found satisfactory. The slide did not involve any recognised phenomenon of liquefaction and was not associated with any unusual external event such as a major earthquake or even a seismic tremor. Therefore, it is not possible to explain the actual events unless some attention is given to the initial stress field. If the value of K could be established from field evidence, a more accurate estimate could be made of the average value of ϕ mobilised during failure. Consequently, the dynamics of the slide could be simulated with much greater confidence.

7.17   AN ALTERNATIVE APPROACH FOR ANALYSIS OF THE VAIONT SLIDE (HENDRON AND PATTON, 1985)

7.17.1   Introduction

As stated earlier, many studies of this catastrophic landslide have been carried out but it has not been easy to explain the most important observations concerning the occurrence, mechanism and the dynamics of this slide. Most investigators have assumed that residual shear strength was operative along the whole of the slip surface with zero cohesion and very low value of the angle of internal friction. Even with the assumption of very pessimistic values of shear strength parameters, some other adverse conditions are required to explain the occurrence of the landslide and its high velocities.

Assuming very high artesian pore water pressures along the rear part of the sliding surface, an interesting approach was outlined by Hendron and Patton (1985). Although it introduces several key assumptions which may be regarded as unrealistic or at least questionable in the light of previous investigators, it deserves to be considered as a serious attempt to explain the landslide. Besides, it is an alternative in stark contrast to the one based on the initial stress approach. Thus the reader should have an opportunity to consider both. Brief introductory references have been made in earlier chapters of this book (sections 1.8, 1.10.6, 2.3.2, 5.6.5, and 5.12.7) to Hendron and Patton's investigation, assumptions and analyses.

7.17.2   2-D static analyses

They first carried out two-dimensional limit (2D) equilibrium analyses on three separate cross-sections of the landslide mass. Significantly the method of (vertical) slices was modified in an unusual way. The inter-slice friction angle was assumed to be have the same value (40°) on every vertical slice boundary (see section 5.6.5). It is analogous to a multi-wedge method in which the inter-wedge boundaries are all vertical and the resultant force on any such boundary has the same inclination to the horizontal (40°). Two alternative distributions of artesian pore water pressure were assumed on the rear part of the slip surface (high and low, corresponding respectively to high and low rainfall). Along the basal part of the slip surface, pore water pressure was considered on the basis of three alternatives in reservoir level (no reservoir, low reservoir and high reservoir).

For two of the three cross-sections analysed, the values of the factor of safety F were significantly below the threshold ($F = 1$) for most of the six cases considered. These results have been summarized in section 5.12.7. Thus the 2D results failed to explain the stability of the landslide prior to reservoir filling or the progress to the condition of critical equilibrium ($F = 1$), prior to the catastrophic change in stability when high reservoir level coincided with high artesian pressures following high rainfall (see section 2.3.2).

7.17.3   3-D static analyses

A three-dimensional (3D) character was postulated for the landslide and justification for this assumption given in terms of the local and regional geology, interpreted from previous detailed investigations of the site. Consequently, it was decided to include three-dimensional (3D) effects in the analysis. A very simplified approach was used to calculate the 3D factor of safety by including the end-resistance at the eastern boundary of the landslide. A friction angle of 36° was assumed along this boundary (see sections 5.6.5 and 5.12.7). Moment equilibrium of the slide body was not considered nor was a rigorous check made of the force equilibrium in the 3D analysis. Nevertheless, the calculated values for the three-dimensional factor of safety were generally sensible. Significantly, the condition of critical equilibrium was predicted for the worst case scenario, the high reservoir-high rainfall case.

It is obvious that pore water and internal friction angle data must have been chosen so as to match a critical equilibrium condition for the most adverse case, high rainfall-high reservoir. These data would be (a) pore water pressure distributions on the rear part of slip surface (b) internal friction angle along the slip surface, (c) the inter-wedge friction angle in 2D method of slices which was modified in an unorthodox manner, and (c) the friction angle along the eastern boundary. Only when this match was obtained, was the method applied to all the cases or combinations of reservoir level and artesian pore water pressure.

The reader should understand that a match of $F = 1$ for the worst case or most adverse case (high rainfall-high reservoir) might also be obtained by considering a number of alternative scenarios or alternative combination of parameters (different pore water pressure distributions with different values for the above three friction angles). The results for 3D values of F as well as 2D values of F are summarized in section 5.12.7.

7.17.4   Analyses for the dynamics of the landslide

Next they carried out analyses for the motion of the landslide mass associated with the decrease of the factor of safety below 1. Based on previous studies of the Vaiont slide, Hendron and Patton (1985) noted that the total horizontal displacement of the slide mass, approx. 400 m, took place in less than a minute and that the maximum velocity of the sliding mass was in the range 20–30 m/sec. As per their static analyses, the shear strength along the sliding surface was already at the residual value represented by the residual friction angle of 12°. Therefore, the observed high velocity of the sliding mass would have resulted from further loss of shear strength caused by other factors or processes. Three contributing factors were proposed by Hendron and Patton (1985) for this loss and supported by calculations.

The first proposed factor was the decrease in inter-slice shear strength angle from 40° to 30°, accounting for an initial acceleration increase of 0.048 g and a maximum velocity increase of about 7 m/sec.

The second proposed factor was a decrease in the 3D contribution at the eastern end of the slide represented by a drop in the angle of shearing resistance along the vertical boundary plane from about 36° to about 25°. This would result in an initial acceleration increase of 0.035 g. The combined effect of the two factors would be an initial acceleration increase of about 0.08 g and a maximum velocity of 12 m/sec, substantially lower than that required for the mass to travel the observed distance in the short time.

The third proposed factor was the heat-generated pore pressures calculated by Anderson (1985). The permeability of the sliding mass is an important factor in the analysis. The lower the permeability, the lower is the rate of movement required for the development of heat-generated pore pressures. It may be noted that such a mechanism of pore pressure increase had been proposed earlier by Romero and Molina (1974), Habib (1976) and Goguel (1978). According to Anderson's calculations, the velocity of the slide increases slowly until displacement reaches 12 m and then velocity increases rapidly, so much so that a 66% loss in strength could occur after a displacement of just 19 m. It would thus seem that the first two proposed contributing factors are the only triggers for the proposed process of strength loss and associated slide dynamics.

7.18   FINAL COMMENT ON THE TWO ALTERNATIVE EXPLANATIONS

7.18.1   Approach based on initial stress field and simulation of progressive failure

The results obtained for the Vaiont case study, on the basis of the 'initial stress' approach, are a vindication of a new analysis method based on a logical development of widely accepted geotechnical concepts. More importantly, the methodology takes into account the observed phenomenon of progressive failure at the site of the Vaiont landslide. Moreover, the basic information available from early investigations of the site is considered without any amendment or manipulation. The reader may refer to Chowdhury (1987b) for further discussion.

The comments made by an expert of the stature of Muller (1977) about the existence of a high stress field, at the site of the Vaiont dam justify the adoption of a method of analysis which takes 'initial stress' into consideration. Even so, the chosen values of K (either $K = 1$, or $K = 2$) are not unreasonably high. Unproven assumptions are not made concerning pore water pressures along the slip surface. Muller's comments have been quoted at the end of section 7.15.

It is interesting to note that Sitar et al. (2005), who used Discontinuous Deformation Analysis (DDA) to analyse the Vaiont slide, commented that their results agreed with those obtained by Chowdhury (1978a) on the basis of the 'initial stress approach'. However, it must be noted that a detailed comparison was not presented. Nevertheless, it is noteworthy that the DDA approach is entirely different from the 'initial stress approach' and yet, it appears from the comments of Sitar et al. (2005) that the results obtained by the two methods are similar.

Inspite of the above claims, one must acknowledge a weakness. This relates to the lack of measured data concerning the initial stress field at the Vaiont site before the occurrence of the landslide. It is also not known if any data concerning ground stresses in the region have been obtained after the catastrophic failure. It is important that attempts be made by researchers to measure initial stresses in the region. In the absence of quantitative data, attempts could at least be made to obtain other evidence of ground stresses, direct or indirect, in order to support the comments of Muller concerning the existence of a high initial stress field at the Vaiont site.

7.18.2   Approach based on assumed high artesian pressures and heat-generated pore water pressures

The approach adopted by of Hendron and Patton offers a reassessment of the site and the data so that limit equilibrium concepts could be used to explain the static stability conditions before the occurrence of the slide and also the conditions corresponding to the instant of critical equilibrium. Yet, there are a number of weaknesses such as the following:

i   The process of progressive failure from stability to critical equilibrium is not recognized by the method.
ii   Assumption of very high artesian pore water pressures is simply unproven and almost in the realm of conjecture.
iii   Modification of the 2D static analysis based on a constant angle of friction at inter-slice boundaries introduces uncertainty as to its correctness within the concept of limit equilibrium. It would be interesting to see the results if a recognized limit equilibrium method were used instead.
iv   Consideration of the dynamics of the landslide is reliant on very unorthodox and unproven concepts such as heat-generated pore water pressures.

Consideration of 3D effects in the static analyses appears reasonable and may be considered as the main strength of the approach. However, the side-shear resistance appears to be disproportionate part of the total shear resistance. One must also question if the 3D analysis method is simplistic. While the overall approach of Hendron and Patton is comprehensive, it needs to be supported by additional evidence. Alternative analyses, more closely following accepted limit equilibrium concepts and widely accepted concepts of dynamics, would be helpful for comparison. The opinion of other experts would be important in reaching a final verdict on this approach. The above points have been developed more fully by Chowdhury (1987b).

Chapter 8

Plasticity and shear band analyses – a brief review

8.1 PLASTICITY

8.1.1 Introduction

There have been many recent developments in the theory of plasticity and some of the basic concepts were summarised in chapter 2. Even when the theory was in a very early stage of development it was found useful for the solution of soil stability problems such as bearing capacity and earth pressure (see for example Terzaghi, 1943). At that stage there were no solutions available for slope stability problems based on plasticity theory. Over the last 50 years, the application of plasticity theory in stability problems has grown significantly and many solutions of definite theoretical value have been obtained. In relation to slope stability problems, the main practical use which has been made of these solutions is to check the validity and accuracy of comparable solution obtained by conventional means. It should be remembered that agreement between two solutions based on somewhat different models does not indicate that either model is necessarily correct in representing the behaviour of a real medium or material. On the other hand, such agreement usually serves to illustrate the extent to which the assumptions made in different solutions produce similar consequences. Therefore, in assessing the value of a method of analysis or a solution, due attention should be given to the validity of the assumptions that have been made in relation to material behaviour and other factors.

On behalf of plasticity theory, it has been claimed with considerable justification that it places the analysis of a certain class of stability problems on a firm and logical footing. Therefore it has immense conceptual appeal and there are continued research efforts to extend the range of its application. Significant practical application in geotechnical engineering has been limited by restrictions on geometrical and loading conditions, material behaviour and the requirement in many cases of homogeneity of the medium. Because of these factors, methods of analysis based on plasticity theory have not been widely adopted in engineering practice to solve slope stability problems. The limitations of limit equilibrium solutions discussed in section 4.1 apply equally to many plasticity solutions. Moreover, at the present time, the range and scope of solutions that can be obtained by limit equilibrium methods far exceeds those that can be obtained on the basis of plasticity theory.

8.1.2 Scope

There is considerable amount of material on plasticity theory and its applications available in the literature at present. Initially this material was restricted to papers and articles scattered over a wide range of journals. Subsequently, several useful books were published (e.g., Sokolovski, 1960, 1965; Harr, 1966; Chen, 1975) which deal with plasticity theory and its application in soil mechanics. These cover classical plasticity theory; limit analysis as well as numerical techniques of solution although there is no book available in which all types of methods are presented together.

Within the scope of this chapter, it is only possible to present a brief overview of the concepts of plasticity and to relevant slope stability. Considering the aims of this book it is not considered desirable to review methods and solutions which are of conceptual as well as practical value. In this brief review it is possible to mention only the significant work. There are several reasons why only brief coverage of different methods is attempted here:

(1) The limited size of this book does not allow space for the derivation of formulae and detailed description of methods of analysis. (2) This book aims at charting a middle course between theory on the one hand and practical realities of slope analysis on the other. (3) Recent books written specially on application of plasticity in soil mechanics are widely available.

8.1.3 Material idealisation and types of solutions

Three basic conditions are required for valid solutions to problems in the mechanics of deformable bodies, namely, (1) stress equilibrium equations, (2) stress-strain relations, and (3) compatibility equations relating strain and displacement. In an elastic-plastic material when the loads are gradually increased three stages may be identified: (1) elastic response (2) contained plastic flow and (3) complete failure or unrestricted plastic flow.

Analyses which are based on plasticity require a particular type of idealisation of material behaviour as discussed briefly in chapter 2. Considering plane strain deformation conditions, plastic strains can be characterised by a dilatancy angle v. This angle which is defined on the basis of strain increments (see Section 2.7) may be compared to the angle ϕ which is defined in terms of stresses at failure. A soil may be regarded as a plastic material with an associated flow rule if $v = \phi$. All real soils have a value of v at peak strength which is significantly less than ϕ and only at the ultimate strength does the value of v approach zero.

A value of $v = \phi$ indicates plastic deformation at constant volume. There is one case in which soil behaviour may be considered to approach the ideal case of $v = \phi$ from initial loading to failure, namely undrained deformation of soft saturated clay. For such a case, '$\phi = 0$' concept is valid and at the same time $v = 0$ because no volume change can occur (due to the extremely low permeability of the clay and the fact that the deformation is rapid).

Because of the departure of real soils from ideal plasticity, non-associated flow rules are sometimes used in which generally a constant value of v lower than ϕ is assumed. A variable value of v decreasing from a maximum value at peak to zero at ultimate strength would, in fact, be more realistic.

Solutions may be obtained by the application of classical plasticity requiring a rigorous analysis. This is not always possible and,therefore, limit analysis solutions are often obtained. In this type of analysis upper bounds or lower bounds or both are obtained for the collapse load. Sometimes the upper and lower bounds are identical indicating that a correct or unique solution to the problem has been obtained. In other cases one has to be content with a possible close bracketing of the solution within two bounds. Classical plasticity solutions are often difficult to obtain and it is fortunate that the development of the finite element method has made numerical solutions possible. Such a solution may require that a loading path be followed to collapse. The load is applied in increments and a finite element analysis carried out to study the effect of each increment. For each incremental step, checks and adjustments are made for the failure criterion and the particular flow rule. The analysis of strain-softening materials is difficult. However, approximate solutions can be obtained by making suitable assumptions with regard to the way in which the strength decreases from peak to residual. Bounds can also be obtained on the basis of solutions for hypothetical plastic materials obeying either the peak or the residual strength of the real material.

8.2 CLASSICAL ANALYSES

8.2.1 Introduction

In this approach for soils, the Coulomb yield criterion is combined with the equations of equilibrium to give a set of differential equations which can be solved to study the stresses at the instant of failure by plastic flow. The equations are transformed to curvilinear co-ordinates so that their directions at every point coincide with the directions of failure planes or slip planes. The Mohr-Coulomb failure criterion is generally used so that at every point the slip lines make an angle of $(45° + \phi/2)$ with the direction of the minor principal stress which varies from point to point. This network of slip lines is called a slip line field and the method is often called the slip line method.

It is not generally possible to obtain closed-form solutions. Sokolovski (1960, 1965) used a numerical technique based on finite-difference approximations to solve a number of stability problems. In this approach the medium is initially assumed to be weightless enabling a preliminary solution to be obtained. Subsequently parameters associated with the solution technique called the method of characteristics are selected so that the solution applies equally well to a medium possessing weight. The solution is obtained for the appropriate boundary conditions in a tabular form and from the characteristics, the slip line field and the surface of discontinuity is finally determined. The stresses within the slip lines may be obtained by interpolation from the nodes of the slip line field.

8.2.2 Critical profile of a slope with loading on the crest

The type of problem concerning the stability of slopes considered by Sokolovski is one in which it is required to determine the critical profile or shape of a slope, the horizontal top surface (or crest) of which may be subjected to an arbitrary loading. A critical profile is one which produces failure of the soil mass corresponding to the strength parameters assumed in the solution. Therefore a slope which is less steep than the critical profile is safe and one which is steeper than the critical profile is unsafe. The profiles usually show marked curvature and are concave upwards.

For the case of a weightless material with a uniform load q per unit area on the crest of the slope (assumed to be horizontal) the slope profile has no curvature and a closed form solution for the uniform inclination α is obtained as follows:

$$\alpha = \frac{\pi}{2} + \frac{\cot\phi}{2}\, \ell n\left(\frac{q}{c\cot\phi}\frac{1-\sin\phi}{1+\sin\phi} \right) \tag{8.1}$$

in which α is the obtuse angle made by the slope with the horizontal (Figure 8.1).

Since the soil mass is assumed to be homogeneous, c and ϕ are constants. Therefore Equation (8.1) predicts constant i.e., uniform inclination of the critical profile. This equation is subject to the condition that $\alpha \geq \pi/2$ and therefore the equivalent normal pressure q must satisfy the condition that:

$$q \geq (c\cot\phi)\frac{1+\sin\phi}{1-\sin\phi} \tag{8.2}$$

Again it appears from examination of Equation (8.1) that the solution is not valid when unit cohesion $c = 0$ for the assumed weightless material. When the medium is considered to have weight, the slope profile and slip lines are all curved and the solution must be obtained numerically. In such cases, Equation (8.1) gives the inclination α_0 of the curved critical slope profile at the crest where the slope meets the horizontal ground surface.

An important special case considered by Sokolovski concerns that in which $\alpha_0 = \pi/2$ i.e., when the slope profile has a vertical tangent where it joins the horizontal ground. For this case he obtained:

$$q = \frac{2c\cos\phi}{1-\sin\phi} \tag{8.3}$$

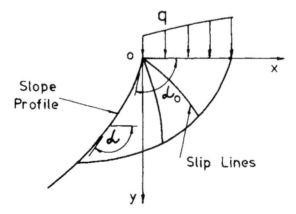

Figure 8.1 Critical slope profile – type of problem considered by Sokolovski (1960, 1965).

Assume that the surface stress q is caused by a uniform soil surcharge of height H_{cr} and unit weight γ. Therefore, we have from Equation (8.3), substituting $q = \gamma H_{cr}$:

$$H_{cr} = \frac{2c}{\gamma} \frac{\cos \phi}{1 - \sin \phi} = \frac{2c}{\gamma} \tan(45° + \phi/2) \tag{8.4}$$

This expression may be considered to represent the critical height of a vertical cut. Comparison with conventional methods shows that Equation (8.4) gives critical height of a vertical cut which is half the value of the critical height predicted on the basis of limit equilibrium calculations (see chapter 4). Recognising this disparity Sokolovski noted that in his approach the surcharge of height H (which is taken to represent the load intensity q) is not considered to be in a state of critical equilibrium as assumed in limit equilibrium calculations. This explanation does not reconcile the different expressions. In fact it is questionable whether the two should be compared at all considering that Sokolovski's approach is concerned with failure below the surcharge of height H which may almost be considered as a problem involving base failure. The determination of critical height of a vertical cut by limit analysis (upper and lower bound techniques) using plane failure and log spiral failure mechanisms is discussed in the next section.

8.2.3 Finding the non-uniform surcharge for a uniform slope of given critical inclination

In general, the solutions concerned with the curvature of the slope profile suggested by Sokolovski are elegant but have little practical value. The reverse problem of finding the non-uniform intensity of surcharge q given a uniform critical slope α has also been tackled. In general, q would vary in intensity along the horizontal crest of the slope. For a weightless material a constant value of q is given by the following expression:

$$q = c \cot \phi \frac{1 + \sin \phi}{1 - \sin \phi} \exp\{(2\alpha - \pi)\tan \phi\} \tag{8.5}$$

in which α is once again the obtuse angle between the horizontal and the slope. More general cases in which the top surface is not considered horizontal have also been considered. These and other solutions including graphical ones have been summarised by Harr (1966).

It is relevant here to note the comment of Chen (1975) that the slip line method ignores the stress-strain relations and that only a partial stress field is generally obtained corresponding to the failed region. A slip line field may be considered acceptable if a kinematically admissible velocity field and a statically admissible stress field can be found for the problem (see section 8.3). Those slip line solutions which consist of a stress solution for the region containing the slip lines and an associated compatible deformation mode are called incomplete solutions and are upper bounds. Complete solutions result when extension of the partial stress solution can be made to the whole body in a statically admissible manner since in that case the slip line solutions are also lower bounds.

8.2.4   Slopes curved in plan

Jenike and Yen (1963) extended Sokolovski's treatment to axisymmetric slopes in homogeneous, isotropic material obeying the Coulomb yield criterion. They considered vertical wells in rock. They found that slopes curved in plan can be made much steeper than straight slopes which have infinite radius of curvature in the horizontal direction. The critical slope inclination increases with lateral constraint which in turn increases with the radius of curvature in a horizontal direction. When the radius of a circular pit decreases with depth, the slopes can be safely steepened with depth for the above reasons.

In discussion, Jenike pointed out that the results must be considered in the light of the fact that only plastic and not elastic behaviour is considered and that the regional stresses are ignored in such analyses. His reference to regional stresses (or initial stresses) is especially pertinent since the release of these stresses may have a dominant influence on the deformations and hence on the behaviour of axisymmetric slopes. They implied that the study of conditions for plastic failure or flow would not be sufficient. This conclusion appears to be in conformity with the strong argument developed in chapter 7 that it is logical to consider the initial stress conditions and then the process of transformation to a simple gravitational stress field and associated changes which may lead to complete slope failure.

It must be noted that Jenike's remarks were made in the context of vertical wells in rock, the problem considered by Jenike and Yen (1963). However, the argument developed in chapter 7 applies to any earth mass in which there is a significant initial stress field.

8.2.5   Uniform slope of soil in which shear strength increases with depth

Booker and Davis (1972) obtained a plasticity solution to the stability of slopes in a soil in which strength increases linearly with depth. This solution corresponds to undrained stability, under '$\phi = 0$' conditions, for a slope in normally consolidated soils in which the ratio of undrained cohesion c to the effective overburden pressure p may be regarded as a constant.

8.2.5.1   Limit equilibrium solution

Gibson and Morgenstern (1962) solved the same problem using a conventional limit equilibrium approach assuming circular failure surfaces. It is useful to consider this solution first. A factor of safety F was obtained as a ratio of resisting and disturbing moments giving (See Figure 8.2):

$$F = \frac{c}{\gamma z \sin^2\alpha \sin^2\lambda} \frac{\{\cot\lambda + \alpha(1 - \cot\lambda\cot\alpha)\}}{\{1 - 2\cot^2\beta + 3\cot\lambda\cot\beta + 3\cot\alpha\cot\lambda - 3\cot\alpha\cot\beta\}} \qquad (8.6)$$

in which z is depth to any point on the slip surface, α is half the central angle of the circular surface, β the slope angle and λ the angle made by the chord of the arc with

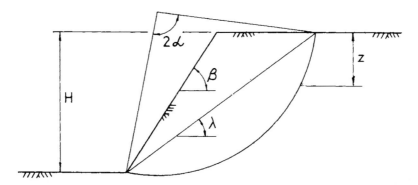

Figure 8.2 Problem analysed by Gibson and Morgenstern (1962) using limit equilibrium approach and by Booker and Davis (1972) using classical plasticity approach. Both solutions are for inhomogeneous cohesive soil in which undrained strength increases linearly with depth. Note that '$\phi = 0$' conditions, considered valid for undrained deformation of soft clay, are assumed.

Table 8.1 Typical values of N [Equation (8.8)].

β	90	53	10	0
N	2	4	11	Infinity

the horizontal. For saturated, normally consolidated fine-grained soils $c/\gamma z$ is a constant given by:

$$\frac{c}{\gamma z} = \left(\frac{c}{p}\right)\left(1 - \frac{\gamma_w}{\gamma}\right) \tag{8.7}$$

Therefore, the factor of safety is independent of the height H of the slope for given slope angle. This result for non-homogeneous soil is most interesting and should be considered in the light of the fact that the factor of safety always decreases with increasing height for all homogeneous cohesive slopes. It was found that an infinity of critical circles passing through the toe or above the toe were possible all of which gave the same minimum value of F. When the slope angle approaches zero the value of F approaches infinity. Taylor (1937) found that F did not approach infinity for homogeneous soils when slope inclination approached zero unless a firm stratum was assumed at some depth.

The critical factor of safety may be considered in terms of a stability factor N, thus:

$$F = N\frac{c}{\gamma z} \tag{8.8}$$

Typical value of N are given above in Table 8.1.

8.2.5.2 *Plasticity solution*

In their plasticity solution to the same problem, Booker and Davis (1972) used the method of characteristics. Combining the equilibrium equations with the failure criterion, hyperbolic equations for the state of stress were obtained which could be represented by characteristics. Equations were then derived to represent the variation in stress. They considered the infinite wedge problem first, the top surface of the wedge being horizontal and the inclined surface representing the slope of infinite height. The condition of failure was interpreted to require that all stresses along any radial line through the apex O (Figure 8.3) increase in proportion to the radial distance. The derived equations were solved with boundary conditions of zero tractions on the surfaces of the wedge, and the kinematic admissibility of the solution was checked. Their solution confirmed that there was only a critical slope angle (or angle of repose) and no critical height. Next they considered the extension of their solution for the finite slope in accordance with the principles of plasticity. This was followed by a check on the kinematic admissibility of the solution which was facilitated by the fact that the stress characteristics are also velocity characteristics when the material deforms plastically at constant volume (as in this $\phi = 0$ case).

From their solution for the finite slope it was found that the limit equilibrium solution is an upper bound to the problem, giving values of unit weight γ to cause failure greater than the value required in the plasticity solution. (In other words for given soil unit weight, limit equilibrium solution gives a lower factor of safety than the one based on plasticity). The difference in the two solutions was less than 10% for slopes steeper than 5°. However, for very flat slopes the difference could be as high as 50%. Considering a practical range of the ratio c/p of 0.15 to 0.4, the range of practical slope inclinations is 6.5° to 24.5° and the slip circle solution cannot be in serious error for this range.

In Equation (8.7) shear strength is assumed to be zero at the surface, i.e., $c = 0$ when $z = 0$. Booker and Davis (1972) suggested how approximate solutions can be obtained for practical cases in which strength increases linearly with depth, starting with a finite value at the ground surface. This can be done by a judicious combination of the limit equilibrium and plasticity solutions to get a close bracketing of the correct solution to the real problem.

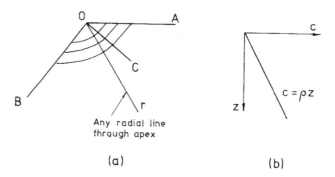

(a)   (b)

Figure 8.3 (a) Infinite wedge problem analysed by Booker and Davis (1972) before finding solution to problem in Figure 8.2. (b) Variation of undrained cohesion with depth assumed in the solution.

An interesting plasticity solution to the problem of mudflows was obtained by Bruiickl and Scheidegger (1973). Profiles were found for both the active and passive modes of failure and the solution for a published case record agreed well with the observed surface profiles.

8.3 LIMIT ANALYSIS

8.3.1 Upper and lower bound theorems

When it is difficult to obtain the exact collapse load directly or to get a classical plasticity solution, it is usual to resort to limit analysis. Plastic limit theorems (Drucker and Prager, 1952) may be used to obtain upper and lower bounds of the collapse load. The lower bound theorem states that for any statically admissible stress distribution unrestricted plastic flow will not occur at a lower load. Therefore the lower bound technique considers only equilibrium and yield and not the deformations or strains. A statically admissible stress field must satisfy the stress equilibrium equations, the stress boundary conditions and must not violate the yield criterion.

In the upper bound technique the external rate of work is equated to the internal rate of dissipation for an assumed mode of deformation also called the velocity field. This assumed mode must satisfy the deformation boundary conditions and the compatibility conditions and is called a kinematically admissible velocity field. The upper bound theorem states that failure by unrestricted plastic flow must have taken place or will take place if a kinematically admissible velocity field can be found. The stresses need not be in equilibrium and the upper bound technique is concerned only with deformations or energy dissipations.

These two theorems of limit analysis may be used to determine the upper and lower bounds to the collapse load for a stability problem. In the case of slopes the critical height (or some other parameter) may thus be bracketed within two bounds.

8.3.2 Example-a vertical slope

8.3.2.1 Upper bound solution with plane failure mechanism

As a simple example, let us consider the limit analysis of a vertical slope (Figure 8.4a). The upper bound may be considered first in terms of a plane failure mechanism. Assuming that failure occurs along a plane at an angle β to the vertical, the rate of work done by gravitational forces is given by multiplying the vertical component of the velocity V (inclined at ϕ to the failure plane) with the weight of the wedge thus:

$$E_1 = \frac{1}{2}\gamma H^2 \tan\beta\, V\, \cos(\phi + \beta) \tag{8.9}$$

The rate of energy dissipation along the discontinuity surface for a Coulomb material is given by the product of the total cohesion and the tangential velocity change as follows:

$$E_2 = cH \sec\beta\, V \cos\phi \tag{8.10}$$

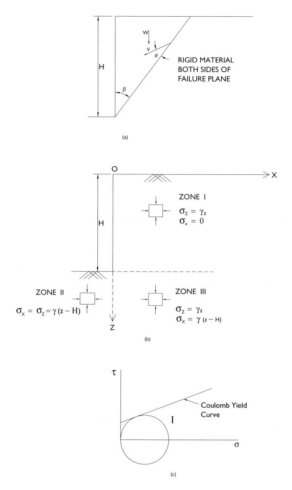

Figure 8.4 Limit analysis of vertical cut in cohesive material: (a) upper bound technique using plane failure mechanism (b) lower bound technique using simple discontinuous stress field (c) yield criterion for lower bound technique.

Equating these two expressions a value of H is obtained which when minimised with respect to angle β gives the critical value of H thus:

$$\beta_{cr} = (45° - \phi/2) \quad \text{and} \quad H_{cr} = \frac{4c}{\gamma}\tan(45° + \phi/2) \tag{8.11}$$

This is the familiar limit equilibrium value implying that the latter is an upper bound unless shown to be exact. The introduction of a tensile crack reduces the critical height by half confirming Terzaghi's (1943) solution for a tensile crack extending the full height of the cut.

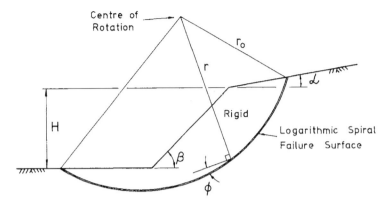

Figure 8.5 Geometry of slope problem analysed by Chen (1975) using logarithmic spiral failure mechanism (upper bound limit analysis technique).

8.3.2.2 Upper bound solution with a rotational failure mechanism

Alternatively, a rotational failure mechanism may be considered assuming the slip surface to be a logarithmic spiral. The justification of a log-spiral surface in terms of plasticity is that, apart from a plane surface, it is the only one which permits a rigid body motion relative to a fixed surface. The log-spiral is, therefore, widely used in limit analysis by the upper bound technique as the plane surface does not give satisfactory results in most problems. However, such a curve and must be of angle ϕ, i.e., it must be of the form $r = r_0 \exp(\theta \tan\phi)$, in which θ is the angle between radious vectors r and r_0 (Figure 8.5). For '$\phi = 0$' conditions, a log-spiral curve becomes a circle.

In limit equilibrium calculations such a log spiral has been found very useful since all resultant forces of reaction along the surface pass through the origin of the spiral and have a zero moment about it, thus simplifying moment equilibrium calculations considerably. The details of calculation with the log spiral mechanism for a vertical cut are lengthy and are not reproduced here. Reference may be made to Chen (1975) who gives the following value of the critical height:

$$H_{cr} = \frac{3.83\,c}{\gamma}\,\tan(45° + \phi/2) \tag{8.12}$$

This is the same value obtained by Fellenius (1927) using the limit equilibrium method. His solution is thus an upper bound unless shown to be exact.

8.3.3 Lower bound solution

A lower bound solution to the vertical cut problem may be obtained by constructing a stress field composed of three zones (Figure 8.4b): a zone subjected to uniaxial compression within the slope (Zone I), a zone of hydrostatic compression beneath the base of the cut (Zone II) and a zone of biaxial compression in between (Zone III). Failure occurs when the Mohr circle representing Zone I meets the yield curve (Figure 8.4c). Therefore:

$$\frac{\gamma H}{2} = c \cos\phi + \frac{\gamma H}{2}\sin\phi \qquad (8.13)$$

Equilibrium is satisfied everywhere and the failure criterion is not violated. Also the stress boundary conditions are satisfied. Therefore the solution gives a lower bound and from Equation (8.13) we have:

$$H_{cr} = \frac{2c}{\gamma}\tan(45° + \phi/2) \qquad (8.14)$$

Note that the assumed discontinuous stresses are not necessarily the actual stresses even when the lower and upper bounds coincide. Equation (8.14) shows that the lower bound is one half the upper bound for the cut without a tension crack but equal to the upper bound for a cut with such a crack for the full height. Thus, in the latter case, the solution is exact. In the former case, the average may be used in which case the maximum error is limited to 33%. The lower bound may be improved by choice of alternate, perhaps more complex stress fields.

8.3.4   Scope of solutions for general cases

Most of the work on slope stability by limit analysis has been done using the upper bound technique (e.g., Chen and Giger, 1971; Chen, 1975; Karal, 1977a, b). Chen (1975) has given the solution for the critical height of a slope defined by angles α and β as shown in Figure 8.5 based on the upper bound theorem. Log spiral surfaces were considered to pass either through the toe or below the toe. He found close agreement between the results given by limit analysis and those given by limit equilibrium methods. Comparison was made with values of $\alpha = 0$ only for which the latter solutions are readily available. Typical values of stability factor $N_s = \gamma H_c/c$ are given in Table 8.2.

In view of the fact that limit equilibrium solutions agree with the upper bound solutions from limit analysis, it is not surprising that the former solutions are considered to be conservative. Few lower bound solutions appear to have been obtained for slopes. The reader may however refer to Lysmer (1970), Chen (1975), Basudhar (1976), Singh and Basudhar (1993a, b) for applications of the lower bound technique of limit analysis to soil stability problems.

Chen (1975) also tabulated values for the case when the crest of the slope is not horizontal, i.e., $\alpha > 0$. No comparable tables or graphs are readily available for this case from the limit equilibrium method. Further, he solved the problems of slope stability in anisotropic, non-homogeneous soil taking into consideration (a) the variation of cohesion with direction and (b) variation of cohesion with depth. He found close agreement between his results for anisotropic soil with those of Lo (1965) who used the ϕ-circle limit equilibrium approach. Chen (1975) also demonstrated the use of the upper bound technique for any non-uniform slope (with a broken inclined face) as well for any slope in a two-layer material.

Table 8.2 Comparison of stability factor $N_s = \gamma H_s/c$ by limit equilibrium and limit analysis (when $\alpha = 0$ in Figure 8.5), after Chen (1975). Permission requested, see page 714, No 42.

		Curved failure surface			Limit analysis
		Limit equilibrium analysis considering			
β	ϕ	Slices	ϕ Circle	Log spiral	Log spiral
90	5	4.19	4.19	4.19	4.19
75	0	4.57	4.57	4.57	4.56
60	25	12.20	12.65	12.82	12.74
45	0	5.88	5.88*	5.88*	5.53*

* Critical surface passes below the toe.

Attention was also given by Chen to different shapes of slip surfaces. From the comparative results of Taylor (1948) using plane, circular and log-spiral failure surfaces for the same problem, it was found by Chen that the log-spiral surface gives the most critical shape as well as the minimum weight W of the sliding mass. The condition of minimum weight was used as a criterion to study the shape of the critical surface of sliding by an optimisation technique based on variational calculus. The results confirmed that the log spiral shape was the most appropriate shape. When $\phi = 0$, the log-spiral becomes a circular surface. As noted earlier, the main advantage of a log-spiral with angle ϕ is that all frictional forces acting on the surface are directed towards the centre of the spiral. Thus the equations of moment equilibrium do not involve any term containing these frictional forces. Therefore it is not necessary to know or to assume the normal stress distribution on the surface of sliding in order to solve the problem statically. In any case, the difference between solutions obtained with circular and log-spiral surfaces is not significant for any arbitrary value of ϕ.

8.3.5 Extension of solutions to more realistic or complex problems

The extension of Chen (1975) solutions to cases with pore water pressure has been demonstrated by Michalowski (1995). The pore water pressure was represented by the simple dimensionless pore pressure parameter r_u which is used in most slope stability charts. Since this parameter is a homogeneous one for the whole slope, realistic representation of spatial variability of pore water pressure has not been considered. It is also important to remember that these solutions do not include consideration of elastic parameters or the initial state of stress or the stress path. Of course, these factors have no influence on the collapse load for a material obeying associated flow rule of plasticity. However, for realistic soil models with non-associated flow rules, these factors must be considered and reference has been made in chapters 2 and 7 to numerical solutions for such cases (e.g., Dounias et al., 1996; Potts et al., 1997). Further attention is given to the use of advanced numerical methods below and in section 8.4.

8.3.6 Possible future extension to modeling of progressive failure

The problem of progressive failure of slope does not appear to have received attention in plasticity and no limit analysis solutions for slopes are available which take account of various concepts or mechanisms of progressive failure. The situation is not much different with regard to other stability problems such as bearing capacity of footings or the pressure on retaining walls, although in some cases progressive development of failure zones has been studied. There is still plenty of scope for further use of limit analysis in stability problems. Capacity to handle progressive failure would certainly be of great value and would pave the way towards making limit analysis a popular working tool.

As discussed in the next section, there has been considerable focus using plasticity models in combination with sophisticated numerical methods for solving problems of progressive slope failure in strain-softening soil (e.g., Dounias et al., 1996; Potts et al., 1997). The requirements of detailed input data may, however, be forbidding. Therefore, many advanced numerical approaches are generally employed for research work only.

8.3.7 Extension of upper bound method

An extension of the upper bound method called the 'energy method' was proposed by Karal (1977a, b). As an improvement to earlier methods which deal only with conditions at failure, he suggested that analyses may be made for design or equilibrium conditions (in addition to those for failure conditions which are usual) by working in terms of mobilised strength parameters $c_m = c/F$ and $\tan\phi_m = \tan\phi/F$. The method allows the inclusion of pore water pressures due to submergence, seepage etc. and takes account of different boundary deformation conditions. Solutions are not restricted to specific geometrical and loading conditions and layered soil media may be tackled provided kinematically admissible mechanisms are constructed. In common with previous upper bound techniques, the method assumes plane strain, ideal plasticity, constant loading during plastic flow and constant degree of shear stress mobilisation (at equilibrium or at failure whichever condition is being considered; this last assumption implies a constant factor of safety for slope problems).

The basic approach is to solve a stability problem by requiring energy equilibrium during plastic flow in a medium. The total rate of work U_1 of external forces during plastic flow is equated to the rate of energy dissipation U_2 within the failure mechanism. From this equation the unknown quantity (which may be factor of safety, external load, critical height of slope, bearing capacity, etc.) is determined. This is repeated for other failure mechanisms to determine the lowest value of the external load or the factor of safety by trial. The quantity U_1 is the sum of two components: (1) The first component is the sum of work done by each external load (external stresses are converted into loads). The work by any load is given as usual by the product of the load and the component of deformation in its direction. (2) The second component is the sum of work done by all body forces e.g., those due to seepage and, earthquake acceleration. The work done by a particular body force is obtained by integrating the product of body force intensity and corresponding displacements over the relevant volume over which the body force acts. The quantity U_1 is given by the product of plastic stress and strain vectors determined by the yield criterion and the flow rule.

The energy method was found to give results close to those obtained by the usual upper bound technique of limit analysis or by the limit equilibrium technique. The method does not enable the determination of approximate stress distribution along shear surfaces or interfaces of slides which is possible in many limit equilibrium methods. It may enable determination of failure mechanisms which give lower factors of safety than those given by conventional procedures, although this has not yet been demonstrated. It must be stated again that this extension proposed by Karal (1977a) does not offer the possibility of tackling problems of progressive failure at least at present. It is also necessary to point out that care is required in the interpretation of equilibrium analyses as proposed by the use of c_m and ϕ_m in place of c and ϕ respectively. This device of using mobilised parameters does not alter the fact that a medium known or considered to be in stable equilibrium is studied by a technique requiring that plastic flow be assumed to occur in the medium.

8.4   PLASTICITY SOLUTION BY FINITE ELEMENTS

8.4.1   Introduction

Numerical methods of stress analysis have been widely used to obtain solutions to different stability problems in soil mechanics on the basis of the theory of plasticity. Of these methods the finite element method is not only the most powerful but also the most versatile. It is, therefore, hardly surprising that this method has replaced other numerical techniques almost completely. The use of the finite element technique enables numerical solutions to be obtained when rigorous or closed-form solutions are difficult to obtain. It enables the solution of problems on the basis of either an associated flow rule or a non-associated flow rule. In such numerical solutions it is possible to take into consideration different yield criteria for the medium under consideration. Behaviour of soil before complete collapse can be studied and the influence of loading path may also be determined.

8.4.2   Strength reduction technique

In applying finite element analysis (FEM) to most geotechnical applications, the load may be applied in increments (the increments becoming very small as colloapse approaches) and the collapse load identified when deformations increase at an excessive rate. For slopes, the strength reduction approach, first introduced by Zienkiewicz et al. (1975), has proved attractive to many investigators (Donald and Giam, 1988; Matsui and San, 1992; Ugai and Leshchinsky, 1995; Dawson et al., 1999). It should be noted, however, that Dawson et al. (1999) did not use FEM but the finite difference method; specifically, the explicit finite difference code FLAC was used. Interestingly enough, the strength reduction safety factors were very close but not exactly equal to limit analysis solutions obtained by Chen (1975) for a wide range of values of parameters including pore pressure ratio, slope angle and dimensionless parameter incorporating unit weight, cohesion and critical height. FEM plasticity solutions have also shown close but not perfect agreement with limit analysis. FEM and FDM solutions are slightly higher than the limit analysis solutions.

8.4.3   Non-homogeneous slopes and realistic material behaviour

It is important to note that, for non-homogeneous slopes, and also in order to incorporate realistic soil models, it is necessary to use one of the advanced numerical methods such as FEM. For instance, Jiang and Magnan (1997) developed the finite element solution based on the constitutive law of plasticity and then used it to analyse several non-homogeneous embankment slopes and compared the results to those obtained by others on the basis of alternative methods (mainly limit equilibrium methods with vertical slices). The agreement was close in most cases, especially where the slip surface was found to be within a narrow shear band interpreted from the velocity fields based on the finite-element analysis. In some cases, the velocity field does not predict a narrow shear band and, therefore, the results are not as close to those based on limit equilibrium. In the latter cases, the stress or strain state below the slip surface is of no consequence and is thus disregarded. However, in the finite element solution based on plasticity, there is a velocity field covering the whole slope. It is important to understand this important conceptual difference although the results are often essentially close though not exactly the same.

8.4.4   Simple and advanced soil models

Generally a perfectly plastic or an elasto-plastic or bilinear stress-strain behaviour is assumed. The exact details of satisfying the requirements of plasticity as specified vary to a large extent although in every case several iterations are required within each loading increment to obtain an acceptable distribution of stresses and strains. Davis and Booker (1973) have emphasised the necessity for checking, for every load increment, that the increment in plastic work in every element is positive. They demonstrated that solutions in which negative plastic work is not allowed to occur converge to the analytical solution better than those in which no check is made for positive plastic work. In discussion, Palmer (1973b) and Smith (1973) questioned if this requirement was really essential but their arguments were advanced from a particular theoretical stand point only.

Zienkiewicz et al. (1975) proposed a visco-plastic model as a realistic one for soil behaviour, and then applied their formulation to the solution of different stability problems in soil mechanics. Both associated and non-associated forms of simple elastic, ideally plastic behaviour were considered. They commented that the usual bounding theorems were not applicable in non-associated forms and that collapse situations predicted by these different from those given by limit theorems. Two slope problems were considered namely, a single stage excavation and a single stage embankment. They used the technique of reducing the values of c and ϕ simultaneously by a factor of N until collapse occurred. In both cases the results agreed closely with alternative solutions by limit equilibrium methods. As stated earlier, this strength reduction technique continues to be popular with researchers and others even three decades after the publication of Zienkiewicz et al. (1975) although several other techniques for modeling slopes to failure have also been used successfully.

8.4.5   A slope in homogeneous soil resting on a rough base

Davis and Booker (1973) studied the problem of a 45° slope with a ratio $E/c = 200$ and $\phi = 30°$, assuming a rough base at a distance from the base of the slope equal to the height H of the slope. They used the associated flow rule as well as a non-associated flow rule with $v = 0$. The values of critical stability factor $\gamma H/c$ were lower than the Taylor limit equilibrium value in both cases. However, the associated flow rule result was closer to the Taylor solution. Lack of close agreement may be due to the kinematic restrictions of the boundaries which must be selected before a finite element analysis is performed. (An infinite extent of soil cannot be considered in this method). Davis and Booker also gave some attention to strain-softening though not in relation to a slope problem or any practical soil stability problem. From a simple example it was shown that in a strain-softening material the loading path has a significant influence on the peak collapse load although the residual load was not different for the two loading paths studied. The analysis of slope problems involving strain-softening calls for further research. Similarly it is necessary to simulate the process of slope formation if plasticity theory is to be extended to realistic situations. By such extensions full advantage can be taken of the versatility of the finite element technique. In incremental studies of embankments and excavations, the influence of initial stress states and history of construction on the behaviour of soil or rock masses can be usefully studied (see chapters 6 and 7).

8.5   SHEAR BAND CONCEPT

8.5.1   Questions relevant to formation and significance of shear bands or slip surfaces

The concept of slip surfaces is an accepted one in soil mechanics and particularly in relation to slopes. It implies that deformation is concentrated in narrow zones which separate regions in which deformations are relatively insignificant. It is of interest to consider the initiation and growth of slip surfaces and the conditions which are favourable to such growth. Such studies seem to be particularly pertinent to overconsolidated clays and clay-shales in which failure is known to be progressive.

Many failures in rock occur along well-defined discontinuities which can be observed or the existence of which can be inferred from field investigations. However, some failures do occur in which slip surfaces do not entirely follow discontinuities. Failures across bedding planes are not uncommon especially in softer rock formations. In soils the shape of slip surfaces is often curved although parts of the surfaces may follow discontinuities and planes of contact between strong and weak layers. Several questions arise:

- How are slip surfaces formed?
- How is the length and shape of these surfaces determined?
- In what manner do slip surfaces influence the mechanism of failure?

These questions cannot be properly answered without an appreciation of the importance of progressive failure. Different concepts of progressive failure have been discussed in chapter 2 and reference to these concepts has been made throughout this book. In this and subsequent sections, a recent approach, which may be referred to as the shear band approach is outlined. This approach is based on the assumption that the growth of slip surfaces is itself a progressive phenomenon.

8.5.2   Some relevant applications reported in the literature

The following paragraphs will, in fact, deal primarily with shear bands in slopes of cohesive soils. Basic mechanisms and field observations of shear band propagation in cohesive soils have been of great interest to researchers for several decades (Bishop, 1967; Bjerrum 1967). An interesting case of field observation of ground movement and progressive failure in Oxford clay was described by Burland et al. (1977). The Selborne cutting stability experiment, a full-scale field trial (Cooper et al., 1998), is another interesting example of careful observation of shear band development. Reference has already been made to advanced numerical analyses of slope performance which enabled the simulation of shear band development at different time stages of a clay slope (e.g., Potts et al., 1997).

Before proceeding to energy approaches that have been used for simulating shear band development in clays and for exploring the scale effect, it is important to consider if shear band development might, in fact, be relevant to cohesionless soils as well.

In that connection, it is interesting to note that evolution of shear band systems in sands behind flexible retaining walls was studied successfully in laboratory experiments (Lesniewska and Mroz, 2000). It is even more interesting that the limit equilibrium approach facilitated the interpretation of results. The plastic softening of soil was expressed in terms of the angle of internal friction (and cohesion, in the general case of cohesive soil) decreasing linearly with soil wedge displacement. It is an extension of the classical Coulomb wedge analysis. The main similarity with slope stability of stiff cohesive soils is that the existence of multiple shear bands is related to the existence of soil softening. The study was mainly applicable to dense sand although a hypothetically looser sand was also considered for comparison in the analyses.

8.5.3   Cases in which internal deformations of soil mass must be considered

Earlier, it was stated that shear band development may be associated with soils where deformation is concentrated in narrow zones and where the rest of the sliding mass may suffer insignificant deformation.

Some notable exceptions in which the sliding mass cannot be assumed to suffer insignificant internal deformations are (1) liquefaction failures in natural soils which are often but not always triggered by seismic events, (2) failures of loose fills (which often include movement of material from underlying natural formations) due to sudden saturation and (3) failures in quick or extra-sensitive clays. In all these cases the sliding mass moves like a viscous liquid and does not retain its original shape or form. Yet a definite surface of slip is formed even in these cases before failure although the post-failure mechanism is different from ordinary slides.

8.6   PALMER AND RICE APPROACH – THE SHEAR BOX PROBLEM

8.6.1   Introduction

There have been several references in soil mechanics literature to some similarities between typical slope stability problems and problems in the field of fracture mechanics (Skempton, 1964; Bishop, 1967). Appreciating the significance of comments relating to these similarities, Palmer and Rice (1973) developed a new approach on the basis of fracture mechanics concepts. They considered a planar slip surface in a given material to be a crack which exhibits a resistance to sliding in accordance with the shear deformation behaviour of the material. The material surrounding the shear band was considered to deform so as to involve only relative sliding and no normal displacement.

They analysed the conditions for the propagation of

- an existing slip surface of finite length in a long shear box, and
- a slip surface starting from a step or cut in a long slope.

8.6.2   Energy balance equation

Consider a soil with peak and residual shear strengths s_p and s_r respectively and the post-peak shear stress-deformation curve shown in Figure 8.6a. From fracture mechanics concepts the area under the curve of shear stress versus relative deformation in the post-peak range is obtained as the following J-integral for any point P in the soil with a shear band in it: (δ_p refers to the relative deformation of P).

$$J_p = \int_0^{\delta_p} \tau(\delta)\, d\delta \qquad (8.15)$$

Consider a point P close to the tip or the end zone of a shear band where relative displacements are large enough to reduce peak strength s_p to residual stress s_r. The integral Equation (8.15) may be divided into the part contributed by the residual stress which equals ($s_r\, \delta_p$) and the remainder which is given by:

$$J_p - s_r\, \delta_p = \int (\tau - s_r)\, d\delta \qquad (8.16)$$

Equation (8.16) represents the hatched area in Figure 8.6a. Define a displacement $\bar{\delta}$ such that:

$$\int (\tau - s_r)\, d\delta = (s_p - s_r)\, \bar{\delta} \qquad (8.17)$$

It is obvious that $\bar{\delta}$ depends on the shape of the post-peak shear stress-deformation curve (Figure 8.6a). From Equation (8.16) and Equation (8.17):

$$J_P - s_r\, \delta_p = (s_P - s_r)\, \bar{\delta} \qquad (8.18)$$

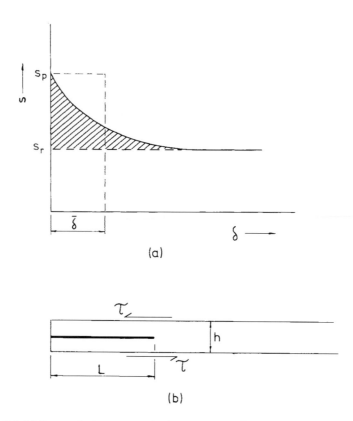

Figure 8.6 (a) Post-peak shear stress-displacement curve for a strain-softening material. (b) Shear band of length L in a long shear box.

Equations (8.16) or (8.18) may be interpreted as an energy balance in which the right hand side represents the energy surplus made available per unit area of advance of the shear band. For stable propagation of any shear band to occur this surplus must just balance the energy due to the excess of the applied shear stress over the residual shear stress along the existing shear band. The shear stresses will depend on the type of problem and the shear resistance would be determined by the given strength parameters for the medium as well as the normal stresses and pore water pressures.

8.7 LONG SHEAR BOX AND INFINITE SLOPE

8.7.1 Long shear box

Consider the soil of thickness h to be in a long shear box and assume that the shear band has developed to a finite length and that the applied shear stress is uniform in the plane of the shear band and equals τ, (Figure 8.6b). From a consideration of the

J integral the left hand side of equation representing the energy due to the excess of the applied shear stress over the residual strength is given as follows on the basis of small strain elastic theory:

$$J_p - s_r \, \delta_p = (h/2G) \, (\tau - s_r)^2 \tag{8.19}$$

in which G is the shear modulus of the soil. From Equations (8.18) and (8.19), the propagation criterion now becomes:

$$(h/2G)(\tau - s_r)^2 = (s_p - s_r) \, \overline{\delta} \tag{8.20}$$

This may be simplified as follows:

$$\frac{\tau - s_r}{s_p - s_r} = \sqrt{\frac{2G}{s_p - s_r} \frac{\overline{\delta}}{h}} \tag{8.20a}$$

The greater the height h of the layer, the smaller the stress τ required for propagation of shear band. This is generally called the 'size effect'. It is easy to show that for stable propagation to occur, h must be greater than a minimum value:

$$h \geq \frac{2G}{s_p - s_r} \, \overline{\delta} \tag{8.21}$$

When the applied shear stress equals the peak strength, simultaneous or runaway failure occurs. Therefore, for progressive failure or propagation of shear band we consider the applied shear stress below that limit leading to Equation (8.21). As Palmer and Rice (1973) pointed out, a huge shear box sample of thickness $h = 1$ metre would be required to study shear band propagation for a soil like London clay (assuming $G/s_p = 50$ and $s_p/s_r = 2$ and $\overline{\delta} = 5$ mm). This may be readily checked from Equation (8.21).

8.7.2   Long slope with a step or cut

Now consider a long slope with a step or cut as shown in Figure 8.7. The cut is assumed to be normal to the slope and a shear band is considered to start from the base of the cut and oriented parallel to the surface of the slope. Considerations of the J-integral of fracture mechanics lead to the following equation (assuming plane strain deformation):

$$J_p - s_r \delta_p = \frac{h(1 - \nu^2)}{2E} \left\{ (\tau_g - s_r)\frac{L}{h} + p \right\}^2 \tag{8.22}$$

in which h is the dimension of the cut, L the length of the shear band required for its propagation, E the modulus of elasticity appropriate to the material of the slope and ν its Poisson's ratio.

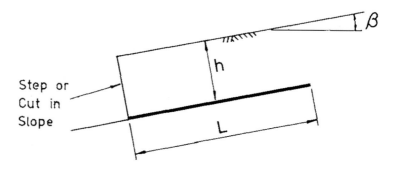

Figure 8.7 Shear band of length L in a slope with a step or cut as shown.

The stresses denoted by τ_g and p are, respectively, the gravitational shear stress along the plane of the shear band and the average normal stress on the face of the cut. These stresses are dependent on the initial stress conditions and the conjugate stress ratio K and can be easily calculated from equations developed in chapter 7. In deriving Equation (8.22), Palmer and Rice assumed the length of shear band to be much greater than the height h of the cut. This is why an average uniform normal stress was considered to act across the cut.

Note that the inclusion of the Poisson's ratio term is appropriate because of the plane strain nature of the problem. Palmer and Rice did not include it in their original equation but in subsequent work (Rice, 1973), that equation was revised to take account of the plane strain nature of the problem.

From Equation (8.18) and Equation (8.22) the propagation criterion becomes:

$$\frac{(\tau_g - s_r)\, L/h + p}{(s_p - s_r)} = \sqrt{\frac{2E}{(1-v^2)}\, \frac{\bar{\delta}}{h}\, \frac{1}{(s_p - s_r)}} \tag{8.23}$$

Simultaneous failure will ensue when τ_g approaches s_p. Therefore the following expression gives the condition for minimum value of h required for progressive failure:

$$\frac{2E}{(1-v^2)\,(s_p - s_r)}\, \frac{\bar{\delta}}{h} < \left\{ \frac{L}{h} + \frac{p}{s_p - s_r} \right\}^2 \tag{8.24}$$

Even when the gravitational shear stress is equal to the residual shear strength, the shear band may propagate because of the energy available due to the release of the stress p acting on the cut in a direction parallel to the plane of the shear band. As stated above a uniform extensional stress is considered along the cut by taking an average value of p. It can be shown that the energy is thus significantly underestimated by about 33% (Chowdhury, 1977c).

8.8   NON-UNIFORM SHEAR STRESS ON BAND

8.8.1   Introduction

In real problems, there is little evidence to suggest that the shear stress along a potential failure can assume only two values i.e., a residual value along the shear band and a peak value outside the shear band. Only when a failure has occurred, does the shear strength approach residual or near residual conditions all along the actual surface of sliding. It is well known that considerable relative deformation is required before residual strength conditions are reached. It is, therefore, unrealistic to consider the shear stresses all along a shear band within a stable slope to equal the residual strength. (Here the word 'stable' is used in the sense that a slide has not occurred). The concepts presented in the previous section may, therefore, be extended to cases in which the shear stress distribution along the shear band is an arbitrary one. Such an extension is possible using a simple energy approach so that there is no need to resort to the *J*-Integral of fracture mechanics.

In the formal approach the zone of transition from peak to residual strength is assumed to be small in relation to the length of the shear band and is referred to as the 'end zone'. Theoretical estimates were made of its size but there was a recognition of the fact that the end zone may, in fact, be large. (See also Palmer 1973a). It is, therefore, of considerable interest to study the influence of the 'end zone' on the propagation criterion. This is achieved below by using an approximate approach rather than a formal one, since there are inherent difficulties in the latter. It is relevant to note that simple and exact analyses were found to compare favourably in basic cases studied by Cleary and Rice (1974) and Rice and Simons (1976).

In the following treatment the distribution of shear resistance or mobilised shear stress along a shear band is considered to be known. This should not be taken to imply that such a distribution can be easily predicted. Here any arbitrary distribution is considered only to study its effect in a qualitative way.

8.8.2   Long shear box

Consider first a long shear box sample as before subjected to shear stress τ. Let the shear band length be L, L_1 being at the residual state (Figure 8.8a) and the strength increasing from residual to peak in an arbitrary manner along the remaining part L_2 of the band. Denoting (L_2/L) by n, the average shear resistance is given by

$$s_{av} = s_r + mn(s_p - s_r) \tag{8.25}$$

in which m depends on the actual distribution of resistance along L_2 and has values between 0 and 1. The driving energy is calculated from the net average shear stress acting along the band. Once again small strain elastic theory is assumed as in the original work of Palmer and Rice (1973). This is always justified since only the strain and deformation of elements outside the shear band is considered. The material above

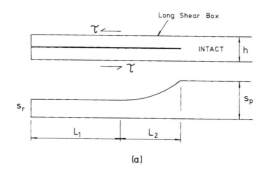

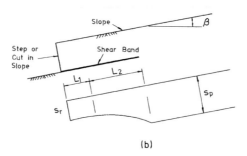

Figure 8.8 Non-uniform shearing resistance along shear band in (a) long shear box (b) long natural slope with cut or step as shown.

the existing shear band is regarded as an overhanging layer which suffers deformation without additional strain. The driving energy is given by:

$$U_D = \frac{h}{2G}(\tau - s_{av})^2 \qquad (8.26)$$

From Equation (8.18) and Equation (8.26) an appropriate propagation criterion is now obtained as follows:

$$\frac{\tau - s_r}{s_p - s_r} = mn + \left\{ \frac{2G\bar{\delta}}{h(s_p - s_r)} \right\}^{\frac{1}{2}} \qquad (8.27)$$

The result in the form of Equation (8.27) is obtained by using Equation (8.18) for the energy released during unit advance of the shear band. It should be noted that Equation (8.18) is the precise expression only when the whole of the shear band is at the residual strength. In the general case considered here, the average shear resistance along the band is greater than the residual and, therefore, an approximation is involved. However, this does not significantly alter the validity of the conclusions or the accuracy of the results.

Equation (8.27) reduces to Equation (8.20a) when $m = 0$ or $n = 0$ corresponding to the case when the shear stress is residual all along the shear band.

8.8.3   Long slope with step or cut

Similar calculations may be made for a slope considering a shear band parallel to the slope surface extending from the base of a cut (Figure 8.8b). The propagation criterion is once again obtained on the basis of small strain elastic theory as follows:

$$\frac{\tau\frac{L}{h}+p}{s_p - s_r} = \left\{ \frac{2E}{1-v^2}\frac{\bar{\delta}}{h}\frac{1}{s_p - s_r} \right\}^{\frac{1}{2}} \tag{8.28}$$

in which

$$\tau = (\tau_g - s_r) - mn\,(s_p - s_r) \tag{8.29}$$

Again, this reduces to Equation (8.23) when $m = 0$ or $n = 0$. Similarly modified forms of Equation (8.21) and Equation (8.24) may be obtained from Equation (8.26) and Equation (8.28) to give the size effect, i.e., the limiting condition for failure to be progressive rather than simultaneous. For example, in the first case:

$$h > \frac{2G}{s_p - s_r}\frac{\bar{\delta}}{(1-mn)^2} \tag{8.21a}$$

For a linear distribution of shear resistance along the entire shear band $n = 1$, $m = 0.5$:

$$h > \frac{8G}{s_p - s_r}\bar{\delta} \tag{8.21b}$$

Comparing this result to Equation (8.21) it is found that the minimum thickness is four times greater in the present case. Therefore, the size effect in modeling progressive failure can be much greater than was revealed by analyses for simpler cases considered in the previous section.

Chowdhury (1977c) also gave consideration to the above problems when the length of the shear box or of the slope is finite. The propagation criterion remains unchanged but simultaneous failure takes place at an average applied stress well below the peak strength and this modifies the size effect significantly depending on the length of the shear box or the slope.

8.8.4   Relatively flat slope – gravitational stress less than residual strength

When the gravitational shear stress along a shear band is less than residual shear strength (as in very flat slopes) the propagation criterion is to be interpreted differently. In fact it only gives an indication of the extent to which a failure surface can develop and numerical examples have been given by Chowdhury (1977c) who also

Table 8.3 Failure surface lengths for two value of $\bar{\delta}$ when
$K = 2$, $\beta = 5°$, $\phi_p = 21.6°$, $v = 0$, $\phi_r = 9.5°$,
$c_p = 62$ kN/m², $c_r = 43$ kN/m², $\gamma = 1600$ kg/m³,
$E = 4790$ kg/m², (after Chowdhury, 1977c).

Product of m and n	h metres	l metres
(a) When $\bar{\delta} = 0$		
0	30	181
0.25	30	130
0.50	30	101
0	3	3.1
0.25	3	2.7
0.50	3	2.4
0	0.3	0.033
0.25	0.3	0.031
0.50	0.3	0.027
(b) When $\bar{\delta} = 10$ mm		
0	30	1.14
0.25	30	0.98
0.5	30	0.86
0	3	1.14
0.25	3	0.98
0.5	3	0.86
0	0.3	
0.25	0.3	No
0.5	0.3	failure

compared his results with those obtained by Christian and Whitman (1969) using a different model of progressive failure (section 8.11). The comparison could only be made for a brittle material with $\bar{\delta} = 0$ because alternative solutions have not been developed for cases when $\bar{\delta} > 0$. Table 8.3 gives maximum failure surface lengths for a typical problem considered also by Christian and Whitman (1969) for two values of $\bar{\delta}$ assuming three different values of slope height and three different values of the product of m and n. Note that a flat slope of 5° inclination is considered.

8.9   SHEAR BAND OF ARBITRARY INCLINATION (AFTER CHOWDHURY, 1978b)

8.9.1   Introduction

Let there be a potential shear plane inclined at any angle α to the horizontal as shown in Figure 8.9a. The driving energy appropriate to the shear band of length L which is at the residual state may be derived as follows:

Consider the deformation of a very small element of length dx just outside the advancing tip of the inclined shear band of length L in Figure 8.9a. The shear stress

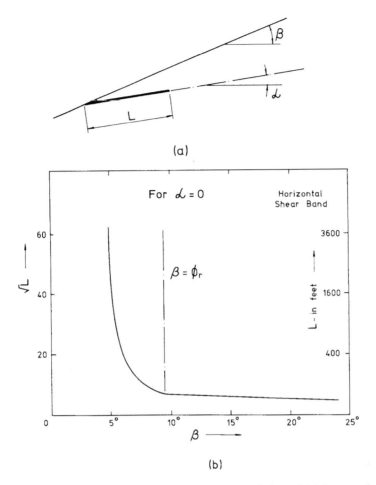

(a)

(b)

Figure 8.9 (a) Shear band of arbitrary inclination in a natural slope. (b) Influence of natural slope inclination on the length of horizontal shear band required for its propagation in a natural slope. Note square root of L is plotted on left and L is in feet – as originally plotted, (after Chowdhury, 1978a, 1977c).

τ and shearing resistance s_r along the shear band are variable because each point has a different depth below the ground surface. (The shear stress and normal stress are directly proportional to the depth below the ground surface and the shearing resistance is linearly related to the normal stress).

8.9.2   Considering the energy balance

Therefore, let us consider a very small length dL of the shear band along which the shear stress and shearing resistance are constant. The net force causing deformation of element of length dx is $(\tau - s_r)\, dL$. Let the deformation of the element be δ_u which is the product of strain ε_x and element length dx. Then the work done during gradual increase of the force by this net amount is given by:

$$\frac{1}{2}\,(\text{Force})(\text{Displacement}) = \frac{1}{2}\,(\tau_\alpha - s_r)\,dL\,\varepsilon_x\,dx \tag{8.30}$$

Assuming small strain elastic theory for the element outside the shear band the strain may be related to the net stress by the modulus E_1. Substituting this in the above expression for work and dividing by the length dx of the element, the energy released is given by $1/2E_1(\tau - s_r)^2\,dL$ per unit length of the element (or per unit length of shear band advance). This is the contribution to driving energy due to small elemental length dL of shear band. For estimating the total driving energy integration may be carried out over the whole length. This yields:

$$U_D = \frac{1}{2E_1}\int_0^L (\tau - s_r)^2\,dL \tag{8.31}$$

The modulus E_1 here is similar to the extension modulus E considered before. It relates the incremental changes in stress and strain of an element outside the advancing tip of the shear band and lying in the plane of the band. In fact, it would be desirable to take a value of the modulus appropriate for plane strain conditions as before. This is accomplished by using a suitable multiplying factor. Therefore, for plane strain, E_1 becomes $E_1/(1 - v^2)$.

8.9.3 The propagation criterion

Equating the driving energy to the energy released during unit advance of the shear band given by Equation (8.18), the following propagation criterion is obtained:

$$\frac{1}{2E_1}\int_0^L (\tau - s_r)^2\,dL = (s_p - s_r)\bar{\delta} \tag{8.32}$$

This may be solved for the length L of the shear band required for its propagation after substitution has been made for normal and shear stresses in terms of variable depth z from (7–28). The integration may be carried out after z is expressed in terms of length L, the inclination of slope surface and inclination of shear band. For the particular case when the shear band is horizontal, i.e., $\alpha = 0$, substitution of shear and normal stresses from (7–19), substitution of z in terms of L and β, and subsequent integration gives the following expression*:

$$L^3A^2/3 - L^2Ac_r + Lc_r^2 = \{(c_p - c_r) + (\tan\phi_p - \tan\phi_r)B\}\,2E_1\bar{\delta} \tag{8.33}$$

---

* The reader may easily derive the corresponding expression for any value of α by substituting for shear and normal stresses from Equation (7.28) in Equation (8.32). This general equation is somewhat lengthy.

in which

$$A = K \gamma \sin^2\beta - \gamma \tan\phi_r \tan\beta(1 + K\sin^2\beta)$$
$$B = \gamma\tan\beta(1 + K\sin^2\beta)L$$

$$(8.34)$$

8.9.4   Results for an example case

The values of length L required for shear band propagation are plotted Figure 8.9b for a typical case in which $c_r = 0$, $c_p = 19$ kN/m², $\phi_r = 9.5°$, $\phi_p = 21.6°$, $\gamma = 1600$ kg/m³, $E_1 = 9580$ kN/m², $v = 0.2$, $K = 2$, $\bar{\delta} = 10$ mm. It is interesting to note that L, the length required for failure propagation, increases sharply when β decreases below ϕ_r. This is understandable because the calculations do not include the effect of a cut and there is no driving force due to stress release caused by excavation. For simplicity shear band propagation is assumed here to initiate at any point on the surface of a natural slope rather than at the base of a cut. For this reason again the length L increases as α increases from 0 to β. It is worth noting that $\alpha = \beta$ is a hypothetical case as the shear band coincides with the surface of the slope for this example of a natural slope without a cut.

The analysis can be further extended to include a cut, arbitrary variation of shear resistance along the inclined shear band in terms of parameters m and n, and the variation of extensional stress p acting along the depth of a cut.

Consideration of the incremental nature of an excavation problem is desirable but presents many difficulties in this type of analysis.

8.10   RATE OF PROPAGATION

Rice (1973) considered the factors which might govern the rate of propagation of shear bands and concluded that dilationally induced suctions could govern the rate of progressive failure of a slope only during the terminal stages of the growth of the shear band. This would involve a time scale of the order of one to several days in typical problems concerning overconsolidated clays. Long-term effects were considered to be explainable in terms of the time-dependent behaviour of the material as a whole as well as due to possible creep effects in the $(\tau - \delta)$ relation. He considered some typical laboratory creep data and estimated that creep effects would require a 10 to 15% increase in average shear stress excess to increase velocity of propagation from an order of 1 m/year to an order of 1 m/day.

Bulk diffusion also influences the rate of propagation. The plane-strain modulus decreases from 4G under completely undrained short-term conditions (assuming $v = 0.5$) to 2.5G for drained conditions (assuming $v = 0.2$). This represents a 37% drop and reduces the driving force term in the energy balance by 21%. Thus the rate of propagation would decrease consequent to initial undrained response due to decrease of driving force energy when drainage occurs. Cleary and Rice (1974) have also discussed time effects and, in particular, the stabilisation of shear faults by coupled deformation-diffusion effects. Further reference is made to rate of propagation in section 8.12.

8.11   A SIMPLE PROGRESSIVE FAILURE MODEL

The problem of progressive failure of a sloping layer of thickness h (Figure 8.10a) discussed in section 8.7 has also been tackled in a different way by Christian and Whitman (1969). However, their aim was not to consider the indefinite propagation of a shear band but only its propagation over a finite length. Also it is valid only for a perfectly brittle material with $\bar{\delta} = 0$ for the stress-strain curve. In their approach, parameters m and n for the actual shear band (Chowdhury, 1977c) are not relevant as the shear band in the slope is considered to be throughout at the residual state. Their proposed model is still of considerable interest and the results agree closely with the Palmer and Rice energy approach for flat slopes in which the gravitational shear stresses are less than residual shear strength. In this solution the pre-peak portion of the shear stress-displacement curve for the shear band was assumed to have a slope of k as shown in Figure 8.10b. Figure 8.10b also shows the brittle nature of strain-softening in the post peak region. From simple equilibrium considerations of a small element and integration of the differential equation, it was shown that first yield occurs if:

$$\frac{p}{s_p} \geq \left(\frac{E}{kh} \right)^{\frac{1}{2}} \tag{8.35}$$

The extent of the failure surface L is given as:

$$\frac{L}{h} = \left\{ -\frac{p}{s_p} + \left(\frac{E}{kh} \right)^{\frac{1}{2}} \right\} \frac{s_p'}{s_r'} \tag{8.36}$$

In these equations s_p' and s_r' are the reduced peak and residual strengths obtained by deducting gravitational shear component ($\gamma h \sin \alpha$) from s_p and s_r respectively.

It is found that if the factor of safety at first yield is greater than one, no yielding takes place. (It can be shown easily that the factor of safety at first yield is given by the ratio of right hand side of Equation (8.35) to its left hand side). As the factor of safety at first yield reduces below one, the length of the failure surface increases. The smaller the factor of safety with respect to the residual strength (in conventional terms) the greater the length of the failure surface. Complete failure occurs when the factor of safety with respect to residual strength (in conventional terms) reduces below one. This might be considered as an indefinite propagation of the failure surface. It might seem contradictory that when the factor of safety against residual strength is greater than one, there is a development of failure. However, one must remember that the release of stress p normal to the cut or step in the slope is acting in addition to the shear stress which is the only driving force in the conventional calculation of the factor of safety.

It may similarly be useful to define a factor of safety for the Palmer and Rice energy calculation (section 8.7) as a ratio of the energy released during unit advance of the shear band and the energy driving the shear band. Thus, in possible future

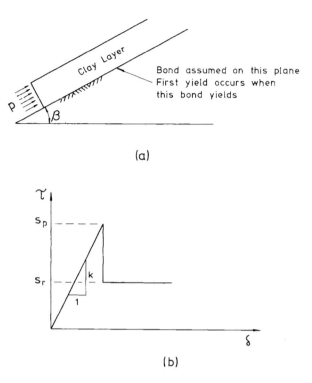

Figure 8.10 (a) Simple progressive failure model considered by Christian and Whitman (1969) in brittle strain softening soil. (b) Shear stress-displacement curve assumed for the model.

developments comparisons could be made with conventional factors of safety. As pointed out in section 8.7, the Palmer and Rice approach gives (a) the length of shear band required for its indefinite propagation when the shear stress is intermediate between peak and residual shear strength values and (b) the length to which a shear band can develop when the shear stress is less than the residual shear strength. When the shear stress equals the peak shear strength there is simultaneous failure and no progressive failure calculation need be made at all.

8.12 APPLICATION OF SHEAR BAND CONCEPTS

Earlier in this chapter energy concepts have been introduced concerning the propagation of shear bands in slopes. These concepts are still in a developing stage but have aroused tremendous interest among geotechnical engineers and researchers. This interest is evident in the discussion following a paper by Rice (1973) during the symposium on plasticity at Cambridge University. The discussion appears in the proceedings edited by Palmer (1973a) and includes a contribution by Burland (1973) in which some evidence of shear band propagation was presented. A cutting in bedded Oxford clay was instrumented and movements were observed during excavation. The measurements which were recorded confirmed the concept of a propagating shear band on which the overlying mass appeared to move as a block. While the theoretical contributions (Palmer and Rice, 1973; Rice, 1973) were based on the assumption of a shallow cut, the example presented by Burland related to a depth of cutting of about 25 metres. Therefore, Rice was reluctant to state that the theoretical model was directly applicable in this case. The precise nature of calculations that would be required to study the propagation of such a shear band may not be the same as suggested in the original model. Perhaps the approximate procedures suggested in this chapter would prove useful. The important thing is that propagation of shear bands has been observed and that there is strong evidence for such propagation in Burland's example. Progress in slope analysis may require a better understanding of how shear bands and slip surfaces are formed. This may be a necessary step towards removing the many uncertainties and difficulties which are encountered in slope analysis. The development of elementary models has alerted research workers and practising engineers alike in this direction and there is no doubt that more case records and measurements will appear in future to clarify the mechanism of progressive failure involving growth of slip surfaces.

It is interesting that Burland presented the same case history again at the 9th International Conference on Soil Mechanics and Foundation Engineering in Tokyo in July, 1977 and complete details were also provided by Burland et al. (1977). The intervening years (1973–77) would have given enough opportunity for the investigators to examine any doubts that might have existed as to the fact of shear band propagation.

Now let us consider another important attempt to apply shear band concepts to real situations. Rice and Simons (1976) examined numerical data based on creep events on the San Andreas fault system in order to understand the basis of stabilisation of these creep movements. They developed the original Palmer and Rice (1973) model further so that speed, slipping length and permeability could be related in a meaningful way. Reported speeds on the fault system ranged between 1 to 10 Km/day and slipping lengths ranged between 0.1 to 10 Km. On the basis of these values and a permeability range representative of fissured and jointed rock masses the theoretical model was able to explain the stabilisation of the creep movements. The calculations are based on the principle that the response of a saturated particulate medium to loading depends on the rate of loading. If excess pore pressures develop faster than they can be dissipated, the response is undrained. If excess pore pressures can dissipate as fast as they are generated the response is drained. When the speed of shear band propagation increases the response tends to be undrained and stiff and this in turn decreases the speed of propagation. That, in essence, explains the stabilisation of creep movements.

Rice and Simons (1976) also considered the rate at which progressive failure occurs in overconsolidated clays. With a typical permeability of $k = 10^{-7}$ cm/sec and a slip surface length of 10 m, speeds in the range 3 m/year to 1 m/day were calculated on the basis of the model. These speeds were considered to be consistent with long-term failures although it was recognised that further study would be required to predict the rate at which slope movements occur. The results so far are only of a qualitative nature and the influence of many other contributing factors must be considered before reliable quantitative data can be obtained concerning the rate of slip surface propagation.

APPENDIX TO CHAPTER 8

C8.1 Slope studies for anisotropic soil

Lo (1965) studied the influence of anisotropy on the stability of slopes in cohesive soil for $\phi = 0$ conditions. He considered only anisotropy due to stress reorientation as discussed in sections 2.9 and in Appendix to Chapter 5. Strength measurements in conventional triaxial tests will invariably be influenced by both types of anisotropy. Therefore, if anisotropic strength parameters from such studies are used, Lo's approach cannot be said to isolate the effects of only one type of anisotropy. The ratio $k = c_h/c_v$ was varied between 0.5 and 1 and was found to have a significant influence on the stability factor $N_s = \gamma H/c_v$. The value of N_s decreased with decreasing value of the anisotropy ratio k in Lo's slip circle solutions for homogeneous soils in which shear strength was assumed to be constant with depth. The influence of anisotropy was less marked in solutions obtained for slopes in inhomogeneous soil in which cohesion increases linearly with depth and was insignificant for steep slopes. Similar results were obtained by Chen (1975) using the upper bound technique of limit analysis. The log-spiral surfaces used in such analysis became circles for these $\phi = 0$ analyses. Excellent agreement between the two types of solutions (limit equilibrium and upper bound limit analysis) is shown below in Table C8.1.

Meyerhof (1965) suggested that approximate solutions could be obtained by using an average cohesion $c = (c_h + c_v)/2$ in isotropic analyses. He also said that anisotropy will influence the shape of slip surfaces which will become elongated in the direction of minimum strength. This in turn will reduce the stability even further than shown by Lo's results.

Matthai and Ranganatham (1968) also studied the influence of anisotropy on the stability factor of a typical slope of height H under $\phi = 0$ conditions assuming circular surfaces of sliding. They varied the ratio k from 2 to 0.2 and found that it has a significant influence on the stability factor. That influence is far greater than the influence of

Table C8.1 Influence of anisotropy ($k = c_h/c_v$) on $N_s = \gamma H/c_v$ assuming constant inclination $f = 55°$ (angle of failure plane with σ_3 direction) and $\phi = 0$: (a) Homogeneous soil, (b) Cohesion increasing linearly with depth (after Lo, 1965; Chen, 1975). Permission requested, see page 714, No 42.

Case	$\beta°$	$k = \dfrac{c_h}{c_v}$	Values of N_s Limit equilibrium Lo (1965)	Limit analysis Chen (1975)
a	50°	1.0	5.68	5.68
		0.7	5.19	5.23
		0.5	4.85	4.95
b	50°	1.0	3.78	3.78
		0.7	3.45	3.45
		0.5	3.17	3.20

the depth factor (ratio of depth to hard stratum and H). The value of $\gamma H/c_v$ decreased from 6.9 to 2.86 as k decreased from 2 to 0.2. Therefore their results show the same trend as those of Lo (1965). However, the type of anisotropy considered is different as they seem to have ignored the value of the orientation of principal stresses and taken the angle θ to be equal to α. Their calculations may be regarded as those for inherent anisotropy. It is interesting that they also found that the critical slip surface becomes flatter with an increase in c_v.

They also proposed a solution to the general problem in which both c and ϕ are anisotropic. However, the proposed solution is based on several oversimplifications. Firstly, a constant ratio K (appropriate to particular stress state, active or passive) was assumed between horizontal and vertical normal stresses. This would be acceptable only for an infinite half-space in which these stresses may be assumed to be principal stresses. When a slope is formed, the ratio of these normal stresses will vary from point to point. Secondly, the vertical normal stress at any depth z was taken equal to γz which is not accurate for a man-made slope (excavation or embankment).

Chapter 9

Earthquake effects and seismic slope analysis

9.1 SEISMIC SLOPE STABILITY AND DEFORMATIONS – AN INTRODUCTION

9.1.1 Aims and scope

9.1.1.1 Introduction

Seismic slope stability is one of the most important areas of geotechnical earthquake engineering. Over the last century there has been an increasing awareness of the adverse impact of earthquakes on slopes, embankments and dams. Catastrophic seismic effects include landslides in natural slopes and the failures of dams and embankments caused either by loss of stability or because of unacceptable magnitude of deformations. Over the last 60 years or so, the response of slopes and earth structures to seismic shaking has attracted tremendous research interest amongst geotechnical engineers. Seismically-triggered failures may be associated with reduction in factor of safety, large deformations and liquefaction phenomena. Research has included the testing of soils under cyclic loading, careful field observations of the nature, location and distribution of failures after earthquakes and detailed studies of individual failures.

9.1.1.2 Ground motion

Seismic activity of sufficient strength to influence the environment or the integrity of structures is called strong ground motion and quantitative description of such motion is necessary for engineering analysis. (Microseismic activity, on the other hand, is mainly of interest to seismologists). Earthquake magnitude and source distance are two of the most important factors which determine ground motion or base rock motion at any particular location. Base rock motion in the form of an acceleration-time relationship or record is the most important seismic data for seismic analysis of a geotechnical structure or a slope. Often, however, the use of the whole of the record may be cumbersome. Therefore, one or more ground motion parameters, derived from the record, are used for assessments of stability and deformation. Typical parameters are peak ground acceleration, duration of motion and predominant period.

9.1.1.3   Site-specific or local slope stability

This chapter is mainly concerned with seismic analysis of slopes and embankments with particular reference to the pseudo-static method and the sliding block approach although reference will also be made to seismic response analyses or dynamic stress analyses. Soil shear strength under seismic conditions is discussed to the extent of its direct relevance to slope analysis. The scope of this chapter, however, does not include detailed discussion of soil stress-strain behaviour under cyclic loading conditions.

9.1.1.4   Regional slope stability

Summaries of research studies and reviews concerning the observed behaviour of natural slopes, embankments and earth dams under seismic conditions are included. An understanding of such behaviour is essential in order to assess the suitability and effectiveness of the various methods of analysis. Catastrophic landslides are associated with earthquakes of relatively high magnitude ($M > 4$) and such landslides can occur tens and even hundreds of kilometres away from the epicentre.

9.1.1.5   Liquefaction

Seismically – induced liquefaction of soils is another very important aspect of geotechnical engineering which can have direct relevance to slope analysis. Only salient aspects of liquefaction which relate to seismic slope stability analysis will be included here. Comprehensive procedures have been developed for assessing the seismic liquefaction potential of soils and for liquefaction-related displacements of level or gently-sloping ground. These topics are outside the scope of this chapter. A lot of research papers have been published concerning empirical approaches for estimating slope deformations. In this chapter, attention will be focused on the concepts and basic methods. Only brief references will be made to empirical equations and charts.

9.1.2   Introducing pseudo-static analysis

A brief introduction of pseudo-static analysis and sliding block analysis is provided below and more detailed discussion is included in later sections.

9.1.2.1   Applying a lateral force in limit equilibrium analysis

Pseudo-static analysis is a tool for simplified evaluation of the seismic factor of safety of a slope. It can be applied to natural or man-made slopes. The earthquake force acting on an element of the slope is represented by a horizontal force equal to the product of the gravitational force and a coefficient, k, the pseudo-static seismic coefficient. Thus the assumed seismic acceleration is k times the gravitational acceleration g ($a = kg$). On a potential sliding mass of weight W the assumed lateral force will be kW.

Analyses performed by several investigators with an inclined seismic force have shown that the inclination can have a significant influence on the value of the factor of safety. The critical (minimum) value of the factor of safety is not necessarily associated with the horizontal direction of the lateral force. In general, a horizontal direction is assumed for the lateral force. There may, however, be situations in which the vertical component of the earthquake force must be taken into consideration.

In the early decades of the development of geotechnical earthquake engineering, most applications were concerned with embankments and dams. However, in recent decades, the pseudo-static approach has also been used for analysis of natural slopes including GIS-based regional landslide hazard analysis.

9.1.2.2   Point of application of lateral force in an analysis

Incorporating the lateral force in an analysis requires a decision as to its point of application. Generally it is applied at the centre of gravity of a potential sliding mass or of a typical vertical slice in any method of slices. Alternatively, the force may be applied at the level of the base of a slice. (Since the seismic acceleration is not constant throughout a potential sliding mass, it is not necessary that the equivalent force is best applied at the centre of gravity of the mass). There can be a significant difference in the result. A well-known example, the analysis of Sheffield Dam, was provided by Seed (1979). With $k = 0.1$ (considered appropriate for an earthquake of magnitude $M = 6.25$ at a distance of 7 miles), the factor of safety was 1.21 when the seismic forces were applied at the base of each slice whereas the factor of safety was 1.32 when the seismic forces were applied at the centre of gravity of each slice. Of course, this dam had failed and pseudo-static analyses did not predict a failure even after the event. The dam failed completely and its failure has been attributed to liquefaction or significant loss of strength of a loose sand layer near the base of the embankment.

9.1.2.3   Additional points about pseudo-static analysis

Considerable uncertainty is associated with the selection of an appropriate value of the coefficient k and this subject is discussed in detail later. A limit equilibrium analysis is performed which includes both the gravitational and earthquake forces acting on the slope above a potential slip surface.

Expressions for the pseudo-static factor of safety for different shapes of slip surface (planar, circular, non-circular) are given in section 9.4. Also the relationship between pseudo-static and static factor of safety for a given planar slip surface is shown to be particularly simple (sub-section 9.4.1).

In general, it is of interest to calculate the minimum pseudo-static value of the factor of safety F_{ss} and to compare it with the static value F before the application of the horizontal earthquake forces. The shape and location of the critical slip surface is, in general, different from that for static loading alone.

The values generally recommended for the seismic coefficient k are discussed in sub-section 9.4.4. Factors influencing the selection of a suitable value are also discussed in detail in that sub section.

It is pertinent to refer to the classical paper of Terzaghi (1950) in which he made significant comments concerning the main assumption implied in using a pseudo-static approach, the values of k which should be used for earthquakes of different severity and the relative seismic stability of slopes in different soil materials. His advice was ignored for decades according to Seed (1979). In most areas of soil mechanics, his advice had always been respected and followed.

The lateral seismic force (kW) on a soil mass (where W is its weight) is assumed to be sustained or permanent, acting only in one direction whereas the earthquake shaking involves a pulsating force. Terzaghi stated that a slope with a pseudo-static factor of safety smaller than 1 may remain stable and one with a factor of safety greater than 1 may fail, depending on the nature of the slope-forming materials He then commented that "The most stable materials are clays with a low degree of sensitivity, in a plastic state, dense sand either above or below the water table and loose sand above the water table. The most sensitive materials are slightly cemented grain aggregates such as loess and submerged or partly submerged loose sand".

By the time of the paper by Seed (1979), considerable research and study had been done and the significance of Terzaghi's comments was fully appreciated by geotechnical engineers and advanced students engaged in the evaluation of seismic stability of slopes and earth dams. Terzaghi's recommendations concerning the value of seismic coefficient k are recalled in sub-section 9.4.4.

9.1.3   Critical seismic coefficient (or yield value of seismic coefficient)

A critical or yield seismic coefficient k_c is that value of k which produces a pseudo-static factor of safety of one. ($F_{ss} = 1$). It is often denoted by k_y as an alternative to k_c. Evaluation of a critical value of k is important for the sliding block approach. This value can be obtained from a plot of k versus factor of safety F. However, a direct numerical solution may be obtained for individual slopes while exact solutions have been derived for simple slopes. The critical acceleration of a slope (also called the yield acceleration) is the product of the critical seismic coefficient and the gravitational acceleration ($a_c = k_c \, g$). It is important to remember that the critical seismic coefficient is related to the static factor of safety of a slope and, therefore, incorporates the influence of all the parameters such as the slope geometry, the soil properties and the pore water pressures. Expressions for critical seismic coefficients are given in Section 9.5.

9.1.4   Introducing Newmark approach of sliding block analysis

The sliding block approach, first outlined by Newmark (1965), provides a method or a set of tools for the evaluation of permanent or irreversible seismic displacement of a slope. Often the displacement computed by this method is called the Newmark displacement or Newmark rigid block displacement. In this context, attention has to be focused on estimating the irreversible or permanent deformations since such deformations have a direct bearing on the continued safety and serviceability of a slope. In contrast, reversible deformations may have little or no implications for slope safety. Many papers have been written concerning sliding block approaches over the last 40 years but the analytical concepts generally follow the original ideas proposed by Newmark (1965).

A potential sliding mass is modeled as a rigid block on a potential sliding plane (Figure 9.1). The block is subjected to a constant gravitational force and transient, time-dependent, earthquake acceleration. As stated earlier the base rock acceleration at any location (the acceleration-time record during an earthquake) is primarily determined by the earthquake magnitude and the source distance.

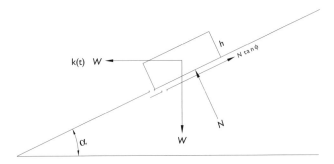

Figure 9.1 A sliding block model: The block represents a potential sliding mass with a slip surface of any shape and k(t) represents the acceleration-time record imparted by earthquake shaking.

The equation for the acceleration of a sliding block and other relevant details are presented in section 9.6. Within the total earthquake duration, the applied acceleration may or may not exceed the yield or critical acceleration which reflects the characteristics of the slope including geometrical and geotechnical parameters. If the yield acceleration is exceeded during any small time step, the block will move and its velocity and displacement may be estimated by integration.

The same can be done for other time steps in which the applied acceleration exceeds the yield acceleration during the acceleration-time history of the earthquake. Consequently the total deformation over the duration of the earthquake can be computed by adding the individual components. The procedure is illustrated in Figure 9.2 (Seed, 1970). For an acceleration pattern similar to that shown in the figure, no displacement will occur until time t_1, when the induced acceleration reaches the critical or yield acceleration for the first cycle, k_{y1}. If it is assumed that the yield acceleration remains constant throughout the first cycle, it may be marked off as shown in Figure 9.2, and the variation in velocity of the sliding mass may be computed by integration over the shaded area. The velocity will continue to increase until time t_2, when the acceleration again drops below the critical value, and the velocity is finally reduced to zero at time t_3, as the direction of acceleration is reversed. The rate of displacement of the sliding mass may then be computed by integration of the velocity-time relationship, as shown in Figure 9.2.

Reference is made, in section 9.7, to empirical approaches for estimating seismic slope deformations. Such estimates are only suitable for regional studies for reasons explained in section 9.7. In such approaches, the ground motion (acceleration-time record pertaining to an earthquake) is represented, for simplicity, by one or more parameters such as the peak acceleration, peak ground velocity and the predominant period.

The Newmark model, in its original form, is a one-dimensional model with assumption of rigid-plastic behaviour of soil. This assumption may lead to errors for assessing the deformation of deep, flexible soil masses and the behaviour of liquefied soil. Accordingly, suitable modifications and extensions have been proposed from time to time. The phenomenon of liquefaction and the concept of residual undrained shear strength of cohesionless soil are considered separately in section 9.3.

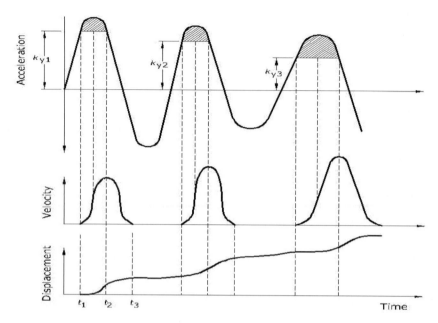

Figure 9.2 Illustrative diagram for estimation of permanent displacement from acceleration-time record (after Seed, 1967, 1970). With permission from ASCE, see page 714, No 28.

An interesting application of the Newmark sliding block model for GIS-based regional landslide hazard analysis has been described by Jibson et al. (1998). The factor of safety at any location was based on the simple "infinite slope" assumption. Calculated Newmark displacements were used as an index to correlate with observed performance during an earthquake in order to estimate the relationship between magnitude of displacement and the likelihood of slope failure. Further reference to this application is made in sub-sections 9.5.2 and 9.11.5.

9.1.5 Three stages of change in stability and permanent deformation

Permanent deformations associated with seismic forces may occur in three stages and a detailed discussion concerning these has been presented, among others, by Ambraseys and Srbulov (1995). Whether one or more of these components of deformation occur depends on the earthquake ground motion as well as on the various slope characteristics and parameters.

The first stage, the co-seismic stage, concerns deformations which occur over the relatively short duration of an earthquake, as explained in section 9.1.4. These deformations depend on the magnitude and duration of the applied earthquake inertia forces in addition to the properties of the slope or embankment and its geometrical configuration. In particular, the undrained shear strengths of the component soils are relevant because the duration of an earthquake is too short for any drainage to occur. Unless otherwise stated, these are the deformations generally estimated by the sliding block method.

The second stage is the immediate post-seismic stage when there are no applied dynamic forces acting on the slope. Deformation and movement during this stage will occur only if the static factor of safety has dropped below one due to a reduction of shear strength to residual along one or more potential slip surfaces. The concept of undrained residual shear strength of cohesionless soils is discussed in a subsequent section. This concept is totally different from the residual shear strength of cohesive soils under static loading, generally denoted by effective stress parameters.

During this second stage of permanent deformation the driving forces will be due to gravity alone. Several site-specific factors will control the speed of movement of the sliding mass, when and where it will stop, and what its factor of safety will be when equilibrium is established.

The third stage of deformations may develop because of a number of phenomena such as generation and migration of excess pore water pressures, filling of cracks by surface or ground water, creep and consolidation processes. The third stage of deformations may not follow immediately after the first or second stages. In fact, there can be considerable time delays associated with the occurrence of such deformations especially if the subsurface conditions are complex. Examples of delayed landsliding under seismic conditions have been documented, among others, by Hutchinson and Del Prete (1985) and D'elia et al. (1985).

Probably the best example of the distinction between second and third stages is the 1971 failure of the upstream face of Lower San Fernando Dam. Analyses reported by Seed (1979) referred to the occurrence of partial drainage from the liquefied zone to dilatant areas and the consequent redistribution of pore water pressure. In turn, the undrained shear strength is reduced in areas where water content has increased. The factor of safety based on undrained strengths immediately after the earthquake was estimated as $F = 1.4$. However, when partial drainage and decrease in shear strength beyond the liquefied zone was considered, the estimate was $F = 0.8$.

The estimation of deformations during the second and third stages will be largely problem-specific and site-specific and, therefore, there is no standard procedure. The principles are, however, the same as applied to general limit equilibrium methods and to the simple dynamics of sliding bodies.

9.2 SOIL BEHAVIOUR UNDER CYCLIC LOADING CONDITIONS

9.2.1 Introduction

During an earthquake, the shear stress on a soil element within a slope increases from static stress to static stress plus dynamic (cyclic) shear stress. Moreover, earthquake shaking may result in a significant loss of shear strength in some types of soil. The increase of shear stress or the decrease of shear strength or both may lead to irreversible strains and deformations within a slope and, under some circumstances, to overall slope failure. The mechanism and type of failure would depend on slope geometry, shear strength of slope materials and other factors.

Again, the likelihood of occurrence of overall failure or of significant deformations would depend on the intensity and duration of the earthquake ground motion as well as on the slope characteristics and material properties. Any acceleration – time history associated with an earthquake reveals a highly variable acceleration over that short duration which, in turn, implies a highly variable applied cyclic shear stress on any soil element within a slope. (Researchers have, however, developed and used methods for estimating the number of equivalent uniform cycles at certain level of applied stress corresponding to specific earthquakes.)

In most laboratory tests on soil samples simulating dynamic conditions, a constant deviator stress is applied cyclically. Considering the hypothetical case of a pulsating or cyclic deviator stress of constant magnitude acting on a slope, the likelihood of failure or of exceeding a certain magnitude of permanent deformation would increase with the increase in the number of cycles. Similarly, as the applied deviator stress is increased, the irreversible strain during a given number of cycles will increase (Seed, 1966; Lee and Seed, 1967; Peacock and Seed, 1968).

An important reason for decrease or loss of shear strength of saturated cohesionless soils under seismic conditions is the development of high excess pore water pressure. During the short time interval of an earthquake, such excess pore water pressures are not dissipated as quickly as they are generated despite the high permeability of cohesionless soils. Rapid dissipation of seismically-induced excess pore water pressures cannot be assumed even in very coarse-grained rockfill especially if there is some percentage of fine-grained materials present.

9.2.2   Cyclic shear strength from laboratory tests

Behaviour of an earth structure under seismic conditions will be controlled by dynamic properties of the component soils. The stress-strain behaviour of cyclically loaded soils differs in important ways from that under static loading conditions. This is a vast subject and here we consider only the main aspects relevant to slope analysis. In particular, soil shear strength parameters to be used in seismic analysis of slopes should be determined from cyclic shear tests. Laboratory tests include the cyclic triaxial test and the cyclic simple shear test. The latter is capable of reproducing earthquake stresses more accurately than the cyclic triaxial test. Static stresses and stress paths appropriate to ground conditions should be applied to soil samples before carrying out the cyclic tests.

The cyclic undrained shear strength of soils decreases with the number of cycles of loading and the failure strain. For soils which undergo only small changes in pore water pressure during undrained loading, Makdisi and Seed (1978) defined the dynamic yield strength as 80% of the undrained strength under static loading. This suggestion was made in connection with a procedure for estimating earthquake-induced permanent deformations in dams and embankments. Significant permanent deformations can occur when the total shear stress (static plus cyclic) exceeds the dynamic yield strength.

9.2.3   Field tests and model tests

There are a number of field tests for measurement or indirect assessment of soil properties under static or dynamic conditions and some of these may prove useful for determining parameters relevant to seismic analysis. For example, the Standard Penetration Test (SPT) has been utilized extensively in geotechnical engineering practice although SPT results (N values) are generally not used for static slope stability assessment.

However, SPT has featured prominently in methods for assessment of seismic liquefaction potential and aspects of seismic slope stability. Standardised and corrected N values from SPT have been correlated to undrained residual shear strength of cohesionless soils under seismic conditions. The concept of residual undrained shear strength of cohesionless soil is discussed in the next section. That value of und rained shear strength is particularly relevant to seismic slope stability analysis if a cohesionless soil layer within a slope is considered to be susceptible to seismically induced liquefaction.

There are also important model tests of great value to geotechnical earthquake engineering especially as research tools. These include 1 g model tests and those performed under higher gravitational accelerations. The most important are Shaking Table tests and Centrifuge tests.

9.2.4   Shear strength parameters for seismic slope analysis

An important issue concerns the type of shear strength parameters to be used in a seismic slope analysis. The choice between total stress and effective stress approach would depend on whether the analysis is for understanding the behaviour during the earthquake or after the earthquake. Again, the immediate post-seismic behaviour will be different from the conditions reached after sufficient time has elapsed for post-seismic equilibrium to be established where failure has occurred. Thus the choice between effective stress and total stress analysis should be considered carefully. Because of the short duration of an earthquake, undrained shear strengths of cohesive soil layers or zones may be relevant and indeed the undrained residual shear strength for those cohesionless soils which have liquefied (see Section 9.3). Thus total stress analyses are generally considered appropriate for the co-seismic stage. However, effective stress analyses may also be carried out in addition to total stress analyses. The lower of the two calculated factors of safety would be adopted for design.

For post-earthquake conditions, it may again be desirable to carry out effective stress analyses in addition to total stress analyses so that the worst-case scenarios can be identified. For a particular slope or dam, analyses may have to be carried out with undrained strengths over parts of a slip surface and drained strengths over other parts of the surface. This would depend on the soil types present and the best estimates of corresponding strengths that are available.

9.2.5   Rate effects on the shear strength along existing slip surfaces

There are cases where landslides with existing slip surfaces were reactivated during earthquakes and the effective residual shear strength parameters were known. In these cases, effective stress back analyses were performed and the inferred residual strength values compared with the measured values. Obviously these were static analyses simulating the post-seismic equilibrium conditions. Researchers have investigated whether the residual shear strength of a slip surface changes during fast or cyclic shearing, the so-called "rate effects". The broad question investigated in such research is the following: "Does the shear strength increase (positive rate effect), decrease (negative rate effect) or stay the same (rate neutral)?" Cohesionless soils or those with a small clay content have been found to be rate neutral whereas other soils may be either rate positive or rate negative. (Tika et al., 1996) The research conducted so far has been limited in scope and has led to the understanding that the rate effect is an independent property and not a consequence of change in pore pressure during fast loading.

9.3   SEISMICALLY-INDUCED SOIL LIQUEFACTION AND RESIDUAL STRENGTH OF COHESIONLESS SOIL

9.3.1   Seismic liquefaction phenomena

As stated above, for saturated cohesionless soils, decrease in shear strength is associated with significant increase in pore water pressure caused by cyclic loading. The pattern of strength decrease depends on the type of soil. Saturated, relatively loose cohesionless soils may be prone to liquefaction, as the pore water pressure during cyclic loading continues to increase. Dense soils exhibit dilatant behaviour and, therefore, are not prone to liquefaction. The factors which influence the likelihood of a soil undergoing liquefaction include the initial void ratio, the confining stresses and the type of ground motion. In a laboratory test, the fast-fluctuating ground motion would be represented by a certain level of applied deviator stress with an equivalent number of cycles corresponding to the particular ground motion.

A comprehensive study of liquefaction failures of slopes caused by earthquakes was presented by Seed (1968). Over a number of years, Seed and his co-workers carried out extensive research work in relation to liquefaction including laboratory tests, numerical modeling, and case studies of actual failures. The conditions under which such failures occur in the field were summarized by Seed (1968). The tremendous importance of minor geological details and of time-histories of ground motion were highlighted. Understanding landslides involving seismically-induced liquefaction requires careful consideration of the complex behaviour of heterogeneous soil deposits during earthquake- shaking.

9.3.2   Liquefaction-related strains and deformations

According to Byrne (1994), the strains required for initial liquefaction are relatively small (say, 0.5%) whereas strains at actual liquefaction may be greater than 5%. The magnitude of post-liquefaction strains depends on the geometry of the slope and the post-cyclic stress-strain properties of the soils within it. Post-liquefaction strains and displacements are not significantly related to the strains prior to liquefaction.

Initial liquefaction is associated with the decrease of effective stress to zero and the soil may lose its stiffness dramatically. As the soil strains further during liquefaction, it dilates and thus the pore water pressure decreases and the soil regains both the stiffness and the strength up to a limiting strain until the residual shear strength value is reached. Thus post-liquefaction behaviour up to the limiting strain can be understood as strain – hardening. The residual strength value is close to the steady state strength of the soil in pre-cyclic, pre-liquefaction, monotonic loading. The concept of undrained residual shear strength is discussed further below.

The basic Newmark model is inadequate for assessing post-liquefaction displacements since it is based on rigid-plastic assumption for soil behaviour while typically 20 to 50 percent strain may be required for mobilizing the residual shear strength after initial liquefaction. Improved computational models including extensions of the Newmark model have been proposed from time to time. Yet, there is no widely recognized model for estimation of post-liquefaction displacements.

Empirical approaches have been proposed for estimating post-seismic failure deformations (as distinct from co-seismic displacements). Several of these empirical approaches have been summarized by Kramer (1996). Significant permanent displacements following liquefaction may occur even for very flat slopes. Detailed discussion of such phenomena, called lateral spreading, is outside the scope of this chapter.

9.3.3 Undrained residual shear strength

In contrast to the concept of residual shear strength for static stability problems which applies only to cohesive soils, the concept of undrained residual shear strength under seismic conditions reflects the behaviour of saturated cohesionless soils. This concept has been invoked to explain the seismic performance of important slopes, embankments and dams. The most well known and frequently analysed case is the 1971 failure of the upstream slope of the Lower San Fernando Dam.

On a theoretical basis, undrained residual strength is considered to be the "steady state strength". This strength is estimated from the results of a series of laboratory tests on soil samples with different initial void ratios. On a plot of initial void ratio versus undrained strength, the steady state line separates dilative states from contractive states (Figure 9.3).

Undrained residual shear strength of cohesionless soils may be obtained in the following ways:

(1) Empirical correlations with corrected N values from SPT tests or, alternatively with cone resistance from Cone penetration tests

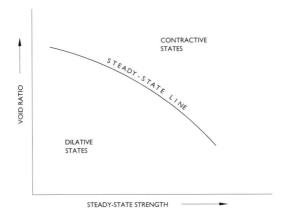

Figure 9.3 Steady-state line in a plot of steady state strength versus void ratio.

(2) Using the initial void ratio preferably measured in the field along with the steady state line obtained from results of laboratory tests at different void ratios

(3) Empirical correlations with initial effective overburden stress

(4) Back calculations from analysis of slope failures in which soil was liquefied before failure

Based on extensive laboratory tests including tests on undisturbed frozen samples of foundation of Duncan dam in British Columbia, Canada, the following indicative values for the ratio of undrained residual shear strength to the initial effective overburden stress have been suggested (Byrne, 1994; Jitno and Byrne, 1995).

Lower bound values (very loose, rounded sand): $s_r/\sigma'_{v0} = 0.087$
Duncan dam foundation, ($N = 13$): $s_r/\sigma'_{v0} = 0.22$ (limiting strain of 22%)
Upper bound value, (dense soils, $N > 15$ or 20): $s_r/\sigma'_{v0} > 0.6$
(For dense soils liquefaction will not occur and the undrained strength will exceed the drained strength).

The N values are the standardized and corrected N values from the SPT test; additional correction factors have been proposed which account for the effect of the percentage of fines present in an otherwise coarse or cohesionless soil.

Field residual shear strength of cohesionless soils has been correlated to the normalised N values from the standard penetration test as reported by Seed and Harder (1990) in the form reproduced in Figure 9.4.

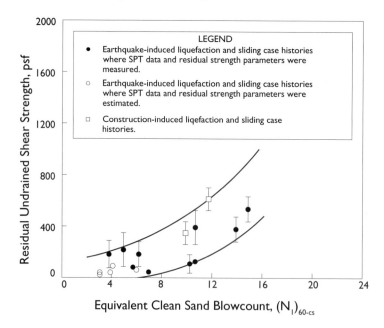

Figure 9.4 Undrained residual shear strength (from case studies) related to corrected N values from standard presentation tests (after Seed and Harder, 1990). Permission requested, see page 714, No 46.

Note: 1psf = 0.04788 kN/m².

The data provided by Seed and Harder (1990) includes both the residual shear strength and the limiting shear strain. For each parameter, they provide a range as well as an average value corresponding to each normalized N value.

9.3.4 Flow liquefaction contrasted with cyclic mobility

Flow failures or flow slides can be sudden and catastrophic and such failures are driven by static shear stresses after flow liquefaction has occurred. Soils susceptible to flow liquefaction are relatively loose soils which plot above the steady state line in Figure 9.3. While very large deformations are usually associated with flow slides following liquefaction, the absence of large deformations in a slide may not necessarily indicate that liquefaction did not occur. Only small areas or pockets within a soil may have liquefied with the result that deformations are of a limited magnitude.

Genuine liquefaction (also termed as flow liquefaction) should be distinguished from cyclic mobility or initial liquefaction. In the former case, the shear stress required for equilibrium is greater than the shear strength of the soil in its liquefied state which is called the undrained residual shear strength. Deformations associated with cyclic mobility or limited liquefaction develop incrementally during an earthquake and are thus caused by both cyclic and static shear stresses. The static shear stress may actually be less than the shear strength of the liquefied soil. The phenomenon of lateral spreading, which can occur on gently sloping or even on level ground, may be triggered by limited liquefaction.

9.4 PSEUDO-STATIC ANALYSIS

9.4.1 Planar slip surfaces

9.4.1.1 Natural slope – "Infinite slope" model

The pseudo-static safety factor F_{ss} for natural slopes may be considered as an indicator of landslide hazard, and it is, therefore, useful to estimate it. The simpler the model for assessing slope stability, the better it is, provided it can be justified based on observation. Thus an "infinite" slope model gets the first consideration. Traditionally such a model was used only for site-specific natural slope applications. However, in recent decades, this model has been used for regional analysis in order to map landslide hazard.

Consider the stability of a natural slope which can be modeled as an "infinite slope" with a potential slip surface parallel to the ground surface. A vertical element of width b and height z, such as in Figure 9.5, is acted upon by its own weight W and a lateral force kW assumed to act horizontally. It is easy to show that the pseudo-static factor of safety is given by the following expression which may be compared to Equation (4.25) for static conditions.

$$F_{ss} = \frac{c' + (\gamma z \cos^2 \beta - k\gamma z \sin \beta \cos \beta - u)\tan \phi'}{\gamma z \sin \beta \cos \beta + k\gamma z \cos^2 \beta} \tag{9.1}$$

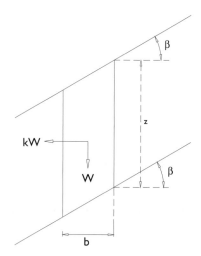

Figure 9.5 Infinite slope analysis.

The following assumptions and other relevant aspects may be noted:

- Only the pre-earthquake pore water pressure u is included in the above expression and thus it is assumed that there is no "excess" pore water pressure generated during earthquake shaking. Assumption of effective drainage, which would ensure zero "excess" pore water pressure during seismic shaking, is only reasonable for very coarse-grained soils such as gravel, and, of course, for dry soils.
- The above expression can be suitably modified if the lateral force is assumed to be inclined to the horizontal.
- The expression, as written above, is based on an effective stress analysis. Marcuson III et al. (1992) state that either a total stress or an effective stress analysis may be used for seismic analysis of embankments and dams. Both short-term (during earthquake-shaking) and long-term (post-earthquake) analyses can be important depending on the type of slope. As discussed in later sections, important slope failures have occurred well after the end of the main shock of a significant earthquake.
- Because of uncertainty concerning the "excess" pore water pressure developed during seismic shaking, total stress analysis may be preferred especially for the short-term conditions.
- To carry out a total stress analysis, replace the effective stress strength parameters by appropriate total stress parameters and remove pore water pressure u from the expression. For existing slopes, such analyses may be based on shear strength parameters from unconsolidated – undrained tests. For new slopes, Duncan and Wright (2005) recommend that shear strength parameters be obtained from consolidated-undrained tests in order to simulate the effects of future consolidation and swell.
- It is assumed that shear strength parameters do not decrease in magnitude during seismic shaking. The post-earthquake strength of soils which liquefy is

significantly reduced to undrained residual values. Also a soil zone which tends to dilate during shearing or failure process would lose strength as water migrates towards that zone.

9.4.1.2 Relationship between pseudo-static factor of safety F_{ss} and static factor of safety F for planar slip surfaces

The pseudo-static factor of safety F_{ss} is obviously related to the static factor of safety F. For simple failure modes (e.g., infinite slope analysis or simple slopes with a planar slip surface) the relationship is explicit considering the same slip surface for both analyses.

For slip surfaces of arbitrary shape, appropriate limit equilibrium models may be used to obtain the relationship numerically. These cases are discussed in the following sections.

As an example, consider a planar slip surface in a simple slope of height H, inclination α and the soil or rock shear strength parameters c and ϕ. The relationship, considering a horizontal inertia force, is:

$$F_{ss} = \frac{F - K \tan \phi}{k \cot \beta + 1} \tag{9.2}$$

in which β is the inclination of the slip surface.

The relationship appears to be independent of cohesion c, slope height H, static pore water pressure u and the unit weight γ of the slope materials. However, the influence of these parameters is included in the static factor of safety, F. The critical seismic coefficient k_c is the value of k when $F_{ss} = 1$. The equation for the critical seismic coefficient is presented in the next section and is applicable to "infinite slope" analysis or to any planar slip surface in a simple slope.

9.4.2 Circular slip surface in saturated soil slope

Consider a saturated clay slope with a potential slip surface of circular shape with radius R and central angle θ (see Figure 9.6). In addition to the weight W, a lateral force kW is assumed to act through the centre of gravity of the potential sliding mass. Let the distance of the force W from the centre of the surface be X and that of the force kW from the centre be Y. Taking moments of resisting forces (based on cohesive shear strength s) and the driving forces, the pseudo-static factor of safety is given by the following expression.

$$F_{ss} = \frac{sR^2\theta}{Wx + kWy} \tag{9.3}$$

This equation may be compared to Equation (5.1) which is applicable to the pre-earthquake static analysis. The relationship between the pseudo-static factor of safety and the conventional static factor of safety considering a given circular slip surface is the following

$$F_{ss} = F\left(\frac{x}{x + ky}\right) \tag{9.4}$$

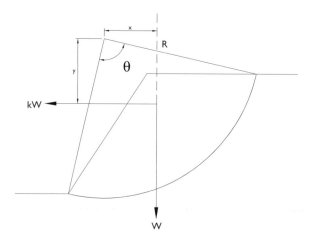

Figure 9.6 Circular slip surface in a slope of saturated clay, "$\phi = 0$" assumption.

The expression for the critical seismic coefficient may be derived by substituting F_{ss} by 1 on the left hand side and k by k_c on the right hand side. This expression is presented in section 9.5.

9.4.3   Slip surfaces of arbitrary shape

A general limit equilibrium solution would be required for a slope with a potential slip surface of arbitrary shape. The choice of limit equilibrium method would be among those discussed in chapter 5. Whatever method is chosen, an additional force corresponding to acceleration kg would have to be applied to each slice or segment of the potential sliding mass. Thus the weight W of a slice or segment acts vertically and the force kW acts horizontally through its centre of gravity. Pore water pressures relevant to the analysis are considered in the same way as for a static slope stability analysis. The same applies for any additional external forces including external water pressures on submerged parts of a slope or embankment.

9.4.4   Seismic coefficient and factor of safety
for pseudo-static analysis

A pseudo-static analysis is considered to be the first or preliminary step in assessment of a slope or earth structure. Minimum values of the factor of safety between 1 and 1.15 have been suggested. If such an analysis shows that the minimum factor of safety is attained, then a Newmark-type sliding block analysis is the next step of assessment. A displacement of 1 metre is considered tolerable for an earth structure such as an embankment or a dam. For landfills, lower tolerable displacements have been suggested (0.15–0.30 metres).

The adoption of an appropriate k value is a matter of experience and judgment. It is of interest to recall Terzaghi's recommendations in his classical paper (Terzaghi, 1950). These are probably the earliest recommendations on the values of the seismic coefficient published by a renowned geotechnical engineer or engineering geologist. He recommended the following values according to the severity of the earthquake:

Severe, Rossi-Forel Scale IX	$k = 0.1$
Violent, destructive, Rossi-Forel scale X	$k = 0.25$
Catastrophic	$k = 0.5$

As an example he mentioned the 1906 San Francisco earthquake as one for which $k = 0.25$ would be appropriate.

During the period 1960–1970, a great deal of attention was given to the importance of selecting a realistic value for k, as briefly outlined in the Appendix to this chapter. The use of dynamic response analysis and pseudo-static stress analysis was also explored. The difficulty in selecting an appropriate value of k must, however, be considered in relation to other uncertainties in any analysis.

Historically, values of k in the range 0.05–0.15 have been adopted for seismic analysis and design of dams in USA even in regions of very high seismic susceptibility such as California. In Japan, which also has high seismic susceptibility, typical values of k less than 0.2 have generally been adopted.

From an ICOLD report, Seed (1979) listed the design criteria for 14 dams in 9 countries. The range of k values used was 0.1 to 0.2 and the range of factors of safety adopted for design was 1.1 to 1.5.

Analysis shows that an appropriate value of k should depend on the height of an embankment and that a value of k varying with embankment depth is more realistic than a constant value (See Appendix to this chapter).

More importantly, the magnitude of peak seismic acceleration associated with the design earthquake should have a significant influence on the choice of value for k.

9.4.4.1   Recommended values or the state of current practice

There are several recommendations in the published literature over the last 30 years. Globally the practice may vary widely although the following values pertaining to USA can be considered as typical. Makdisi and Seed (1978) recommended a minimum pseudo-static factor of safety of 1.5 based on a soil strength reduction factor of 0.8 and the following values of acceleration $a = kg$ associated with two different values of earthquake magnitude M.

$a = 0.1$ g, for $M = 6.5$, (implying $k = 0.1$)
$a = 0.15$ g, for $M = 8.25$, (implying $k = 0.15$)

Hynes-Griffin and Franklin (1984) recommended a seismic coefficient based on half of the peak seismic acceleration, $a = 0.5\ a_{max}$. They stipulated further that, if the calculated factor of safety on this basis was considered adequate, dynamic analysis should not be required. Kavazanjian et al. (1997) suggested a minimum pseudo-static factor of safety of 1, also based on a soil strength reduction factor of 0.8 and the following values of 'a', expressed as a proportion of the peak horizontal acceleration (a_{max}) on soil sites:

$a = 0.17\,a_{max}$, if dynamic response analysis is also to be performed for the slope or earth structure.

$a = 0.5\,a_{max}$, if dynamic response analyses is not to be performed for the slope or earth structure.

9.4.5 Beyond pseudo-static analysis

The following points sum up the current practice

1   For most slope problems, analyses with a pseudo-static approach can prove to be useful for assessment of stability provided a suitable value is adopted for the seismic coefficient based on past experience, analysis, earthquake magnitude and engineering judgment.

2   The assessment of deformations based on a Newmark sliding block approach is most desirable. The basis for such estimation is discussed further in the following sections, 9.5–9.7.

3   For important structures such as embankments and dams, and especially where one or more zones consist of saturated cohesionless soils, a dynamic response analyses would be carried out to obtain detailed information about the effects of earthquake shaking. Further reference to the basis for this type of analysis and its application is made in section 9.9. In particular, such analyses can provide detailed information about the variation within an embankment of seismically induced accelerations, stresses and permanent displacements. Appropriate dynamic soil testing would be carried out to determine the behaviour of soil elements at different locations under the estimated dynamic stresses applied on top of the initial static stresses. Moreover, assessments would be made of the liquefaction potential of the vulnerable soil layers or zones in the earth structure and its foundation (section 9.9).

9.5   CRITICAL SEISMIC COEFFICIENT

9.5.1   Introduction – the range of methods and solutions

As stated earlier, the critical or yield acceleration is that which reduces the factor of safety of a slope to unity ($F = 1$) consistent with a condition of critical equilibrium. The associated seismic coefficient is called the critical or yield seismic coefficient. Thus the critical seismic acceleration may be expressed as the product of the critical seismic coefficient k_c and the gravitational acceleration, g.

Estimation of this parameter is necessary for proceeding with a Newmark (sliding block) analysis for estimating displacements as will become clear in the next section (section 9.6). It is related to the static factor of safety F, the relationship depending on the shape of the slip surface, i.e., the failure mechanism. Thus k_c is an indirect measure of the stability of a slope under static conditions. Explicit solutions can be derived for planar slip surfaces and the relevant equations are presented later in this section (see sub-section 9.5.2).

Limit equilibrium solutions with log-spiral slip surfaces have also been found to be convenient to obtain k_c using an effective stress analysis and a numerical solution (Prater, 1979; Lighthall, 1979).

Kinematic limit analysis has also been used for deriving solutions based on the log-spiral mechanism and very interesting results were presented by Crespellani et al. (1998).

The extension of the upper bound limit analysis approach (upper bound method) to multiblock model for a slope subjected to seismic excitation using both associative and non-associative flow rules has been presented by Michalowski (2007).

For slip surfaces of arbitrary shape and for problems involving several soil layers as well as arbitrary variations of pore water pressure, a general limit equilibrium solution will be required. The outline of a direct solution is presented in sub-section 9.5.4.

More sophisticated approaches, such as Non-linear Finite Element method or Finite Difference method can also be used to determine the critical acceleration or factor of safety of slopes along with the permanent displacements as well. The use of such methods will generally not be justified within the context of pseudo-static or sliding block approaches. The simpler methods mentioned in this chapter are considered good enough for estimating the critical seismic coefficient.

9.5.2   Critical seismic coefficient for slip surfaces of planar or log spiral shapes

9.5.2.1   Planar slip surface, horizontal earthquake force

An explicit relationship can be derived for a simple planar shape of slip surface, the location of which is known. For example, translational landsliding for long natural slopes is often analysed using the 'infinite slope' approach. (The assumptions are that the slip surface is approximately parallel to the ground surface and that the sliding layer is of shallow depth). The equation for the critical seismic coefficient can be written in the following form when the earthquake force is considered to act horizontally.

$$k_c = (F-1)\frac{\tan\beta}{1+\tan\beta\tan\phi} \tag{9.5}$$

Where β is the inclination of the ground surface (also that of the planar slip surface).

The above relationship is also valid for a plane wedge failure mechanism with plane slip surface passing through the toe and having a known inclination β.

9.5.2.2   Numerical solutions using a log spiral slip surface and a planar slip surface

Numerical solutions for minimum value of k_c have been derived for a simple slope considering

i   A plane failure mechanism passing through the toe for which the optimum inclination β is not known in advance, and

ii A log spiral failure mechanism passing through the toe. Reference is made in subsection 9.7.5 to the solution of Crespellani et al. (1998).

The ratio of k_c (plane) to k_c (log spiral) was found to be always greater than 1 and, as critical equilibrium for a given slope is reached (F approaching 1), the ratio increases to infinity. The assumption of a plane failure mechanism for a simple slope, therefore, leads to an underestimation of displacements with respect to the assumption of log special failure mechanism.

9.5.2.3   *Planar slip surface, earthquake force parallel to slip surface and ground surface*

Another simple equation for the critical seismic coefficient applies when the earthquake force (acceleration) is assumed to act parallel to the slip surface

$$k_c = (F - 1) \sin \beta \tag{9.6}$$

An "infinite slope" model is the simplest that can be used for natural slopes either to estimate the factor of safety or to estimate critical acceleration and hence Newmark displacement. Yet, it can be very useful not only for site-specific analysis but also for regional analysis as demonstrated by Jibson et al. (1998, 2000). Reference to this application was made earlier in sub-section 9.1.4 (see also 9.11.5). Incidentally, in that application, the lateral force was assumed parallel to the sliding block and hence Equation (9.6) was used rather than Equation (9.5).

9.5.3   Critical seismic coefficient for circular slip surface

For the general slope stability problem with a slip surface of circular or arbitrary shape, several numerical solutions are obtained using an appropriate method of limit equilibrium analysis. Each solution will correspond to one assumed value of the seismic coefficient k. By plotting F against k, the critical value of k (which corresponds to $F = 1$) can be found.

For a given slip surface of circular shape and considering a saturated clay soil, the expression for critical seismic coefficient as a function of the static factor of safety, obtained by substituting $F = 1$ in Equation 9.4, is the following. (See also Figure 9.6.)

$$k_c = \frac{x}{y}(F - 1) \tag{9.7}$$

9.5.4   Critical seismic coefficient for homogeneous slope considering slip surface of arbitrary shape

Several numerical solutions have been proposed within the framework of limit equilibrium As an example, a direct numerical solution for the critical seismic coefficient, proposed by Sarma (1988), is summarized below:

A slope with an arbitrary slip surface is shown in Figure 9.7. Assume that the normal stress distribution on the slip surface can be expressed by

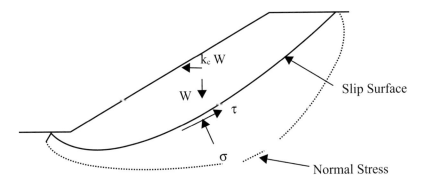

Figure 9.7 Geometry of a slip surface in a slope and a possible normal stress distribution (after Sarma, 1988).

$$\sigma_n = \lambda q + u \tag{9.8}$$

where q is a known function representing the effective stress, λ is an unknown constant to be determined from the solution, and u is the pore water pressure.

Assume that under the action of the total weight W and the lateral seismic force $k_c W$, and with the assumed normal stress distribution, the potential sliding mass is in limiting equilibrium. The Mohr-Coulomb failure criterion is

$$\tau_f = c' + (\sigma_n - u)\tan\phi' \tag{9.9}$$

The following equations relate to the vertical and horizontal equilibrium of the potential sliding mass

$$\int \left[\sigma_n + \tau\frac{dy}{dx} \right] dx = W \tag{9.10}$$

$$\int \left[\tau - \frac{d\sigma_n}{dx} \right] dx = k_c W \tag{9.11}$$

The solution depends on the assumed function q. The following expression for q was found by Sarma (1988) to give satisfactory results, particularly when the slip surface is the one giving the smallest critical acceleration.

$$q = [(\gamma h - u)\cos\phi' - c'(\sin\beta + \sin\phi')]\frac{\cos\phi'}{1 + \sin\beta\sin\phi'} \tag{9.12}$$

where $\beta = 2\alpha - \phi'$
γh = overburden pressure at the point on the slip surface, and
u = pore water pressure at the same point.

9.6   SLIDING BLOCK SOLUTION FOR PERMANENT DISPLACEMENTS

9.6.1   The Newmark approach

As stated in Section 9.1, an approach originally proposed by Newmark (1965) and based on the analogy of a rigid block on an inclined plane has proved to be a very important and versatile tool for estimating permanent displacements of slopes. It has been used successfully for assessments concerning both man-made and natural slopes. It is a one-dimensional dynamic analysis based on the assumption that the potential sliding mass behaves as a rigid body.

The calculation of permanent seismic displacements of such a block is based on the fact that, when the applied seismic acceleration is bigger than the critical acceleration, the block will move down along the slip surface. The magnitude of displacement will depend on the amplitude of the applied acceleration, how often the accelerations exceed the critical and for what duration. Newmark considered three cases: (a) a slope with a potential slip surface of circular shape, (b) block sliding of an embankment along a horizontal slip surface in its foundation and (c) a slope with a planar slip surface. For each of these cases he derived a simple equation for the yield seismic coefficient (yield acceleration as a proportion of gravitational acceleration).

If yield acceleration is larger than the applied acceleration throughout an earthquake, permanent displacement will not occur. However, if the yield acceleration is exceeded at some point after the start of an earthquake, there is a net driving force or net driving acceleration acting on the potential sliding mass. By double-integration the resulting displacement of the block relative to the sliding plane can be calculated.

For a block on a horizontal plane subjected to a single acceleration pulse, Newmark (1965) showed that the maximum displacement is proportional to the square of the velocity and depends on the ratio of yield acceleration to the applied acceleration. He then considered the displacement resulting from the shaking of a block caused by each of four different earthquake ground motions (acceleration – time records). From the results he concluded that displacement was a function of peak ground acceleration (PGA) and peak ground velocity (PGV) as well as the yield or critical acceleration.

9.6.1.1   Basic equation for acceleration of a block

The acceleration of a rigid block moving on an inclined plane of inclination β may be expressed in the following form:

$$a = \frac{\cos(\phi - \beta)}{\cos\phi} [k(t) - k_c] g \qquad (9.13)$$

in which $k(t)$ represents the applied acceleration-time history and ϕ is the friction angle relevant to the interface between the rigid block and the inclined plane. This simple equation has been successfully applied to slopes with different translational and rotational failure mechanisms.

Sarma (1975) suggested a method for determining the angle of inclination of the equivalent sliding plane corresponding to a curved slip surface. A simple way to understand this is to consider the force polygon representing the potential sliding mass above a slip surface of arbitrary shape. The force resultant for this polygon represents the inclination of the sliding plane in the sliding block model.

Double integration of the equation is, of course, required to calculate the deformations. In the standard Newmark method, both the static factor of safety and the critical acceleration are assumed to remain constant for the duration of the earthquake. Possible decrease of these parameters during seismic shaking is considered in sub-sections 9.6.3 and 9.8.8.

As stated earlier, total stress analysis is generally considered appropriate for stability and deformation assessment under co-seismic conditions. Thus undrained shear strength parameters of the soils comprising the slope may be used in the limit equilibrium analyses if total stress approach is considered appropriate. For any soil layer which has liquefied or is considered potentially liquefiable during the earthquake, the residual undrained shear strength would be appropriate.

9.6.1.2   Software for implementing the Newmark method

Researchers at the United States Geological Survey have developed appropriate software (Jibson and Jibson, 2003) for implementing the Newmark method which is available on the web and is in the public domain. Readers may refer to the following website for conducting rigid-block analysis and simplified decoupled analysis: (courtesy, R.W. Jibson, personal communication, March 2009). http://earthquake.usgs.gov/resources/software/slope_perf.php

9.6.1.3   Extensions of the Newmark model

The assumption of a potential sliding mass as a rigid body is quite acceptable for slopes formed in rock or in relatively stiff soil. According to a study dealing with a modified Newmark model for compliant slopes (Kramer and Smith, 1997), the rigid body assumption provides good estimates of the permanent displacements of relatively thin or stiff failure masses but tends to overestimate deformations of thick and/or soft failure masses. For landfills, this overestimate may be a factor of two. On the other hand, for natural slopes, any overestimation of deformations based on the rigid block model is unlikely to be significant.

Analysis using multi-block sliding model shows that for small displacements, Newmark's single sliding block model is sufficiently accurate while for large displacements, it may not be so (Chlimintzas, 2003).

As outlined below in sub-section 9.6.3, for strain-softening soils and for soils which are susceptible to increase in excess pore pressure during earthquake shaking, an interactive, incremental time-step procedure has been proposed in order to account for a variable critical seismic coefficient. On the basis of a constant value of k_c, permanent deformations would be significantly underestimated.

Comparisons carried out by Miles et al. (1999) shows that different models may forecast notably different levels of slope performance. Therefore, it is important to have access to a range of analysis tools in order to assess the range of deformations

Table 9.1 Probable upper bound displacements for embankment dams subjected to earthquakes of magnitude $M = 6.5$. (Little or no strength loss is assumed in the computations.) (After Seed, 1979). With permission, see page 714, No 30.

	Crest acceleration	k_m	*Factor of safety with alternative assumptions*		
			$F_{ss} = 1.15$ for $k = 0.05$ (15% strength loss) $k_y = 0.05$	$F_{ss} = 1.15$ for $k = 0.1$ (15% strength loss) $k_y = 0.10$	$F_{ss} = 1.15$ for $k = 0.1$ (no strength loss) $k_y = 0.15$
Probable upper bound of accelerations for most earth dams	1.0 g	≈0.4	≈4.0 ft	≈1.8 ft	≈1.0 ft
	0.75 g	≈0.3	≈2.7 ft	≈1.2 ft	≈6.0 in
	0.50 g	≈0.2	≈1.7 ft	≈6.0 in	≈1.0 in
	0.25 g	≈0.1	≈6.0 in	0	0

Note: 1 ft = 30.48 cm (0.3048 m) and 1 in = 2.54 cm, k_m = Effective peak acceleration coefficient.

Table 9.2 Probable bound displacements for embankment dams subjected to earthquakes of magnitude $M = 8.25$; little or no strength loss is assumed in the computations. (After Seed, 1979). With permission, see page 714, No 30.

	Crest acceleration	k_m	*Factor of safety with alternative assumptions*		
			$(F_{ss}) = 1.15$ for $k = 0.1$ (15% strength loss) $k_y = 0.10$	$F_{ss} = 1.15$ for $k = 0.15$ (15% strength loss) $k_y = 0.15$	$F_{ss} = 1.15$ for $k = 0.15$ (no strength loss) $k_y = 0.20$
Probable upper bound of accelerations for most earth dams	1.00 g	≈0.4	≈17 ft	≈7 ft	≈3 ft*
	0.75 g	≈0.3	≈10 ft	≈3 ft*	≈8 in*
	0.50 g	≈0.1	≈3 ft*	≈4 in*	0*
	0.25 g	≈0.1	0*	0*	0*

* Acceptable performance. Note: 1 ft = 30.48 cm (0.3048 m) and 1 in = 2.54 cm, k_m = Effective peak acceleration coefficient.

that may be expected. In this regard a spatial decision support system (SDSS) has been proposed by them.

9.6.2   Typical estimated values of seismic displacement

Seed (1979) compiled the results of computations made by his research group and a number of other researchers. These computations were based on the basic Newmark model and considering peak seismic accelerations for representative forms of ground motion. (Empirical correlations between calculated sliding block displacement and significant ground motion parameters are discussed in the next section, Section 9.7).

Seed tabulated the probable upper bound displacements for embankment dams subjected to earthquake magnitudes of 6.5 and 8.25 ($M = 6.5$ and $M = 8.25$). These tables are reproduced above (Tables 9.1 and 9.2).

The estimates are based on the assumption that the slope forming materials would not lose more than 15% of their original strength as a consequence of earthquake shaking. Such an assumption is considered to be valid for many clays, dense saturated sands and clayey sands. The critical or yield acceleration was assumed to remain constant during earthquake shaking.

Seed (1979) concluded that:

- Where the crest accelerations are less than 0.75 g, computed displacements of an embankment are within acceptable limits if the embankment is designed to safely withstand an inertia force of 0.1 g to 0.15 g.
- Provided that a soil does not suffer significant strength loss or develop large pore water pressures during earthquake shaking, a value of $F_{ss} = 1.15$ would be considered adequate for $(M = 6.5$ with $k = 0.1)$ as well as for $(M = 8.25$ with $k = 0.15)$.

Thus, progress in research and the use of sliding block analysis has shown that a pseudo-static approach can be adequate for embankment analysis under certain conditions. However, in important projects, it would be advisable to supplement the pseudo-static assessments with sliding block and dynamic analyses.

9.6.3 Considering variable critical seismic coefficient

If soil shear strength decreases significantly during earthquake shaking, the assumption of constant critical acceleration coefficient will prove to be unconservative.

Since some soils suffer a loss in shear strength during earthquake shaking, both k_c and static factor of safety F should, in general, be considered functions of time during an earthquake. This effect can be significant for cohesionless soils in which pore water pressure increases during cyclic loading.

$$k_c = k_c(t)$$
$$F = F(t)$$
(9.14)

For cohesionless soils in which significant strength loss is associated with increase in excess pore water pressure, the estimation of excess pore pressure due to seismic shaking is essential for tracking the decrease in the critical seismic coefficient at any time during the earthquake duration. The sliding block model can then be extended into a more comprehensive method by adopting an interactive incremental time-step procedure in which iterative limit equilibrium analyses must be made at each time step and the varying value of the critical seismic coefficient used successively over the complete acceleration-time history (Chowdhury 1995, 1996). The limit equilibrium analyses would obviously have to be carried out within an effective stress framework and this is discussed in section 9.8.8. Such a comprehensive approach can provide a valuable perspective concerning the seismic response of slopes and embankments comprising saturated cohesionless soil in one or more zones.

Sarma and Jennings (1980) proposed the concept of dynamic pore pressure coefficients under earthquake loading conditions. They analysed published experimental data from different sources and found that the following simple equation could be used to estimate excess pore water pressure Δu from the results of cyclic triaxial tests.

$$\frac{\Delta u}{\sigma'_{3c}} = A_n \frac{\Delta \sigma_1}{\sigma'_{3c}} \tag{9.15}$$

in which $\Delta \sigma_1$ is the increment of cyclic major principal stress, σ'_{3c} is the minor principal consolidation stress and A_n is a pore water pressure coefficient appropriate to n cycles of loading.

Based on their analysis, the following relationship between A_n and A_1 was also proposed:

$$A_n^{\frac{1}{2}} = A_1^{\frac{1}{2}} + \beta \log n \tag{9.16}$$

in which A_1 is the pore water pressure coefficient for one cycle of loading and β is another soil parameter.

In case results of cyclic simple shear tests were to be used (instead of the results of cyclic triaxial tests) the following alternative equation was proposed:

$$\frac{\Delta u}{\sigma_{vo'}} = A_n \frac{\Delta \tau}{\sigma_{vo'}} \tag{9.17}$$

in which $\Delta \tau$ is the increment of cyclic simple shear stress and $\sigma_{vo'}$ is the effective vertical overburden stress on the sample.

9.7   EMPIRICAL/REGRESSION EQUATIONS FOR PERMANENT DISPLACEMENTS

9.7.1   Introduction and scope of equations from regression analysis

Predictive models for earthquake-induced sliding displacement, based on empirical or regression equations have been proposed from time to time. In each case a number of earthquake ground motion records (acceleration-time histories) are used as a basis for calculating displacements. The calculated displacement values are correlated to the yield acceleration and to one more significant ground motion parameters such as peak ground acceleration (PGA), peak ground velocity (PGV), Arias Intensity, predominant period etc.

Typical equations based on research during the period (1988–1998) are presented in the following sub-sections. Some are based on just one or two ground motion parameters. However, Sarma and Koukoulis (2004), among others, pointed out that sliding block displacements depend on many factors. Therefore, use of just a single descriptor of earthquake ground motion, such as peak acceleration, would lead to an empirical equation of low accuracy.

Empirical equations utilizing Arias Intensity are considered preferable to those utilizing other parameters such as peak ground acceleration and predominant period. This is because Arias Intensity combines both the amplitude and frequency content of ground motion. Arias Intensity is obtained by integration of the square of the acceleration over the entire duration of an earthquake rather than the duration of strong motion. Thus it is independent of the method used to define the duration of strong motion.

Jibson (2007) used 2270 strong motion recordings from 30 earthquakes and the predictive relationships were developed from 875 values of calculated displacement evenly distributed between four values of the yield acceleration. Saygili and Rathje (2008) carried out analyses based on 2000 acceleration-time records and found that the combination of PGA and PGV results in the smallest standard deviation in calculated displacement compared to any other pair of ground motion parameters. If Arias intensity is included as a third ground motion parameter, standard deviation is reduced further.

The regression equations presented by Jibson (2007) predict Newmark displacement in terms of (i) critical acceleration ratio, (ii) critical acceleration ratio and earthquake magnitude, (iii) Arias intensity and critical acceleration, and (iv) Arias intensity and critical acceleration ratio. While these equations are well constrained to fit the data, they have standard deviations of 0.5 log units. This implies that the range defined by "one standard deviation either side of the mean" spans about an order of magnitude.

The question, therefore, arises

"What is the role of regression models in seismic slope analysis?"

According to Jibson (2007), regression models should be used for region-scale seismic landslide hazard mapping or for rapid preliminary screening of sites, but not for site-specific design. In region-scale assessment and mapping of seismic landslide hazards, the dynamic stability of the grid cells in a map area are estimated and compared. Thus assessing relative hazard is the main concern and it is appropriate to do this comparison based on mean values of displacement. Of course, local and regional judgment, based on past experience, can be used to ensure that the absolute hazard categories are realistic."

In summary, regression models can be very useful for rapid assessment of expected level of seismic displacement of slopes and embankments. Such models can also be used in probabilistic seismic hazard analysis for sliding displacement.

9.7.2   An equation based on (i) the ratio of critical seismic coefficient and peak ground acceleration coefficient and (ii) the predominant period

Sarma (1988) proposed the following equation in which the acceleration-time history is represented by just two ground motion parameters, the peak ground acceleration and the predominant period:

$$\log\left[\frac{1}{C}\frac{4u}{k_m g T^2}\right] = 1.07 - 3.83\frac{k_c}{k_m} \tag{9.18}$$

where,

$$C = \frac{\cos(\phi - \beta)}{\cos \phi}$$

ϕ = average angle of friction on the slip surface;
β = slope angle of the equivalent plane slip surface;
T = predominant period of the acceleration record;
k_c = critical acceleration of the slip surface;
k_m = peak acceleration of the record;
u = final displacement with the block sliding in down-slope direction only;
g = acceleration due to gravity. The dimension of g determines the dimension of u.

9.7.3   An equation based only on the ratio of critical seismic coefficient and peak ground acceleration coefficient

Ambraseys and Menu (1988) proposed the following equation based only on one ground motion parameter, namely, the peak ground acceleration.

$$\log[u_{cm}] = 0.90 + \log\left[\left(1 - \frac{k_c}{k_m}\right)^{2.53}\left(\frac{k_c}{k_m}\right)^{-1.09}\right] \tag{9.19}$$

9.7.4   An equation based on Arias intensity and critical seismic acceleration

To facilitate large numbers of analyses associated with regional hazard mapping, empirical regression equations have been developed by researchers for particular regions. Thus double integration can be avoided and the numerical process is simplified considerably. For example, for the Los Angeles (California) region, the Newmark displacement D_N (cm) was expressed as a function of Arias intensity I_a (in metres per second and the critical seismic acceleration a_c in g's (Jibson et al., 1998)) as follows:

$$\log D_N = 1.52 \log I_a - 1.993 \log a_c - 1.546 \tag{9.20}$$

Arias intensity is a single numerical measure of an acceleration-time record calculated by integrating the squared acceleration values over the entire duration (not limited to the period of strong motion). It has the unit of a velocity.

For the same region (Los Angeles), the Arias Intensity was related to earthquake magnitude M and source distance R (Wilson and Keefer, 1985) as follows:

$$\log I_a = M - 2 \log R - 4.1 \tag{9.21}$$

9.7.5   Seismic Destructiveness Potential Factor and its use in numerical analyses

A term 'Seismic Destructiveness Potential Factor' has also been defined by the ratio of the Arias intensity I_a and the square of the number of zero crossings per second of the accelerogram (Araya and Saragoni, 1984):

$$P_D = \frac{I_a}{v_0^2} = \frac{\pi}{2g} \frac{\int_0^{to} a^2(t)dt}{v_0^2} \tag{9.22}$$

The displacement of a rigid block on a horizontal plane is a function of P_D and the critical seismic coefficient k_c. For a slope with given geometry and a specified failure mechanism an appropriate correction factor can then be applied (Crespellani et al., 1998). Based on 310 earthquake records, the authors obtained two regression equations for permanent deformation of a rigid block with confidence levels of 50% and 90% respectively, denoted as s_{50} and s_{90}.

This approach highlighted several aspects of permanent deformation analysis.

Firstly, displacements associated with a plane failure mechanism are constant along the plane but those associated with a curved failure mechanism vary significantly along the slip surface.

Secondly, the critical seismic coefficient for a rotational failure mechanism is smaller than that for a plane failure mechanism. Consequently the displacements corresponding to a rotational failure mechanism are greater than those for a plane failure mechanism.

Thirdly, the displacement ratio, s (curved)/s (plane), can be even greater than the corresponding k_c ratio. For further elaboration of the merits of this approach, the reader may refer to Chowdhury (2001).

9.8   DYNAMIC ANALYSES

9.8.1   Introduction

As stated in the previous sections, earthquakes impose cyclic loading on slopes and embankments and generate alternating stresses. Therefore, any existing tensile stresses may be increased to unacceptable levels and existing compressive stresses may become tensile. Limitations of pseudo-static analyses are now widely recognized. By using dynamic analyses, more realistic information can be gained about the response of earth slopes and structures to earthquake shaking. In addition to giving information on the time histories of stresses, natural frequencies and the effects of damping, it is possible to estimate equivalent seismic coefficient. Moreover the nonlinear behaviour of earth structures can be simulated.

However, dynamic analyses can be significantly more complex. Moreover, carrying out such analyses requires additional data such as the values of dynamic soil properties.

The first vibratory studies of earth dams were made on the assumption that a dam could be considered as a vertical one-dimensional shear beam of triangular shape. Only shearing deformations were considered and the assumption was made that these were uniformly distributed over horizontal planes. Finite-difference studies of Ishizaki and Hatakeyama (1962) showed that the shear beam type of approach is inadequate for predicting the stresses away from the central parts of the dam.

Clough and Chopra (1966) extended the finite element method of analysis to dynamic problems and considered a homogeneous dam on a rigid foundation. Chopra (1967) made further two-dimensional response analyses and compared the results with those obtained from the assumption of a one-dimensional shear beam or shear wedge. He found significant differences in mode shapes. He also found significant normal and vertical stresses and resulting deformations which differ considerably from the pure shear deformations assumed in the shear wedge approach. The results of the latter are independent of side slopes but in the finite element analyses steeper slopes were found to lead to greater stresses.

The values of seismic co-efficient determined by a shear wedge approach were 10 to 20% greater than those computed by finite element analysis. Chopra did point out the limitation that the analysis at that stage was based on linearly elastic response and that inelastic deformations and the yielding process were not considered. However, the finite element method is versatile and there has been very rapid progress in connection with dynamic studies relating to embankments. By the mid 1970s, dams were already being studied using non-linear dynamic finite element analyses, e.g., a study of the Hawkins Dam by Lee and Roth (1977).

9.8.2   Basic concepts and equations

The essential features of a dynamic finite element analysis are as follows:

Consider the motion of a slope with respect to a stationary reference or base and assume a finite element subdivision of the slope into elements connected by nodal-points. The slope is subjected to inertia forces due to base acceleration $a(t)$ given by the following for any nodal point:

$$R(t) = -M\,a(t) \tag{9.23}$$

The nodal mass M is obtained by lumping at each node the appropriate proportion of the mass of each element surrounding that node. Let the nodal displacement be r. Then its equation of motion is:

$$M\ddot{r} + C\dot{r} + Kr = R(t) \tag{9.24}$$

in which C is the coefficient of viscous damping, K the appropriate stiffness and dots indicate differentiation with respect to time. In matrix form, we can write for the whole assemblage of elements:

$$[M]\,\{\ddot{r}\} + [C]\,\{\dot{r}\} + [K]\,\{r\} = \{R(t)\} \tag{9.25}$$

in which $[M]$, $[C]$ and $[K]$ are the matrix of mass, damping and stiffness respectively and the load matrix is obtained by considering both the horizontal and vertical components of the earthquake acceleration.

The undamped free vibration mode shapes and the corresponding natural frequencies of vibration are first determined by the solution of the usual characteristic value problem and the normal co-ordinates of the system related to nodal co-ordinates. The equations of motion are then reduced to n normal mode equations (Clough and Chopra, 1966). These equations are solved for the normal co-ordinates and finally the dynamic displacements $\{r\}$ are determined at discrete intervals of time. From these the dynamic element stresses and, therefore, the nodal point stresses are obtained.

A certain percentage of critical damping is assumed in the solution in each mode. Appropriate computer programs have been developed to carry out dynamic analyses by finite elements and are continually being refined and improved. In view of the variety of such programs it is essential that the basis for any particular program and the assumptions on which it is based are carefully studied before the programme is actually used. Finn and Khanna (1966) analysed dams with or without permeable cores on flexible foundations. A dynamic analysis will give the variation of dynamic displacements and stresses with time at any given point in the slope. It has been found that the response of an earth bank depends on its fundamental period in relation to the frequency distribution of an earthquake in addition to other obvious factors. Therefore specification of design earthquake requires attention not only to its magnitude but also its frequency content.

Knowing the stresses at a point in a slope before an earthquake, a suitable consolidation or confining stress for laboratory shear tests can be selected. Knowing the dynamic stresses due to earthquake at the same point and their variation, a range can be selected for cyclic loading of the specimen in such tests. From the dynamic strains which have accumulated at the end of such cyclic shear tests, the deformations of the dam during an earthquake can be studied. The selection of points in the slope or earth dam to which such tests should correspond, and of the types of shear tests which are suitable for them, has been discussed by Seed (1968). In order that a dynamic analysis may be meaningful it must be used in conjunction with shear test data obtained from experiments which take into consideration the location of the slip surface as well as the type of cyclic loading.

9.8.3   Example of analyses for a failed dam

Seed (1968) made a comparison (Table 9.3) of various methods to study the failure of Sheffield Dam in terms of the seismic co-efficient required to cause failure (see also Seed et al., 1969 and Seed, 1973).

Table 9.3 Analytical results for Sheffied Dam failure (after Seed, 1968). With permission from ASCE, see page 714, No 29.

Method	Seismic co-efficient to cause failure for critical slip surface in the probable failure zone	Notes on ground motion
Pseudo-static with strength parameters from static consolidated-undrained tests (total stress)	0.21	Max. ground acceleration during earthquake about 0.15 g. Duration of shaking about 15 seconds
Dynamic analyses using test data from cyclic loading anisotropically consolidated-undrained triaxial compression test (10 cycles)	0.19	Response analysis indicated about 10 cycles with seismic co-efficient of 0.15 for slides extending to base of embankment
Dynamic analyses using test data from cyclic loading simple shear tests (10 cycles)	0.11	—

The success of analyses which were based on cyclic loading simple shear tests were attributed to two factors:

1   The initial condition of near-zero shear stress and high normal stress on near horizontal planes (corresponding to near horizontal probable failure plane in the dam) could be simulated in such shear tests before cyclic loading was applied, and
2   The principal stress re-orientation occurring on these planes during earthquake could be considered in simple shear tests but not in triaxial tests.

It was noted that in cyclic loading simple shear tests representative of the actual stress conditions, failure of the soil sample always developed by liquefaction. This was consistent with the development of failure by liquefaction in the Sheffield Dam borne out by dynamic response analyses. The zone of liquefaction along the base of the embankment increased in length from less than half of the base after 2 seconds of motion to nearly the entire length of the base of the cross-section after 10 seconds of ground motion. (See also Seed, 1973.) The critical failure surface was found by analysis to be along the base of the dam (also considered to be the most probable location on the basis of post failure observations).

9.8.4   Other procedures developed and used in the 1970s

For some further insight of early developments concerning dynamic analysis procedures it is useful to refer briefly to the studies of Hawkins Dam made by Lee and Roth (1977). The Berkeley (University of California) programme QUAD 4 was used to calculate the response of the maximum section of the dam (divided into 8 elements) to each of the selected earthquake motions.

Irregular field stress-time histories were converted into equivalent uniform cyclic stress-time history corresponding to laboratory test data. The number of equivalent uniform cycles of some average cyclic stress intensity that would have the same damaging effect on the soil (e.g., cause the same strain) as the actual irregular stress-time history were thus determined. Non-linear modulus and damping properties were based on undrained shear strength data. Core and shell zones were given same properties because under cyclic loading all soils had been found to behave in a similar manner.

Pre-earthquake static stresses were determined from static linear elastic finite element program which was considered satisfactory from past experience. Seepage forces were included in the static stress analysis of this hydraulic fill dam. These were based on a flow net drawn on the assumption of homogeneous isotropic soil. Local factors of safety were calculated for each finite element as a ratio of (1) cyclic strength of soil measured in the laboratory and converted to field conditions (cyclic stress on failure plane at failure) and (2) the equivalent average uniform cyclic shear stress calculated by QUAD 4. Both these stresses refer only to the seismic part of the shear stress and the static gravity stresses were not included in this ratio. Calculations were based on cyclic strength data defined by stresses required to cause 5% single amplitude cyclic strain in the laboratory triaxial test. This criterion was considered as a satisfactory definition of failure from past experience. (Other approaches involving the concept of strain potential have also been used). Contours were plotted of the local seismic factors of safety F_i and of the local cyclic strain potentials corresponding to $F_i = 1$. Both alternative approaches give a reasonable idea of the seismic stability.

A third approach was also used in which a single overall factor of safety along a potential slip surface was determined. This was obtained as the ratio of 'a' and 'b' defined as follows:-

'a' is sum of the products of length of slip surface in each element and cyclic strength of soil corresponding to that element including the strength component due to pre-earthquake static stresses, and

'b' is the sum of the products of length of slip surface in each element and the total driving shear stress which includes the pre-earthquake static shear stress.

In this case the shear stresses were considered in the direction of the potential slip surface in each element. (Note that for local factors of safety horizontal direction was assumed as the failure plane direction irrespective of element location). Estimates of permanent deformations that may occur during selected ground motions were also made in accordance with procedure developed by Lee (1974). Effects on factors of safety, arising from modifications of the dam to stop downstream seepage, were also studied.

9.8.5   The Seed-Lee-Idriss procedure for dams or embankments which include saturated cohesionless materials

By 1979, the research group at University of California at Berkeley, under the leadership of Professor H.B. Seed, had developed a comprehensive approach for seismic analysis of dams or embankments. Such a comprehensive procedure was considered to be warranted, in particular, if saturated cohesionless soils were included amongst the embankment-forming materials. As outlined by Seed (1979), a number of steps need to be followed. Considering such a project task as multi-disciplinary, involving geotechnical engineers, geologists and seismologists, the steps required may be summarized as follows:

- Determine the cross-section of the dam before the earthquake and carry out a static stress analysis using, for instance, the finite element method (FEM).
- Estimate the maximum time history of base excitation to which a dam and its foundation might be subjected.
- Estimate dynamic properties of soils comprising the dam and the variation of parameters such as bulk modulus, shear modulus and damping characteristics with strain (non-linear characteristics).
- Estimate dynamic stresses induced in the embankment using, for instance, dynamic finite element analysis.
- From a number of tests on soil specimens subjected to initial static stresses plus induced dynamic stresses, determine development of strains and generation of excess pore water pressures. The number of tests should be sufficient to represent all important locations in the embankment.
- From the above results, evaluate the factor of safety against failure during or after the earthquake.

Table 9.4 Predicted performance based on dynamic analysis procedure compared to observed performance (after Seed, 1979). With permission, see page 714, No 30.

Dam	Date of earthquake	Maximum acceleration	Predicted performance	Actual performance	Reference*
Sheffield	1925	0.2 g	Failure by sliding	Failure by sliding	Seed et al., 1971
Lower San Fernando	1971	0.5 g	Major upstream slide	Major upstream slide	Seed et al., 1973
Upper San Fernando	1971	0.5 g	No failure; large downstream movement	No failure; large downstream movement	Serff et al., 1976
Dry Canyon	1952	0.1 g	Small deformation; some cracking	Small deformation; some cracking	Lee and Walters, 1972
Lower Franklin	1971	0.2 g	No damage	No damage	Seed et al., 1973
Silver Lak	1971	0.2 g	No damage	No damage	Seed et al., 1973
Fairmont	1971	0.2 g	No damage	No damage	Seed et al., 1973
Chabot	1906	0.4 g	No damage	No damage	Makdisi et al., 1978

*Note that the references in this column were cited in the original paper (Seed, 1979) but are NOT cited in the Reference List at the end of this book. The reader may look up these references from Seed's original paper.

- If the factor of safety is satisfactory, assess the total deformations from the strains.
- In all steps incorporate knowledge and judgement based on past performance of embankments and dams in other earthquakes.

Seed (1979) acknowledged criticism by colleagues and other experts that the above procedure was cumbersome. He cited several research papers by different authors which discussed the use of simplified versions of the procedure. He commented, in part, as follows:

"Some engineers have commented that the dynamic analysis procedure I have proposed for cohesionless soils is too sophisticated ... I do not see the procedure in this light – but simply as a series of steps which forces the engineer to consider the essential elements of the problem ...".

A comparison of the results of dynamic analyses of a number of dams published in the period 1971–1978 (predicted performance) with the observed performance of those dams was summarized by Seed (1979) and the table is reproduced here (Table 9.4).

9.8.6 Analysis of Lower San Fernando Dam – Seed's approach

As an example of the application of dynamic analysis, Seed presented the following results for the Lower San Fernando Dam. The time-history of acceleration in the base rock is shown in the base diagram of Figure 9.8. The computed history of crest acceleration is shown in the upper diagram of the same figure. The zones of liquefaction failure in the dam after 10.5, 13.5 and 15 seconds of earthquake shaking are shown in the middle diagram of Figure 9.8.

The observed/inferred slip surface within the dam with estimated spatial distribution of undrained shear strength at the end of the earthquake is shown in Figure 9.9. As shown in the figure, the limit equilibrium factor of safety was estimated using a total stress approach. The estimated value was found to be 1.4 ($F = 1.4$). Thus failure during the earthquake or at the end could not be explained on the basis of a sophisticated dynamic analysis procedure. On the observed evidence it was also concluded that the actual failure occurred some time after the end of the earthquake.

According to Table 7 in Seed (1979), strong motion of the main shock of the San Fernando earthquake was completed at 14 seconds with only a small tilting of the dam crest. It was at 40 seconds after the start of the main shock, and following four

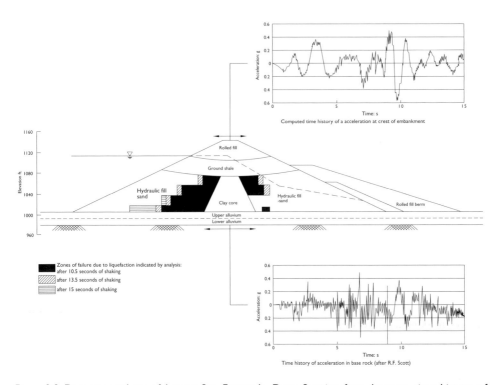

Figure 9.8 Dynamic analysis of Lower San Fernando Dam: Starting from bottom, time history of acceleration at base, liquefied zones in dam and acceleration of crest (after Seed, 1979). With permission, see page 714, No 30.

Note: 1 ft. = 0.3048 m.

aftershocks, that slide movements at the crest started. It was 90 seconds from the start that the main slide movement ended (instrument tilted about 26°). Further tilting to 37° occurred during the following 10 days.

Therefore, a progressive process of redistribution of excess pore water pressure within the dam was postulated by Seed. Such redistribution was considered to have caused water to migrate from the liquefied zone to nearby areas of soil dilation. Thus it was postulated that the undrained shear strength of those areas was reduced. Estimates of the redistributed undrained shear strength are shown in Figure 9.10. On this basis, the factor of safety was found to be well below 1 ($F = 0.8$). Thus failure occurring a short time after the earthquake could be explained. This particular paper (Seed,

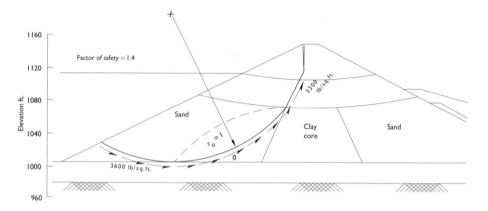

Figure 9.9 Stability of Lower San Fernando Dam immediately after earthquake. With permission, see page 714, No 30.

Note: undrained loading of all zones; shear resistance drops to zero where $r_u = 1$ (pore pressure ratio defined with respect to submerged unit weight of soil)-after Seed (1979). 1 ft. = 0.3048 m and 1 lb/sq. ft. = 0.04788 kN/m².

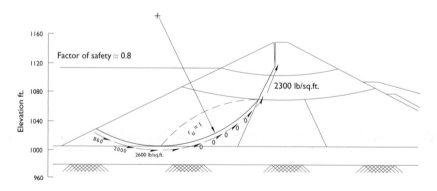

Figure 9.10 Stability of Lower San Fernando Dam immediately after earthquake motions stop. With permission, see page 714, No 30.

Note: Undrained loading of all zones; shear resistance drops to zero where $r_u = 1$ (pore pressure ratio defined with respect to submerged unit weight of soil)-after Seed (1979). 1 ft. = 0.3048 m and 1 lb/sq. ft. = 0.04788 kN/m².

1979) does not include details of how the redistributed values of undrained shear strength were estimated. For full details, the reader must refer to previous publications of Seed and his research team.

In these figures the pore pressure ratio $r_u = 1$ is shown for the liquefied zone. This is because Seed's definition of the ratio was pore pressure divided by product of submerged unit weight and soil depth. Thus the effective stress of a submerged soil element would reduce to zero when the excess pore pressure due to seismic shaking was equal to the product of soil depth and submerged unit weight. If the conventional definition of pore pressure based on total saturated unit weight was used, excess pore pressure ratio would be about 0.5.

9.8.7 Alternative explanation for failure of Lower San Fernando Dam

According to Marcuson III et al. (1992), this case study was re-evaluated during the period 1985–1989, and provided the critical data point in evaluating post liquefied residual strengths. The occurrence of the slide was explained again by a total stress type of analysis and on the basis of the steady state procedure for the liquefied soil zone. This implies that undrained residual strength was applicable within the whole of the liquefied zone which differs sharply from the assignment of zero undrained shear strength to a significant part of the slip surface in Seed's analysis. Yet Marcuson III et al. (1992) commented:

> "This study shows that both the steady state procedure and the Seed procedure would have predicted that the dam would slide as a result of seismic shaking".

The implication of failure occurring after an earthquake was highlighted with the comment that "the failure should be treated as a static problem using strengths that have been degraded as a result of seismic shaking and pore pressure build up."

The general procedure for dynamic analysis was summarized by Marcuson III et al. (1992) as a series of steps which are very similar to those outlined by Seed more than a decade earlier. However, it is important to remember that there are significant differences as regards assigning the undrained strengths to be applied to cohesionless soil and especially to the zones assessed to have undergone liquefaction.

In one of the steps it is stated that either total stress or effective stress approach may be used in limit equilibrium analysis (after the dynamic response has been evaluated). The following comment is of particular interest "… if a total stress approach is used, one should use both the drained and undrained strength parameters; whichever yields the lower factor of safety governs." This may be a useful advice from a practical perspective but a rational explanation would have been of great interest.

More importantly, it is interesting to note that an effective stress analysis was not applied to an important case study such as the failure of the Lower San Fernando Dam either by Seed and co-workers or by others such as Marcuson III et al. (1992).

Therefore, the results of a new approach, based on degradation of the critical seismic coefficient during earthquake shaking, are presented in the following section. The limit equilibrium part of this analysis uses an effective stress approach.

9.8.8   Effective stress approach for analysis of Lower San Fernando Dam

The traditional Newmark (sliding block) approach is based on the assumption that the critical seismic coefficient remains constant during an earthquake. This may be a reasonable assumption in some cases but not for others. If earthquake shaking is strong enough to generate high pore water pressures within some sections of a slope or dam and, in particular, if liquefaction occurs, the average shear strength along a potential slip surface would decrease significantly. Consequently, the static factor of safety and the critical seismic coefficient would also decrease significantly. In his important state-of-the-art paper, Seed (1979) clearly implied that a constant value of the critical seismic coefficient is only an assumption. Thus the results obtained on this basis, for cases such as the Lower San Fernando dam, must be considered with a careful exercise of engineering judgment.

For an effective stress analysis of a slope or embankment which incorporates saturated cohesionless soil in one of its zones, it is important to be able to estimate the excess pore water pressure developed during seismic shaking and also the value of the critical seismic coefficient. Both may vary with time depending on the soil properties and the intensity of shaking. Therefore an incremental time-step procedure must be adopted with a sufficiently small time-step.

Equation (9.13) for acceleration of the slope must be updated simply to incorporate a time-dependent k_c as defined in Equation (9.14). If the value of the dynamic pore water pressure coefficient (sub-section 9.6.3) is known for the saturated cohesionless soil, pore water pressure may be estimated by using Equations (9.15) to (9.17), for the appropriate stress increments applicable to a particular stage of analysis.

An effective stress approach for a time-dependent analysis, with particular reference to the Lower San Fernando Dam has been developed (Dawei, 1994; Chowdhury, 1995, 1996). The steps used in the procedure are illustrated by the following flowchart (Figure 9.11).

Different soil zones of the dam and a potential slip surface are shown in Figure 9.12 and the corresponding soil properties, based on Lee et al. (1975), are shown in Table 9.5. Amongst these zones, Zone 2 was the one which liquefied prior to the occurrence of the slide. Therefore, the initial estimate of the effective friction angle for that zone may have been an overestimate. However, the original published value was used in these analyses.

The acceleration-time history to be used in the sliding block model was generated as per procedures described by Dawei (1994) to match the published 15 seconds record which is reproduced in Figure 9.8.

Based on analysis of published data reported by Sarma and Jennings (1980), the following values of A_n ($n = 1$ to $n = 5$) were considered to apply:

Lower San Fernando Dam: $A_1 = 0.67$ and $A_5 = 1.35$
Upper San Fernando Dam: $A_1 = 1.25$ and $A_5 = 2.56$

Thus it was considered desirable to use values in the range 0.67–2.8 in the analyses. $A_1 = 0.67$ was kept the same for all analyses and only A_5 was varied in the range 1.6–2.8.

It is of interest to note that, for some soils, values as high as $A_5 = 7$ have been interpreted by Sarma and Jennings (1980) from the data published by prominent researchers.

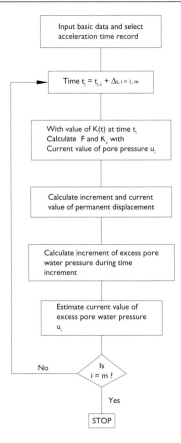

Figure 9.11 Effective stress analysis procedure using variable critical seismic coefficient in a sliding block analysis.

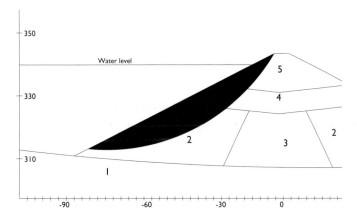

Figure 9.12 Cross-section showing different soil zones and a potential slip surface.

Table 9.5 Soil properties in different zones shown in Figure 9.12 (from Lee, et al., 1975).

Zone	γ (kN/m³)	c' (kN/m²)	ϕ' (Degrees)	c_u (kN/m²)
1	17.3	0	38	–
2	20.5	0	37	–
3	19	–	–	81.4
4	20	0	33	–
4	19	–	–	81.4

Table 9.6 Results of effective stress analysis for Lower San Fernando Dam (sliding block model assuming variable critical seismic acceleration) considering predicted critical slip surface (Chowdhury, 1995, 1996).

Dynamic PWP parameter	F	k_c
Before earthquake $A_1 = 0$, $A_n = 0$	2.04	0.36
$A_1 = 0.67$, $A_n = 1.6$	1.49	0.16
$A_1 = 0.67$, $A_n = 2.4$	1.19	0.07
$A_1 = 0.67$, $A_n = 2.6$	1.1	0.04
$A_1 = 0.67$, $A_n = 2.8$	Failure*	Failure*

* Time to failure, $t_c = 14.55$ seconds.

Table 9.7 Results of effective stress analysis for Lower San Fernando Dam (sliding block model assuming variable critical seismic coefficient) considering observed slip surface.

Dynamic PWP parameters	F	k_c
Before earthquake $A_1 = 0$, $A_n = 0$	2.29	0.48
$A_1 = 0.67$, $A_n = 1.6$	1.55	0.20
$A_1 = 0.67$, $A_n = 2.4$	1.21	0.04
$A_1 = 0.67$, $A_n = 2.6$	Failure*	Failure*

* Time to failure, $t_c = 14.535$ seconds.

Analyses were carried out with (1) the critical slip surface located by a search procedure incorporate in the computer program, and (2) the observed slip surface as reported in the literature. The factor of safety values are shown in Tables 9.6 and 9.7. Results concerning variation of excess pore pressure with time and increase of permanent displacement with time are not presented here.

The results of these analyses demonstrate that a sliding block analysis incorporating a time-dependent critical seismic coefficient can be used successfully. Moreover, the estimation of the critical seismic coefficient can be made logically and rationally in terms of effective stress analysis. It is perhaps fortuitous that failure occurs close to the end of the duration of input motion.

Moreover, the magnitude of the dynamic pore pressure coefficient required to cause failure, though well within the range of values for the two San Fernando dams (the Upper and the Lower), is greater than the values quoted for the Lower San Fernando dam by Sarma and Jennings (1980). Obviously there must be a significant variability in the data which is not captured by a single set of values.

Considering the uncertainties about soil parameter variability, the best one can conclude is that the results of such an effective stress approach must be used with careful exercise of engineering judgement. In important cases, such an approach could be a useful addition to other procedures and tools discussed in this chapter.

9.9   OCCURRENCE OF EARTHQUAKE-INDUCED LANDSLIDES

9.9.1   Landslides related to some major earthquakes – key findings

Earthquakes may cause significant failures and movements of natural slopes, embankments, earth dams and excavations. Many landslides triggered by earthquakes have resulted in major disasters. A recent example relates to landslides associated with the Pakistan earthquake of October 8, 2005 ($M = 7.6$) which caused enormous economic loss, infrastructure damage, social disruption and loss of life in the tens of thousands. For many historical earthquakes, landslides are responsible for a high proportion of the total losses. For example the proportion of loss due to landslides during the 1964 Alaska earthquake was estimated to be more than 50% of the total (Wilson and Keefer, 1985). Hundreds of large landslides associated with the 1920 Haiyuan earthquake (Ningxia Province, China) caused more than 100,000 deaths (Close and McCormick, 1922). More than 50% of all deaths caused by large earthquakes ($M > 6.9$) in Japan in the period 1964–1980 were caused by landslides (Kobayashi, 1981).

The occurrence of landslides triggered by earthquakes differs in significant respects from rainfall-induced landslides. These differences include landslide types, mechanisms, locations and frequencies. Relatively high earthquake magnitude ($M >$ about 4) is a key determinant of the occurrence of widespread landsliding. Research in high seismicity areas concerning earthquake-induced landslides include a study of landslide size, spatial distribution, landslide type and other features in relation to earthquake size which has been found to be the dominant parameter.

A key paper (Keefer, 1984) included a database from 40 earthquakes covering the period 1811–1980. This research has been extended for the period 1980–1997 in a study including 36 earthquakes worldwide (Rodriguez et al., 1999). The related regions include a variety of topographical, geological and climatic settings. The first study concluded that, in general, the smallest earthquakes likely to cause landslides are those with moment magnitude $M = 4$. Even in areas highly susceptible to slope failure only a few landslides may occur from an earthquake with $M < 5$. In contrast, earthquakes with $M > 7.5$ typically trigger thousands or tens of thousands of landslides.

However, one should pause and reflect on the fact that even such broad findings are limited in scope. For example, such visual observations do not reveal sub-surface shear movements or permanent displacements, which may indicate significantly reduced slope stability at specific locations where catastrophic landsliding has not occurred. Quite clearly these subsurface movements, rarely recorded, would have considerable relevance to assessment and management of landslide susceptibility, hazard and risk in the future.

The most abundant landslide types resulting from earthquakes are rock falls, rock slides and fast-moving disrupted soil-rock slides. Less abundant landslide types include slower-moving and deeper-seated slumps and block slides, large and complex rock avalanches, soil avalanches, soil fills, slow earth flows, fluid, fast moving soil flows and landslides caused by liquefaction. The last of these include lateral spreads and sub-aqueous landslides and occur mostly in gently sloping alluvial flood plains, coastal areas and offshore.

Relationships were plotted by Keefer (1984) for the following against earthquake magnitude (both surface wave and moment magnitude): (a) Total area affected by landslides, (b) Maximum epicentral distance and (c) Maximum distance to fault plane projections. These relationships were plotted separately for the following: (a) Disrupted slides, (b) Coherent slides and (c) Spreads and flows. Note that such plots do not take into account the susceptibility of the region to landslides in general. As expected, the relationships show considerable scatter. However, in each case an upper bound was easy to determine.

The analysis of data from the 1999 study confirmed the findings of the earlier (1984) study except that the maximum area affected was even greater than shown by the 1984 study. The 1999 study showed that, in exceptional cases, highly susceptible slopes may slide after quite distant seismic events and that even very small size earthquakes can trigger landslides under particular circumstances. In discussing the findings of the 1999 study, and how research may be extended further, it has been suggested that rainfall-induced landslide hazard should be studied at the same time as earthquake-induced landslide hazard.

For example, comparison of landsliding caused by (a) the great Indian earthquake of 12 June 1897 and (b) the Assam earthquake of 15 August 1950 shows the combined effect of both rainfall and earthquake. Both earthquakes are of similar magnitudes (about 8.6) and occurred in the same region of Assam, India. The 1897 earthquake occurred just before the monsoon season while the 1950 earthquake occurred in the middle of monsoon. The second earthquake caused landslides over an area in excess of 35000 km^2 as estimated by Sarma (pers. com., 2006) from a map produced by Mathur (1953). The 1897 earthquake did not result in such widespread landsliding although spectacular landslides did occur as a consequence of both events. A summary of the effects of the 1897 earthquake is found in Richter (1958).

9.9.2   Some empirical relationships between earthquake magnitude *M*, landslide volume *V*, and landslide area *A*

Returning now to the research concerning landslide volume and distribution, wide scatter of the various relationships between magnitude and parameters such as volume and area of landslides was to be expected. Moreover, the presence of extreme outliers was also noted in the 1999 study. These may indicate unusual situations such as quick clay landslides and also the effect of multiple earthquakes and the simultaneous arrival of different phases of seismic waves.

The following linear regression equation between landslide volume in cubic metres and earthquake moment magnitude M has been proposed (Keefer and Wilson, 1989).

$$\text{Log}_{10}\ V = 1.44\ M - 2.34 \tag{9.26}$$

This linear regression equation was based on data from ten earthquakes in North and South America, India, New Zealand and New Guinea. Based on data from fifteen historical earthquakes the following equation was reported in a subsequent paper (Keefer, 1994).

$$\text{Log}_{10} V = 1.45\ M - 2.50 \tag{9.27}$$

It is clear that there is little difference between this and the 1989 relation. These relations have also been presented in a modified form, M being replaced by the seismic moment, M_0. However, the modified relationships need not be presented here. The total volume does not include the contribution of liquefaction-induced landslides because these volumes are difficult to estimate.

From an analysis of data from 37 earthquakes the average area A of landslide occurrence in an earthquake has been related to earthquake size as follows (Keefer and Wilson, 1989)

$$\text{Log}_{10}\ A = M - 3.46\ (5 < M < 9.2) \tag{9.28}$$

The overall distribution is not uniform and more than 95% of landslides triggered by an earthquake are concentrated in less than half of the total area. For example, an "average" $M = 8$ earthquake would trigger landslides over an area of 35,000 km² but most landslides would occur within an area of 17,500 km² (Keefer, 1994).

For a specific region, the number of earthquakes N of magnitudes greater than or equal to M per unit time is of the standard form:

$$\text{Log}_{10} N = a - b\ M \tag{9.29}$$

where a and b are coefficients to be determined empirically.

Combining this relation with the mean landslide volume versus M relation, the mean rate of earthquake-induced landslide material V can be determined for a particular region. For example, the rate for Peru was calculated to be: 1.7×10^8 m³/year.

On this basis, a systematic study of the importance of seismic landsliding to long-term slope erosions and slope failure hazard was included in the 1994 study (Keefer, 1994). Three measures were proposed: the rate of earthquake-triggered landslide volume, comparison of this rate with erosion rate from other processes and its comparison with the erosion rate from fluid sediment discharge. Applied to twelve seismically active regions, the analysis revealed significant regional variations.

9.9.3   Summary of a subsequent study (Keefer, 2007)

The findings of a most recent study, reported by Keefer (2007), are concerned with landslides caused by ten relatively large earthquakes (magnitude ranging from

$M = 5.6$ to 8.4) which occurred between 1989 and 2004. In some respects, the recent study confirmed trends noted from previous studies of historical earthquakes summarized above. However, there were some differences, anomalies and unexpected effects.

For example, the landslide concentrations associated with the Loma Prieta earthquake (California, October 1989, $M = 6.9$) were found to diminish with distance from the earthquake source whereas for the St. George earthquake (Utah, September 1992, $M = 5.6$) and Tecoman earthquake (Mexico, January 2003, $M = 7.6$), individual landslides or high landslide concentrations occurred at relatively large distances from the source.

For the Denali Fault earthquake (Alaska, November 2002, $M = 7.9$), landslides were restricted to zones much smaller than indicated by general trends.

For the Racha earthquake (Georgia, April 1991, $M = 7$), landslide movements occurred after substantial time delays.

The Loma Prieta, Northridge (California, January 1994, $M = 6.7$) and Denali Fault earthquakes revealed a wider range of hazards than was considered plausible from past studies.

The severity of landsliding and ground failure due to the Southern Peru earthquake (June 2001, $M = 8.2–8.4$) was such as to produce a shattered landscape.

9.9.4 Topographic amplification effects

Seismic ground accelerations are often amplified depending on the local site conditions as well as on the topography. The former is called site amplification and concerns the influence of local soil conditions (the depth and stiffness of each of the surface soil layers). This effect is widely recognized by geotechnical and earthquake engineers. For example, enormous damage to buildings and infrastructure during the Mexico earthquake was associated with the amplification of ground motion due to the soft soils of Mexico city. In contrast, the importance of topographic amplification effects is not as widely known in spite of research over more than two decades.

Numerical analysis approaches such as finite element, finite-difference and boundary element methods have been used for analysis of topographic amplification and a brief review has been presented by Tabesh and Chowdhury (1997). Using the finite-difference program FLAC, some time-domain analyses were carried out, for example, problems representing homogeneous and non-homogeneous escarpments (Chowdhury and Tabesh, 1998). The results showed that the presence of a valley has little effect on the ground response of an otherwise level area. On the other hand, the presence of a mountain results in significant amplification of the displacement response.

As an example of observed field effects, several landslides in the coastal bluffs of the Pacific Palisades during the 1994 Northridge earthquake have been attributed to topographic amplification. Severe damage to houses on the top of a bluff was concentrated within about 50 metres (one slope height) of the slope crest. Response analyses using 2D visco-elastic frequency domain GCTB (Generalised Consistent Transmitting Boundaries) analyses was able to explain the spatial distribution of the damage and the topographic amplification was estimated to be in the range 52–76% (Ashford and Sitar, 1998).

The response of a slope is often influenced by the direction of wave propagation and wave inclination relative to a slope. For example, during the 1989 Loma Prieta earthquake, massive failures occurred on spurs from ridges but there was no failure associated with nearby cliffs. There are many instances in different parts of the world of landslides occurring with greater frequency on one side of a valley or ridge relative to the other side.

Where analyses have been carried out and compared with observed topographic effects, it has been suggested that analyses may significantly underestimate observed amplifications "which mostly range from 2 to 10 and up to as much as 30" (Ashford et al., 1997). However, topographic amplification may, in some cases, be offset by reduced site amplification (Ashford and Sitar, 1997).

9.10 EFFECT OF EARTHQUAKES ON EARTH DAMS AND EMBANKMENTS

9.10.1 Examples of dams that failed during earthquakes

9.10.1.1 Early comments on dam safety

It is regarded as fortunate that few major earth dams have been subjected to very severe shaking during earthquakes. Only a small number of earth dams have failed completely. However, a large number of earth dams have suffered significant damage. Sherrard (1967) made the following pertinent comments:

- Confidence in our ability to build safe dams is derived primarily from the satisfactory performance of literally hundreds of large dams and thousands of small ones. Hence in order to guide and support design procedures for dams under ordinary conditions of performance, there is available literally thousands of 'dam-years' of experience with dams of all kinds under all conceivable circumstances all over the world and, in addition, a large volume of measurements with instruments.
- The equivalent experience available concerning the probable behaviour of dams shaken by earthquakes is relatively so much smaller as to be insignificant. Judgments on the future performance of dams can, of course, be facilitated by analyses and considerable reliance was placed on the pseudo-static approach for many years.
- Experience has shown, however that a pseudo-static factor of safety greater than 1 does not ensure stability or indicate satisfactory performance. This was made clear by Terzaghi (1950) in his classical paper. However, his advice was ignored for decades as pointed out by Seed (1979).

9.10.1.2 Comparison of analysis results for four dams

Seed (1979) presented selected results of pseudo-static analyses for four dams which failed as a consequence of earthquakes. These include Sheffield Dam (1925 earthquake), Lower and Upper San Fernando Dams (1971 earthquake) and a tailings Dam in Japan (1978 earthquake). The cross-sections of three of the dams with slip surfaces

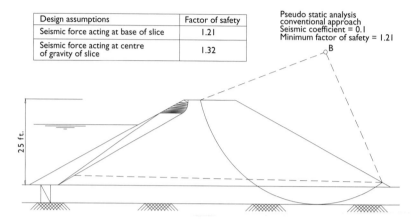

Design assumptions	Factor of safety
Seismic force acting at base of slice	1.21
Seismic force acting at centre of gravity of slice	1.32

Pseudo static analysis
conventional approach
Seismic coefficient = 0.1
Minimum factor of safety = 1.21

Figure 9.13 Pseudo-static analysis of embankment stability during earthquake – Sheffield Dam (after Seed, 1979). With permission, see page 714, No 30.

Note: 1 ft. = 0.3048 m.

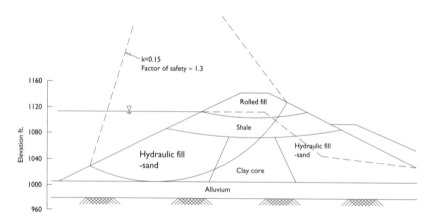

Figure 9.14 Pseudo-static analysis of embankment stability – Lower San Fernando Dam (after Seed, 1979). With permission, see page 714, No 30.

Note: 1 ft. = 0.3048 m.

considered in pseudo-static analysis are shown below (Figures 9.13 to 9.15). The table showing k values and corresponding calculated factors of safety is also presented and are reproduced below (Table 9.8).

9.10.2   Example of a dam surviving a strong earthquake

A dam may not fail due to a fortunate combination of circumstances even during a strong earthquake. For example, Sherrard (1967) commented in relation to the Hebgen

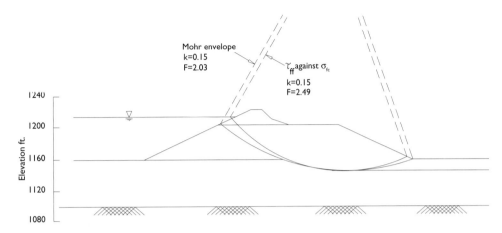

Figure 9.15 Results of pseudo-static analysis of embankment stability – Upper San Fernando Dam (after Seed, 1979). With permission, see page 714, No 30.

Note: 1 ft. = 0.3048 m.

Table 9.8 Summary of pseudo-static analysis results for four dams which failed (after Seed, 1979). With permission, see page 714, No 30.

Name of Dam	k	F	Nature of failure due to earthquake
Sheffield Dam	0.1	1.2	Complete failure
Lower San Fernando Dam	0.15	1.3	Upstream slope failure
Upper San Fernando Dam	0.15	≈ 2 to 2.5	Downstream shell and crest slipped about 6 ft. downstream
Tailings Dam, Oshima Island, Japan	0.2	≈ 1.3	Failure with release of tailings

Note: 1 ft = 30.48 cm.

Lake earthquake of 1959 (magnitude $M = 8.6$) "Almost every dangerous effect of an earthquake was present: major faulting, large deformations of the earth's crust, strong earth shaking, landslides and a major rockfall; an extremely fortunate array of conditions prevented a complete failure of the Hebgen dam in Montana. With such a large reservoir the failure would have been a disaster even in that sparsely populated area".

The fortunate circumstances were:

1   The main Hebgen fault was located on the valley wall several hundred feet from the dam and did not run down the centre of the stream channel as faults more commonly do.
2   By a fortunate coincidence the rock foundation of the dam sank 9.7 ft. at the same time that the 20 mile-long reservoir went down an average of more than 10 ft.

If only the dam had sunk, failure by overtopping would have been certain.

3   The block of foundation rock moved without tilting. Some tilting or differential displacement causing a large fissure would probably have resulted in a piping failure.

4   Landslides occurred away from the right abutment although the topography and materials at the landslide sites were similar to that at the right abutment. A landslide at this location would have led to rapid piping and breach through the abutment.

5   The massive rockslide occurred 7 miles downstream of the dam. If it had occurred on the upstream side into the reservoir, a wave would have been generated as at the Vajont dam (Muller, 1964) and failure could have occurred by overtopping. In fact, the location of the rockslide had been considered as an alternative site for the dam.

6   The spillway which was damaged during the earthquake did not have to be used before it was repaired. If a flood had occurred before repairs could be completed, complete failure could result.

According to Seed (1973) there were other fortunate circumstances. For example, the main fault movement adjacent to the dam was in a vertical direction indicating that the main inertia forces were in that direction. Horizontal inertia forces have a much greater influence on embankment stability than vertical inertia forces. Inspite of this, there was significant slumping of the upstream slope of Hebgen dam. Seed examined settlement data to conclude that the crest settlement due to slumping on the upstream side of the dam amounted to as much as 8% of the height. (Settlements of the extent observed in the downstream slope were assumed to be due to consolidation of the foundation materials and not due to shear deformations. The difference between upstream and downstream settlements was attributed to shear deformations). While slumping of this magnitude did not prove critical for Hebgen dam, it could be a major hazard for many other dams. Had the direction of fault movement been more conducive to shear displacements, Hebgen dam might have failed completely.

9.10.3   Failure modes and earthquake resistant design

An earth dam may fail due to an earthquake in many ways (Sherrard et al., 1963) e.g., (1) disruption by major fault movement in the foundation, (2) overtopping of the dam due to failure of spillway or outlet works, (3) overtopping of dam due to slides or rockfalls into the reservoir, (4) overtopping of dam due to seiches in the reservoir, (5) piping failure due to cracks induced by the ground motions, (6) loss of free board due to differential tectonic ground movements, (7) sliding of the dam on weak foundation materials, (8) slope failures induced by ground motions.

Earthquake resistant design requires that many precautions be taken to avoid most of the possible types of failures. Such measures as may be taken require experience and sound judgement and are not necessarily dependent upon a specific type of slope analysis, e.g., (Seed, 1973): (1) Location of the dam in an area in which there are no active faults, (2) provision of ample free board to allow for slumping of slope or subsidence of dam, (3) use of wide transition sections of filter materials which are not vulnerable to cracking, (4) use of wide cores of materials which are capable of self healing in the event cracking should develop, 5) careful examination of the stability of slopes adjoining the reservoir, (6) measures to be taken for handling overtopping that may result from seiches or slope failures into the reservoir.

Good design measures based on experience, judgement and careful planning may provide adequate protection against the first six types of failures considered above. However, a method of analysis would still be required to evaluate the possibility of slope failures and sliding along weak foundation materials. Qualitative judgements in respect of these aspects of earthquake design must be backed by adequate quantitative information. The main types and methods of analysis have already been described in the preceding sections of this chapter namely pseudo-static, sliding block and dynamic approaches.

9.11 ROLE OF PROBABILISTIC ANALYSIS

9.11.1 Numerous uncertainties

Assessment of seismic landslide hazard involves a number of uncertainties. These include:

1 Spatial and temporal variability of geotechnical parameters
2 Uncertain failure mechanisms and the assumptions associated with geotechnical models
3 Systematic uncertainty due to limited data from site investigation and due to the choice of site investigation and testing methods
4 Uncertainties associated with the ground motion including site and topographical amplification effects

9.11.2 Probability of failure conditional on earthquake occurrence

In view of these uncertainties accurate prediction of slope performance on a deterministic basis is generally difficult. It is, therefore, desirable to carry out probabilistic analysis in which the geotechnical parameters are treated as distributions rather than as constants. The probability of failure p_F would then be an indicator of landslide susceptibility/hazard. It could be defined on the basis of the dynamic factor of safety F_{dy}, given a value of seismic acceleration or seismic coefficient or acceleration-time history relevant to the particular earthquake magnitude and distance from the source as

$$p_F = P\,[F_{dy} < 1] \tag{9.30}$$

It could alternatively be defined on the basis of the permanent deformation s exceeding a specified value s_1:

$$p_F = P\,[s > s_1] \tag{9.31}$$

The estimation of these probabilities can be facilitated by adopting appropriate limit equilibrium and sliding block models. A convenient and simplified approach for deformation-based probabilities of failure would be to use one of the regression equations for deformation as the performance function, if such an equation applicable to a given region is available.

9.11.3   Probability of failure over the design life of a slope

Each of the values obtained from the above equations represents a probability of failure or of unacceptable magnitude of deformation conditional upon earthquake occurrence. Therefore, such a value needs to be multiplied by the probability of earthquake affecting the site over the design life of the slope or earth structure under consideration.

Such a probability may be obtained by first calculating the annual probability of earthquake occurrence and then the probability of occurrence over the design life of the slope, using a suitable probability model. For example, a Poisson's distribution might be suitable for such a calculation.

9.11.4   Estimating annual probability of earthquake occurrence

Calculating earthquake probability requires identification of the faults historically associated with earthquake occurrences in the region and the maximum size or magnitude of earthquake associated with each of these faults. Using the appropriate magnitude recurrence relationship, the annual probability can be calculated for each fault. The next step is to calculate the probability for the particular time period (design life) in respect of each of these faults. The contribution of all the faults to the overall probability of failure at the site can be calculated by following relevant probability concepts.

9.11.5   Probability of landsliding based on observation and calculated values

Considerable uncertainty is associated with failures of natural slopes triggered by earthquakes. For earthquakes of relatively large magnitude, landslides may cover very large areas. Thus it is hardly feasible to make individual, site-specific, detailed calculations (deterministic or probabilistic) for hundreds or thousands of slopes that might be considered important in a region. Therefore, it is more appropriate to combine a simple calculation model on a generic basis and validate the results based on experience and assessment of observational data from previous events.

An 'infinite slope' model for the static factor of safety (and hence the critical acceleration) was combined with a Newmark sliding block analysis by Jibson et al. (1998, 2000). An innovative definition of the probability of failure was proposed. This definition correlates calculated values of displacement with observations in the field. The estimated probability was used for the preparation of digital probabilistic seismic landslide hazard maps.

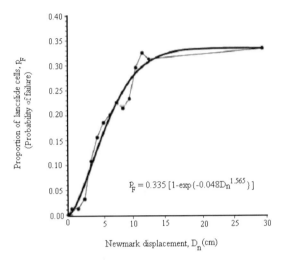

$$P_F = 0.335 \, [1 - \exp\{-0.048 D_n^{1.565}\}]$$

Newmark displacement, D_n (cm)

Figure 9.16 Proportion of landslide cells as a function of Newmark displacement. Data are indicated by dots with a connecting line; the bold line is the best fit of the Weibull function shown in the figure. (after Jibson et al., 1998, 2000). With permission, see page 714, No 31.

In their analysis, Jibson et al. (1998, 2000) subdivided their study area into 10 m × 10 m cells. Displacements were then calculated for all the cells using the Newmark model. Calculated displacements of all the cells were compared with the inventory of landslides triggered by the Northridge earthquake. The full range of calculated displacements for all cells was separated into different displacement categories (e.g., 1–2 cm, 2–3 cm, 3–4 cm etc.). Cells located in landslide source areas were identified along with their calculated displacement category. The probability of failure associated with a particular displacement was defined as the cumulative proportion of landslide cells in all displacement categories up to that particular displacement.

Landslide failure probability was plotted against displacement category. (See Figure 9.16). The curve shows a monotonic increase of the defined probability of failure with displacement up to an upper limit. This shape of the cumulative probability curve reflects the brittle nature of most failures typical of the region considered. The curve flattened out at a deformation about 15 cm with no further increase in the failure probability beyond about 0.27 or 27%.

As stated above, the generated curve was used for producing seismic landslide hazard maps showing spatial variation of landslide probability. The methodology could be used for any set of ground-shaking conditions but recalibration would be required if it was used for a different region.

The 'infinite slope' model, used as a basis for calculating the permanent displacements, facilitated GIS-based regional mapping tasks. However, the inherent uncertainties and limitations of this choice must, however, be recognized. The importance of the correct failure mechanism must be emphasized. As stated in sub-section 9.5.2, a curved failure mechanism may lead to deformations significantly greater than a plane failure mechanism.

There are, of course, considerable difficulties in predicting or anticipating the right failure mechanisms and their variability in the region of interest. Moreover, methods and techniques need to be extended further so that a two-dimensional analysis procedure could be integrated with a GIS-based approach in a regional hazard assessment task.

9.11.6   Increase in existing landslide hazard due to earthquakes

How one may estimate earthquake-related increase in landslide hazard of a site with known prior failure probability has been considered in a different way by Christian and Urzua (1999). Their approach may be summarized as follows.

The probability of failure p_F is related to the reliability index β, the relationship depending on the probability distribution of the factor of safety F. Considering a specified value of prior probability p_F and assuming a reasonable value for σ_F, the standard deviation of the factor of safety F, the expected value of static factor of safety F was determined. The relationship between F_{dy}, the factor of safety during an earthquake and F was determined on the basis of a pseudo-static approach. Knowing the expected value of F, the expected value of F_{dy} was calculated.

The corresponding values of reliability index and probability of failure were calculated under dynamic (pseudo-static conditions) for values of acceleration a_h and amplification factor A relevant to the site. The authors (Christian and Urzua, 1999) obtained a curve showing the relationship of p_F to the product Aa_h (amplified acceleration).

They also considered the earthquake recurrence rate for a given site (for which detailed data were available) to obtain the overall (combined) landslide probability including earthquakes of different return periods at the site, based on a numerical integration procedure. The authors concluded that, for a reasonable range of parameters, the increase in probability of landsliding was only 10 to 20% above the pre-existing probability. This was less than the assumed uncertainty associated with the pre-existing landslide ($\sigma_F = 30\%$). The authors were trying to explain how some significant landslide sites do not fail during earthquakes whereas both major and minor failures due to earthquakes at many sites do occur frequently.

One must, of course, be careful in interpreting this type of conclusion too narrowly. This may lead to generalisation which is not warranted. Although the analysis process is systematic and elegant, it appears to be associated with a circular argument. The initial failure probability is assumed on the basis of observation/historical data whereas the probability associated with earthquakes is based partly on the assumed value under static conditions and partly on a calculation process and using a plane failure mechanism. It would be interesting to research the issue further by using a systematic and consistent calculation process for both static and seismic conditions and considering both plane and curved failure mechanisms.

APPENDIX TO CHAPTER 9

C9.1 Some discussions during the period (1960–1973) concerning the seismic coefficients

C9.1.1 Factors influencing pseudo-static factor of safety

Procedures for pseudo-static limit equilibrium analysis appear to differ widely (Seed, 1973). For example:

1 Shear strength data may be used from drained or undrained tests and shear tests may be triaxial compression tests or plane strain compression tests with either isotropic or anisotropic consolidation of the soil specimens before shearing.
2 Shear strength may be taken from Mohr envelopes or from relationships between the shear stress on the failure plane at failure (τ_{ff}) and normal stress on the failure plane before the earthquake (σ_{fc}).
3 Inter-slice or inter-wedge forces may be assumed to be either horizontal or inclined.
4 The pseudo-static force on each slice may be applied either at the centroid of each slice or at the base of each slice.
5 The seismic force may or may not be considered in determining the effective normal stress on the base of each slice.
6 The location of the critical sliding surface during an earthquake may either be taken as that for the static analysis, or it may be determined separately with inclusion of the pseudo-static force.

The influence of this wide range of choices on the computed factor of safety F may outweigh any variations that are considered in the seismic co-efficient k. Seed (1973) referred to preliminary design studies concerning Oroville dam in California, and pointed out that changes of 130% in k may be offset simply by making small and generally acceptable changes in the value of inter-wedge force inclination δ (e.g., zero inclination or that equal to developed friction angle) or in the value of ϕ (e.g., plane strain value rather than triaxial value).

In one case, k was varied from 0.1 to 0.23 but in each case $F = 1.10$ was obtained by making acceptable changes in δ and ϕ.

In another case, value of F with $k = 0.2$ was higher than its value with $k = 0.1$. In the first case ϕ was taken as plane strain value and $\delta = \phi$, while in the second case ϕ was taken as triaxial value and $\delta = 0$.

It is obvious that there are potential dangers in placing undue faith in the precise value computed for the factor of safety. Important decisions have to be made concerning the analytical details and the value of seismic coefficients and the designer must be thoroughly familiar with details of

1 Soil testing procedures,
2 Different methods of stability analysis,
3 Seismic effects.

Judgment and experience are necessary for the assessment of hazard and for decisions concerning design.

In addition to limit equilibrium analysis, Seed (1966) also considered the use of static stress analysis in which pseudo-static lateral forces are included.

C9.1.2   Estimating seismic coefficient based on visco-elastic response analysis

During the period 1960–1970, it was also suggested that the value of k be based on visco-elastic response analyses. An embankment was assumed to consist of a series of infinitely thin horizontal slices, connected by linearly elastic shear springs and viscous damping devices and subjected to a uniformly distributed base motion.

The seismic co-efficient at any depth was taken as one of the two following alternatives:

1   As the square root of the sum of the squares of the seismic coefficients for peak response in the first four modes, or
2   As the maximum value at that depth for anyone of the modal distributions (Ambraseys, 1960).

Seismic co-efficient variation with depth, at any instant during an earthquake, was determined by dynamic analysis (See also Krishna, 1962). The co-efficient evaluated in this manner varied from a maximum at the crest of an embankment to near zero at its base.

A procedure for computing the inertia forces directly for individual slide masses was proposed by Seed and Martin (1966). This procedure was later used by Ambraseys and Sarma (1967) for developing curves giving the value of seismic co-efficient for soil wedges of different configurations and depths in embankments of different heights.

Visco-elastic response analyses are useful for assessing dynamic forces induced in embankments during earthquakes although there are limitations in the procedure which assumes an embankment as a series of horizontal slices and considers viscous rather than hysteretic damping. Different methods of determining seismic coefficients were compared by Seed and Martin (1966) and Seed (1973).

C9.1.3   Seismic coefficients related to inertia forces

Consider a potential sliding mass of weight W and assume that at any time the stress distribution due to an earthquake has been determined throughout an embankment by a dynamic response analysis (e.g., by using the finite element approach). Horizontal and vertical inertia forces on the sliding mass $F_h(t)$ and $F_v(t)$ respectively at the instant t may be calculated by a summation of the normal and shear stresses on the boundary of the potential sliding mass. The equivalent seismic coefficients $k_h(t)$ and $k_v(t)$ are then given by the following equations:

$$k_h(t) = F_h(t)/W$$
$$k_v(t) = F_v(t)/W$$

$$(C9.1)$$

The equivalent maximum seismic co-efficient is highest for assumed potential sliding masses which are small and located towards the top of an embankment. As the assumed sliding mass increases in size and includes lower parts of the embankment, the co-efficient decreases. The co-efficient increases as the total height of an embankment decrease, assuming a sliding mass extending the same proportion of height of the embankment. Increase in shear wave velocity of the material increases the co-efficient. As an example Seed and Martin (1966) found the co-efficient to be 0.25 for an embankment 150 ft. (45.72 m) high and only 0.1 for an embankment 450 ft. (137.16 m) high, assuming sliding mass extending the full height in each case, same shear wave velocity of 1000 fps (304.8 m/second, or 30480 cm/second) and the application of the same earthquake loading (EI Centro Earthquake). These results illustrate the need for rational procedures for the selection of pseudo-static co-efficient k.

Chapter 10

Probabilistic approaches and reliability analyses

10.1 BASIC PROBABILISTIC APPROACH FOR SLOPES

10.1.1 Introduction

In chapter 3 the topic of uncertainties was introduced and the broad types identified as natural variability, systematic uncertainties and model error. Neglecting uncertainties in slope analysis is an important limitation of the conventional deterministic approach. In consequence, the conventional 'factor of safety' is often not a reliable indicator of slope performance. A probabilistic approach, on the other hand, allows for the systematic analysis of uncertainties and for their inclusion in evaluating slope performance. Important geotechnical parameters such as shear strength parameters and pore water pressures may be regarded as random variables, each with a probability distribution, rather than deterministic values or constants. Consequently, the factor of safety F of a slope under specified conditions must also be regarded as a random variable with a probability distribution. In chapter 3, the terms 'reliability index' and 'probability of failure' or 'the probability of inadequate performance' were first introduced as performance indicators within a probabilistic framework. Evaluating these indicators complements the evaluation of a conventional factor of safety and enhances the assessment of slope reliability.

Thus we start this chapter with the simplest and most obvious advantage of a probabilistic approach or reliability analysis within a probabilistic framework. This is to complement a deterministic analysis by incorporating uncertainties associated with the performance of the geotechnical structure or facility to be analyzed.

Let us recall the definitions of reliability index and probability of failure first introduced in chapter 3. The reliability index is defined by the following simple equation [see also Equation (3.1)].

$$\beta = \frac{\bar{F} - 1}{\sigma_F} = \frac{E[F] - 1}{\sigma_F} \tag{10.1}$$

where the expected or mean value of F is denoted by $\bar{F}$ and the standard deviation of F is denoted by σ_F.

Thus, reliability index is the safety margin $(F - 1)$ standardized in terms of the standard deviation of F.

The reliability index may also be written in terms of the mean of F and its coefficient of variation (c.o.v.), i.e., V_F which is the ratio of standard deviation and the mean. Thus, standard deviation is the product of $\overline{F}$ and V_F.

The probability of failure is the probability that F is less than 1, expressed as follows [see also Equation (3.2a)]:

$$p_F = P\left[F < 1\right] \tag{10.2}$$

This may be evaluated by integrating the probability density function (PDF) of F between the appropriate limits. Alternatively, it is represented by the area of the PDF curve between the appropriate limits. (See Figure 10.1.)

For a given probability distribution function (PDF) of F, the probability of failure is a unique function of the reliability index.

Based on the assumption of a Normal or Gaussian distribution for F,

$$p_F = \Phi\left(-\beta\right) \tag{10.3}$$

where Φ is the cumulative distribution function (CDF) of the standard Normal distribution. These CDF values are widely tabulated (see Table C3III.1 in Appendix 3 to Chapter 3). From such a table, the area of the PDF corresponding to any value of the standardized variable (often called standard Normal variate) can be read. In this case the reliability index with a negative sign is the variate.

Apart from the use of tables of CDF, several alternative ways for evaluating probability corresponding to the standard Normal distribution are listed in section 10.5.5.

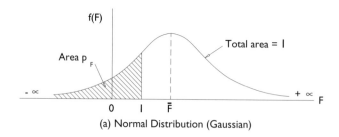

(a) Normal Distribution (Gaussian)

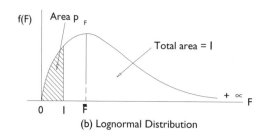

(b) Lognormal Distribution

Figure 10.1 (a) Normal (Gaussian) and (b) lognormal probability distributions, the hatched area representing, in each case, the probability that the factor of safety is less than 1 (usually called the 'probability of failure').

Student Exercise 10.1

For mean factor of safety varying between 1 and 2.5 and assuming several constant values of standard deviation of F, say, $\sigma_F = 0.1$, 0.2, 0.3, 0.4, plot the relationship between reliability index and mean factor of safety as a family of curves, one for each constant value of standard deviation of F. These will, in fact, be straight line relationships.

Student Exercise 10.2

For mean factor of safety varying between 1 and 2.5 and assuming several constant values of coefficient of variation of F, say, $V_F = 0.1$, 0.2, 0.3, 0.4, plot the relationship between reliability index and mean factor of safety as a family of curves, one for each constant value of the coefficient of variation of F. Why are these plots not linear?

Student Exercise 10.3

Using probability tables for CDF of the standard Normal distribution plot the relationship between reliability index and probability of failure, varying the reliability index from 0.5 to 3 and using a log scale for the probability of failure.

Student Exercise 10.4

Assuming suitable values for the mean factor of safety and standard deviation, plot a family of curves, each based on a constant standard deviation, relating mean safety factor to probability of failure.

In subsequent sections, we will discuss the pros and cons of assuming a Normal distribution or a lognormal distribution for F. Moreover, we will give considerable attention to the analysis of uncertainties and the estimation of the mean and standard deviation of F.

For the present, let us assume that these statistical parameters of F have been evaluated and let us consider some simple numerical examples to illustrate the advantages of a simple reliability approach and of using a probabilistic framework.

10.1.2   Numerical examples

EXAMPLE 10.1

Consider a slope with a conventional deterministic factor of safety $F = 1.1$ and compare with a reliability approach based on a mean value $\bar{F} = 1.1$ and a standard deviation of $\sigma_F = 0.1$.

Solution
$F = 1.1$ implies a conventional safety margin of 10% which does not reflect the uncertainties that might be associated with slope performance. The value of F is based on a constant value of each of the parameters on which it depends. The variability and thus

the overall uncertainty associated with the value of each parameter is thus ignored in calculating the value of F. Therefore it will not represent the reliability of the slope accurately.

Consider now a reliability approach within a probabilistic framework. Consider F as a random variable or stochastic parameter with mean value $F = 1.1$ and a standard deviation of 0.1 (this implies a coefficient of variation (c.o.v.) of F, $V_F = 9.1\%$). Then the reliability index from Equation (10.1) above is $\beta = 1$.

Further, consider a Normal or Gaussian distribution of F. Then, based on Equation (10.3) above, the probability of failure i.e., the probability that $F < 1$, may be read from the widely tabulated values of cumulative standard normal distribution (Table C3III.1) (Later in this chapter, in Section 10.5.5, attention will be drawn to alternative form of such tables which is more convenient for our purposes).

We find the probability of failure p_F to be about 16%. The two results (β and p_F) reflect both the mean trend of F and the uncertainty associated with it. Therefore, the results are more meaningful than the conventional deterministic value of the factor of safety by itself.

EXAMPLE 10.2

In the above example, the mean factor of safety is increased from 1.1 to 1.2 without any change to the standard deviation. Calculate the reliability index and probability of failure and comment on the results.

Solution
With a mean F of 1.2 and a standard deviation of 10% (note that now this value implies a c.o.v., $V_F = 8.3\%$), the reliability index $\beta = 2$, and the probability of failure p_F is about 2.2 %.

Thus we note that the reliability index has doubled and the probability of failure has decreased by a factor of about 7.2 (about 86%) although the mean factor of safety increased by only about 9.1%.

EXAMPLE 10.3

Calculate the values of standard deviation and c.o.v. of the factor of safety which are associated with each of the following cases:

(a) Reliability index, $\beta = 1.1$. Mean factor of safety, $\overline{F} = 1.1$
(b) Reliability index, $\beta = 1.2$. Mean factor of safety, $\overline{F} = 1.2$

Solution
(a) Using Equation (10.1), we have standard deviation, $\sigma_F = 0.091$ and c.o.v. of F, $V_F = 8.26\%$
(b) Using Equation (10.1), we have standard deviation, $\sigma_F = 0.167$ and c.o.v. of F, $V_F = 13.9\%$

EXAMPLE 10.4

In a region affected by periodic landsliding, zones of different degrees of landslide hazard have been identified. Landsliding is often associated with increase of pore water pressure during and after intense rainstorms. For a zone where the hazard is classified as "moderate to high", it is proposed to limit the probability of failure of the natural slopes to a maximum of 0.01 or 1%. At one location, A, the mean factor of safety is about 1.4 associated with a standard deviation of 0.15. At another location, B, the mean factor of safety is 1.26 associated with a standard deviation of 0.15. Compare the two sites in terms of the proposed limit on probability of failure. Also comment on the desirable approach to analysis for planning remediation.

Solution

Location A
The reliability index is $\beta = 2.67$. From tabulated values, the probability of failure, based on Normal distribution, is $p_F = 0.38\%$, well below the 1% maximum requirement. Therefore, this site does not require any remediation.

Location B
The reliability index is $\beta = 1.73$. From tabulated values, the probability of failure based on normal distribution is $p_F = 4.18\%$, higher than the 1% maximum requirement. Therefore, remediation is needed for this site.

Suggested approach to analysis for planning remediation

The following questions must be asked and appropriate steps carried out:

1   Based on local experience in the area, what mechanism of failure is appropriate? Is an 'infinite slope model' appropriate? If not, do failures occur on slip surfaces of curved shape or of bi-planar shape?
2   Choose the performance function (factor of safety equation) accordingly.
3   Note that long-term stability analysis with effective stress parameters would be appropriate in this case.
4   Based on previous case records including back-analyses which are the significant random variables in this case? In some cases, cohesion may be so small as to be of negligible significance. The internal friction angle will always be important in such cases. Pore water pressure will be the other most significant parameter. The slip surface location may also be subject to uncertainty.
5   Mean and standard deviation of each parameter must be estimated before carrying out the analysis.
6   This analysis will reveal the parameters which dominate the mean of F and the standard deviation of F.
7   Usually, in such cases, factor of safety can be improved significantly by reducing pore water pressure through drainage measures, surface and sub-surface.

8   An observational approach will help to monitor the fluctuation of pore water pressure before and after the installation of remedial drainage works.

9   Notwithstanding the above, results of detailed analysis and site conditions may point to an alternative approach for remediation. Cost-benefit comparison of alternatives may help in selecting the best approach for remediation.

EXAMPLE 10.5

This example refers to a case study concerning stability of spoil pile (waste dump) in a strip coal mining operation (an example of relatively high failure probabilities).

A bi-planar slip surface with a two-wedge failure mechanism has been established in many spoil pile failures in Queensland, Australia. Many deterministic and some probabilistic studies, based on such a failure mode, have been carried out from time to time. Nguyen and Chowdhury (1984) carried out a probabilistic study using the three alternative numerical methods mentioned later in this chapter (see section 10.4). In this study, the height of the spoil pile was in the range 38 – 80 m, pitward spoil slope inclination 30° – 42°, and, floor inclination (base angle) 2° – 8°. For floor material, the mean cohesion was in the range 0 – 50 kPa and, for the spoil pile, in the range 50 – 200 kPa. Moreover, based on the available data and published evidence from relevant sources, the coefficient of variation was taken as 35% for cohesion.

The internal friction angle range was 10° – 30° for floor and 15° – 40° for spoil pile. Again, based on data and published evidence from elsewhere, the coefficient of variation was taken as 15%.

Solution and selected results

A number of results were obtained for the probability of failure and its relationship to the mean safety factor in each case. Obviously the precise relationship between F and p_F will depend on the slope height, particular shear strength values, slope geometry and pore water pressures, if any. The probability of failure increased with increasing slope angle and was, in fact, a somewhat non-linear function of the pit-side slope angle. On the other hand, the increase in failure probability with increase in base inclination was a linear relationship.

A typical set of results showed that as the mean factor of safety increased from 1.15 to 1.35, the probability of failure decreased from 15% to 2.5%. In other words a 17% increase in the mean factor of safety decreased the failure probability by about 83%.

Thus a reliability approach within a probabilistic framework provides more meaningful outcomes concerning slope performance, which will facilitate more rational and effective decision-making strategies. Moreover, valuable new insight may be gained from detailed analysis of uncertainties related to shear strength and other soil properties as discussed below.

EXAMPLE 10.6

This example refers to a case study of embankment design (performance governed by undrained shear strength and influenced by both systematic and spatial uncertainty): an example of relatively low failure probabilities.

As an example of how valuable new insight can be gained from detailed analysis of uncertainties related to soil properties, it is useful to refer briefly to some results of a detailed case study concerning embankment design involving single or multi-stage construction and potential slip surfaces of curved shape [dikes on soft clay associated with the James Bay hydroelectric project (Christian et al., 1994)]. The foundation soils consisted of marine clay overlying lacustrine clay. Although a number of other variables were included in the analysis, expected values and uncertainties of the undrained shear strength of these clays had a dominant effect on the outcome of reliability analysis within a probabilistic framework.

Three cases were considered for construction of the embankment (a) Single stage with height $H = 6$ m, (b) single stage with $H = 12$ m and (c) multi-stage with $H = 23$ m. Careful analysis was required of both systematic and spatial components of the uncertainty in undrained shear strength. These two types of uncertainty are discussed in Sections 10.6. Reference to selected results is made here but some additional illustrative calculations will be presented in section 10.6.

Solution and selected results

The complete analysis gave the following values for reliability index β of embankments of different heights: 1.84 for $H = 6$ m, 2.66 for $H = 12$ m and 3.69 for $H = 23$ m., the respective mean factor of safety values being $F = 1.5$ for $H = 6$ m, $F = 1.45$ for $H = 12$ m and $F = 1.43$ for $H = 23$ m.

Corresponding to the reliability index values, the calculated values of probability of failure were 0.033 ($H = 6$ m), 0.004 ($H = 12$ m) and 0.0001 ($H = 23$ m). Thus the highest embankment has the lowest probability of failure. This seemingly puzzling outcome stems from the fact that spatial uncertainty decreases as the length of failure surface, which is proportional to H, increases. Lower uncertainty implies lower standard deviation and, therefore, higher reliability index and thus lower probability of failure.

One approach to design may be to require lower target failure probability as embankment height increases. On this basis, setting the target probabilities of failure as 0.01 (for $H = 6$ m), 0.001 for $H = 12$ m and 0.0001 for $H = 12$ m, the required mean factors of safety were calculated by Christian et al. (1994) as 1.63 ($H = 6$ m), 1.53 ($H = 12$ m) and 1.43 ($H = 23$ m).

Alternatively, a single target probability of failure may be chosen and the required value of mean safety factor calculated.

The authors of the paper fixed the target probability of failure at $p_F = 0.001$ and calculated the mean factor of safety required for each alternative embankment height. The required values of the mean factor of safety were, $F = 1.84$ for the first case ($H = 6$ m), $F = 1.53$ for the second case ($H = 12$ m) and $F = 1.36$ for the third case ($H = 23$ m). The relevant information is summarized in Table E10.1.

At first glance these results may seem puzzling. Within a deterministic framework, the expectation would be of a lower factor of safety required for a smaller height of embankment, just the opposite of what is revealed by probabilistic analysis.

As stated above, the results reflect the fact that, due to averaging effects, spatial uncertainty along the slip surface reduces as the length of the slip surface increases (The length of slip surface increases with increase in H). In this case study, the spatial

Table E10.1 Reliability calculations extracted from Christian et al. (1994) concerning embankments (dikes) of different heights.

Height H in metre	$\bar{F}$	β	σ_F	$\bar{F}$ required for different p_F	$\bar{F}$ required for $p_F = 0.001$ or $\beta = 3.10$ for all cases
6	1.5	1.84	0.27	1.63 (Target $p_F = 0.01$)	1.84
12	1.45	2.66	0.17	1.53 (Target $p_F = 0.001$)	1.53
23	1.43	3.69	0.116	1.43 (Target $p_F = 0.0001$)	1.36

Note: The differences in $\bar{F}$ required are small if target p_F is varied according to height. Differences in $\bar{F}$ required are larger if there is a single target p_F.

component of uncertainty in undrained shear strength was almost eliminated for the $H = 23$ m embankment. The total uncertainty is the highest for $H = 6$ m and lowest for $H = 23$ m.

EXAMPLE 10.7

This example refers to a case study of an excavated slope that failed as a consequence of a design decision to save costs (performance governed by undrained shear strength of soil).

During the construction of a new Lighter Aboard Ship (LASH) terminal at the Port of San Francisco, a 30 m high slope was excavated in San Francisco Bay mud with a 0.875(H):1(V) inclination instead of 1:1 considered to be satisfactory based on past experience in the same soil. This steeper slope was a cost saving measure (cost reduction estimated at US$200,000). In the event, a 75 m long section of the slope failed and later a second failure occurred over a length of 60 m. The total length of slope was 600 metres. Thus the proportion of failure was 22.5%.

Solution and selected results
• Duncan (2000) revisited the case in order to perform a reliability analysis. The factor of safety was estimated to be 1.17. With a flatter 1:1 slope, the factor of safety was estimated as 1.25. The most significant contributor to the standard deviation of factor of safety was the undrained shear strength of the Bay mud. The unit weight of Bay mud was also a contributor to a lesser extent. The standard deviation of the factor of safety was 0.18. (c.o.v. about 16%). Based on a lognormal distribution of F, Duncan estimated failure probability as 18% and concluded, in view of the slope failure, that this was too high a value.

Incidentally this value of 18% is close to the failed percentage of the total excavation length (22.5%). However, such an agreement should be disregarded as fortuitous. (For different ways of defining probability of failure refer to section 10.3 and especially item 4).

Based on a Normal distribution, the reliability index is close to 1 and the probability of failure is about 16% which is not significantly lower than the result based on lognormal distribution.

- It is of interest to consider the calculated values if a flatter 1:1 slope had been excavated. Analysis of such slope was found to yield an estimated mean factor of safety, $F = 1.25$. In this case the reliability index, based on the same estimated standard deviation, is 1.39. The probability of failure is about 8% (Normal distribution assumption) and, on the basis of logNormal distribution, the probability of failure is about 6%.

The question arises "Even with the flatter slope of 1:1 inclination, with estimated probability of failure between 6 and 8%, would the design in this case have been safe enough?"

The U.S. Army Corps of Engineers and many other agencies use $F = 1.5$ for long-term stability of slopes. However, there seem to be little guidance as to the guidelines for F values for short-term stability. And there are no guidelines about the target failure probability. Later in this chapter, in section 10.13, guidelines for target probabilities of failure are suggested for the first time. The reader will find that, according to those guidelines, failure probability levels lower than 6–8% range are considered appropriate for slopes greater than 30 m high.

One can also look at this from a cost-benefit point of view. The construction cost associated with an increase in design factor of safety must be compared to the reduction in the expected cost of failure. This is given by a product of the reduction in probability of failure associated with more reliable design multiplied by cost of failure. With 18% estimated failure probability, it was concluded that a more reliable design (1:1 slope) would have been better (The cost of excavating the mud and providing the extra sand fill was approximately the same as the estimated savings from excavating steeper slopes).

Question: With a 6–8% probability of failure, would the expected failure cost still be too high? If so, it could be argued that slope inclinations flatter than 1:1 should have been adopted for the excavation.

10.1.3 Aspects of probabilistic analysis covered in published work – a sample

The merits of probabilistic analyses in geotechnical engineering have been identified by many researchers over the last few decades. In many routine situations the use of a probabilistic approach may be considered desirable but not essential. However, this is a simplistic view based on an incomplete understanding of the role and the range of benefits of a probabilistic approach. Depending on the goals of analysis in a particular project, the use of a probabilistic approach may, in fact, be considered essential. Moreover, broad new perspectives for assessing safety and reliability can be gained by adopting a probabilistic framework and examples are given in section 10.3.

There are many references in the literature to alternative formulations, calculation procedures and applications of probabilistic analysis to typical geotechnical problems, including books such as Harr (1987), and Baecher and Christian (2003). Reference is made below to a few recent publications to give the reader some idea of the broad range of geotechnical problems to which reliability analysis has been applied successfully. Other successful applications are mentioned in the next paragraph and elsewhere in this chapter and in other chapters. Duncan (2000, 2001) presented very useful guidance for adoption of probabilistic analysis in geotechnical practice. A spreadsheet approach has been suggested by Low (1996). An approach for probabilistic analysis based on the finite-element method has been outlined by Xu and Low (2006). Christian (2004) has drawn attention to conceptual and practical issues concerning several geotechnical applications. Babu and Murthy (2005) carried out reliability analyses of unsaturated soil slopes. The reliability of braced excavations in clay against basal heave has recently been analyzed by Goh et al. (2008).

For slope stability, in particular, there are a number of publications dealing with advanced applications such as reliability associated with a progressive failure modes and system reliability. As a sample of the many publications which include discussion of significant basic issues in analysis, overview of trends in practice as well as innovative applications, attention of readers is drawn to Chowdhury (1984, 1985, 1986, 1987a, 1988, 1992), Christian et al. (1992, 1994), Christian and Baecher (2001), Nguyen and Chowdhury (1984, 1985), Chowdhury et al. (1987, 2004), Chowdhury and Xu (1992, 1994, 1995), Chowdhury and Zhang (1993), Duncan (2000, 2001) and Christian (2004). Several of the ideas and methods presented in these publications will be discussed briefly in the following sections of this chapter. However, we start with the elements of a basic probabilistic analysis relevant to slope reliability.

10.2   ELEMENTS OF A BASIC PROBABILISTIC APPROACH

10.2.1   Recalling the basic resistance – load probability model

Let us summarize the basis of this model introduced in the Appendix II to Chapter 3. The analysis of an engineering structure involves consideration of the relationship between resistance or capacity, R, and load or demand Q. The factor of safety may be defined as the ratio, $F = R/Q$ and the safety margin as, $SM = (R - Q)$. In a probabilistic analysis, one or both of R and Q may be regarded as random variables, each with a probability distribution, rather than as constants or single-valued parameters, as in deterministic analysis.

Consequently, the safety margin and the factor of safety are also random variables and each has a probability distribution. From basic probability theory one can evaluate the mean (expected value) and standard deviation of SM from the means (expected values) and standard deviations of R and Q.

The resistance-load model, however, is unsuitable for slope stability in general. Slope stability models based on the concept of limit equilibrium have proved to be successful and are, therefore used widely.

10.2.2   Probabilistic approach based on general limit equilibrium models of slope stability

For slope stability problems, the factor of safety is generally a function involving several parameters, some of which are regarded properly as random variables and others treated as constants. For example, the shear strength parameters are often treated as random variables and the geometrical parameters as constants. More importantly, the factor of safety, F, is not an explicit function of the basic parameters considering recognized methods of slope stability analysis for slip surfaces of circular and non-circular shapes. Based on probability concepts, the first two statistical moments of F (its mean or expected value and variance which is the square of the standard deviation) must be calculated from the statistical moments of all the basic random variables. However, there are several convenient numerical approaches for evaluating the statistical moments as outlined in section 10.4. Once the statistical moments of F and/or its probability distribution have been determined, one can proceed with the calculation of reliability index and the probability of failure.

10.2.3 Probability distribution of a function of several variables such as the factor of safety, F

For some relatively simple functions of random variables, the statistical moments of the function (expected value and variance) can be derived exactly from basic probability concepts. For example, the expected value or mean of the sum of several independent (uncorrelated) variables is the sum of the expected values of the variables. Also, the variance of the sum is the sum of the variances of independent (uncorrelated) variables.

Similarly, for some relatively simple functions of one or more variables, probability distributions have been derived in closed form. For non-linear functions, such as the factor of safety F from most limit equilibrium methods, it is necessary to use a numerical approach to obtain the statistical moments.

An assumption may have to be made about the probability distribution of F before proceeding further to calculate the probability of failure. Among the widely used numerical methods, only the Monte Carlo Simulation method (MSM) aims at generating the probability distribution of F numerically. The choice of a distribution for F will be considered further in Section 10.5.

Before proceeding to numerical methods for basic probabilistic analysis in section 10.4, let us look at the big picture concerning perspectives and benefits offered by adopting a probabilistic framework for analysis.

10.3 THE BIG PICTURE – ROLE AND BENEFITS OF A PROBABILISTIC APPROACH

To gain a broad perspective and to appreciate the wider benefits of adopting a probabilistic framework for slope analysis, one must look well beyond the definition and evaluation of new performance indicators. Replacing 'conventional factor of safety' by 'reliability index' and/or 'probability of failure' or 'probability of unsatisfactory performance' is just the most obvious and well-recognized advantage. With a probabilistic perspective, significant questions can be asked about the performance of individual slopes and sloping regions.

To support that statement, some examples are given below. This is not an exhaustive list and the readers are encouraged to think of other examples to add to this list.

1   The recognition that any slope has some probability of failure or of inadequate performance, however small, is implicit in a probabilistic approach. On the other

hand, within a deterministic framework, a computed factor of safety greater than 1 ($F > 1$) implies successful performance without qualification.

It may be argued that the higher the magnitude of F, the greater is the reliability and the smaller its probability of failure. Yet the scale of this decrease can only be gauged by probabilistic analysis. This involves identifying and quantifying uncertainties and then including them in assessment of reliability.

For example, consider the increase in the mean safety factor of a slope from 1.2 to 1.4, the coefficient of variation being 10% in both cases. The reliability index increases from 1.67 to 2.86. Assuming a Normal distribution for F, the probability of failure decreases by almost three orders of magnitude from 4.7% to 0.0021%.

2   Slope stability changes with time and, in most cases, this is an adverse change. A realistic assessment of long-term performance is feasible within a probabilistic framework. For example, the pore water pressure at a site may increase with time reducing the mean factor of safety from 1.2 to 1.1, the coefficient of variation remaining at 10% in both cases. The reliability index would decrease from 1.67 to 0.91. Moreover, based on Normally distributed F, the probability of failure would increase almost fourfold from 4.7% to 18.1%.

3   The incorporation of time with calculated probabilities of failure is often important. There is no widely accepted procedure for incorporating time with calculated probabilities of failure. This is obviously because time is not a variable in widely accepted geomechanics models of slope stability. In fact, this important issue of time has been left out of consideration from even key papers and even the most recent reviews of practice, such as Whitman (1984), Duncan (2000) and Christian (2004). Yet, for risk estimation, it is recognized that estimation of 'an annual failure probability' would be required rather than just 'a probability of failure'. For example, one can see this from the well known Whitman diagram (Whitman, 1984) relating hazard (probability) to consequences (loss of life, economic loss) for different engineering applications.

If the factor of safety F were defined as a time-dependent performance function, then it would be feasible to calculate a time-dependent probability of failure as an indicator of performance. This is rarely done in practice.

On the other hand, the term 'annual probability of failure' is often based on analysis or interpretation of observational data rather than on reliability calculations within a probabilistic framework. Such a temporal probability may be interpreted as the inverse of the recurrence interval of multiple slope failures. However, strictly speaking, these values are statistical frequencies rather than probabilities. Again, this fact is not emphasized in the geotechnical engineering literature. Let us consider two examples, the reactivation of a single landslide site and the occurrence of widespread landsliding within a region.

A particular landslide site may reactivate every 10 years implying an annual recurrence probability of 0.1(10%).

In terms of a region, widespread landsliding may occur, on an average, once in every 40 years implying a hazard of extensive landsliding with an annual probability of 0.025 (2.5%). Only a probabilistic perspective enables us to present and evaluate such information.

4   Consider slope stability of a long embankment, or a long road, or a long railway cutting. Within a probabilistic framework, one can address questions concerning potential failure of a certain magnitude. For example,

"What is the probability of failure involving greater than 20 m of a specific embankment or cutting, anywhere along its length?"

This is different from evaluating the probability of failure at a particular location along the embankment or cutting. For example, the probability of failure at a location A of a 1000 m long embankment may be 2%. This does not mean that 20 m length of embankment is likely to fail, in the event that failure does occur. A different type of probabilistic calculation will be required to estimate the probability that 20 m length of this 1000 m long embankment will fail.

5   Consider several potential problem locations along a road. At one location, there is the potential of a shallow translational slide; at another location, there is the potential of a deep-seated rotational failure; and at a third location, there is the potential of debris slide coming down from part of the slope above the road.

Different lengths of road are involved at these locations. The performance of the road as a whole has to be evaluated. A probabilistic framework allows the assessment of failure probabilities associated with each location mentioned above. These probabilities can then be integrated to estimate the overall probability of road closure which may be caused by at least one of these failures occurring.

In contrast, while a deterministic framework enables calculation of the factors of safety at the three locations, it is not feasible to estimate a combined factor of safety for the section of road which includes these three locations.

6   Due to constraints on time and resources, qualitative assessments along roads and railway lines are often required before detailed investigations can be made and quantitative parameters can be evaluated. For example, the operation of road or railway line may have been disrupted by occurrence of landslides after a major rainstorm. Alternatively, an earthquake may have triggered a number of landslides. Restoring traffic as soon as possible after such a landslide-triggering event is extremely important. Clearly a probabilistic framework is most appropriate although the assessments have to be qualitative in the immediate aftermath of the failures.

Thus qualitative assessments are made in the first instance, based on visual observation and guided by past experience and professional judgment. For example, according to Ko Ko et al. (2004), hazard level of sites may be characterised in the following five categories of failure likelihood (or probability); the proposed annual probability of failure is shown in paranthesis:

- Very High (>0.2),
- High (0.2 – 0.02),
- Medium (0.02 – 0.002),
- Low (0.002 – 0.0002), and
- Very Low (<0.0002).

Degrees of consequence may also be defined in specific categories. The next step is to assess risk using a likelihood-consequence matrix. A consistent guide to a qualitative, site specific, assessment of hazard and risk for different types of slopes has been outlined (Ko Ko, 2001; Ko Ko et al., 2004).

After a significant landslide triggering event, qualitative analysis of hazard and risk facilitates prioritization of sites for remediation and detailed investigation. For instance, sites with hazard or risk category 'Very High' may be remedied first followed by sites in the category 'high' and so on. Such priority list will thus facilitate decision-making.

Once detailed investigations are carried out at important sites along the length of the road or railway line and sufficient data become available, quantitative analyses may be carried out to complement and update the qualitative probabilistic assessments.

Concepts of landslide hazard and risk are explored further in sections 10.13 to 10.15.

7   Regional studies of slope performance require identification of zones or sub-regions with different levels of landslide susceptibility. A probabilistic framework allows such assessments to be made using either a qualitative or a quantitative approach. Such probabilistic assessments can be extremely valuable although the estimated probabilities may be relative rather than absolute values. Aspects of a comprehensive regional study of landslide susceptibility and hazard are outlined in chapter 11.

8   Slope performance is a function of several parameters: observed, measured or assumed. Moreover, the selected model for the slope performance function may envisage events or assumptions associated with probabilities.

Consider a natural slope for which a conventional factor of safety has been evaluated with given values of shear strength parameters and pore water pressures as $F = 1.3$. For the same slope the probability of F being less than 1 has been evaluated as 0.05.

The pore water pressure within the slope fluctuates in accordance with the magnitude and intensity of rainfall. The pore water pressure assumed for the calculation of factor of safety and probability of failure was associated with a rainfall event with an annual probability of 0.2.

One must also ask the question, "What is the probability that the occurrence of this rainfall event over the relevant catchment leads to the assumed pore water pressure within this slope?"

Let that probability be 0.7.

Within a probabilistic framework, the concept of conditional probability allows assessment of the overall probability of inadequate performance to be evaluated simply as the product of these three probabilities, i.e., 0.05, 0.2 and 0.7. Thus the probability of failure is, $p_F = 0.7\%$.

Alternatively, if the annual probability of the rainstorm event is much higher at 0.9, while other probabilities remain the same, the probability of failure is, $p_F = 3.15\%$.

Thus, the estimated probability of failure requires consideration of the probability of associated events, in addition to the use of a reliability calculation based on conventional slope model. The value of $F = 1.3$ in itself has limited value in assessing whether the slope reliability is acceptable. This is because the question about slope performance is framed in restrictive terms within a deterministic framework than it is within a probabilistic one.

9   Occurrence of an earthquake of certain magnitude within a region is associated with a recurrence interval and hence a temporal probability. Consequently, it can be very useful to assess seismic safety of slopes within a probabilistic framework.

10 Systematic assessment of hazard and risk is now regarded as an important part of geotechnical engineering. Such assessments involve the identification of an event or hazard, the estimation of likelihood (probability) of that event, the identification of elements at risk, and the estimation of the vulnerability of those elements. Thus hazard and risk associated with the performance of slopes can only be estimated within the framework of probability. In this connection, it is very important to define or specify levels of risk which may be considered "acceptable" or "tolerable" and, in the absence of sufficient data from case studies, this is no easy task.

In an important paper, Whitman (1984) presented a risk diagram as a plot of annual probability of failure (y-axis) vs. consequence of failure in dollars and/or lives lost (x-axis). Based on historical and other data on probability of failure and consequences of failure, he sketched on this diagram the approximate location of different applications such as geotechnical foundations, dams, slope stability, mining etc. He also located two lines or boundaries on the diagram based on information concerning acceptable or tolerable risk levels in different applications:

The region below the lower boundary was designated as a region of 'acceptable risk'.

The region above the upper boundary was designated as the region of 'unacceptable risk'.

The region in between the two boundary lines was designated as the region of 'marginally acceptable risk'. Probability vs. consequence diagrams have gained wide acceptance during the last two decades.

Whitman (1984) also outlined various methods and approaches for risk assessment for several types of geotechnical projects. Invariably all those methods require probabilistic evaluations.

11 Considering the potential for progressive failure along a slope, one can ask the following type of question: "If failure has progressed from the toe of a slope (location A) to another location B above the toe, what is the probability that complete failure will occur?"

A probabilistic framework allows the question to be answered based on the available data. On the other hand, the question cannot even be asked within a deterministic framework because, any value of F greater than 1 implies that the probability of failure is zero (complete reliability) and any value of F smaller than 1 implies certainty of failure.

For further discussion of probability of progressive failure along a slip surface refer to section 10.9. For a discussion of the probability of successive failures and systems reliability refer respectively to sections 10.7 and 10.8.

10.4 NUMERICAL METHODS FOR EVALUATING STATISTICAL MOMENTS OF FACTOR OF SAFETY OR FOR SIMULATING ITS PROBABILITY DISTRIBUTION

Only three most commonly used numerical methods are mentioned here. These are:

- First Order Second Moment Method (FOSM)
- Point Estimate Method, or Rosenblueth Method (PEM)
- Monte Carlo Simulation Method (MSM)

The first two methods enable the approximate calculation of the first two statistical moments (mean or expected value and the standard deviation or its square, the variance) of the factor of safety, F. From those moments, one can then obtain the reliability index and the probability of failure. (Higher statistical moments may also be calculated but are, in general, not required for most practical problems). The third numerical method enables the direct simulation of the probability distribution function, PDF, of F. Then, from the PDF, one can obtain the basic statistical parameters, the reliability index and the probability of failure.

Only the simplest versions of the three methods have been introduced here. In each case, refinements have been proposed over the last two or three decades in order to improve the accuracy and range of application of the methods. However, it has been found that, for all practical purposes, all three basic methods work well for slope stability problems.

10.4.1 First Order Second Moment Method (FOSM)

The expression for performance function F may involve a number of basic parameters, some of which are to be regarded as random variables. Any such function may be expanded as a Taylor series. In this method, only the first order terms are included and other terms are neglected. From the basic definition of first two statistical moments, relatively simple expressions for the expected value of F and its variance are obtained. A complete presentation of the method may be found in any text on applied probability, such as, Ang and Tang (2007). It turns out that the expected value of F is simply the value of the function with mean values for each basic parameter. The expression for the variance of F consists of two summation terms, a variance term and a covariance term, both including the partial derivatives of the function with respect to the variables evaluated at the mean values of those variables. If all the variables are independent (uncorrelated), the covariance term can be neglected. If any two variables are correlated, the relevant correlation coefficient must be known. The details and relevant mathematical expressions are included in most books on applied probability. These are summarized in Table 10.1. For the slope stability problems, noting the terminology used here for the performance function, the variable y in these equations represents the factor of safety F and the variables x represent the parameters on which F depends in accordance with the adopted slope stability model.

It is quite obvious that the FOSM method is straightforward and is applicable for slope stability models in which F is an explicit function of the variables and where partial derivatives of F can be evaluated. Otherwise it is much better to use the other

Table 10.1 Equations of FOSM method which is based on Taylor series expansion of a function of several variables.

If the function $y = g(x_i)$ is differentiable with respect to all variables x_i, it is possible to derive the various moments of y by a Taylor series expansion around the mean

$$\bar{y} = g(\mu_{x_1}, \mu_{x_2}, \ldots, \mu_{x_n})$$

Benjamin and Cornell (1970) gave the following mathematical expressions for the first and second moments:

$$m_1 = E[y] = \mu_y$$

$$\approx g(\mu_{x_1}, \mu_{x_2}, \ldots, \mu_{x_n}) + \frac{1}{2}\sum_{i=1}^{n}\sum_{j=1}^{n} \frac{\partial^2 g}{\partial x_i \, \partial x_j}\bigg|_{\mu_{x_1}, \mu_{x_2}, \ldots, \mu_{x_n}} \times \sigma_{ij}$$

In the FOSM method the second order terms are neglected. Thus,

$$m_1 \approx g(\mu_{x_1}, \mu_{x_2}, \ldots, \mu_{x_n})$$

$$m_2 = E[(y - \mu_y)^2]$$

$$\approx \sum_{i=1}^{n}\sum_{j=1}^{n} \frac{\partial g}{\partial x_i}\bigg|_{\mu_{x_1}, \mu_{x_2}, \ldots, \mu_{x_n}} \frac{\partial g}{\partial x_i}\bigg|_{\mu_{x_1}, \mu_{x_2}, \ldots, \mu_{x_n}} \times \sigma_{ij}$$

where σ_{ij} is the covariance between x_i and x_j which becomes the variance when $i = j$, i.e., σ_{x_i} considering the notation used for the standard deviation. When all the variables x_i ($i = 1$ to n) are independent,

$$\sigma_{ij} = 0 \quad \text{for } i \neq j$$

$$\sigma_{ii} = \sigma_{x_i}^2 = E[(x_i - \mu_{x_i})^2]$$

whence

$$m_2 = \sigma_y^2$$

$$= \sum_{i=1}^{n} \left(\frac{\partial g}{\partial x_i}\bigg|_{\mu_{x_1}, \mu_{x_2}, \ldots, \mu_{x_n}} \times \sigma_{x_i} \right)^2$$

two methods outlined in this section, namely, the Point Estimate Method (PEM) or the Monte Carlo Simulation Method (MSM).

It needs to be emphasized that for a rigorous reliability analysis, the first order approximations of the first and the second moments must be evaluated at a point on the failure surface $g(x) = 0$. When this is done, the FOSM method is referred to as the Hasofer-Lind method (Hasofer and Lind, 1974). It is also known as the Advanced Second Moment (ASM) method in the literature. When the first order approximations are evaluated at the mean values of the basic variates, the method is often referred to as the Mean-Value First Order Second Moment (MFOSM) method (Hassan and Wolff, 1999) or simply, the Taylor Series Expansion method (Duncan, 2000). The method has been popular due to its simplicity although reservations have been expressed in regard to its accuracy (Ang and Tang, 1984).

10.4.2 Point Estimate Method or Rosenblueth method (PEM)

In this method, proposed by Rosenblueth (1975), discrete values of the performance function are evaluated at the mean values of the basic variables, at values one standard deviation above the mean value and at values one standard deviation below the mean values. Computer-based slope stability evaluations of this type would be quite convenient. From these values, the statistical moments of the performance function are obtained by using very simple equations involving the addition of 2 terms if there is just one random variable, 4 terms if there are 2 random variables, 9 terms if there are 3 random variables (in general, there are 2^n terms to be added where n is the number of variables). Correlations between variables can be taken into consideration provided the covariance or the correlation coefficient between each pair of variables is known or assumed.

The equations for a function of two random variables are shown in Table 10.2. For slope stability problems, considering the terminology adopted here for the performance function, y represents the factor of safety, F, and the variables x represent the geotechnical parameters on which F depends. The derivation of corresponding equations for a function of 3 or more variables has been demonstrated by Nguyen and Chowdhury (1985).

The estimation of higher statistical moments of the performance function has also been demonstrated by Nguyen and Chowdhury (1984, 1985). This refers to the

Table 10.2 PEM method (Rosenblueth method for a function of 2 variables).

When y is a function of two variables x_1 and x_2, the first moment and the second central moment, or expected value of y and $(y - \mu_y)^2$ respectively, can be estimated as

$$m_1 = E[y] = \mu_y$$
$$\approx P_{++} y_{++} + P_{+-} y_{+-} + P_{-+} y_{-+} + P_{--} y_{--}$$

and

$$m_2 = E[\{y - E(y)\}^2] = \sigma_y^2 = E[y^2] - (E[y])^2$$
$$\approx P_{++} y_{++}^2 + P_{+-} y_{+-}^2 + P_{-+} y_{-+}^2 + P_{--} y_{--}^2 - m_1^2$$

where the coefficients P are

$$P_{++} = P_{--} = 0.25(1 + \rho_{x_1,x_2})$$
$$P_{+-} = P_{-+} = 0.25(1 - \rho_{x_1,x_2})$$

(ρ_{x_1,x_2} is the correlation coefficient between x_1 and x_2. If x_1 and x_2 are independent, then $\rho_{x_1,x_2} = 0$ and $P_{++} = P_{--} = P_{+-} = P_{-+} = 0.25$.)

Furthermore,

$$y_{++} = y(x_{1+}, x_{2+})$$
$$y_{+-} = y(x_{1+}, x_{2-})$$

etc. $y(x_{1+}, x_{2-})$ means that the value of function y is evaluated at

$$x_{1+} = \mu_{x_1} + \sigma_{x_1}$$
$$x_{2-} = \mu_{x_2} - \sigma_{x_2}$$

third and fourth moments in addition to the first moment (expectation or mean) and the second moment (variance or the square of standard deviation). A statistical coefficient relating to the shape of a probability distribution known as skewness is the third moment while another coefficient denoted as kurtosis is the fourth moments. The values of these coefficients can help establish the shape of a generated probability distribution. Often the distribution of a function of two or more Normally distributed variables is also Normal.

Extensions to improve the efficiency of PEM have been suggested by several researchers. For example, a modified Point Estimate Method for calculating the reliability of slopes was proposed by Li (1992). The method requires $(n^2 + 3n + 2)/2$ evaluations of the performance function with n correlated random variables. Thus it is more efficient than the Rosenblueth method for those situations where the number of random variables exceeds $3(n > 3)$.

10.4.3   Monte-Carlo Simulation Method (MSM)

This method has been known and used for several decades and is included in most books on applied probability. Discrete values of each variable are randomly selected from its probability distribution. Using a set of such discrete values a value of the performance function F is then obtained. This process is repeated many times. Typical number of simulations may range from a 100 to a 1000. With modern computing power, the computing effort is not a significant factor in the choice of method of analysis. However, relative to this method, the PEM method, even with four random variables, requires a much smaller number of calculations of F. From a large number of values of F generated, using randomly selected values of the continuous variables, a probability distribution of the performance function is obtained. The accuracy of the results increases as the number of simulations is increased. Application of MSM to geotechnical engineering and its extension to correlated variables has been demonstrated by Nguyen and Chowdhury (1984, 1985). With a reasonably large number of simulations, the first two statistical moments as well as the third and fourth moments can be estimated with a high degree of accuracy.

Detailed presentation of Monte Carlo Simulation may be found in applied probability texts such as Ang and Tang (2007). The latter has included several numerical examples which make use of commercial software.

10.4.4   Summing up – comparison of results from use of different methods

For the estimation of first and second moments, the PEM method (Rosenblueth method) has been shown to be as accurate as the FOSM method and the MSM method. One advantage of the PEM method over the FOSM method is that partial derivatives of the performance function F need not be evaluated. Secondly, this method is convenient to use even if F is a non-explicit function of the basic parameters as is the case for most recognized methods of limit equilibrium involving slip surfaces of arbitrary shape. Since Nguyen and Chowdhury (1984, 1985) have shown that the PEM method can be used for estimating the third and fourth statistical moments, we may ask the question, "How accurate are those values?"

Let us refer to the problem tackled by Nguyen and Chowdhury (1985) concerning the time required for water table draw-down near a box cut of an open strip coal mine in which the permeability and the storage coefficients were regarded as correlated stochastic variables. In this case, the third and fourth moments estimated by PEM method were found to decrease in accuracy in comparison to the Monte-Carlo simulation method, as the correlation coefficient increased above 0.7. However, it was concluded that the values were approximated better by PEM in comparison to the MSM method.

As stated above, all the three numerical methods have been found to provide reliable and comparable results. However, for the reasons stated above, the PEM method is straightforward, involves much less computing effort than the MSM method and, arguably better than the other two.

Sometimes the accuracy of results is emphasized unduly and in this respect the following comments of Duncan (2001) are appropriate:

"In view of the uncertainties involved in tests, test interpretation, deterministic models, and probabilistic analyses, values of geotechnical probability, no matter how computed, will seldom be highly accurate".

Duncan (2001) then goes on to quote the answer of Dr Ralph B. Peck to a question asked of him at a workshop on risk analysis (organized by Corps of Engineers in 2000). The question was about the approach he would recommend to obtain the final results in a case where the calculated probability of failure was (4.65×10^{-4}). Dr Peck replied "I would disabuse myself of the idea of reporting a probability of failure to three significant figures, especially as the exponent might even be in question!"

10.5   ESSENTIAL QUESTIONS AND ELEMENTARY CALCULATIONS FOR PROBABILISTIC ANALYSIS

10.5.1   Select random variables: which parameters are significant?

Assessing the performance of a slope or an earth structure requires consideration of a number of factors such as the potential failure modes, the geometry of slope, location of discontinuities, the geotechnical properties and the pore water pressures. From this and other relevant information, an appropriate slope stability model can be developed. The outcome of deterministic analysis is a value of the conventional factor of safety F which is obtained without considering the uncertainties associated with the significant parameters in the model. In order to obtain a more meaningful and accurate measure of potential slope performance, the use of a probabilistic approach may be considered desirable or essential. One must, therefore, decide which parameters to treat as random variables and how to estimate the statistical parameters of each such stochastic variable. One may also decide, on the basis of available data and from experience, what type of probability distribution should be assumed for each variable.

10.5.1.1   Two statistical moments of each variable

At the very least two statistical moments of each random variable are to be quantified. These are (1) the expected value or mean and (2) the variance which is the square of the standard deviation. In a slope stability problem, shear strength has to be considered along a slip surface. Considering the mean of a strength parameter over the whole of a slip surface (the global mean), the spatial uncertainty with respect to that mean will decrease as the length of the slip surface increases. For example, the calculated value of standard deviation of undrained shear strength from a limited number of test results will be an overestimate of standard deviation of that strength for a slope reliability calculation unless the reduction due to the averaging effect over the length of the slip surface is considered. In absence of sufficient data, the reduction will have to be based on judgment. Analysis of uncertainties is discussed further in section 10.6.

10.5.2   Statistical moments of F: which numerical methods are to be used?

First identify significant parameters, evaluate uncertainties and estimate the statistical parameters for each variable. Next, estimate expected value of the factor of safety F and the associated overall uncertainty in F, using one of the methods mentioned in the previous section.

As stated earlier, all the three methods provide reasonably accurate results. Where F is an explicit function of the variables the FOSM method may be used especially if the partial derivatives of F can be evaluated. For cases where F is a non-explicit function of the variables, it is better to use one of the other two methods although PEM is preferable because, when the number of variables is reasonably limited, the number of calculation of F is much smaller than that for the MSM method. As the number of variables n increases, the computing effort required for the PEM method (which increases as 2^n) may approach or even exceed that for the MSM method (Li's method, however requires less computing effort). So MSM method may be adopted in preference to PEM for a large number of variables. Moreover, there may be other good reasons for adopting the Monte Carlo simulation (MSM) method. For example, assessing the actual shape of the PDF for F may be important.

10.5.3   Alternative definition of reliability index: is a simple definition of reliability index good enough?

A more elaborate definition of reliability index has been suggested and this leads to more complex formulation of what has been called the invariant reliability index or non-linear reliability index. There are frequent discussions on this more complex approach in the literature. A detailed formulation and interpretation has been provided, among others, by Chowdhury and Xu (1992) who compared the results for reliability index calculated on the basis of either a simple definition or an advanced formulation. The differences were negligible for practical purposes. More recently, Goh et al. (2008) carried out reliability assessments of the stability of braced excavations in clay against basal heave. They also found negligible difference in results based on either a linear analysis (four random variables, simple definition of reliability index) or nonlinear analysis (five or seven random variables and a complex definition of reliability index).

Thus, based on all available evidence, the simple definition of reliability index given by Equation (10.1) is adequate and will lead to accurate assessment of reliability and probability of failure for all practical purposes.

10.5.4   Meaning of probability of failure as usually defined

If a probability distribution of F is assumed, one may evaluate the 'probability that the factor of safety F is less than 1', using Equation (10.2). This probability is often termed the 'probability of failure' and the use of that term may sometimes be misleading. For example, a slope may suffer very limited movement if and when critical equilibrium is reached but may be far from approaching catastrophic failure. Therefore, the alternative term "probability of unsatisfactory performance" is sometimes suggested.

The reader must remember that the calculation refers to 'the probability that the factor of safety is less than one' regardless of the notation or terminology that may be used in the literature.

Where probability calculation is intended for the event of catastrophic failure, that intention should be specifically mentioned. A more stringent criterion may have to be specified to define the event of catastrophic failure, as different from F being less than 1.

Again, if the calculation of probability refers to a particular time-frame such as 'annual', that qualification should be mentioned. Similarly, if the calculated probability is conditional on a particular event, those particulars should be specified.

10.5.5   Options for evaluating probability of failure based on the assumption that F follows a normal probability distribution

The FOSM and PEM methods do not enable the determination of the PDF of F. Therefore, the assumption of a PDF is necessary. Consider first the calculation of probability of failure based on Normal distribution.

There are several options for calculation:

1   The CDF values of a standard normal distribution are widely tabulated in books. From such a table, the probability value appropriate to the calculated reliability index may be found. (see appendix to chapter 3 for such a table).
2   Duncan (2001) has provided a chart from which the probability of failure may be obtained directly given the mean and the coefficient of variation of the factor of safety F, assuming that F follows a Normal or Gaussian distribution. Earlier, he had provided a similar chart on the assumption that F follows a lognormal distribution (Duncan, 2000). Note that, in those charts, the mean or expected value of F is denoted as the most likely value (MLV) of F.
3   Use of software is another option and, for accurate calculations, this is the best option. For example, one may use the function NORMDIST in MS Excel.
4   CDF is also a library function in the mathematical software packages such as MATLAB.

Note: In the second edition of the well known book on probability concepts in engineering, Ang and Tang (2007) have included a chapter on computer-based numerical and simulation methods in probability. In their examples, reference is made to the use of commercial software such as Mathcad, Matlab, Mathematica and to spreadsheet software such as MS Excel and Visual Basic.

10.5.6 Probability distribution of F: which PDF to assume for F, Normal or Lognormal?

Sometimes objections are expressed about the assumption of a Normal distribution for F. Such a distribution implies the possibility of negative F values which is a serious conceptual drawback. However, it has been argued (Christian and Baecher, 2001) that

- the likelihood of negative values is very small, and
- that use of a Normal distribution for the factor of safety has merit on other grounds. For example, studies have shown that many of the variables (such as soil properties) individually follow Normal distributions. Hence, the Central Limit Theorem has been invoked to argue that the assumption of a Normal distribution for F is justified.

From a practical standpoint, the accuracy of tabulated or calculated values must be queried. At relatively high values of the reliability index, the calculated probability is dominated by the middle of the PDF and is, therefore, insensitive to the complete shape of the distribution. However, as the reliability index decreases, the calculated value of the probability of failure is dominated by the tail of the distribution and is, therefore, very sensitive to the full shape of the distribution. Thus, both from a conceptual and a practical perspective, an improved choice of PDF for F is highly desirable.

It is arguable that one should obtain both values, one based on the Normal distribution and the other based on lognormal distribution. By studying the a wide range of values of probability of failure from the charts developed by Duncan (2000, 2001), it was clear that, in some cases, Normal distribution gave higher value and, in other cases, log Normal distribution gave higher values. Therefore, it is incorrect to generalize that one or the other assumption is conservative in relation to the other.

10.5.7 Probability of failure based on Lognormal distribution

The choice of a Lognormal distribution for F is often considered to be preferable to that of a Normal distribution since there is no implication of negative values of F and also because the tail of the distribution is less dominating. To facilitate the calculation of probability of failure based on log-Normal distribution for F it is useful to calculate the log-Normal reliability index as follows.

$$\beta_{LN} = \frac{\ell n\left[\frac{\bar{F}}{\sqrt{1+v^2}}\right]}{\sqrt{\ell n\left(1+v^2\right)}} \tag{10.4}$$

in which v represents the coefficient of variation of F, or V_F, i.e.,

$$v = \frac{\sigma_F}{\bar{F}} = V_F \tag{10.5}$$

The probability of failure may then be calculated from the CDF of a standard normal distribution from tabulated values or from software as mentioned above.

Moreover, as stated earlier in this section, Duncan (2000) has tabulated the probability of failure (the probability that the factor of safety is less than one) as a function of the two statistical parameters, mean or expected value of F, which he calls a most likely value (MLV) of F, and the coefficient of variation of F. These two tables (one for normal distribution and the other for lognormal distribution) are reproduced for ready reference at the Appendix to this chapter.

10.5.8 Estimating standard deviations of basic variables

In order to calculate the coefficient of variation of F, one must first estimate the mean and standard deviation of each of the significant variables and then, based on the relevant slope stability model, calculate the mean and standard deviation of F, using the alternative methods described in section 10.4. The coefficient of variation of F is then the ratio of its standard deviation to its mean.

How is the standard deviation of each significant variable to be estimated? The detailed analysis of uncertainty in a parameter or variable is discussed in section 10.6. For the present, we just consider total uncertainty in a variable to be represented by an estimate of its standard deviation. As will become clear in section 10.6, this is a simplification of the real situation since geotechnical uncertainty often has different components. In some situations, this simplification may be justified but in others, more detailed analysis is necessary to separate systematic and spatial components because they have to be treated differently. For the simplified approach, one may use the following alternatives for estimating the standard deviation of a geotechnical variable.

1   If sufficient data about a parameter x is available from observations and/or laboratory tests and/or previous case records, basic equations of statistics will enable the estimation of the mean and the standard deviation.

2   Alternatively, there may be published values or ranges of the coefficient of variation of some geotechnical parameters. Such published values may provide a guide, especially if these refer to a particular region or a particular soil deposit. One would adopt this approach of estimation based on judgement and published values, only in the absence of sufficient data of good quality.

3   Reference has already been made in chapter 3 to another alternative for estimation of standard deviation of any variable in the absence of data. This alternative is the use of a "Three Sigma Rule" (Dai and Wang 1992; Duncan 2000) on the basis that 99.73% of all values of a normally distributed variable are located within three standard deviations on either side of the mean. Thus the standard deviation is taken as one sixth of the difference between the highest and the lowest conceivable values of the variable. In a discussion of Duncan (2000), Christian and Baecher (2001) showed, from statistical principles, that the expected range of values in a sample of 20 observations is 3.7 times the standard deviation and in a sample of 30 observations the factor is 4.1. Thus the three sigma rule would give an underestimate since it is based on a factor of 6. Based on judgement, therefore, one may use either a factor of 4 or a factor of 6.

Duncan (2000) also demonstrated the use of a "graphical three sigma rule" for three cases, namely: preconsolidation pressure decreasing with depth, undrained shear strength increasing with depth and shear strength envelope as a function of effective normal stress. Once again, a factor of 4 or a factor of 6 may be used based on judgement.

10.5.9 Final comment

The methods for calculating reliability index and probability of failure presented above are simple and straightforward and so are the approximate methods proposed for estimating uncertainties associated with geotechnical parameters. For slope stability problems, it is important to consider the reduction in uncertainty of shear strength along slip surfaces. As the length of slip surface increases, the spatial uncertainty in shear strength decreases due to the effect of averaging. In the absence of detailed data, the reduction must be based on judgement. Analysis of uncertainties is considered further in section 10.6 below.

10.6 UNCERTAINTY COMPONENTS AND ISSUES FOR UNCERTAINTY ANALYSIS

10.6.1 Introduction

For natural slopes as well as for built-up or engineered slopes such as embankments, excavations and dams, the uncertainties in geotechnical properties are usually the most important. Such uncertainties have both spatial and systematic components. A third source of uncertainty is model error.

Systematic uncertainty includes statistical error in the mean due to (i) insufficient number of tests or observations (small sample size) and (ii) bias in measurement methods.

Spatial uncertainty includes real spatial variability as well as random testing error or noise.

Both systematic uncertainty and real spatial variability must be taken into consideration in an analysis after the noise is eliminated.

It is also important to consider the model error in an analysis. This may be done by using another random variable 'e', representing model error, as a multiplying factor in the performance function. Alternatively, it may be done by adding an error term to the performance function. In either case, estimates of the expected value of 'e' and of its variance would be required to carry out the uncertainty analysis.

In addition to geotechnical uncertainties with respect to soil properties, there may be temporal uncertainties. For example, the variability of pore water pressure with time may be of key importance in evaluating the long-term performance of natural slopes.

Finally one must consider external loads in slope stability problems. Uncertainty in the magnitude and frequency of external loads acting on slopes must also be considered, where appropriate. For instance, assessing the performance of slopes during earthquake shaking would involve such considerations.

10.6.2   Spatial variation of a geotechnical parameter

First of all it is important to identify random testing errors or noise and eliminate it from consideration. Then what remains of spatial uncertainty is the real spatial variation which must be taken into consideration in an analysis. How this may be done in a practical case has been explained by Christian et al. (1992, 1994).

Over relatively short distances, the value of a geotechnical parameter may vary far more from the mean value than it does if averaged over relatively long distances. Thus, estimating the standard deviation of a geotechnical parameter requires careful analysis of data. If the spatial fluctuation of a geotechnical parameter is rapid, measurements made at locations separated by relatively large distances would be misleading as to the nature of fluctuation of the parameter. A rapidly fluctuating parameter is said to have a small autocorrelation distance. Alternatively, it may be a very uniform parameter so that fewer measurements made at widely separated points are sufficient to judge its fluctuation. Such a parameter is said to have a large autocorrelation distance.

Understanding this issue is central to correctly estimating the average uncertainty over regions of different extent. For example, considering a parameter such as shear strength over a potential slip surface, its spatial variability will be averaged over the length of the slip surface. Thus the effects of spatial variability on the reliability index will be reduced as the length of the slip surface increases. Reduction factor for the variance of a parameter is a function of the distance or length. The modeling of this reduction function is not easy because detailed data may not be available on the spatial variability of the parameter. Some idealization is required for modeling the spatial variability.

For example, Tang et al. (1985) used a triangular auto-correlation function from which the reduction factor with increasing distance was calculated.

A different type of reduction function was used by Vanmarcke (1977a,b) who first introduced a random field model for spatial variability.

Christian et al. (1994) estimated the reduction factor for undrained shear strength of soft clay as the ratio $2r/L$ in which r is the autocorrelation distance and L the slip surface length considered.

10.6.2.1   Considering a case study

Let us recall the example (Christian et al., 1994) concerning embankment (dike) stability first cited in section 10.1 (Example 10.6 dealing with dikes founded on soft clay, for the James Bay hydraulic project). In that example, factors of safety for embankments with three different heights were compared. The most important variables were the undrained shear strengths of two foundation soils. The target failure probability in each case was the same. Higher factor of safety was required for embankment of lower height for achieving the same target probability of failure.

Consider, for the same case study, the significance of averaging effect on the shear strength variability due to slip surface length. (Note that the slip surface length increases as the embankment height H increases.) A multiplying factor (reduction factor) was estimated for reducing the associated variance component of the undrained shear strength.

The multiplying factors were 0.7 for $H = 6$ m, 0.2 for $H = 12$ m and 0.07 for $H = 23$ m. The reliability index values after this reduction in variance were 1.84 for $H = 6$ m, 2.66 for $H = 12$ m and 3.69 for $H = 23$ m (see Table 10.3).

If the reduction due to averaging of the spatial variability had not been made, the reliability would have been seriously underestimated especially for the higher embankments. The calculated values without reduction of spatial uncertainty would be 1.66, 1.76 and 2.5 respectively for $H = 6$, 12 and 23 m. Thus the probabilities of failure would have been seriously overestimated (see Table10.3).

10.6.3 Length of slope failure – insight provided by spatial variability

Considerations of spatial variability may help one to understand and analyze the relative likelihood of small or large failures. For example, a small slope failure (short length of slope or embankment) may be more likely than a large failure (large length of slope or embankment) because in the latter case spatial variability will be reduced significantly due to averaging.

The length of slip surface being proportional to slope height, failure of a slope of small height may be more likely than failure of a slope of large height with nearly the same design factor of safety.

Further discussion is presented in section 10.12 of this chapter concerning the modeling of spatial variability and its implications for estimating the likely extent or length of failure of a long embankment.

Table 10.3 Calculations concerning variance due to systematic and spatial uncertainty for embankments (dikes) of different height: (a) data extracted from Christian et al. (1994), (b) reliability index calculations based on different assumptions.

(a) Data of systematic, spatial and total variance for embankments (dikes) of different height

1	2	3	4	5	6
Height H	Systematic variance	Spatial variance	Correction factor	Corrected spatial variance (3×4)	Total variance $(2 + 5)$
6 m	0.0243	0.0704	0.7	0.0493	0.0736
12 m	0.0199	0.0459	0.2	0.0092	0.0291
23 m	0.0122	0.0176	0.007	0.0012	0.0134

(b) Reliability index calculations based on different assumptions

			β values on incorrect assumption		
H	$\bar{F}$	β	No correction for spatial averaging	Systematic uncertainty ignored	All uncertainty considered spatial
6 m	1.5	1.84	1.66	2.27	1.94
12 m	1.45	2.66	1.76	4.73	3.94
23 m	1.43	3.69	2.5	12.34	9.35

10.6.4   Systematic uncertainty of a geotechnical parameter

Systematic uncertainty or error is important regardless of the spatial extent. Thus its influence will be equally important for short or long embankments or whether the slip surface length is small or large. Systematic uncertainty may be regarded as the uncertainty in the location of the mean trend of a parameter. In contrast, spatial variation may be regarded as the scatter of the parameter about the mean trend. As stated earlier, there are two components of systematic uncertainty, statistical error in the mean and measurement bias. One well known statistical method estimates the variance of the mean or expected value of a parameter x as the ratio of the variance of the parameter and the number of sampling observations (sample size), n.

$$V\left(E\left[x\right]\right) = V\left(\bar{x}\right) = V\left(x\right)/n \tag{10.6}$$

Taking square roots on both sides the equation can be written in terms of standard deviations. Thus the standard deviation of the expected value of the parameter is the ratio of the standard deviation of the parameter and the square root of n, the number of sampling observations, n.

The estimate of measurement bias would be guided by accumulated experience and a multiplying factor may be introduced which is regarded as a random variable. As a well-known example, the interpretation of shear vane test results includes such a multiplying factor. The idea of a multiplying factor on an important geotechnical variable, based on statistical analysis of data, is part of an established practice.

This is best illustrated by the well known 'Bjerrum correction factor' for undrained shear strength of clay. Based on a number of back analyses of failed slopes in clay, Bjerrum (1972, 1973) proposed a statistical correlation between a correction factor μ to be applied to vane shear strength measured from field vane tests s_{FV} and the plasticity index of the clay. Thus the equation for mobilized shear strength s is written as: $s = \mu\, s_{FV}$.

At very low plasticity index, the correction factor (μ) is above 1 (approaching 1.2). But, the correction factor decreases as plasticity index increases, and can be as low as 0.6. The important point is that the correction curve is drawn from a set of data with huge scatter. Thus in probabilistic analysis one would have a mean value and a standard deviation of the correction factor.

10.6.4.1   Considering a case study again

Considering again the embankment stability case study cited earlier (Christian et al., 1994), systematic component of uncertainty was found to be significant for all cases. Neglecting the systematic component of uncertainty would lead to significant overestimate of reliability (significant underestimate of probability of failure) for all three cases of embankment heights (refer to Table 10.3). The values are 2.27 for $H = 6$ m, 4.73 for $H = 12$ m and 12.34 for $H = 23$ m.

Thus, neglecting the systematic uncertainty leads to overestimate of reliability. Estimated reliability increase sharply with increase in embankment height, being a gross overestimate for embankment with $H = 23$ m.

What about the consequences if all the uncertainty was erroneously considered as spatial uncertainty (systematic and spatial lumped together)? In that case the reduction factors would be applied to the total uncertainty and thus overall uncertainty would be less than the actual case where systematic uncertainty was included in full. Obviously, the reliability would be overestimated although not to the extent resulting from neglect of systematic component considered above (refer again to Table 10.3). The calculated values for reliability index are, 1.94 for $H = 6$ m, 3.94 for $H = 12$ m and 9.35 for $H = 23$ m.

Consider these numbers in comparison to the values based on treating the spatial and systematic components separately which, as quoted above, were: 1.84, 2.66 and 3.69 respectively for embankment heights of 6, 12 and 23 m.

Student Exercise 10.5

Using the information given in Table10.3(a), calculate the values of reliability index for the various options listed in the top row of Table 10.3(b) and check the calculated values in the other rows of the same table.

10.6.5   Summing up

Analysis of geotechnical uncertainty involves several significant issues requiring a complete understanding of the spatial and systematic components of uncertainty in each parameter. Accurate uncertainty analysis is possible only if detailed data are available. Where such data are lacking, judgment must be exercised in the selection of standard deviations of geotechnical parameters. For example, if the standard deviation of a shear strength is expected to be in a certain range, lower values in that range will be applicable to relatively longer slip surfaces and higher values in the range will be applicable to relatively shorter slip surfaces. Such considerations are necessary to obtain meaningful results from reliability analysis within a probabilistic framework. Reference to discussion and closure (Duncan, 2001) is strongly recommended for the reader seeking well-informed but diverse opinions on components of uncertainty. This discussion refers to the paper of Duncan (2000).

10.7   PROBABILITY OF SUCCESSIVE FAILURES

10.7.1   Introduction

One failure along a slope may be followed by another although the time interval between such successive failures can vary greatly. Moreover, one or both of two successive failures may involve either limited movement or catastrophic failure. In the latter case, whole or part of the volume of material involved in the slope failure may move away from the exposed slope face.

It is of great interest to ask the question "If a failure occurs along a relatively shallow slip surface, will it be followed by another failure along a relatively deeper slip surface"? If the question is framed within deterministic terms, an attempt to answer it is fraught with difficulties. Consider just two issues. Firstly, if the calculated factor of safety for the shallow slip surface is greater than 1, consideration of the first failure is a contradiction of the safety indicated by $F > 1$.

Secondly, if the factor of safety associated with the deeper slip surface is smaller than that associated with the shallow one, the question of failure occurring first on the shallow slip surface does not arise.

On the other hand, if the question is asked within a probabilistic framework, there is a probability of failure associated with each potential slip surface. The answer to the probability of one failure being followed by another can be provided by invoking the concept of conditional probabilities and using the conditional probability theorem.

If weak discontinuities such as joints, faults or existing slip surfaces exist in a slope, the assessment of performance is associated with potential failure modes which include these surfaces. Otherwise the focus is on determining the location of the critical slip surface by computational techniques which minimize F, the factor of safety. In deterministic studies, the factor of safety associated with a critical slip surface is then determined. In probabilistic studies also, one may determine the reliability index and probability of failure with respect to the deterministic critical slip surface. Alternatively, one may determine a critical slip surface which minimizes the reliability index or maximizes the probability of failure (e.g., Zhang, 1989; Bhattacharya et al., 2003). In some instances, the respective critical slip surfaces defined in these two ways may be very close in shape and location but not in other cases.

10.7.2   Formulation in terms of safety margins along two discontinuities within a slope

Referring to Figure 10.2, denote the safety margin along a potential slip surface A as SM_A and along another potential slip surface B at a deeper level as SM_B. In a rock mass, joint planes or faults are often the potential slip surfaces.

In a soil slope, the potential slip surfaces are often of arbitrary shapes. Considering the location, material composition and geometry of a particular slope, a decision can be made whether to choose circular or non-circular shapes for the analyses. The expressions for safety margin for successive slip surfaces can then be developed based on geometrical parameters and the important variables such as shear strength parameters.

Failure probabilities associated with each of the potential slip surfaces may be denoted by P_A and P_B respectively. Then, one can write

$$P_A = P(SM_A \leq 0) \tag{10.7}$$

$$P_B = P(SM_B \leq 0) \tag{10.8}$$

The probability of failure along both A and B may be denoted by $P_{A \text{ and } B}$. Then, one can write

$$P_{A \text{ and } B} = P(SM_A \leq 0 \text{ and } SM_B \leq 0) \tag{10.9}$$

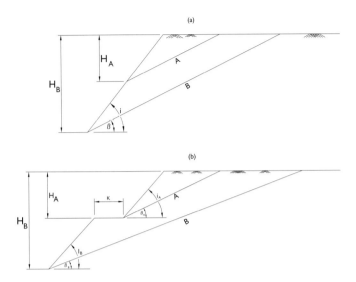

Figure 10.2 Planar slip surface along discontinuities in rock (a) simple slope and (b) a slope with a bench or berm.

This is called the joint probability of the two safety margins. If the probability distribution of the individual safety margins is considered to be Normal, the two safety margins together may be considered to follow a joint Normal distribution. The marginal distributions of such a joint distribution are also normal (see Appendix I to Chapter 3, Ang and Tang, 2007).

Denote by P_{AB}, the successive failure probability, i.e., the probability that failure occurs along B, given the failure along A. This is a conditional probability which is the ratio of the joint probability that safety margin along both A and B is less than or equal to zero and the probability that the safety margin along A is less than or equal to zero. Then, by invoking the conditional probability theorem,

$$P_{AB} = \frac{P(SM_A \leq 0 \text{ and } SM_B \leq 0)}{P(SM_A \leq 0)} \tag{10.10}$$

Thus it is necessary to evaluate the probabilities of failure implied in the numerator and in the denominator of this expression. These probabilities must be evaluated accurately to avoid numerical errors especially when the ratios of very small numbers are involved in the calculations. The use of tabulated values is therefore, inadvisable for such computations.

Estimating the probability of failure associated with a single safety margin falling to zero or below means evaluating the integral of the Normal probability density function from minus infinity to zero (if working in terms of factor of safety F rather than the safety margin, the limits of integration would be from minus infinity to 1).

The Normal PDF of the two safety margins may be expressed by the following equations:

$$f_{SM_A} = \frac{1}{\sqrt{2\pi} s_A} \exp\left(-1/2\, Z_A^2\right) \tag{10.11}$$

$$f_{SM_B} = \frac{1}{\sqrt{2\pi} s_B} \exp\left(-1/2\, Z_B^2\right) \tag{10.12}$$

in which S_A and S_B are the standard deviations of SM_A and SM_B respectively, and Z_A and Z_B are the standard normal variates given by:

$$Z_A = \frac{SM_A - \overline{SM}_A}{S_A}, \quad Z_B = \frac{SM_B - \overline{SM}_B}{S_B} \tag{10.13}$$

Thus the probabilities of failure are given by

$$P_A = \int_{-\infty}^{0} f_{SM_A}(x)\, dx = F_{SM_A}(0) \tag{10.14}$$

$$P_B = \int_{-\infty}^{0} f_{SM_B}(x)\, dx = F_{SM_B}(0) \tag{10.15}$$

Estimating the probability associated with both safety margins being less than zero requires double integration of the joint density function from minus infinity to zero and this is discussed below.

10.7.3   Joint normal distribution

A joint normal distribution of two variables x and y involves five independent parameters, the mean and standard deviation of each variable and the correlation coefficient, r, between them. Graphically, it is represented by Figure 10.3 and expressed mathematically as follows:

$$f_{SM_A, SM_B} = \frac{1}{2\pi S_A S_B \sqrt{1-r^2}} \exp\left[-\frac{1}{2(1-r^2)} \left(Z_A^2 - 2r Z_A Z_B + Z_B^2\right)\right] \tag{10.16}$$

in which the correlation coefficient between the safety margins r is

$$r = r_{AB} = r_{SM_A SM_B}$$

Thus the statistical moments of SM_A and SM_B must first be evaluated followed by the coefficient of correlation, r of SM_A and SM_B. For these calculations the statistical parameters of each the random variables (such as cohesion and friction angle) must be known and also the coefficient of correlation between the random variables.

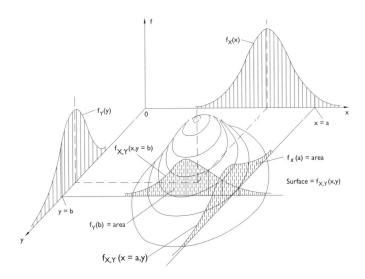

Figure 10.3 Joint and marginal probability distribution functions of two continuous random variables
x and y.

Thus the probability of both safety margins being less than zero is given by

$$P_{A \text{ and } B} = \int_{-\infty}^{0} \int_{-\infty}^{0} f_{SM_A, SM_B}(x, y) \, dxdy = F_{SM_A, SM_B}(0,0) \tag{10.17}$$

10.7.4 Trend of results for probability of successive failure along rock discontinuities

At the outset it must be mentioned that the calculations of probabilities should be based on accurate numerical integration of the probability distribution function of individual and joint safety margins within the required limits of integration. Use of approximate, tabulated values will lead to error because the calculations of conditional probabilities often involve the division of two very small quantities.

The conditional probability of failure occurring on a deeper slip surface given that the first failure has occurred on a shallow slip surface, can be several orders of magnitude greater than those associated with the individual slip surfaces. The correlation coefficient of safety margins along two parallel joints is always very high especially with the assumption of the same statistical moments of shear strength parameters (cohesion and coefficient of internal friction). This is a consequence of assuming statistically homogeneous shear strength.

Independent variation of the coefficient of variation of cohesion or of coefficient of internal friction or of the correlation coefficient between the two can have significant influence on the probability of successive failure. As each parameter increases, the successive failure probability generally increases, approaching unity at very high values of the independent variable. The complete formulation and results are presented by Chowdhury (1986).

Where parallel discontinuities in a rock slope are assumed to have different shear strength variables, the formulation and results have been presented by Chowdhury (1987a). The value of the coefficient of correlation between the cohesions along each joint was found to have a significant influence on the calculated value of successive failure probability. The coefficient of correlation between the coefficients of internal friction also was found to have a significant effect on the probability of successive failure, but to a lesser extent than the correlation coefficient between cohesions along the two surfaces. For some analyses, assumption was made of the removal of all material above the first surface after first failure. Alternative analyses were based on the assumption that the material was not removed although slip occurred. Results were significantly dependent on such alternative assumptions.

10.7.5 Trend of results for probability of successive failures in a soil slope

The formulation of equations and the results of analyses for a statistically homogeneous slope were reported by Chowdhury (1985). For an example problem (Figure 10.4), the expected value of cohesion was assumed as 23.94 kPa, the expected value of coefficient of internal friction (tan ϕ) as $\mu = \tan \phi = 0.78$ (further $\gamma = 18.84$ kN/m³) and coefficients of variation of 0.5 or 50% were assumed for both cohesion and the coefficient of internal friction. The coefficient of correlation between these two variables was assumed to be 0.2. The calculated probability of failure along a shallow slip surface A was 3.3% and along a deeper slip surface B was 2.4%. Assuming that the soil mass above slip surface A would have been removed if failure along A occurred, the probability of progression to failure along slip surface B was considered. This was found to be 49.5%, an order of magnitude greater than the individual failure probabilities.

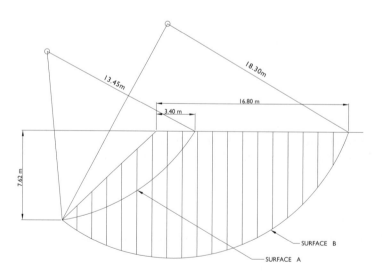

Figure 10.4 Two curved slip surfaces in a 45° soil slope and the subdivision into vertical slices.

However, the trend of results varied significantly with differences in assumed values of the variables. For example, assuming the coefficient of variation of friction angle to be small, 0.1 rather than 0.5 (while keeping that for the cohesion as 0.5), the probabilities of failure were extremely small and the progression probability negligible for increasing values of coefficient of variation of cohesion up to about 0.5, even at a value of V_c as high as 0.8, the progression probability was only 1.48%.

On the other hand if V_μ was assumed as 0.5, the progression probability was 96% even at V_c of 0.2, decreasing with increase in V_c to 19.1% at $V_c = 0.5$.

The probabilistic approach for successive failures presented by Chowdhury (1985) was invoked to explain cases of soil slope failure in which the size of the failure was much larger than that predicted from deterministic analysis on the basis of the concept of a critical slip surface. It was argued that such large slides are, in fact, a consequence of multiple failures which have occurred in quick succession reflecting, among other possible factors, the high correlation of the safety margins of potential slip surfaces adjacent to each other. In support of this contention, reference was made to a well-documented case history, the failures at Kimola canal discussed by Leonards (1983). Due to the speed with which such successive failures may occur in some cases, an observer arriving soon after the event would see only the final shape and extent of the failed mass. In the first instance, it would seem to be the result of a single failure. On reflection and analysis, it may, however be easier to appreciate the retrogressive nature of the failure process.

10.8 SYSTEMS RELIABILITY

Instead of considering the reliability or probability of failure to be associated with a single surface such as the critical slip surface, it may be more realistic to consider a number of slip surfaces within such a slope. Thus the slope may be regarded as a system for which the calculation of systems reliability is appropriate. Usually upper and lower bounds of the system are calculated on this basis. Extending the published work of others, equations for systems reliability appropriate to multiple slip surfaces were developed by Chowdhury and Xu (1995) who also analyzed several examples or case studies.

The first case study concerned the undrained stability of a heterogeneous slope with three clay layers of different mean shear strength and a top layer of sand (Figure 10.5). This represents the Congress Street Cut (Ireland 1954, Tang et al., 1976, Skempton and Hutchinson, 1969). The shear strength was assumed to be fully cohesive with relatively high values of coefficient of variation on the basis of data provided by previous researchers. The system was considered to consist of 12 slip surfaces of circular shape. Of these, 6 slip surfaces were tangential to the base of layer 3, the lowest clay layer 3 m thick, and the other 6 tangential to the interface of this layer with layer 2, 6 m thick. Considering each group of 6 slip surfaces separately, the upper and lower bounds of failure probability coincided exactly with that associated with the corresponding critical slip surface (26.6% for layer 2 and 27.4% for layer 3). On the other hand, considering the whole system together, both the failure probability associated with the critical slip surface and the lower bound failure probability was 27.4% but the upper bound failure probability was significantly greater

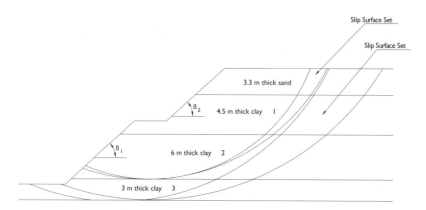

Figure 10.5 Cross-section of the Congress Street Cut.

at 44.7%. Corresponding mean safety factors associated with the critical slip surfaces were: 1.118, 1.109 and 1.109. Thus the systems reliability approach provides a new insight and leads to a conservative result.

Further study with different strength parameters showed that the upper bound systems failure probability was less different from the lower bound if the assumed coefficients of variation of shear strength were smaller for each of the clay layers.

Other examples studied by Chowdhury and Xu (1995) included soil layers with both the cohesive and frictional components of shear strength and different slope geometries. One case was of an embankment on soft soil. In another case, the system of slip surfaces included a bounding planar slip surface as well as a set of surfaces of circular shape. The results obtained in each of the examples confirmed that the upper bound failure probability of the whole system is much higher than the lower bound.

The formulation and application of the system reliability approach considering slip surfaces of arbitrary shape (non-circular) was presented by Chowdhury and Xu (1994). The difference between upper and lower bound failure probabilities was again highlighted.

10.9   PROBABILITY OF PROGRESSIVE FAILURE ALONG A SLIP SURFACE

10.9.1   Basic model considering local safety margins

Methods of slope analysis, based on the concept of limit equilibrium, generally include the implicit assumption that failure, if it occurs, will be simultaneous at all points along a potential slip surface. This is the reason that the local factor of safety at any point is considered equal to the global factor of safety. A basic probabilistic approach, based on the limit equilibrium model will, therefore, seek to estimate a single value of reliability index and corresponding value of probability of failure for a given potential slip surface. However, it is now widely recognized that failure along a slip surface may progress from the toe or from the crest or from any other point. Therefore, one can consider one such mode of failure progression, and attempt to estimate the probability that failure will progress from one segment of a slip surface to an adjacent segment.

In order to facilitate this type of calculation, Chowdhury and A-Grivas (1982) defined the performance function as local safety margin of a segment of a slip surface (the base of a vertical slice in conventional limit equilibrium analysis). The probability of failure of any segment was then estimated as the probability that local safety margin is equal to or less than zero. Two adjacent safety margins were considered to be governed by a joint probability distribution. The distributions of individual safety margins were considered Normal and of two adjacent safety margins as joint Normal. The expected value of each safety margin and its standard deviation was easily estimated.

The expression for the correlation coefficient of two adjacent safety margins was determined from basic definitions of covariance and correlation. Based on the conditional probability theorem, the transition probabilities (probability of progression from slice i to slice $i + 1$) were then estimated as explained in Section 10.7 for estimating the probability of failures along multiple slip surfaces. The local failure probabilities of different segments may be very small. In an example problem considering 9 slices or segments of the slip surface, the values were 0.7% for slice 1 near the toe, 0.04% for slice 3 and 4.5% for slice 9 near the crest.

The transition probability matrix for the example problem (failure mode assumed was from toe to crest of slope) revealed a wide range of values of the probability of failure progression. These values were one or more orders of magnitude greater than the local failure probabilities. For example the calculated value was 87% for progression from slice 1 to 2 and 19% for progression from slice 7 to 8.

This initial model of the probability of progression along a slip surface led to the further work on probability of successive failure along multiple slip surfaces, of planar shape as well as of curved shape. This work has been described by Chowdhury (1985, 1986, 1987a) and discussed briefly in section 10.7.

However, as regards the progression of failure along a slip surface, the need for a more elaborate model became obvious. Such a model is discussed below.

10.9.2   Advanced model for probability of sliding by progressive failure

A more sophisticated model was developed by Chowdhury et al. (1987) considering a slope in a brittle strain-softening soil. Thus, if failure has already progressed through a segment A of the potential slip surface, then it may be assumed that the shear strength along that segment would have reduced from peak value to the residual value. As the failure progresses from one end of the slip surface to the other, it is implied that the operational shear strength, over the whole of the slip surface, falls to the residual shear strength (see Figures 10.6 and 10.7).

The main aim of this model was to determine the effect of a progressive failure on the overall or global probability of failure along a given potential slip surface. In other words, the question to be answered is: "How does the progressive failure probability compare with the simultaneous failure probability?" This probability was also denoted as the probability of sliding in order to avoid confusion with the probability of progressive failure encompassing several segments but not the whole of a slip surface.

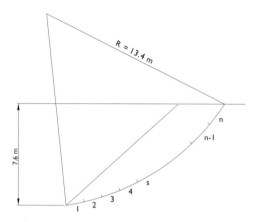

Figure 10.6 Geometry of soil slope.

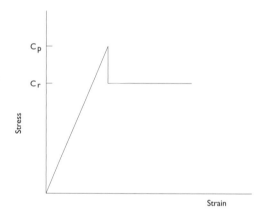

Figure 10.7 Stress-strain curve for strain-softening soil.

Of course it was acknowledged that the probability of sliding would be dependent on the mode of progression assumed such as "from toe to crest" or "from crest to toe" or "from an interior point in either direction".

The safety margin of any slip surface segment or a group of such segments was defined as the difference of shear strength (resisting force) and the applied shear stress over those elements. However, it was recognized that the shear stresses may be based on the results of a stress analysis such as FEM as an alternative to gravitational stresses calculated simply as the components of slice weights. Three potential slip surfaces are shown in Figure 10.8 and alternative stress distributions along two of these in Figure 10.9.

To introduce further complexity in this model, the spatial variability of shear strength was taken into consideration on the basis of the model proposed by Vanmarcke (1983), the random field model. Both systematic and spatial uncertainties

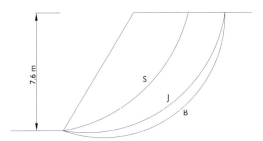

Figure 10.8 Three potential slip surfaces within a slope. (after Chowdhury et al., 1987). With permission, see page 714, No 32.

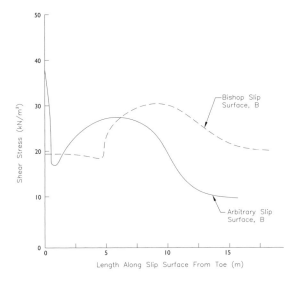

Figure 10.9 Shear stress distributions along slip surfaces B and S. (Terzaghi and Peck, 1967). With permission, see page 714, No 32.

were included. The random field model applies to the spatial uncertainty which decreases with increasing length of slip surface.

The most interesting feature of this model is the manner in which the failure progression is modeled. The event of failure at any given stage *i* (say arrival of progression and thus strain-softening to segment *i* on the slip surface) encompasses the safety margin of all the segments from the initiation of that mode (say beginning at the toe of the slope) being equal to or less than zero. The next event would consider the safety margin of (*i* + 1) segments from toe. Thus individual failure probability at any stage *i* involves the combined safety margin of *i* segments, all at residual shear strength. To consider progression to the next segment *i* + 1, we consider safety margin of *i* segments at residual shear strength and the (*i* + 1) th segment still at peak strength. Each event of failure considered separately lead us to the associated calculation of probability of failure. Then considering the two as joint failure events, the joint failure probability can be calculated. Next, using the conditional probability theorem, the conditional probability of each pair of events is calculated. Finally, the progressive failure probability consisting of more than two adjacent events is calculated as an intersection of the successive conditional events.

Once all the conditional probabilities between pairs of events are multiplied, the outcome of the product of these quantities is the sliding probability. For a brittle strain-softening slope, this implies that the whole of the slip surface is at the residual strength. A calculated sliding probability applies only for the particular mode of progression assumed for that calculation, for example, the progression from toe to crest.

The example solved by Chowdhury et al. (1987) consists of a purely cohesive slope in strain-softening soil. This corresponds to the short-term slope stability in saturated clay under undrained conditions. Results were obtained both for an arbitrary slip surface S and for a critical slip circle based on the Bishop simplified method B. Sliding probabilities were obtained for each of the following assumptions as to failure mode: (a) Conventional – all peak (b) Conventional – all residual (c) Progressive from toe (d) Progressive from crest (e) Progressive from an internal point (f) Progressive – all peak (g) Progressive – all residual.

Typical results are shown in Figure 10.10 and it may be noted that the results for any progressive failure mode stabilize to a constant value after the number of slices increases to about 50.

The mode (e) defined above, i.e., 'progressive from an internal point' was the critical progression mode with a sliding probability of 3% (Slip surface S) and 5% (Slip surface B) although for S, the 'progressive from toe' also gave the same value as 'progressive from an internal point' perhaps because of stress concentration at the

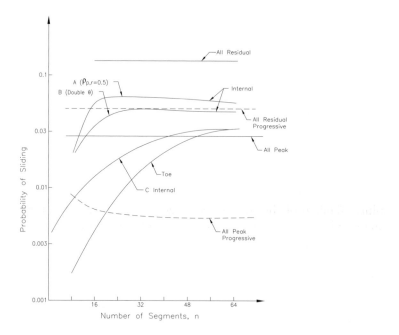

Figure 10.10 Probability of sliding (progressive) as a function of number of segments (after Chowdhury et al., 1987). With permission, see page 714, No 32.

toe. 'Progressive all residual' gave high probability values, 5%, for slip surface S and 10.2% for slip surface B.

Conventional sliding probabilities were much higher for the Bishop critical slip circle B (3.9% and 17% for 'all peak' and 'all residual' cases respectively, than for the arbitrary slip surface S (2.9% and 10.3% for 'all peak' and 'all residual' cases respectively).

In conclusion, the results for probability of sliding do not follow a simple pattern because of so many variables and because of the complexity of the model which incorporates not only the concept of failure progression but also spatial variability of shear strength as well as assumed brittle strain-softening characteristics for the soil slope.

10.9.3 Further development of the model for probability of sliding by progressive failure

This work was further extended by Tang et al. (1985) to model (a) the effect on sliding probability of soil brittleness and (b) the probable length of the failure surface which occurs as a consequence of progressive failure.

For example, as the ratio of residual shear strength to peak strength decreased, there was a significant increase in the sliding probability. For a strength ratio of about 0.85 the probability was about 0.01 whereas for a strength ratio of about 0.55 the probability was about 0.1.

The modeling of probable failure length along the slip surface was also demonstrated. Thus a discrete probability distribution of failure length was developed from the formulation and from such a distribution the expected failure length can be estimated.

The shape of the discrete probability distribution of failure length and thus the magnitude of the expected failure length will depend on (a) the values of the statistical parameters of peak and residual shear strength, (b) the location of the slip surface, (c) the shear stress distribution along the slip surface, and (d) the mode of failure progression assumed in the modeling process.

10.10 SIMULATION OF SLIDING PROBABILITY OF A PROGRESSIVELY FAILING SLOPE

It has been stated earlier that probabilistic analysis can provide good insight concerning the performance of a slope. We have seen that this includes the consideration of progressive modes of potential failure in contrast to consideration of simultaneous failure. While probabilistic analysis is generally not suited to prediction of failure, it can provide insight into the failure process through simulation of increasing probability of sliding. Such a scenario is briefly presented in this section.

We have already noted that, for a slope with a potential slip surface, there is a sliding probability associated with a particular progressive failure mode. This may correspond to a stage in the life of this slope when no part of the slope may have actually failed. Considering a slip surface with n segments, the number of segments actually failed is zero. If we imagine that inclinometers are placed along the slip surface in each segment, none of the inclinometers would detect lateral movement signifying failure. Let this initial calculated probability of sliding based on progressive model be denoted by PS(0).

Consider that at some stage the first segment of the slip surface actually fails. For example, if the mode of progression is from toe to the crest, it would be the first segment. Then the probability of failure associated with that segment is 1 and the probability of sliding for the whole slope will be higher than before and may be denoted by PS(1). By the time i segments have actually failed, the probability of sliding of each of those slices is 1.0 and the probability of sliding of the whole slope increases further and let the value be denoted by PS(i). By the time failure approaches the last of the n slices or segments, the sliding probability denoted by PS(n) approaches and then becomes equal to 1.0 which is the value that must be associated with actual occurrence of sliding.

It is thus of interest to simulate the shape of the increase from the initial value of PS(0) to the final value of PS(n) which approaches and then becomes equal to 1.0.

Chowdhury (1992) demonstrated the simulation of this process of increasing probability of sliding. It is logical to consider an appropriate mode of progressive failure in such a simulation. Sliding probability is plotted as a function of the proportion of failed slip surface. The initial point on the curve depends on a number of factors including the variables and the assumptions in the model. The shape of the curve is also dependent on a number of factors. Experience has shown that it is dominated by the shape of the slip surface.

Two simulations for the clay slope analyzed by Chowdhury et al. (1987) and Tang et al. (1985) are shown in Figures 10.11 and 10.12. If shear stress along the slip surface is assumed to be gravitational, the sliding probability remains relatively low and constant for much of the simulation process (Figure 10.11). On the other hand, if FEM stress distribution is assumed, the sliding probability increases rapidly from the very beginning of the simulation. This is a significant difference and points to the need for using a stress distribution which is realistic.

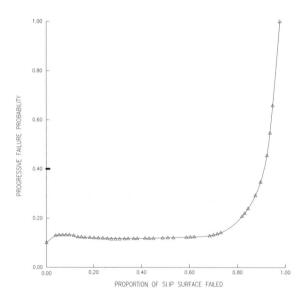

Figure 10.11 Sliding probability in a progressively failing slope as a function of failed proportion of slip surface B of Figure 10.8 with gravitational stress distribution, after Chowdhury (1992). With permission, see page 714, No 33.

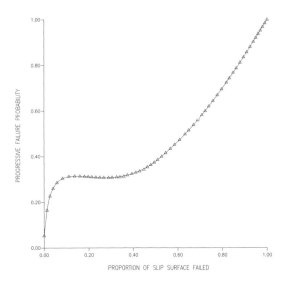

Figure 10.12 Sliding probability in a progressively failing slope as a function of the failed proportion of slip surface B of Figure 10.8 with FEM stress distribution, after Chowdhury (1992). With permission, see page 714, No 33.

It is important to note that this model (Chowdhury, 1992) requires the formulation of joint probabilities of two events associated with safety margins as discussed in the previous section.

A simpler approach was proposed by Chowdhury and Zhang (1993) in which joint probabilities need not be calculated. The performance function is based on the safety margin as before. The event of failure of a group of slices is defined on the basis that the total safety margin of that group of slices falls to zero. The associated failure probabilities can then be estimated without considering the intersection of conditional probabilities. For a progressively failing slope, the curve of sliding probability as a proportion of the slip surface is again plotted. The shape and location of the curve is very similar to that based on the elaborate bivariate model used by Chowdhury et al. (1987) and Chowdhury (1992). However, the initial point in the simulation curve is usually found to be rather different from that calculated on the basis of the more elaborate model.

On the whole, the simpler simulation model (Chowdhury and Zhang, 1993) can facilitate a good understanding of the failure process of a slope system within a probabilistic framework with a reasonable degree of accuracy. Therefore, for the type of simulation exercises discussed here, the simpler model is recommended without reservation.

10.11   BAYESIAN UPDATING

10.11.1   Introduction

Bayes' theorem is one of the most useful theorems in probability and can be derived from the theorems of total probability and conditional probability. Bayes' theorem is often used as a tool for updating the initial probability of an event (prior probability) on the basis of additional information or data that becomes available. The updated probability is often termed the posterior probability. Once a probabilistic assessment has been made in connection with the performance of a slope or a landslide, observation of the slope or site may lead to significant additional information. For instance, the event of failure or of survival at any stage in the life of a slope, after the initial probability calculation was made, can be significant for updating the reliability or probability of failure.

10.11.2   Updating the reliability of an open-cut mining slope

Zhang (1989) analyzed the reliability of an open-pit mining slope at various stages (increasing depth of the mining excavation from 15 m to 90 m). He then formulated the equations for Bayesian updating in such a way that, if the slope had not failed in the previous stage, the posterior or updated probability of the next stage could be evaluated. The significance of survival is that the updated failure probability is lower and thus the reliability is higher.

Uncertainty in shear strength was the basis for probabilistic analysis. In the developed model, the mean or standard deviation or both of the shear strength parameters could be regarded as the random variables which could be updated on the basis of additional information such as the survival of the excavated slope.

Calculations were made for two different pore water pressure conditions, one more adverse than the other. If the excavated slope in the early stages of excavation survives inspite of an adverse pore water pressure condition, the increase in updated reliability is even higher than that achieved for the less adverse pore water pressure conditions. The results obtained for the example problem confirmed this expectation.

For example, assuming that the piezometric surface draws down as excavation proceeds (for a fractured rockmass with high permeability this is a reasonable assumption) and based on survival of the 65 m deep excavation, the probability of failure of the 90 m deep excavation decreased from about 18% (prior) to about 16% after updating.

For the next alternative scenario, a more adverse assumption concerning the ground water condition was made. It was assumed that high rainfall saturated the slope during the excavation of the stage from 40 m depth to 65 m depth and still the slope survived. The calculated failure probability of the 90 m excavation was found to be updated from 18% (prior) to 10.9% (Chowdhury and Zhang, 1989). This is a significant further reduction as compared to the first assumption of pore water pressure condition.

10.11.3   Back-analysis through reliability updating

Back-analysis is an important tool in slope stability and slope engineering and is firmly based in deterministic geomechanics. It is generally assumed that back-analysis within a probabilistic framework is not feasible. This seems to be a reasonable point of view because the occurrence of failure represents a deterministic rather than a probabilistic outcome.

However, new insight can be gained by considering back-analysis as an exercise in reliability updating. For example, deterministic back-analysis enables an estimate of the mean or average shear strength along a slip at the time of slope failure. However, nothing can thus be learnt about the variance of the shear strength. Moreover, significant uncertainty may be associated with the mean value of the shear strength itself. Consequently, it is important to try and update the mean shear strength as well. Therefore, the use of a probabilistic framework seems desirable and, in fact, the use of Bayesian approach has been found to be successful (Zhang, 1989; Zhang and Chowdhury, 1989; Chowdhury et al., 2004).

A formulation was developed for using the Bayesian approach for updating the shear strength of a failed slope. The formulation included two alternatives: updating carried out only once or updating carried out twice. For the latter case, the second stage involved an additional simplifying assumption about the conditional probability in accordance with failure having occurred (Zhang, 1989).

The model was applied to a well known case study, the Congress Street Cut (Figure 10.5), the first paper on which was published in 1954 (Ireland, 1954). Since then, a number of researchers have studied it including Skempton and Hutchinson (1969), Yuceman et al. (1973) and Tang et al. (1976). It is a layered slope with three horizontal relatively soft clay layers and a top layer of sand. The whole system rests on a stiff to very stiff clay.

The shear strength of each clay has, in previous analyses, been considered as purely cohesive corresponding to the short-term stability of undrained saturated clay slopes.

Based on initial values of mean and coefficient of variation of cohesion of each of the three layers provided by Yuceman et al. (1973), the mean value of F was 1.16 and the probability of failure negligible. Obviously, this does not accord well with the fact that the slope failed. Updating process provided revised values of mean cohesion so that the probability of failure was 99.34% with the corresponding mean factor of safety of 0.94.

A further step of updating was also carried out which changed the shear strength again and yielded a probability of failure close to 1.0 with a mean safety factor of 0.95.

The calculations were repeated with a different set of initial values of the shear strength parameters provided by Skempton and Hutchinson (1969). The initial mean factor of safety was 1.48 and the probability of failure negligible. After first updating, the values of mean safety factor and probability of failure were respectively 0.98 and 74.9%. After second updating, the values were respectively 0.98 and close to 100%.

This exercise was a successful demonstration that back-analysis, incorporating a Bayesian approach within a probabilistic framework, can prove very useful. More research is, of course, very desirable, and should include the analysis of a number of well-documented case histories.

10.12   RELIABILITY ANALYSIS FOR A THREE-DIMENSIONAL SLOPE PROBLEM

A probabilistic approach to a specific problem of three-dimensional limit equilibrium slope stability was developed by Vanmarcke (1977b). A long embankment of constant cross-section was assumed for analysis (Figure 10.13). Consideration was given to the uncertainty attributable to the natural variability of strength mobilised along the failure surface. However, it was assumed that the load and strength characteristics do not vary along the embankment axis and that the failure surface is cylindrical and extends along the axis for a finite length b (Figure 10.13b).

An expression for the 2-D factor of safety for this problem, based on a deterministic approach, is given by Equation (5.1a) in section 5.12.2. This conventional factor of safety, applicable under '$\phi = 0$' conditions only, is easy to modify for 3-D analysis of an embankment of length b, assuming the cross-section of the potential sliding mass to be constant. The total shearing resistance in the equation for 3-D factor of safety has two terms, one for the shear resistance over the curved surface of the cylindrical mass, and another for shearing resistance over the plane surfaces at the two ends of the cylinder.

Vanmarcke took the 3-D expression for the factor of safety as a basis for his probabilistic calculations. He found that failure involving either very short lengths or very long lengths (very small or very large values of b) was highly improbable. Figure 10.14a shows the variation of mean factor of safety with the failure length b. The variation of the probability density function for different failure lengths is

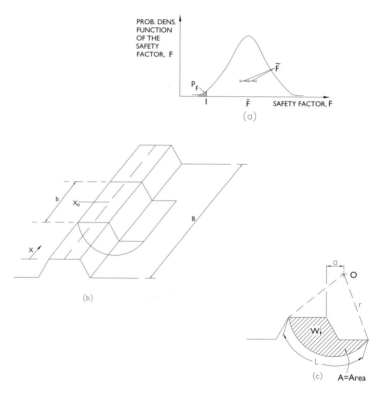

Figure 10.13 Problem of three-dimensional embankment slope stability considered by Vanmarcke: (a) Probability density function of the safety factor F, (b) View of embankment and failure area, (c) Cross section of sliding mass assumed to be constant (after Vanmarcke, 1977b). With permission from ASCE, see page 714, No 34.

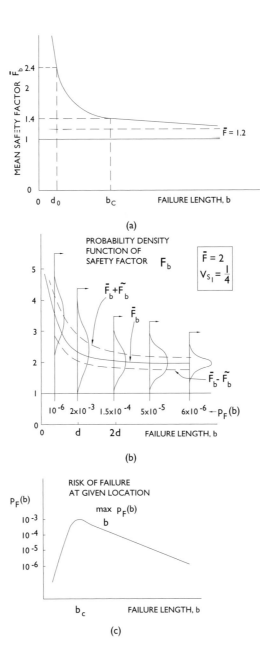

Figure 10.14 (a) Mean safety factor plotted against failure length *b*. (b) Probability density function of factor of safety for different failure lengths. For each value of *b*, probability of failure is the area under probability density function for values of factor of safety less than 1, i.e. values $(F_b < 1)$. (c) Probability of failure versus width of failure area (after Vanmarcke, 1977b). With permission from ASCE, see page 714, No 34.

shown in Figure 10.14b. At any value of the failure length the probability of failure is given by the area of the corresponding curve (PDF) below $F_b = 1$. Finally, Figure 10.14c shows the variation of the probability of failure with the magnitude of b. Thus there is a critical failure length for such a problem. For details of obtaining this critical length the reader is directed to the original paper which also calculates the risk that a failure will occur anywhere along an embankment of given total length. It appears that the length of the embankment has a significant influence on the risk of failure because there is a term in the expression for risk of failure which is linear in embankment length. Vanmarcke's work exemplifies the potential of probabilistic approaches in dealing with slope stability problems. It is significant that the problem is treated both in a three-dimensional and probabilistic framework. It is interesting that the mean safety margin (corresponding to the most probable failure length) was found by Vanmarcke to be about twice as large as that predicted by plane strain analysis.

10.13   TARGET FAILURE PROBABILITIES

10.13.1   Introduction

When using traditional deterministic analysis for a slope, a geotechnical engineer is expected to ask the question:

"What is the acceptable minimum value or range for the factor of safety F in this case?"

While the importance of specifying acceptable values of F is acknowledged in technical reports and publications, there are few widely accepted guidelines. Reference was made in the early chapters of this book to some local or national trends concerning acceptable values of F (see sub-section 3.2.5). Some organizations may have their own internal guidelines.

Moving on to reliability analysis within a probabilistic framework, it is similarly important to consider the questions:

"What is the acceptable minimum value or range for the reliability index?", and "What is the acceptable maximum value of the probability of failure?"

There are no guidelines available concerning acceptable values for different types of slopes. There may be occasional references in research papers such as the values for natural slopes suggested by Chowdhury and Flentje (2003). These suggested values are reproduced at the end of this chapter as Table C10.3.

It is considered highly desirable to make relevant suggestions about target failure probabilities in this book about constructed and excavated slopes. Before doing so, it seems important to make a point about the terminology. The term 'target values' is perhaps preferable to 'acceptable values' because of lack of sufficient experience and data. Thus the extent to which calculated values of reliability and failure probability are comparable to actual or observed values is very uncertain. For example, there are few slopes whose performance, at specific stages of their lives, has been compared to the results of associated probabilistic analyses. Moreover, data are even more scarce about the whole-of-life performance of slopes considered together with associated probabilistic studies.

Of course, there is more data available about engineered structures like power plants and dams. Thus it is of interest to mention here that, the US Department of energy considers 1 in 100,000 as the target mean annual probability of exceedance for civilian nuclear power plants. For dams, a target annual failure probability of 1 in 10,000 has sometimes been mentioned (as a lower bound). It is useful and thought provoking to quote Peck (1980) in this regard:

"From a probabilistic point of view, it is logical to assume a base level of probability of failure of 1 in 10,000 (10^{-4}) per dam year. There is no reason, however, why engineers should be satisfied to consider such a failure rate as the norm. Dams should be designed and constructed not to fail, even if a probability of failure is incorporated into a cost-benefit analysis. Since we know where the great weaknesses lie, we should be able to devise the means for applying judgment to avoid these weaknesses. If we succeed we should be able to justify a base level of failure no more than 1 in 100,000 (10^{-5}) per dam year. Such an improvement is now within the state-of-the-art. Its achievement does not depend on the acquisition of new knowledge..."

10.13.2 Suggested target values of reliability index and failure probability for slopes

Based on personal experience of probabilistic analysis and the limited information presented in the literature, suggested target values of reliability index and probability of failure are presented in Table 10.4 for built-up and excavated slopes. A range of values corresponds to each range of slope height. With more experience and the publication of more case studies, it might be possible to consider embankment slopes differently from excavated slopes.

For convenience, the estimated mean factors of safety which correspond to particular values of reliability index, considering three different values of the coefficient of variation of F, are shown in Table 10.5. The reader should pay close attention to the notes below the two tables because of references to short-term and long-term stability analyses and the spatial averaging effects on uncertainties.

Table 10.4 Suggested target reliability index (β) and probability of failure (p_F) for built-up and excavated slopes.

Height of slope (m)	Reliability index β	Probability of failure p_F (%)	Annual p_F for an assumed life span of 50 years (%)
<10	1.0–1.5	15–5	0.3–0.01
10–20	1.5–2.0	5–1.0	0.1–0.02
20–30	2.0–2.5	1.0–0.5	0.02–0.01
>30	2.5–3.0	0.5–0.1	0.01–0.002

Notes: (1) Having due regard to slope type (e.g., excavated slope or embankment) and other pertinent factors, there may be significant differences between short-term and long-term reliability of a slope. A decision maker (geotechnical engineer) may either (a) choose different target values for short-term and long-term conditions, or (b) take the minimum of the calculated reliability values and compare that to the suggested target range.
(2) See Table 10.5 below for the values of mean factor of safety required to achieve a given reliability index for different values of coefficient of variation of factor of safety.

Table 10.5 Mean factor of safety $\bar{F}$ required to achieve different values of reliability index β for different values of coefficient of variation of factor of safety V_F.

β	$\bar{F}$ for $V_F = 20\%$	$\bar{F}$ for $V_F = 15\%$	$\bar{F}$ for $V_F = 10\%$
3.0	2.5	1.82	1.43
2.5	2.0	1.60	1.33
2.0	1.67	1.43	1.25
1.5	1.43	1.29	1.18
1.0	1.25	1.18	1.11

Note: Due to spatial averaging one can expect lower total V_F for higher slopes associated with longer slip surfaces. This factor should be considered carefully in decision-making about required values of F.

10.13.3   Discussion and limitations

1   What about factors left out of formal analysis?

Uncertainties considered in formal reliability analysis of slopes relate to parameters relevant to the basic slope mechanisms and models. However, other significant uncertainties are not considered in these analyses. For example, uncertainties in pore water pressure and shear strength parameters including systematic and spatial components are included. Considerations of model error and bias may also be included as far as possible. However, there may be significant uncertainties with regard to factors such as (a) construction quality and (b) likelihood of internal erosion and piping within a slope.

These uncertainties, which may have a significant influence on slope performance, are generally not included in formal geotechnical analysis, deterministic or probabilistic. Consequently such factors are not included in Table 10.4. Target values of reliability index would have to be higher and those of probability of failure would have to be lower in order to cover these additional uncertainties. However, further development in reliability analysis is required before such revisions can be made with sufficient credibility.

Fortunately, there are different techniques available for assessing the effect of such factors on slope reliability. The use of 'event trees' and 'fault trees' has been advocated from time to time and the reader would benefit greatly from examples presented by Whitman (1984) concerning the safety of dams.

2   Why bother about target values of reliability and probability of failure when the level of risk (concerning economic loss, individual human safety etc.) is the key issue?

In addition to probability of occurrence of failure, the factors which influence the level and acceptability of risk significantly are the following:

Type of risk (human fatality, injury, economic loss, environmental damage)
Perception of risk
The number and location of elements at risk
The economic value of each element
The vulnerability of each element
(Refer to further discussion in Section 10.14).

The design and management of slopes and earth structures is often guided by costs of construction and maintenance as well as the consequences of failure. Thus the assessment of hazard and risk often assumes importance as part of an overall design and management strategy. In some instances, only the economic risk may be important while in other cases, the risk to human safety may be the critical factor. The subject of risk assessment is, therefore, considered briefly in the next section. Reference will be made to the use of probabilities in seeking to minimize total cost and the need for guidelines on the minimum annual risk of fatality.

Therefore, a question arises here:

"Why have target values on reliability index and probability of failure, if, what really matters, is total cost including the expected cost of potential failure and the annual risk of fatality?"

The answer to this is that both approaches are important. Reliability studies must be sufficient on their own which includes target values against which the results of analysis can be checked. If risk studies are made, expected costs of failure and risk to human safety must be considered even if the results of reliability analyses are considered to be adequate.

3 Are risk studies routinely made? Will a risk study always follow on from a reliability study?

It is important to note that risk studies involve a lot more work such as identifying and classifying assets or elements at risk and estimating the potential for destruction or damage to those assets. Thus risk studies are not made routinely for individual slopes or for geotechnical projects in which slope analysis is a component. Therefore, it is important that reliability analysis for a slope within a probabilistic framework be carried out as a complete exercise in itself.

It is also important to note that estimates of likelihood or probability in risk studies are not always based on formal probability calculations. Alternatives include the use of historical data concerning frequency assessment and subjective judgment based on the experience of professionals. An interdisciplinary approach involving both geoscientists and geotechnical engineers is very useful for making such estimates and decisions. Validating such alternatives through formal probabilistic analysis is highly desirable although it may not always be feasible especially in regional studies.

10.14 HAZARD AND RISK CONCEPTS AND SITE-SPECIFIC ASSESSMENTS

10.14.1 The basic terminology

The terms hazard and risk are used in many areas of life and human endeavor such as the natural environment, trade and investment, economic development, human health and safety, engineered structures, transport and other infrastructure, damaging events (rainstorms, floods, earthquakes, cyclones etc.). A characteristic feature of hazard and risk in any particular application is, of course, uncertainty with regard to the contributing factors or causes. The definition and usage of the terms may differ from one application to another. Therefore, it is appropriate to limit attention here to slopes, earth structures and associated phenomena such as landslides. For slopes and landslides, it is important to distinguish between first occurrence and reactivation or renewal of movement. The hazard and risk may be quite different for the two different failure stages or phenomena.

Hazard may be regarded as a threat of economic loss, and/or a threat to human safety (death, injury) and/or a threat to the quality and safety of the environment. The most important aspects of hazard are the probability of its occurrence (also called likelihood) and its magnitude. As stated earlier, the dominant feature is uncertainty.

In relation to slopes and sloping areas, there may be uncertainty relating to location of failure occurrence (where?), the timing of occurrence (when?), the magnitude (how large? how much deformation or movement or travel distance? how fast?) and the frequency (how often?).

The terms "failure susceptibility" or "landslide susceptibility" are often used to denote the probability of occurrence of a slope failure or landslide. In connection with landslides, the term "landslide susceptibility" is often used.

It may be important to distinguish between primary hazard event and secondary hazards, follow-on hazards and post-event hazards. For instance, an earthquake (primary hazard) may trigger one or more landslides (secondary hazards). The debris from a significant landslide (primary hazard) may block a river or stream forming a landslide dam (secondary hazard).

The basic questions concerning a potential hazard of slope failure or landslide are:

What is the probability? How large is the potential failure? What kind of mechanism of failure? Will the deformation be limited and slow or will it occur catastrophically? What is the potential travel distance?

Risk may be regarded as the potential for adverse consequences related to particular hazard or hazards. It is therefore necessary to consider what assets and elements are at risk from a slope or landslide hazard and to assess the value and vulnerability of each of those assets. The first basic question with regard to risk concerns the expected economic loss. In this regard, quantification of risk involves the product of probability of event and the expected value of loss and damage which is the product of value and vulnerability of the asset. Thus,

RISK = Probability × Adverse Consequences
= Probability × Expected Loss and Damage

The second basic question with regard to risk is "What is the probability of loss of human life?"

This probability is a product of the hazard probability, the impact probability and the vulnerability of individuals.

Vulnerability of a particular asset or element is the degree to which harm or damage will occur to that asset or element. This may be expressed as a factor varying from 0 to 1, the same limits which apply to probability. Assessment of vulnerability requires consideration of a number of factors and the choice of values is likely to be dominated by subjective judgment.

10.14.2   Types of risk and risk assessments

As stated earlier, one must distinguish between risk to life and safety, economic risk and environmental risk. Moreover, it is also important to distinguish between individual risk and societal risk and between voluntary and involuntary risk. In connection with slopes and landslides, it is important to distinguish between site-specific and regional risk and between qualitative, semi-quantitative and quantitative assessments.

As an example of qualitative definitions of the terms such as likelihood (hazard), consequence and risk, the reader may refer to AGS (2000). There are qualitative risk assessment guidelines developed by different organizations around the world and some of these may have been published in the literature.

A recent example is the work of Ko Ko et al. (2004) to which reference has already been made in section 10.3 along with his proposed qualitative hazard categories .These are repeated below for the convenience of the reader.

- Very High (>0.2),
- High (0.2–0.02),
- Medium (0.02–0.002),
- Low (0.002–0.0002), and
- Very Low (<0.0002).

Degrees of consequences were also proposed in specific categories.
Risk was then defined in terms of a matrix of likelihood and consequence.

10.14.2.1   Qualitative site – specific approach

During a site inspection, different attributes of a slope are allocated relative scores or weights based on experience and judgment. This exercise is carried out separately for likelihood and consequence and separately for economic loss and human safety.

Based on total scores for each of likelihood and consequence, risk level may be determined as per the guidelines already set up. The procedure is different in some respect for each type of slope (e.g., natural slope, embankment, excavation etc.) In this way, a consistent guide to a qualitative, site specific, assessment of hazard and risk for different types of slopes has been outlined by Ko Ko (2001) and published in summary by Ko Ko et al. (2004).

An effort was made to validate the results of such studies for several sites within a study area.

10.14.2.2   Quantitative site-specific approach

In cases where detailed analysis has been carried out and likelihood and consequence can be quantified, the risk levels may be estimated quantitatively. Some numerical examples are presented in sub-section 10.14.4 after considering acceptable or tolerable risk levels below.

10.14.3   Acceptable or tolerable risk levels

The perception of risk amongst individuals and groups varies widely depending on the type or source of the risk as well as on the level of awareness and exposure. Most people have little or no personal exposure to risks associated with the failures of engineered structures such as major buildings, bridges and dams. The situation is similar with regard to natural slopes, embankments and excavated slopes. Even in urban areas affected by periodic landsliding, the understanding and perception of landslide risk to individuals may vary widely.

One may start with a general principle concerning acceptable or tolerable risk. The level of risk from a project or facility to an individual or society which may be accepted or tolerated should be inversely proportional to the adverse consequences of failure. However, the level of acceptability or tolerance of risk also depends on risk awareness or perception and also on whether the risk is voluntary or involuntary. For example, people engaged in adventurous sporting or recreational activities are likely to accept much higher levels of risk from those activities than they would in pursuing other facets of their lives.

From time to time, researchers have collected and analyzed data concerning risk of death from natural causes, traffic accidents, plane crashes, disease, industrial disasters, and from a number of voluntary and involuntary activities. Thus, the order-of-magnitude variation in risk levels can be compared. Against that background, acceptable or tolerable risk levels with regard to engineered structures and natural hazards such as landslides can be considered. For example, it would be unnecessary to require that annual risk of death from slope failure be lower than the annual risk of death from ordinary activities such as walking, driving a car or traveling by air.

A research methodology which can contribute to developing risk guidelines for specific structural or geotechnical applications is to survey people about risk perception and acceptance. For example, in regions affected by landsliding, people could be surveyed about awareness, perception and acceptability or tolerance of risk (a) within the residential subdivisions, and (b) while traveling along the roads and railway lines within the region.

Another methodology is to study failures of a particular type of engineered structure and associated fatalities. The results can provide guidance about annual failure probabilities as well as on annual risk levels associated with that type of structure. Such work has been done about dam failures and, therefore, published guidelines can be found in the literature. The individual risk criteria proposed by ANCOLD (1994) concerning dams include the following[*]:

- As an average over the population, an objective risk level of 1 in a million (1 in 1000,000) per exposed person per year

---

[*] ANCOLD (1994)[*] includes $f-N$ curves which define comparative societal risk criteria. For example, frequency (events per facility per year > N) as a function of N, the number of fatalities. At $N = 1$, frequency may vary from 1 in 1000 to 1 in 10,000. The risk levels drop dramatically to a millionth of those levels as number of deaths increase by three orders of magnitude. On these types of graphs, acceptable and unacceptable regions are usually shown with an ALARP region in between.

[*] It should be noted that, in the last 15 years, extensions and updates of 1994 guidelines have been published by ANCOLD.

- For the person most at risk, an objective risk level of 1 in hundred thousand (1 in 100,000) per exposed person per year
- For existing dams, a limit of 10 times the objective values was proposed subject to:-

  a The principle of ALARP (As Low as Reasonably Practicable) with regard to risk levels
  b The revised risk level should be regarded as tolerable only if further risk reduction is impracticable.

In comparison to data on dams, collecting and analyzing regional and global data on slope failures and landslides presents enormous difficulties. Records, if kept, are rarely continuous and the number of reactivations of failure may be unknown. The variation in velocity and magnitude of movement of different types of slope failures can extend over many orders of magnitude. At the lower end, movement may be so small that it is impossible to define the occurrence and timing of failure. As the velocity increases, travel distance can vary widely. Moreover, data will tend to be available only on catastrophic failures.

It is therefore not surprising that few attempts have been made to suggest universal guidelines about acceptable or tolerable risk concerning slopes and landslides. One attempt, obviously influenced by the emerging practice concerning dam safety, has led Fell and Hartford (1997) to propose the following:

Existing slopes: tolerable risk for loss of individual life is 1 in 10,000 for the person most at risk, and 1 in a million (1 in 1000,000) for the average person at risk.

New slopes: tolerable risk for loss of individual life is 1 in 100,000 for the person most at risk, and 1 in a million (1 in 1000,000) for the average person at risk.

10.14.4 Calculations and simple examples concerning risk

10.14.4.1 Economic risk

Consider that the failure probability of a slope or the occurrence of probability of a landslide is p and that the only asset at risk has an economic value E and a vulnerability V. Then the Risk R is a product of these three values as follows:

$$R = p \times E \times V \tag{10.18}$$

Now consider that there are several assets at risk from this single potential landslide. Let the economic values of the assets be $E1$, $E2$, $E3$ etc. with respective vulnerabilities $V1$, $V2$, $V3$ etc.

Then the Risk R is given by the sum of the products of E and V multiplied by the probability p as follows:

$$R = p\,(E1\,V1 + E2\,V2 + E3\,V3 + \cdots) \tag{10.19}$$

Now consider a section of road and the potential failure of several slopes in that section. Multiple slope failures may, for instance, be triggered by a significant rainstorm event.

Each slope failure or landslide might impact several assets or elements which are at risk. Some assets may be impacted by more than one landslide.

The risk associated with each of these landslides may be assessed respectively as $R1$, $R2$, $R3$, etc., using their respective failure probabilities and the associated sum of the products of asset values and vulnerabilities. Then the total risk, RT, associated with the potential slope failures and landslides, is:

$$RT = R1 + R2 + R3 + \cdots$$

(10.20)

EXAMPLE 10.8

There are two potential slope failures to consider along a section of road. Slope A has a failure probability of 0.02 and slope B has a failure probability of 0.05. There are two assets at risk from failure of slope A with values of $150,00 and $50,000 and respective vulnerabilities of 0.1 and 0.5. There are three assets at risk from slope B with values of $100,00, $70,000 and $140,000 with respective vulnerabilities of 0.01, 0.2 and 0.4 respectively. Estimate the economic loss associated with each potential failure and the total expected loss.

Solution
Using Equation (10.19),

$RA = 0.02 \ (150,000 \times 0.1 + 50,000 \times 0.5) = \$800$
$RB = 0.05 \ (100,000 \times 01 + 70,000 \times 0.2 + 140,000 \times 0.4) = \$3550$

Thus, from Equation (10.20),

$RT = \$4350$

We note that the risk associated with slope B is the dominant component.

EXAMPLE 10.9

There is a proposal to adopt certain remedial measures in order to reduce the probability of failure of slope B of Example 10.8 to 0.02. The estimated cost of remediation is about $18000. The risk to human safety from the failure of slope B is considered to be negligible whether the slope is remediated or not. Is remediation justified on economic grounds? Assume that the costs associated with road restoration, which are additional to the losses from impact on assets, are the same whether remediation is carried out or not.

Solution
From Equation (10.19),

The estimated loss after remediation RBr is

$RBr = 0.02(100.00 \times 0.01 + 70,000 \times 0.2 + 140,000 \times 0.4) = \$1420$

Total cost including cost of remediation (RT) is

$RT = 18,000 + 1420 = \$19,420$

This is significantly greater than the estimated loss without remediation which is $3550. Therefore, from a simple economic perspective, the proposed remediation is not justified.

10.14.4.2   Risk to an individual (risk of loss of life)

Quantitative assessment of risk to human safety is difficult. In particular, while considering the risk associated with catastrophic landslides, it is very difficult to estimate how many lives are likely to be lost. Risk to an individual may be considered in terms of the annual probability of loss of life or injury. A great deal of subjective judgement is required to make such estimates especially if there is limited previous experience to learn from.

The following equation, first proposed by Morgan et al. (1992), is a reasonable basis for estimating the annual risk to an individual [for instance, the annual probability of individual loss of life, $R(\text{In})$]. The equation is written in terms of a product of the probability of the hazard and several conditional probabilities as follows:

$$R(\text{In}) = P(H)\, P(S|H)\, P(T|S)\, V(L|T) \tag{10.21}$$

Considering the right hand side of the equation (10.21), the first term from the left is the probability of the occurrence of the hazard (slope failure, landslide), the second term is the probability of spatial impact by the landslide on the asset (an individual or a house occupied by the individual), given the occurrence of the hazard, the third term is the probability of temporal impact (the presence of the individual at the time of the landslide in the zone of impact within or outside the house), given that the spatial impact has occurred, and, the fourth or the last term is the vulnerability of the individual, given that the temporal impact has occurred.

EXAMPLE 10.10

The probability of failure of a slope resulting in a potential landslide is estimated to be 0.02. A residential house is located only about 10 metres directly downhill from the slope and is expected to be impacted by the potential landslide resulting from a failure of the slope. Slope failures in this region are known to occur after severe rainstorms by a mechanism of sliding along relatively steep slip surfaces and such failures occur catastrophically with considerable travel distance. It is known that the house is occupied by a retired couple. Calculate the individual risk to the occupants of the house. Is this risk tolerable?

Solution
The probability of spatial impact may be regarded as at least 0.9, given the location of the house in relation to the slope and in the direct path of the landslide. The probability of temporal impact is also likely to be high considering that, in addition to occupation during the night, the retired couple are likely to spend a significant proportion of the day in the house. A value of 0.7 seems appropriate. Finally, the vulnerability of the couple must be estimated. As the couple are living in a known landslide area, they may take some heed of warnings especially as there might be warnings concerning severe rainstorms and a time lag between the worst part of the storm and the occurrence of a landslide. Even so, a vulnerability of 0.6 seems appropriate because, the occupants of the house may not keep themselves informed, and may be taken unawares during the night.

Thus the annual risk to individual life (Equation 10.21) is

$R(\text{In}) = 0.02 \times 0.9 \times 0.7 \times 0.6 = 0.00756$, or approximately, 0.8%

The tolerable annual risk to an individual is generally much lower, say, less than 0.0001 or 0.01%.

The estimated risk is almost 1% which is two orders of magnitude higher than the minimum annual tolerable risk.

It is, therefore, concluded that the individual risk to the occupants of this house is too high.

10.15   REGIONAL ASSESSMENT OF HAZARD AND RISK

10.15.1   Introduction

Regional studies for landslide hazard and risk assessment are extremely useful for the development and implementation of risk management strategies. Such studies also facilitate the planning of the extent and intensity of development in sloping areas. The results of such studies are often consolidated and presented as maps of landslide susceptibility and hazard. In some cases risk maps may also be developed. The framework of GIS (Geographical Information Systems) has revolutionized the speedy and efficient development of such maps including the associated processes of analysis and synthesis of data concerning a variety of factors that contribute to hazard and risk. In chapter 11 of this book, different aspects of a regional landslide study in an urban area are summarized

GIS is a versatile tool which facilitates the collection, organization, verification, quality control, analysis and synthesis and display of a data or information concerning a particular region or phenomenon. Often the final maps are obtained from a synthesis of base maps, representing the spatial distribution of each contributing or influencing factor such as geology, existing landslides, slope inclination, significant geotechnical properties, vegetation, extent of development, elements at risk from landsliding etc. GIS-based methods can handle considerable volume and variety of spatial and temporal data. More importantly, GIS based analyses and maps can be updated frequently and conveniently in the light of additional data and new information.

10.15.2   Purpose

The basic purpose of such a regional study is:

i   to understand the occurrence of landsliding against the background of geographical, geological, geotechnical and climatic and other factors.
ii   to study the factors which contribute to landslide susceptibility, hazard and risk and the uncertainties associated with each of these factors.
iii   to facilitate knowledge and understanding of spatial and temporal variability of hazard and risk within the region.
iv   to identify and demarcate areas or sub-regions with different degrees of landslide susceptibility, hazard and risk. For example, susceptibility categories may be described as: 'very high', 'high', 'medium', 'low' and 'very low'. Each category

might be associated with a range of likelihood or probability. For example, 'very high' susceptibility or hazard category may be defined as that with an annual probability greater than 0.2 or a return period of less than 5 years.

In achieving these goals, the methods used by geoscientists and geotechnical engineers are governed by certain important assumptions as outlined below.

10.15.3 Key assumptions in regional studies

The key assumptions implicit in a modern landslide hazard and risk assessment process are (Varnes, 1984; Hutchinson, 1995):

i landslides will always occur in the same geological, geomorphological, hydrogeological and climatic conditions as in the past.
ii the main conditions that cause landsliding are controlled by identifiable physical factors.
iii the degree of hazard can be evaluated.
iv all types of slope failure can be identified and classified.

10.15.4 Defining the scope

The extent and scope of a regional study will be determined by the specific and detailed aims and objectives for a particular region, the resources allocated to achieve those aims and the time-frame envisaged for completing the study. For example, landslide risk management often has a very high priority in well-populated urban areas with a history of losses associated with landsliding. Relevant local, regional and national authorities should allocate appropriate resources for hazard and risk studies applicable in the short to medium-term and also for long-term studies.

The following are among the various elements that may be incorporated in the assessment process or the overall study:

i Development of topographic maps at a scale appropriate to the scope and purpose of the study.
ii Compiling a geological database and the development of detailed maps of geology. Again the scale of the maps would be appropriate to the scope and detailed objectives of the study.
iii Compiling a comprehensive landslide inventory and the development of detailed maps showing the distribution of existing landslides and the categories of landslides such as slides, flows, falls etc. As stated for topography and geology, the scale for these maps will be appropriate to the purpose of the study.
iv Extent and intensity of forest cover or vegetation.
v Depth of soil cover, significant geotechnical properties, water table depth and other relevant factors.
vi Digital elevation model from which data concerning local topographic features can be derived to be used for the purpose of modeling susceptibility.
vii Geotechnical models appropriate to the types of landslides observed in the region and expected in the future.

viii Models for assessing hazard and risk based on all the data. For example, one may develop a computer intelligence model which makes use of the previous landsliding history (locations, frequency etc.) for predicting or projecting what might happen in the future.

An example of quantitative modeling of landslide susceptibility and hazard is summarized in chapter 11 of this book.

10.15.5   Qualitative and quantitative approaches for regional analysis

Regional susceptibility and hazard assessment methods may be qualitative or quantitative. However, the way in which methods are classified is somewhat subjective and some methods may be best described as semi-quantitative. Of course, a quantitative approach requires availability of good quality data with minimal reliance on subjective judgment.

For every method, qualitative or quantitative, one must ask the question as to whether relative or absolute susceptibility and hazard are being assessed. The final outcomes are presented invariably as maps of susceptibility and hazard, showing zones in a number of categories depending on the needs of the project and the project goals.

For example, the degree of landslide susceptibility may be classified in five categories as "very high", "high" "moderate", "low" and "very low. If a quantitative method has been used, it may be useful to specify the magnitude of likelihood associated with each of these descriptions.

10.15.5.1   Qualitative methods

Fully qualitative methods rely mostly on subjective judgment. The input data may be based on assessments made during field visits and, in some cases, supported by aerial photo interpretation. Field geomorphological analyses fall into this category. In such methods, the geoscientist carries out an assessment during site inspection based on expertise and previous experience preferably that obtained in regions similar to the study area in question. The final maps for landslide susceptibility and hazard would then be obtained directly from such field assessments. Of course, assessed gradations of susceptibility or hazard are relative rather than absolute.

Another qualitative approach consists of combining or overlaying of different index maps which are available for the study area or which have been specifically prepared for the qualitative assessment. Such synthesis or combination of information from index maps (for example, slope map, geology map, geomorphic map and land use map) may be carried out with or without weighting of the influencing factors. In any case, if weights are attributed, the basis will be purely subjective. Again, the final maps will display relative rather than absolute susceptibility and hazard.

10.15.5.2   Quantitative methods

Quantitative methods include statistical analyses (bivariate statistical analyses or multivariate statistical analyses), neural networks, knowledge based approaches and, of course, geotechnical engineering approaches (deterministic or probabilistic). Description of these different methods is outside the scope of this chapter. However, a brief comment about using geotechnical engineering approaches for regional studies is relevant to this book. A factor of safety approach for a regional study can be easily facilitated within a GIS framework. For example, the "infinite slope" model is often very helpful for the analysis of slopes and especially for assessing the potential for shallow sliding. Just like any other data concerning the study area, the important parameters in an "infinite slope" model (slope inclination, slip surface depth, soil unit weight, pore water pressure, shear strength parameters, etc.) can be attributed to individual pixels within a GIS model for the study area. Thus a factor of safety map can be developed as the susceptibility map or as the basis for such a map.

Similarly, with a GIS framework for a regional study, it is feasible to use a simple probabilistic approach associated with a geotechnical model such as the 'infinite slope' model.

However, it is also important to highlight the fact that other approaches such as knowledge-based methods can provide a different kind of insight and may prove to be more advantageous than geotechnical engineering approaches. The latter are, after all, more suited for site-specific studies, having been developed for that purpose. Aspects of a knowledge-based approach developed for an urban area subject to periodic landsliding are summarized in chapter 11.

10.15.6 Role of an observational approach – monitoring of slopes and landslides

Observational methods have always been considered very important in geotechnical engineering. In particular, the instrumentation and monitoring of embankments, earth dams, excavations, natural slopes and landslides can prove to be very useful.

Monitoring of data can facilitate (a) better understanding of failure mechanisms (b) improving design (c) preventive and remedial measures (d) decisions concerning early warning systems.

The 'observational method in applied soil mechanics' proposed by Professor Ralph B. Peck became widely accepted. However, it was meant to be a methodology for modifying and improving design during construction. With recent advances in geotechnical engineering including the application of new concepts and methods such as probabilistic methods, hazard and risk assessment, the GIS framework etc, it is important to extend the scope of the observational method. For instance, an observational approach or strategy can be very useful for updating hazard and risk assessments and for a dynamic approach to risk management.

With accelerating progress in modern communication and computer technologies, the development of real-time or near real-time monitoring methods for slopes and landslides has been facilitated. Consequently, real-time communication of data and making of decisions is feasible. When faced with landslide triggering events, risk management can be carried out in near real time. More details of landslide monitoring including continuous or real-time monitoring are presented in chapter 11.

10.16   ADDITIONAL NUMERICAL EXAMPLES

EXAMPLE 10.11

The reliability of a natural slope is to be estimated for full seepage conditions which are associated with heavy rainfall. The mean pore water pressure ratio under such conditions is considered to be 0.5 although pore pressures in this region can vary significantly from the mean. (Artesian conditions have frequently been encountered in some parts of this region while, in other parts, the top flow line may be below the ground surface even after very heavy raunfall). The potential slip surface is assumed to be approximately parallel to the ground surface and, therefore, an "infinite slope" model is considered appropriate for stability assessment. The slope parameters are as follows. These may be regarded as most likely or mean values. Slope inclination, $i = 12°$ Bulk unit weight of soil above potential slip surface, $\gamma = 19.62$ kN/m^3. Potential slip surface depth, $z = 4$ m. Cohesion along potential slip surface, $c' = 4.8$ kN/m^2. Angle of internal friction along slip surface, $\phi' = 20°$ (tan $\phi' = 0.364$). Estimate the reliability index assuming

(a) c' as the only random variable (b) tan ϕ' as the only random variable (c) pore pressure ratio, r_u as the only random variable, and (d) slip surface depth z as the only random variable. Assume the coefficient of variation of the random variable as 0.2. Use direct equations for statistical moments of F (mean and variance) where appropriate. However, use also the numerical methods, namely First Order Second Moment (FOSM), and Point Estimate Method (PEM).

Solution
Given data:

Mean Values: $z = 4.0$ m, $c' = 4.8$ kN/m^2, tan $\phi' = 0.364$, $\gamma = 19.62$ kN/m^3, $r_u = 0.5$.

For an infinite cohesive slope subjected to seepage parallel to the slope surface, the factor of safety can be obtained from [Equation (4.25)]. Substituting $u = r_u \gamma z$ in Equation (4.25),

$$F = \frac{c' + \gamma z (\cos^2 i - r_u) \tan \phi'}{\gamma z \sin i \cos i} \qquad \text{[E10.1]}$$

Case (a): c' is the only random variable

Method I: Using direct equations for statistical moments
The above Equation (E10.1) can be rewritten as

$$F = \frac{c' + K_1}{K_2} = \frac{1}{K_2} c' + \frac{K_1}{K_2} \qquad \text{[E10.2]}$$

where, K_1 and K_2 are constants (independent of c') whose numerical values are

$$K_1 = \gamma z (\cos^2 i - r_u) \tan \phi'$$
$$= (19.62)(4.0)(\cos^2 12° - 0.5)(0.364)$$
$$= 13.0485 \text{ kN/m}^2$$

and,

$$K_2 = \gamma z \sin i \cos i$$
$$= (19.62)\,(4.0)\,(\sin 12° \cos 12°)$$
$$= 15.96 \text{ kN/m}^2$$

Now, in Equation (E10.2), F being a liner function of c', the mean or expected value of F is given by

$$E[F] = \frac{1}{K_2}\mu_{c'} + \frac{K_1}{K_2} \text{ [See Chapter 3 and Ang and Tang (2007), pp. 180–183]}$$

$$= \frac{1}{15.96}(4.8) + \frac{13.0485}{15.96} = 1.1183$$

And, the variance of F is given by,

$$V[F] = V\left[\frac{1}{K_2}c' + \frac{K_1}{K_2}\right]$$

$$= \frac{1}{K_2^2}V_{c'}$$

whence,

$$\sigma_F = \frac{1}{K_2}\sigma_c'$$

$$= \frac{1}{15.96}(0.2)(4.8) = 0.06015$$

Thus, Reliability Index,

$$\beta = \frac{E[F]-1}{\sigma_F}$$

$$= \frac{1.1183-1}{0.06015}$$

$$= 1.967$$

Method 2: Using mean-value first order second moment method (MFOSM)

In this method, from Taylor-series expansion, (see Table 10.1) the mean or expected value of F is given by,

$$E[F] = F(\mu_z, \mu_{c'}, \mu_{\tan\phi'}, \mu_{r_u}, \gamma) \tag{E10.3}$$

Thus, substituting the mean values in Equation (E10.1),

$$E[F] = \frac{4.8 + (19.62)(4.0)(\cos^2 12° - 0.5)\,(0.364)}{(19.62)(4.0)\sin 12° \cos 12°}$$

$$= 1.1183 \text{ (as in the solution using Method 1).}$$

Again, from Taylor-series expansion for un-correlated variables, (Table 10.1) the variance of F is given by,

$$V[F] = \sum_{j=1}^{n} \left(\frac{\partial F}{\partial X_j} \right)^2 \sigma_{x_j}^2$$

$$= \left(\frac{\partial F}{\partial c'} \right)^2 \sigma_{c'}^2 \text{ (in this case).}$$

(E10.4)

From Equation (E10.2), $\partial F / \partial c' = 1/K_2$
In the MFOSM method, the partial derivates are evaluated at the mean values of the concerned random variables. Thus,

$$\frac{\partial F}{\partial c'} = \frac{1}{K_2} = \frac{1}{15.96}$$

Then,

$$V[F] = \left(\frac{1}{15.96} \right)^2 (0.96)^2$$

$$= (0.6015)^2$$

whence, $\sigma_F = 0.06015$, and

$$\beta = \frac{1.1183 - 1}{0.06015} = 1.967$$

Note that the values of $E[F]$, σ_F and β are identical with those obtained from direct equations, which should be the case for linear performance functions like Equation (E10.1).

Method 3: Using the point estimate method
From Rosenbleuth method (see Table 10.2) involving a single random variable, assuming skewness as zero or negligible (the distribution of X is symmetric), the points of estimation (x_+, x_-) and the weights $(P_+$ and $P_-)$ are given by

$$x_+ = \mu_x + \sigma_x$$
$$x_- = \mu_x - \sigma_x$$
$$P_+ = P_- = 0.5$$

In the present case with c' as the only random variable,

$$x_+ = \mu_{c'} + \sigma_{c'} = 4.8 + 0.96 = 5.76$$
$$x_- = \mu_{c'} - \sigma_{c'} = 4.8 - 0.96 = 3.84$$

The corresponding values of F are obtained from Equation (E10.1) as:

$$F_+ = 1.179 \quad \text{and} \quad F_- = 1.058$$

From Rosenbleuth's general expression

$$E[F^m] = P_+ F_+^m + P_- F_-^m \tag{E10.5}$$

It follows that,

$$
\begin{aligned}
E[F] &= P_+ F_+ + P_- F_- \\
&= 0.5(1.179 + 1.058) = 1.1185
\end{aligned} \tag{E10.6}
$$

$$
\begin{aligned}
E[F^2] &= P_+ F_+^2 + P_- F_-^2 \\
&= 0.5\,(1.179^2 + 1.058^2) = 0.5\,(1.390 + 1.119) \\
&= 1.255
\end{aligned} \tag{E10.7}
$$

$V[F]$ is then obtained from

$$
\begin{aligned}
V[F] &= E[F^2] - \{E[F]\}^2 \\
&= 1.255 - 1.1185^2 \quad \text{[See Ang and Tang (2007), p. 90]} \\
&= 1.255 - 1.251 \\
&= 0.004
\end{aligned} \tag{E10.8}
$$

when, $\sigma_F = 0.06325$, and

$$\beta = \frac{1.1185 - 1}{0.06325} = 1.874$$

Case (b): tan ϕ' is the only random variable

Method 1: Using direct equations for statistical moments
Equation (E10.1) can be rewritten as

$$F = \frac{K_1}{K_3} + \frac{K_2}{K_3} \tan \phi' \tag{E10.9}$$

where, $K_1 = c' = 4.8 \text{ kN/m}^2$

$$
\begin{aligned}
K_2 &= \gamma z \,(\cos^2 i - r_u) \\
&= (19.62)\,(4)\,(\cos^2 12° - 0.5) \\
&= 35.85
\end{aligned}
$$

$$K_3 = \gamma z \sin i \cos i$$
$$= (19.62)\,(4)\,\sin 12° \cos 12°$$
$$= 15.96$$

As explained before in the solution for Case (a),

$$E[F] = \frac{K_1}{K_3} + \frac{K_2}{K_3}\mu_{\tan\phi'}$$
$$= \frac{4.8}{15.96} + \frac{35.85}{15.96}(0.364)$$
$$= 0.0075 + 0817632$$
$$= 1.1183$$

and

$$V[F] = \left(\frac{K_2}{K_3}\right)^2 V_{\tan\phi'}$$

whence,

$$\sigma_F = \left(\frac{K_2}{K_3}\right)\sigma_{\tan\phi'}$$
$$= \left(\frac{35.85}{15.96}\right)(0.0728)$$
$$= (2.2462)\,(0.0728)$$
$$= 0.1635$$

and,

$$\beta = \frac{1.1183 - 1}{0.1635}$$
$$= 0.723$$

Method 2: Using MFOSM method
As in the solution for Case (a),

$$E[F] = 1.1183$$

and,

$$V[F] = \left(\frac{\partial F}{\partial(\tan\phi')}\right)^2 \sigma^2_{\tan\phi'}$$

From Equation (E10.9),

$$\frac{\partial F}{\partial(\tan\phi)} = \frac{K_2}{K_3}$$

Thus,

$$V[F] = \left(\frac{K_2}{K_3}\right)^2 \sigma^2_{\tan\phi'}$$

whence,

$$\sigma_F = \left(\frac{K_2}{K_3}\right)\sigma_{\tan\phi'}$$
$$= (2.2462)(0.0728)$$
$$= 0.1635$$

Therefore,
Reliability Index,

$$\beta = \frac{1.1183 - 1}{0.1635}$$
$$= 0.723$$

Method 3: Using PEM
As in case (a),

$$x_+ = \mu_{\tan\phi'} + \sigma_{\tan\phi'} = 0.364 + 0.0728 = 0.4368$$
$$x_- = \mu_{\tan\phi'} - \sigma_{\tan\phi'} = 0.364 - 0.0728 = 0.2912$$

The corresponding values of F are obtained from Equation (E10.1) as:

$$F_+ = 1.282 \text{ and } F_- = 0.955$$

Then, from Equation (E10.6),

$$E[F] = P_+ F_+ + P_- F_-$$
$$= 0.5(1.282 + 0.955) = 1.118$$

and, from Equation (E10.7)

$$E[F^2] = P_+ F_+^2 + P_- F_-^2$$
$$= 0.5(1.282^2 + 0.955^2)$$
$$= 1.278$$

From Equation (E10.8),

$$V[F] = E[F^2] - \{E[F]\}^2$$
$$= 1.278 - (1.118)^2 = 0.0281$$

Therefore, $\sigma_F = \sqrt{0.0281} = 0.1676$ and Reliability Index,

$$\beta = \frac{1.118 - 1}{0.1676}$$
$$= 0.704$$

Case (c): r_u is the only random variable

Method I: Using direct equation for statistical moments
Equation (E10.1) can be rewritten as

$$F = \frac{K_1 + K_2 - K_3\, r_u}{K_4}$$
$$= \frac{K_1 + K_2}{K_4} - \frac{K_3}{K_4} r_u$$

(E10.10)

Proceeding as in the previous cases (a) and (b) of linear performance functions, we obtain

$$E[F] = \frac{K_1 + K_2}{K_4} - \frac{K_3}{K_4}\mu_{r_u}$$
$$= \frac{4.8 + 27.332}{15.96} - \left(\frac{28.567}{15.96}\right)(0.5)$$
$$= 2.013 - 0.895$$
$$= 1.118$$

$$V[F] = V\left[\frac{K_1 + K_2}{K_4} - \frac{K_3}{K_4} r_u\right]$$
$$= \left(-\frac{K_3}{K_4}\right)^2 V_{r_u}$$

$$\therefore \sigma_F = \frac{K_3}{K_4}\sigma_{r_u}$$
$$= \left(\frac{28.567}{15.96}\right)(0.1)$$
$$= 0.17183$$

Thus, the Reliability Index,

$$\beta = \frac{1.118 - 1}{0.17183}$$
$$= 0.687$$

Method 2: Using MFOSM method
As in the solution for Case (a) and Case (b),

$$E[F] = 1.1183$$

and

$$V[F] = \left(\frac{\partial F}{\partial r_u}\right)^2 \sigma_{r_u}^2$$

From Equation (E10.10),

$$\frac{\partial F}{\partial r_u} = -\frac{K_3}{K_4}$$

Therefore,

$$\sigma_F = \frac{K_3}{K_4}\sigma_{r_u} = \frac{28.567}{15.96}(0.1)$$
$$= 0.17183$$

Thus,
The Reliability Index,

$$\beta = \frac{1.1183 - 1}{0.17183}$$
$$= 0.687$$

Method 3: Using PEM
As in Case (a) and Case (b),

$$x_+ = \mu_{r_u} + \sigma_{r_u} = 0.5 + 0.1 = 0.6$$
$$x_- = \mu_{r_u} - \sigma_{r_u} = 0.5 - 0.1 = 0.4$$
$$F_+ = 0.939, \ F_- = 1.297$$
$$E[F] = 0.5(0.939 + 1.297)$$
$$= 1.118$$
$$E[F^2] = 0.5(0.939^2 + 1.297^2)$$
$$= 1.282$$

Therefore,

$$V[F] = 1.282 - 1.118^2 = 0.0321$$
$$\sigma_F = 0.1791$$

and,

$$\beta = \frac{1.118 - 1}{0.1791}$$
$$= 0.6588$$

Case (d): z is the only random variable

For this case, Equation [E10.1] can be suitably written as

$$F = \frac{K_1 + K_2 z}{K_3 z} = \frac{K_2}{K_3} + \frac{K_1}{K_3}\left(\frac{1}{z}\right)$$ (E10.11)

where, substituting the mean values, $K_1 = 4.8$, $K_2 = 3.262$ and $K_3 = 3.99$

Unlike cases (a), (b) and (c), in this case F is a nonlinear function of the basic variate, z.

For a general function of a random variable X, say, $Y = g(X)$, the exact moments of Y may be obtained as

$$E(Y) = \int\limits_{-\infty}^{\infty} g(x) f_X(x) dx$$

and,

$$V(Y) = \int\limits_{-\infty}^{\infty} [g(x) - E(Y)]^2 f_X(x) dx$$

It is obvious that, to obtain the mean and variance of the function Y with the above relations, it is necessary to have information on the density function $f_X(x)$ which may not be known in many applications. Even when $f_X(x)$ is known, the integrations indicated above may be difficult to perform [see Ang and Tang, (2007) p. 183], and will not be attempted here.

For such problems, therefore, numerical methods like MFOSM and PEM are quite useful for finding approximate mean and variance of the function Y.

Method 1: Using MFOSM method

As before, $E[F] = 1.1183$ and

$$V[F] = \left(\frac{\partial F}{\partial z}\right)^2 \sigma_z^2$$

From Equation (E10.11),

$$\frac{\partial F}{\partial z} = -\frac{K_1}{K_3}\frac{1}{z^2} = -\frac{4.8}{3.99}\left(\frac{1}{4^2}\right) = -0.0752$$

Therefore,

$$V[F] = (0.0752)^2\,(0.8)^2 = 0.003618$$

and

$$\sigma_F = 0.06015$$

Thus,
The Reliability Index,

$$\beta = \frac{1.1183 - 1}{0.06015}$$
$$= 1.967$$

Method 2: Using point estimate method
As before,

$$x_+ = \mu_z + \sigma_z = 4 + 0.8 = 4.8$$
$$x_- = \mu_z - \sigma_z = 4 - 0.8 = 3.2$$
$$F_+ = \frac{4.8 + 3.262\,(4.8)}{3.99\,(4.8)} = 1.068$$
$$F_- = \frac{4.8 + 3.262\,(3.2)}{3.99\,(3.2)} = 1.193$$

$$E[F] = 0.5\,(1.068 + 1.193) = 1.1305$$
$$E[F^2] = 0.5\,(1.068^2 + 1.193^2) = 1.282$$
$$V[F] = 1.282 - (1.1305)^2 = 0.00397$$

Therefore,

$$\sigma_F = \sqrt{0.00397} = 0.063$$

and

$$\beta = \frac{1.1305 - 1}{0.063} = 2.071$$

EXAMPLE 10.12

Work out the above example (Example 10.11) assuming (a) c' and $\tan \phi'$ as random variables (b) c' and r_u as random variables (c) $\tan \phi'$ and r_u as random variables (d) z and c' as random variables. For each of the random variables, assume a coefficient of variation of 0.2.

Solution

Case (a): c' and $\tan\phi'$ as random variables

Method 1: Using direct equations for statistical moments
For this case the factor of safety given by equation (E10.1) can be rewritten as

$$F = \frac{c' + K_1 \tan \phi'}{K_2} = \frac{1}{K_2} c' + \frac{K_1}{K_2} \tan \phi'$$

(E10.8)

where,

$$K_1 = \gamma z (\cos^2 i - r_u) = (19.62)\,(4)\,(\cos^2 12° - 0.5) = 35.85$$

and

$$K_2 = \gamma z \sin i \cos i = (19.62)(4)\sin 12° \cos 12° = 15.96$$

The expected value of F is given by

$$E[F] = \frac{1}{K_2} E[c'] + \frac{K_1}{K_2} E[\tan \phi']$$

$$= \frac{1}{15.96}(4.8) + \frac{35.85}{15.96}(0.364)$$

$$= 0.30075 + 0.8176$$

$$= 1.1183$$

Now, considering c' and $\tan \phi'$ (i.e., ϕ') as uncorrelated, the variance of F is given by

$$V[F] = \left(\frac{1}{K_2}\right)^2 V_{c'} + \left(\frac{K_1}{K_2}\right)^2 V_{\tan \phi'}$$

$$= \left(\frac{1}{K_2}\right)^2 \sigma_{c'}^2 + \left(\frac{K_1}{K_2}\right)^2 \sigma_{\tan \phi'}^2$$

$$= \left(\frac{1}{15.96}\right)^2 (0.96)^2 + \left(\frac{35.85}{15.96}\right)^2 (0.0728)^2$$

$$= 0.003618 + 0.02674 = 0.03036$$

Therefore,

$$\sigma_F = 0.1742$$

and

$$\beta = \frac{F[F] - 1}{\sigma_F}$$

$$= \frac{1.1183 - 1}{0.1742} = 0.679$$

Method 2: Using MFOSM method

Substituting the mean values of c' and $\tan \phi'$ in Equation (E10.12),

$$E[F] = \frac{4.8}{K_2} + \frac{0.364 K_1}{K_2}$$

$$= \frac{4.8 + 0.364 \ K_1}{K_2}$$

$$= \frac{4.8 + 0.364(35.85)}{15.96}$$

$$= 1.1183$$

The variance $V[F]$ is calculated from the Equation (E10.13)

$$V[F] = \sum_{j=1}^{2} \left(\frac{\partial F}{\partial X_j} \right)^2 \sigma_{x_j}^2$$

$$= \left(\frac{\partial F}{\partial c'} \right)^2 \sigma_{c'}^2 + \left(\frac{\partial F}{\partial \tan \phi'} \right)^2 \sigma_{\tan \phi'}^2$$

$$= \left(\frac{1}{K_2} \right)^2 \sigma_{c'}^2 + \left(\frac{K_1}{K_2} \right)^2 \sigma_{\tan \phi'}^2 \qquad \text{(E10.13)}$$

$$= \left(\frac{1}{15.96} \right)^2 (0.96)^2 + \left(\frac{35.85}{15.96} \right)^2 (0.0728)^2$$

$$= 0.003618 + 0.02674 = 0.03036$$

Therefore,

$$\sigma_F = \sqrt{0.03036}$$

$$= 0.1742$$

and

$$\beta = \frac{1.1183 - 1}{0.1742} = 0.679$$

Method 3: Using PEM

In the Rosenblueth procedure for n variables, 2^n points are selected so that the value of each variable is one standard deviation above or below its mean.

For two variables X_1 ($=c'$) and X_2 ($=\tan \phi'$), the four points are:

$$\begin{aligned}
x_{++} &= (\mu_{X_1} + \sigma_{X_1}, \mu_{X_2} + \sigma_{X_2}) \\
&= (\mu_{c'} + \sigma_{c'}, \mu_{\tan \phi'} + \sigma_{\tan \phi'}) \\
&= (4.8 + 0.96, 0.364 + 0.0728) \\
&= (5.76, 0.4368)
\end{aligned}$$

Similarly,

$$\begin{aligned}
x_{+-} &= (5.76, 0.2912) \\
x_{-+} &= (3.84, 0.4368) \\
x_{--} &= (3.84, 0.2912)
\end{aligned}$$

Corresponding to these four points, the four values of Factor of safety are:

$$\begin{aligned}
F_{++} &= 1.342 \\
F_{+-} &= 1.015 \\
F_{-+} &= 1.222 \\
F_{--} &= 0.895
\end{aligned}$$

With these four F – values,

$$\begin{aligned}
E[F] &= 0.25(1.342 + 1.015 + 1.222 + 0.895) = 1.1185 \\
E[F^2] &= 0.25\,(1.342^2 + 1.015^2 + 1.222^2 + 0.895^2) \\
&= 0.25\,(1.8 + 1.0302 + 1.493 + 0.801) = 1.28105
\end{aligned}$$

and

$$V[F] = 1.28105 - 1.1185^2 = 0.0300$$

Therefore,

$$\sigma_F = 0.1732$$

and

$$\beta = \frac{1.1185 - 1}{0.1732} = 0.684$$

Case (b): c' and r_u as random variables

Method 1: Using direct equations for statistical moments

For this case Equation (E10.1) can be suitably re-written as

$$F = \frac{c' + K_1 - K_2 r_u}{K_3} = \frac{K_1}{K_3} + \frac{c'}{K_3} - \frac{K_2}{K_3} r_u \qquad (E10.14)$$

where,

$$K_1 = \gamma z \cos^2 i \tan \phi' = (19.62)(4) \cos^2 12° (0.364)$$
$$= (78.48)(0.9568)(0.364) = 27.3318$$
$$K_2 = \gamma z \tan \phi' = (19.62)(4)(0.364)$$
$$= (78.48)(0.364) = 28.567$$
$$K_3 = \gamma z \sin i \cos i = 15.96$$

As demonstrated in Case (a),

$$E[F] = \frac{K_1}{K_3} + \frac{1}{K_3} \mu_{c'} - \frac{K_2}{K_3} \mu_{r_u}$$
$$= \frac{27.3318}{15.96} + \frac{1}{15.96}(4.8) - \frac{28.567}{15.96}(0.5) = 1.1183$$

and,

$$V[F] = \frac{1}{K_3^2} \sigma_{c'}^2 + \left(\frac{K_2}{K_3}\right)^2 \sigma_{r_u}^2$$
$$= \frac{1}{15.96^2}[0.96^2 + (28.567)^2(0.1)^2]$$
$$= \frac{1}{254.72}[0.9216 + 8.1607] = 0.0357$$

Therefore,

$$\sigma_F = \sqrt{0.0357} = 0.1888$$

and

$$\beta = \frac{1.1183 - 1}{0.1888} = 0.626$$

Method 2: Using MFOSM method
Substituting the mean values of c' and r_u in Equation (E10.14)

$$E[F] = \frac{4.8 + K_1 - K_2(0.5)}{K_3}$$

$$= \frac{4.8 + 27.3318 - 28.567(0.5)}{15.96} = 1.1183$$

The variance $V[F]$ is calculated from the Equation (E10.13)

$$V[F] = \sum_{j=1}^{2} \left(\frac{\partial F}{\partial X_j}\right)^2 \sigma_{x_j}^2$$

$$= \left(\frac{\partial F}{\partial c'}\right)^2 \sigma_{c'}^2 + \left(\frac{\partial F}{\partial r_u}\right)^2 \sigma_{r_u}^2$$

$$= \left(\frac{1}{K_3}\right)^2 (0.96)^2 + \left(-\frac{K_2}{K_3}\right)^2 (0.1)^2 = 0.0357$$

Therefore,

$$\sigma_F = \sqrt{0.0357} = 0.1888$$

and

$$\beta = \frac{1.1183 - 1}{0.1888} = 0.626$$

Method 3: Using PEM
Following the steps mentioned while solving for Case (a), the four points of estimation are:

$$x_{++} = (\mu_{x_1} + \sigma_{x_1}, \mu_{x_2} + \sigma_{x_2})$$
$$= (\mu_{c'} + \sigma_{c'}, \mu_{r_u} + \sigma_{r_u})$$
$$= (4.8 + 0.96, 0.5 + 0.1)$$
$$= (5.76, 0.6)$$

Similarly,

$$x_{+-} = (5.76, 0.4)$$
$$x_{-+} = (3.84, 0.6)$$
$$x_{--} = (3.84, 0.4)$$

Corresponding to these points the values of the factor of safety are:

$F_{++} = 0.999$
$F_{+-} = 1.357$
$F_{-+} = 0.878$
$F_{--} = 1.237$

Then,

$E[F] = 0.25\,(0.999 + 1.357 + 0.878 + 1.237)$
$\qquad = 1.117$

and

$E[F^2] = 0.25\,(0.999^2 + 1.357^2 + 0.878^2 + 1.237^2)$
$\qquad = 1.285$

Thus,

$V[F] = 1.285 - 1.117^2 = 0.0373$
$\therefore\ \sigma_F = \sqrt{0.0373} = 0.1932$

Finally,

$\beta = \dfrac{1.117 - 1}{0.1932}$
$\quad = 0.606$

Case(C): tan ϕ' and r_u as random variables

Method 1: Using direct equations for statistical moments
For this case Equation (E10.1) can be suitably re-written as

$$F = K_1 + K_2 \tan \phi' - \frac{1}{K_3} r_u \tan \phi' \qquad (E10.15)$$

where

$K_1 = \dfrac{c'}{\gamma z\,\sin i\,\cos i} = \dfrac{4.8}{15.96} = 0.3008$
$K_2 = \cot i = \cot 12° = 4.7046$
$K_3 = \sin i\,\cos i = \sin 12°\cos 12° = 0.2034$

Equation (E10.15) indicates a non-linear performance function of the basic variates tan ϕ' and r_u. For the reasons stated in the solution of Example 10.11(d), it is rather difficult to solve this problem using direct integration, and will not be attempted here.

Method 2: Using MFOSM method

Substituting the mean values of the basic variates, $\tan \phi'$ and r_u, in Equation (E10.15),

$$E[F] = 0.3008 + (4.7046)\,(0.364) - \frac{1}{0.2034}\,(0.5)\,(0.364)$$

$$= 1.1183$$

and,

$$V[F] = \sum_{j=1}^{2} \left(\frac{\partial F}{\partial X_j} \right)^2 \sigma_{x_j}^2$$

$$= \left(\frac{\partial F}{\partial \tan \phi'} \right)^2 \sigma_{\tan \phi'}^2 + \left(\frac{\partial F}{\partial r_u} \right)^2 \sigma_{r_u}^2$$

The partial derivatives are

$$\frac{\partial F}{\partial \tan \phi'} = K_2 - \frac{1}{K_3} r_u = 4.7046 - \frac{0.5}{0.2034}$$

$$= 2.2464$$

and

$$\frac{\partial F}{\partial r_u} = -\frac{1}{K_3} \tan \phi' = -\frac{1}{0.2034}(0.364) = -1.7896$$

Thus,

$$V[F] = (2.2464)^2 \,(0.0728)^2 + (-1.7896)^2 \,(0.1)^2$$

$$= 0.587$$

and,

$$\sigma_F = \sqrt{0.0587} = 0.2424$$

Therefore,

$$\beta = \frac{1.1183 - 1}{0.2424}$$

$$= 0.4880$$

Method 3: Using PEM

In this case the four points of estimation are:

$$x_{++} = (\mu_{\tan\phi'} + \sigma_{\tan\phi'}, \mu_{\tan\phi'} + \sigma_{\tan\phi'}) = (0.4368, 0.6)$$
$$x_{+-} = (\mu_{\tan\phi'} + \sigma_{\tan\phi'}, \mu_{\tan\phi'} - \sigma_{\tan\phi'}) = (0.4368, 0.4)$$
$$x_{-+} = (\mu_{\tan\phi'} - \sigma_{\tan\phi'}, \mu_{\tan\phi'} + \sigma_{\tan\phi'}) = (0.2912, 0.6)$$
$$x_{--} = (\mu_{\tan\phi'} - \sigma_{\tan\phi'}, \mu_{\tan\phi'} - \sigma_{\tan\phi'}) = (0.2912, 0.4)$$

The corresponding F values are:

$$F_{++} = 1.0675$$
$$F_{+-} = 1.497$$
$$F_{-+} = 0.812$$
$$F_{--} = 1.0983$$

Then, the moments of F are obtained as:

$$E[F] = 0.25\,[1.0675 + 1.497 + 0.812 + 1.0983] = 1.1187$$
$$E[F^2] = 0.25\,[1.0675^2 + 1.497^2 + 0.812^2 + 1.0983^2] = 1.3115$$

Thus,

$$V[F] = 1.3115 - 1.1187^2 = 0.0600$$

and

$$\sigma_F = 0.245$$

Finally,

$$\beta = \frac{1.1187 - 1}{0.245} = 0.4845$$

Case (d): c' and z are random variables

For this case the Equation (E10.1) can be suitably re-written as

$$F = K_1 + \frac{c'}{K_2 z} \qquad\qquad\qquad\qquad (E10.16)$$

where,

$$K_1 = \frac{(\cos^2 i - r_u)\tan\phi'}{\sin i\,\cos i} = \frac{(\cos^2 12° - 0.5)(0.364)}{\sin 12°\cos 12°} = \frac{0.1663}{0.2034} = 0.8174$$

and

$$K_2 = \gamma \sin i \, \cos i = (19.62) \sin 12° \cos 12° = 3.9907$$

Method 1: Using direct equations

Equation (E10.16) being nonlinear in c' and z, solution using direct integration is difficult, as discussed earlier, and will not be attempted here.

Method 2: Using MFOSM method

Substituting the mean values of the basic variates, c' and z, in Equation (E10.16)

$$E[F] = 0.8174 + \frac{4.8}{3.9907(4.0)} = 1.1183$$

The variance,

$$V[F] = \sum_{j=1}^{n} \left(\frac{\partial F}{\partial x_j} \right)^2 \sigma_{x_j}^2$$

$$= \left(\frac{\partial F}{\partial c'} \right)^2 \sigma_{c'}^2 + \left(\frac{\partial F}{\partial z} \right)^2 \sigma_z^2$$

The values of the partial derivatives evaluated at the mean values of the basic variables are

$$\frac{\partial F}{\partial c'} = \frac{1}{K_2 \, z} = \frac{1}{(3.9907)(4.0)} = 0.0626$$

$$\frac{\partial F}{\partial z} = -\frac{c'}{K_2} \frac{1}{z^2} = -\frac{4.8}{(3.9907)(4.0)^2} = -0.0752$$

Thus,

$$V[F] = (0.0626)^2 \times (0.96)^2 + (-0.0752)^2 \times (0.8)^2$$
$$= 0.0072307$$

Then,

$$\sigma_F = \sqrt{0.0072307} = 0.08503$$

and,

$$\beta = \frac{1.1183 - 1}{0.08503} = 1.3913$$

Method 3: Using PEM

In this case, the four points of estimates are:

$$x_{++} = (\mu_{c'} + \sigma_{c'}, \mu_z + \sigma_z) = (5.76, 4.8)$$
$$x_{+-} = (\mu_{c'} + \sigma_{c'}, \mu_z - \sigma_z) = (5.76, 3.2)$$
$$x_{-+} = (\mu_{c'} - \sigma_{c'}, \mu_z + \sigma_z) = (3.84, 4.8)$$
$$x_{--} = (\mu_{c'} - \sigma_{c'}, \mu_z - \sigma_z) = (3.84, 3.2)$$

The corresponding F values are:

$$F_{++} = 1.1181$$
$$F_{+-} = 1.2540$$
$$F_{-+} = 1.0179$$
$$F_{--} = 1.1181$$

The moments of F are then obtained as:

$$E[F] = 0.25\,(1.1181 + 1.2540 + 1.0179 + 1.1181)$$
$$= 1.127$$
$$E[F^2] = 0.25\,(1.1181^2 + 1.2540^2 + 1.0179^2 + 1.1181^2)$$
$$= 1.2772$$
$$V[F] = 1.2772 - 1.127^2$$
$$= 0.007071$$
$$\sigma_F = \sqrt{0.007071} = 0.08409$$

Therefore,

$$\beta = \frac{1.127 - 1}{0.08409} = 1.51$$

EXAMPLE 10.13

Work out Example 10.11 assuming (a) c', $\tan \phi'$ and r_u as random variables, and (b) z, c' and r_u as random variables. For each of the random variables, assume a coefficient of variation of 0.2.

Case (a): c', $\tan\phi'$ and r_u as random variables

Method 1: Using direct equations for statistical moments

In this case, in the performance function [Equation E10.1] the term involving $r_u \tan \phi'$ introduces nonlinearity and hence, for reasons stated earlier, solution using direct equations for statistical moments will not be attempted.

Method 2: Using MFOSM
Re-writing Equation (E10.1) as

$$F = \frac{c'}{K_1} + \frac{(K_2 - r_u)\tan\phi'}{K_3} \qquad\qquad \text{[E10.17]}$$

where,

$$K_1 = \gamma z \sin i \, \cos i = (19.62)\,(4)\,(\sin 12°)\,(\cos 12°) = 15.96$$
$$K_2 = \cos^2 i = \cos^2 12° = 0.9568$$
$$K_3 = \sin i \, \cos i = \sin 12° \cos 12° = 0.2034$$

Then,

$$\frac{\partial F}{\partial c'} = \frac{1}{K_1} = \frac{1}{15.96} = 0.06266$$

$$\frac{\partial F}{\partial \tan\phi'} = \frac{K_2 - r_u}{K_3} = \frac{0.9568 - 0.5}{0.2034} = 2.246$$

$$\frac{\partial F}{\partial r_u} = -\frac{\tan\phi'}{K_3} = -\frac{0.364}{0.2034} = -1.7896$$

Now, from Equation (E10.17),

$$E[F] = \frac{4.8}{K_1} + \frac{(0.9568 - 0.5)\,(0.364)}{K_3}$$
$$= 1.1183$$

$$V[F] = \sum_{j=1}^{3} \left(\frac{\partial F}{\partial x_j}\right)^2 \sigma_{x_j}^2$$

$$= \left(\frac{\partial F}{\partial c'}\right)^2 \sigma_{c'}^2 + \left(\frac{\partial F}{\partial \tan\phi'}\right)^2 \sigma_{\tan\phi'}^2 + \left(\frac{\partial F}{\partial r_u}\right)^2 \sigma_{r_u}^2$$

$$= (0.06266)^2\,(0.96)^2 + (2.246)^2\,(0.0728)^2 + (-1.7896)^2\,(0.1)^2$$

$$= 0.0623$$

Therefore, $\sigma_F = \sqrt{0.0623} = 0.2496$ and
Reliability Index,

$$\beta = \frac{1.1183 - 1}{0.2496}$$
$$= 0.474$$

Method III: Using PEM
In this case, there are 2^3 or 8 points of estimation which are as follows:

$$x_{+++} = (\mu_{c'} + \sigma_{c'}),(\mu_{\tan\phi'} + \sigma_{\tan\phi'}),(\mu_{r_u} + \sigma_{r_u}) = 5.76, 0.4368, 0.6$$

$$x_{++-} = (\mu_{c'} + \sigma_{c'}),(\mu_{\tan\phi'} + \sigma_{\tan\phi'}),(\mu_{r_u} - \sigma_{r_u}) = 5.76, 0.4368, 0.4$$

$$x_{+-+} = (\mu_{c'} + \sigma_{c'}),(\mu_{\tan\phi'} - \sigma_{\tan\phi'}),(\mu_{r_u} + \sigma_{r_u}) = 5.76, 0.2912, 0.6$$

$$x_{-++} = (\mu_{c'} - \sigma_{c'}),(\mu_{\tan\phi'} + \sigma_{\tan\phi'}),(\mu_{r_u} + \sigma_{r_u}) - 3.84, 0.4368, 0.6$$

$$x_{--+} = (\mu_{c'} - \sigma_{c'}),(\mu_{\tan\phi'} - \sigma_{\tan\phi'}),(\mu_{r_u} + \sigma_{r_u}) = 3.84, 0.2912, 0.6$$

$$x_{---} = (\mu_{c'} - \sigma_{c'}),(\mu_{\tan\phi'} - \sigma_{\tan\phi'}),(\mu_{r_u} - \sigma_{r_u}) = 3.84, 0.2912, 0.4$$

$$x_{-+-} = (\mu_{c'} - \sigma_{c'}),(\mu_{\tan\phi'} + \sigma_{\tan\phi'}),(\mu_{r_u} - \sigma_{r_u}) = 3.84, 0.4368, 0.4$$

$$x_{+--} = (\mu_{c'} + \sigma_{c'}),(\mu_{\tan\phi'} - \sigma_{\tan\phi'}),(\mu_{r_u} - \sigma_{r_u}) = 5.76, 0.2912, 0.4$$

The corresponding F values are obtained as:

$F_{+++} = 1.8948$

$F_{++-} = 1.3835$

$F_{+-+} = 2.3243$

$F_{-++} = 1.7745$

$F_{--+} = 2.2040$

$F_{---} = 1.5495$

$F_{-+-} = 1.2632$

$F_{+--} = 1.6698$

The weights are taken as $1/2^3 = 1/8 = 0.125$
Thus,

$$E[F] = 0.125[\Sigma F]$$
$$= 1.3913$$

and

$$E[F^2] = 0.125[\Sigma F^2]$$
$$= 2.6643$$

Variance

$$V[F] = E[F^2] - \{E[F]\}^2$$
$$= 2.6643 - (1.3913)^2$$
$$= 0.7285$$
$$\sigma_F = \sqrt{0.7285} = 0.8535$$

Finally,
Reliability Index

$$\beta = \frac{E[F]-1}{\sigma_F}$$

$$= \frac{1.3913-1}{0.8535} = 0.4585$$

Case (b): z, c' and r_u as design variables
Equation (E10.1) can be re-written as

$$F = \frac{c' + \gamma z(\cos^2 i - r_u)\tan\phi'}{\gamma z \sin i \, \cos i}$$

$$= \frac{c' + \gamma z \cos^2 i \, \tan\phi' - \gamma z r_u \tan\phi'}{\gamma z \sin i \, \cos i}$$

$$= \cot i \, \tan\phi' + \frac{c'}{(\gamma \sin i \, \cos i)z} - \left(\frac{\tan\phi'}{\sin i \cos i}\right)r_u \qquad \text{(E10.18)}$$

$$= K_1 + \frac{c'}{K_2 z} - K_3 r_u$$

where,

$$K_1 = \cot i \, \tan\phi' = (\cot 12°)\,(0.364) = 1.7125$$
$$K_2 = \gamma \sin i \, \cos i = (19.62)\,(\sin 12°)\,(\cos 12°) = 3.99$$
$$K_3 = \frac{\tan\phi'}{\sin i \, \cos i} = \frac{0.364}{\sin 12° \cos 12°} = \frac{0.364}{0.2034} = 1.7896$$

Method I: Solution by direct equation
Like case (a), in this case the term $c'/k_2 z$ introduces nonlinearity in the performance function (E10.18) and therefore, solution by direct integration will not be tried.

Method II: Solution using MFOSM
The partial derivatives are obtained as:

$$\frac{\partial F}{\partial z} = -\frac{c'}{K_2 z^2} = -\frac{4.8}{(3.99)\,(4)^2} = -0.07519$$

$$\frac{\partial F}{\partial c'} = \frac{1}{K_2 z} = \frac{1}{(3.99)\,(4)} = 0.06266$$

$$\frac{\partial F}{\partial r_u} = -K_3 = -1.7896$$

Now from Equation (E10.18)

$$E[F] = K_1 + \frac{4.8}{K_2(4)} - K_3(0.5)$$

$$= 1.7125 + \frac{4.8}{(3.99)(4)} - 1.7896(0.5)$$

$$= 1.1183$$

and

$$V[F] = \sum_{j=1}^{3} \left(\frac{\partial F}{\partial x_j} \right)^2 \sigma_{x_j}^2$$

$$= \left(\frac{\partial F}{\partial z} \right)^2 \sigma_z^2 + \left(\frac{\partial F}{\partial c'} \right)^2 \sigma_{c'}^2 + \left(\frac{\partial F}{\partial r_u} \right)^2 \sigma_{r_u}^2$$

$$= (-0.07519)^2 (0.8)^2 + (0.06266)^2 (0.96)^2 + (-1.7896)^2 (0.1)^2$$

$$= 3.61826 \times 10^{-3} + 3.61845.6 \times 10^{-3} + 0.0320267$$

$$= 0.03926$$

Therefore,

$$\sigma_F = 0.19815$$

and,
   The Reliability Index,

$$\beta = \frac{1.1183 - 1}{0.19815}$$

$$= 0.597$$

Method III: Using PEM
The eight points of estimation are:

$$x_{+++} = (\mu_z + \sigma_z), (\mu_{c'} + \sigma_{c'}), (\mu_{r_u} + \sigma_{r_u}) = (4.8, 5.76, 0.6)$$
$$x_{++-} = (\mu_z + \sigma_z), (\mu_{c'} + \sigma_{c'}), (\mu_{r_u} - \sigma_{r_u}) = (4.8, 5.76, 0.4)$$
$$x_{+-+} = (\mu_z + \sigma_z), (\mu_{c'} - \sigma_{c'}), (\mu_{r_u} + \sigma_{r_u}) = (4.8, 3.84, 0.6)$$
$$x_{-++} = (\mu_z - \sigma_z), (\mu_{c'} + \sigma_{c'}), (\mu_{r_u} + \sigma_{r_u}) = (3.2, 5.76, 0.6)$$
$$x_{--+} = (\mu_z - \sigma_z), (\mu_{c'} - \sigma_{c'}), (\mu_{r_u} + \sigma_{r_u}) = (3.2, 3.84, 0.4)$$
$$x_{---} = (\mu_z - \sigma_z), (\mu_{c'} - \sigma_{c'}), (\mu_{r_u} - \sigma_{r_u}) = (3.2, 3.84, 0.4)$$
$$x_{-+-} = (\mu_z - \sigma_z), (\mu_{c'} + \sigma_{c'}), (\mu_{r_u} - \sigma_{r_u}) = (3.2, 5.76, 0.4)$$
$$x_{+--} = (\mu_z + \sigma_z), (\mu_{c'} - \sigma_{c'}), (\mu_{r_u} - \sigma_{r_u}) = (4.8, 3.84, 0.4)$$

The Corresponding F values are:

$F_{+++} = 0.939$

$F_{++-} = 1.297$

$F_{+-+} = 0.839$

$F_{-++} = 1.090$

$F_{--+} = 0.939$

$F_{---} = 1.297$

$F_{-+-} = 1.448$

$F_{+--} = 1.197$

Then,

$$E[F] = 0.125 \sum F = 0.125 \times 9.047865$$
$$= 1.131$$

and

$$E[F^2] = 0.125 \sum F^2 = 0.125 \times 10.553270$$
$$= 1.319$$

Variance,

$$V[F] = E[F^2] - \{E[F]\}^2$$
$$= 0.0398$$
$$\sigma_F = \sqrt{0.0398} = 0.1996$$

Therefore,
The Reliability Index,

$$\beta = \frac{E[F] - 1}{\sigma_F}$$
$$= 0.656$$

EXAMPLE 10.14

Often some uncertainty is associated with the assumed model of slope stability. Thus the estimated F may have to be multiplied by a correction factor, e, in order to account for the uncertainty or the imperfection. Therefore, the performance function is the product eF in which both e and F are random variables. Estimate the reliability index for Example 1 with c, $\tan \phi$ and r_u as the random variables plus the model error represented by e as the additional random variable. Consider two cases:

(a) when mean of $e = 1$, and, the standard deviation of $e = 0.2$ (thus coefficient of variation is also 0.2) (b) when mean of $e = 1.1$, and the standard deviation of $e = 0.22$ (thus coefficient of variation is also 0.2).

Solution

In this case the performance function is given by

$$g = eF - 1 \tag{E10.19}$$

where F is given by Equation [E10.1] and e is an additional random variable. Considering that c', $\tan \phi'$ and r_u are the random variables in F, this problem is one of four random variables.

Method I: Using MFOSM

Substituting the expression for F from Equation [E10.17] of the Example 10.13 Case (a), we have,

$$g = e\left[\frac{c'}{K_1} + \frac{(K_2 - r_u)\tan \phi'}{K_3}\right] - 1 \tag{E10.20}$$

where,

$$K_1 = 15.96, \ K_2 = 0.9568 \text{ and } K_3 = 0.2034$$

From Equation (E10.19),

$$E[g] = E[e] \, E[F] - 1 \tag{E10.21}$$
$$= \mu_e \, E[F] - 1$$

The partial derivatives are worked out as:

$$\frac{\partial g}{\partial e} = \frac{c'}{K_1} + \frac{(K_2 - r_u)\tan \phi'}{K_3} = 1.1183$$

$$\frac{\partial g}{\partial c'} = \frac{e}{K_1} = \frac{e}{15.96} = 0.0627 \, e$$

$$\frac{\partial g}{\partial \tan \phi'} = \frac{e \, (K_2 - r_u)}{K_3} = \frac{e \, (0.9568 - 0.5)}{0.2034} = 2.2458 e$$

$$\frac{\partial g}{\partial r_u} = -\frac{e \tan \phi'}{K_3} = -\frac{0.364 \, e}{0.2034} = -1.7896 e$$

Case (a): $\mu_e = 1.0$, $\sigma_e = 0.2$
Since $\mu_e = 1.0$, from Equation (E10.21)

$$E(g) = E[F] - 1 = 1.1183 - 1 = 0.1183$$

Substituting in the above expressions, the values of the partial derivatives at the mean values of the corresponding variables are:

$$\frac{\partial g}{\partial e} = 1.1183, \quad \frac{\partial g}{\partial c'} = 0.0627, \quad \frac{\partial g}{\partial \tan \phi'} = 2.2458 \quad \text{and} \quad \frac{\partial g}{\partial r_u} = -1.7896$$

Now,

$$V[g] = \sum_{j=1}^{4} \left(\frac{\partial g}{\partial X_j} \right)^2 \sigma_{x_j}^2$$

$$= (1.1183)^2 (0.2)^2 + (0.0627)^2 (0.96)^2 + (2.2458)^2 \times (0.0728)^2 + (-1.7896)^2 (0.1)^2$$

$$= 0.112403$$

Therefore,

$$\sigma_g = 0.3353$$

and,

The Reliability Index,

$$\beta = \frac{E[g]}{\sigma_g} = \frac{0.1183}{0.3353}$$

$$= 0.3528$$

Case (b): $\mu_e = 1.0$; $\sigma_e = 0.2$
From Equation (E10.21),

$$E[g] = (1.1)(1.1183) - 1 = 1.2301 - 1 = 0.2301$$

From the expressions for partial derivatives derived earlier, by putting $e = 1.1$,

$$\frac{\partial g}{\partial e} = 1.1183$$

$$\frac{\partial g}{\partial c'} = (0.0627)(1.1) = 0.06897$$

$$\frac{\partial g}{\partial \tan \phi'} = (2.2458)(1.1) = 2.4704$$

$$\frac{\partial g}{\partial r_u} = (-1.7896)(1.1) = -1.96856$$

Thus,

$$V[g] = (1.1183)^2 (0.22)^2 + (0.06897)^2 \times (0.96)^2 + (2.4704)^2 (0.0728)^2$$
$$+ (-1.96856)^2 \times (0.1)^2$$
$$= 0.06053 + 0.004384 + 0.03234 + 0.03875$$
$$= 0.136006$$

and $\sigma_g = 0.3688$

Finally,

The reliability index

$$\beta = \frac{E[g]}{\sigma_g}$$

$$= \frac{0.2301}{0.3688}$$

$$= 0.624$$

Method 2: Using PEM

In this case there are 2^4 i.e., 16 points of estimation with a common weight value, $P = 1/2^4 = 0.0625$, as the random variables are uncorrelated.

Case (a): $\mu_e = 1.0$, $\sigma_e = 0.2$

Table E10.2 shows the calculations with g evaluated at 16 points. The first column indicates the point numbers. The second, third, fourth and fifth columns give the values of c', tan ϕ', r_u and e at each point. Columns 6, 7 and 8 give the values of F, g, (from Equation E10.20) and g^2 at each point.

Table E10.2 Results from PEM for Example 10.14 Case (a).

Point (1)	c'(2)	tan ϕ' (3)	r_u (4)	e (5)	F (6)	g (7)	g^2 (8)
1	5.76	0.4368	0.6	1.2	1.3526	0.6231	0.388254
2	5.76	0.4368	0.6	0.8	0.9017	−0.2786	0.077618
3	5.76	0.4368	0.4	1.2	1.8679	1.2415	1.541322
4	5.76	0.4368	0.4	0.8	1.2453	−0.0038	1.44E05
5	5.76	0.2912	0.6	1.2	1.0461	0.2553	0.065178
6	5.76	0.2912	0.4	1.2	1.3897	0.6676	0.44569
7	5.76	0.2912	0.4	0.8	0.9264	−0.2588	0.066977
8	3.84	0.2912	0.4	0.8	0.8302	−0.3358	0.112762
9	3.84	0.2912	0.4	1.2	1.2453	0.4944	0.244431
10	3.84	0.2912	0.6	0.8	0.6011	−0.5191	0.269465
11	3.84	0.4368	0.4	0.8	1.1491	−0.0808	0.006529
12	3.84	0.4368	0.6	0.8	0.8055	−0.3556	0.126451
13	5.76	0.2912	0.6	0.8	0.6974	−0.4421	0.195452
14	3.84	0.4368	0.4	1.2	1.7236	1.0683	1.141265
15	3.84	0.2912	0.6	1.2	0.9017	0.082	0.006724
16	3.84	0.4368	0.6	1.2	1.2082	0.4498	0.20232
						$\Sigma = 2.6074$	$\Sigma = 4.8905$

$E[g] = 0.0625 \ \Sigma g = (0.0625) \ (2.6074) = 0.16296$

$E[g^2] = 0.0625 \ \Sigma g^2 = (0.0625) \ (4.8905) = 0.30566$

$V[g] = E[g^2] - \{E[g]\}^2 = 0.27911$

$\sigma_g = \sqrt{V[g]} = 0.5238$

Reliability Index, $\beta = \dfrac{E[g]}{\sigma_g} = 0.30846$

Case (b): $\mu_e = 1.1$ and $\sigma_e = 0.22$

As described for Case (a), calculations are done in a Tabular form and presented in Table E10.3

Table E10.3 Results from PEM for Example10.14 Case (b).

Point (1)	c′ (2)	tanϕ′ (3)	r_u (4)	e (5)	F (6)	g (7)	g^2 (8)
1	5.76	0.4368	0.6	1.32	1.4878	0.9639	0.929103
2	5.76	0.4368	0.6	0.88	0.9919	−0.1272	0.01618
3	5.76	0.4368	0.4	1.32	2.0547	1.7123	2.931971
4	5.76	0.4368	0.4	0.88	1.3698	0.2055	0.04223
5	5.76	0.2912	0.6	1.32	1.1507	0.5189	0.269257
6	5.76	0.2912	0.4	1.32	1.5286	1.0178	1.035917
7	5.76	0.2912	0.4	0.88	1.0191	−0.1032	0.01065
8	3.84	0.2912	0.4	0.88	0.9132	−0.1964	0.038573
9	3.84	0.2912	0.4	1.32	1.3698	0.8082	0.653187
10	3.84	0.2912	0.6	0.88	0.6612	−0.4181	0.174808
11	3.84	0.4368	0.4	0.88	1.2639	0.1123	0.012611
12	3.84	0.4368	0.6	0.88	0.886	−0.2203	0.048532
13	5.76	0.2912	0.6	0.88	0.7671	−0.3249	0.10556
14	3.84	0.4368	0.4	1.32	1.8959	1.5027	2.258107
15	3.84	0.2912	0.6	1.32	0.9919	0.3093	0.095666
16	3.84	0.4368	0.6	1.32	1.329	0.7543	0.568968
						Σ = 6.5149	Σ = 9.1913

$E[g] = 0.0625 \, \Sigma g = (0.0625)(6.5149) = 0.4072$
$E[g^2] = 0.0625 \, \Sigma g^2 = (0.0625)(9.1913) = 0.5744$
$V[g] = E[g^2] - \{E[g]\}^2 = 0.4086$
$\sigma_g = \sqrt{V[g]} = 0.6392$

Reliability Index, $\beta = \dfrac{E[g]}{\sigma_g} = 0.6370$

Table C10.1 Probabilities that factor of safety is smaller than 1.0, based on lognormal distribution of factor of safety (after Duncan, 2000). With permission from ASCE, see page 714, No 35.

F_{MLV}	Coefficient of variation of factor of safety (V_F)														
	2%	4%	6%	8%	10%	12%	14%	16%	20%	25%	30%	40%	50%	60%	80%
1.05	0.8%	12%	22%	28%	33%	36%	39%	41%	44%	47%	49%	53%	55%	58%	61%
1.10	0.00%	0.9%	6%	12%	18%	23%	27%	30%	35%	40%	43%	48%	51%	54%	59%
1.15	0.00%	0.03%	1.1%	4%	9%	13%	18%	21%	27%	33%	37%	43%	48%	51%	56%
1.16	0.00%	0.01%	0.7%	3%	8%	12%	16%	20%	26%	32%	36%	42%	47%	50%	56%
1.18	0.00%	0.00%	0.3%	2%	5%	9%	13%	17%	23%	29%	34%	41%	45%	49%	55%
1.20	0.00%	0.00%	0.13%	1.2%	4%	7%	11%	14%	21%	27%	32%	39%	44%	48%	54%
1.25	0.00%	0.00%	0.01%	0.3%	1.4%	4%	6%	9%	15%	22%	27%	35%	41%	45%	51%
1.30	0.00%	0.00%	0.00%	0.06%	0.5%	1.6%	3%	6%	11%	17%	23%	31%	37%	42%	49%
1.35	0.00%	0.00%	0.00%	0.01%	0.2%	0.7%	1.9%	4%	8%	14%	19%	28%	34%	40%	47%
1.40	0.00%	0.00%	0.00%	0.00%	0.04%	0.3%	1.0%	2%	5%	11%	16%	25%	32%	37%	45%
1.50	0.00%	0.00%	0.00%	0.00%	0.00%	0.04%	0.2%	0.7%	3%	6%	11%	19%	27%	32%	41%
1.60	0.00%	0.00%	0.00%	0.00%	0.00%	0.01%	0.05%	0.2%	1.1%	4%	7%	15%	22%	28%	38%
1.70	0.00%	0.00%	0.00%	0.00%	0.00%	0.00%	0.01%	0.06%	0.5%	2%	5%	12%	19%	25%	34%
1.80	0.00%	0.00%	0.00%	0.00%	0.00%	0.00%	0.00%	0.01%	0.2%	1.2%	3%	9%	16%	22%	31%
1.90	0.00%	0.00%	0.00%	0.00%	0.00%	0.00%	0.00%	0.00%	0.08%	0.65%	2%	7%	13%	19%	29%
2.00	0.00%	0.00%	0.00%	0.00%	0.00%	0.00%	0.00%	0.00%	0.03%	0.36%	1.3%	5%	11%	17%	26%
2.20	0.00%	0.00%	0.00%	0.00%	0.00%	0.00%	0.00%	0.00%	0.01%	0.10%	0.56%	1.3%	8%	13%	22%
2.40	0.00%	0.00%	0.00%	0.00%	0.00%	0.00%	0.00%	0.00%	0.00%	0.03%	0.23%	1.9%	5%	10%	19%
2.60	0.00%	0.00%	0.00%	0.00%	0.00%	0.00%	0.00%	0.00%	0.00%	0.01%	0.09%	1.1%	4%	7%	16%
2.80	0.00%	0.00%	0.00%	0.00%	0.00%	0.00%	0.00%	0.00%	0.00%	0.00%	0.04%	0.66%	3%	6%	13%
3.00	0.00%	0.00%	0.00%	0.00%	0.00%	0.00%	0.00%	0.00%	0.00%	0.00%	0.02%	0.39%	1.8%	4%	11%

Note: F_{MLV} = factory of safety computed using most likely values of parameters (mean values).

Table C10.2 Probabilities that factor of safety is smaller than 1.0, based on normal distribution of factor of safety (After Duncan, 2001). With permission from ASCE, see page 714, No 35.

F_{MLV}	Coefficient of variation of factor of safety														
	2%	4%	6%	8%	10%	12%	14%	16%	20%	25%	30%	40%	50%	60%	80%
1.05	0.9%	11.7%	21.4%	27.6%	31.7%	34.6%	36.7%	38.3%	40.6%	42.4%	43.7%	45.3%	46.2%	46.8%	47.6%
1.10	0.0%	1.2%	6.5%	12.8%	18.2%	22.4%	25.8%	28.5%	32.5%	35.8%	38.1%	41.0%	42.8%	44.0%	45.5%
1.15	0.0%	0.1%	1.5%	5.2%	9.6%	13.9%	17.6%	20.7%	25.7%	30.1%	33.2%	37.2%	39.7%	41.4%	43.5%
1.16	0.0%	0.0%	1.1%	4.2%	8.4%	12.5%	16.2%	19.4%	24.5%	29.1%	32.3%	36.5%	39.1%	40.9%	43.2%
1.18	0.0%	0.0%	0.6%	2.8%	6.4%	10.2%	13.8%	17.0%	22.3%	27.1%	30.6%	35.1%	38.0%	40.0%	42.4%
1.20	0.0%	0.0%	0.3%	1.9%	4.8%	8.2%	11.7%	14.9%	20.2%	25.2%	28.9%	33.8%	36.9%	39.1%	41.7%
1.25	0.0%	0.0%	0.0%	0.6%	2.3%	4.8%	7.7%	10.6%	15.9%	21.2%	25.2%	30.9%	34.5%	36.9%	40.1%
1.30	0.0%	0.0%	0.0%	0.2%	1.1%	2.7%	5.0%	7.5%	12.4%	17.8%	22.1%	28.2%	32.2%	35.0%	38.6%
1.35	0.0%	0.0%	0.0%	0.1%	0.5%	1.5%	3.2%	5.3%	9.7%	15.0%	19.4%	25.8%	30.2%	33.3%	37.3%
1.40	0.0%	0.0%	0.0%	0.0%	0.2%	0.9%	2.1%	3.7%	7.7%	12.7%	17.0%	23.8%	28.4%	31.7%	36.0%
1.50	0.0%	0.0%	0.0%	0.0%	0.0%	0.3%	0.9%	1.9%	4.8%	9.1%	13.3%	20.2%	25.2%	28.9%	33.8%
1.60	0.0%	0.0%	0.0%	0.0%	0.0%	0.1%	0.4%	1.0%	3.0%	6.7%	10.6%	17.4%	22.7%	26.6%	32.0%
1.70	0.0%	0.0%	0.0%	0.0%	0.0%	0.0%	0.2%	0.5%	2.0%	5.0%	8.5%	15.2%	20.5%	24.6%	30.3%
1.80	0.0%	0.0%	0.0%	0.0%	0.0%	0.0%	0.1%	0.3%	1.3%	3.8%	6.9%	13.3%	18.7%	22.9%	28.9%
1.90	0.0%	0.0%	0.0%	0.0%	0.0%	0.0%	0.0%	0.2%	0.9%	2.9%	5.7%	11.8%	17.2%	21.5%	27.7%
2.00	0.0%	0.0%	0.0%	0.0%	0.0%	0.0%	0.0%	0.1%	0.6%	2.3%	4.8%	10.6%	15.9%	20.2%	26.6%
2.20	0.0%	0.0%	0.0%	0.0%	0.0%	0.0%	0.0%	0.0%	0.3%	1.5%	3.5%	8.6%	13.8%	18.2%	24.8%
2.40	0.0%	0.0%	0.0%	0.0%	0.0%	0.0%	0.0%	0.0%	0.2%	1.0%	2.6%	7.2%	12.2%	16.5%	23.3%
2.60	0.0%	0.0%	0.0%	0.0%	0.0%	0.0%	0.0%	0.0%	0.1%	0.7%	2.0%	6.2%	10.9%	15.3%	22.1%
2.80	0.0%	0.0%	0.0%	0.0%	0.0%	0.0%	0.0%	0.0%	0.1%	0.5%	1.6%	5.4%	9.9%	14.2%	21.1%
3.00	0.0%	0.0%	0.0%	0.0%	0.0%	0.0%	0.0%	0.0%	0.0%	0.4%	1.3%	4.8%	9.1%	13.3%	20.2%

Note: F_{MLV} = factor of safety computed using most likely values of parameters. Where table values are boldface, value of p_F computed assuming normal distribution is greater than value of P_f computed assuming lognormal distribution. Where table values are lightface, normal p_F is smaller than the lognormal p_F.

Table C10.3 Suggested target values, reliability index and failure probability of natural slopes – suggested values (Chowdhury and Flentje, 2003). With permission, see page 714, No 36.

Slope type and location	Potential failure mode	Potential consequences	Minimum reliability index	Maximum failure probability
Wooded/forested slopes, moderate to steep inclination, colluvium or residual soil cover	Shallow sliding, limited movement or just slope deformation without overall failure	No elements at risk, no potential for debris flow formation	1.0	15%
Slopes of low to moderate inclination in which high pore water pressures can develop, forested or cleared sloping areas	Slow-moving slides, shallow to deep-seated, relatively flat slip surfaces	No potential for catastrophic failure without warning signs. Progressive action during successive rainstorms may induce complete failure over time; no elements at risk	1.5	5%
Relatively steep slopes with high relief in forested or cleared areas, slopes near natural gullies, colluvium or residual soil cover	Shallow sliding with rapid movement and potential for large travel distances	Significant potential for debris flow formation during intense storms, considerable travel distance; elements at low to moderate risk of damage	2.0	1%
Slopes in which high pore pressure can develop; near urbanised areas	Sliding with rapid movement, shallow to deep slip surfaces with relatively steep inclination	Elements at moderate to high risk of damage or destruction from landsliding	2.5	0.5%
Slopes in which high pore pressures can develop; very close to properties in urbanised areas	Sliding with rapid movement Shallow to deep slip surfaces with relatively steep inclination	Elements at high to very high risk of destruction from landsliding	3.0	0.1%

Chapter 11

Case studies of urban slope stability

11.1 AIMS OF THIS CHAPTER

The main aims of this chapter are the following:

1 Introduce briefly several aspects of urban slope stability, with particular reference to three sites, in the Illawarra region of New South Wales, Australia. Knowledge concerning regional aspects such as topography, geomorphology and geology is essential to gain an understanding of the behaviour of slopes in a region and for obtaining a better perspective of the role of stability analysis. Moreover, knowledge concerning the occurrence, location and history of landsliding in a region can be valuable. Fortunately, a comprehensive Landslide Inventory (slope instability database) has been developed for this region during research that was initiated in 1993 at the University of Wollongong (UoW), New South Wales, Australia.

2 Introduce and present the key features of a Landslide Inventory for the region and refer briefly to the GIS-based maps of geology and landslides.

3 Provide illustrative examples of limit equilibrium slope stability analysis using commercially available software and to answer questions concerning the relationship between shear strength, pore water pressure and factor of safety for three sites. All the three slopes discussed in this section have a history of landsliding associated with significant rainfall. The analyses presented here are best described as parametric back-analyses of individual slope failures or landslides induced by rainfall through the mechanism of pore water pressure increase. There are, of course, differences in local geology and topography between the three landslide sites.

4 Outline briefly the role of rainfall as an important factor for landsliding in the region, and the approach used for determining rainfall thresholds. In order to assess or estimate the rainfall thresholds for widespread landsliding to occur, it is necessary to analyse previous events of widespread landsliding associated with major rainfall events. For example, different durations of a rainfall event have different average rainfall intensities.

5 Introduce briefly the process concerning the regional assessment of landslide susceptibility and hazard and the development of relevant maps.

6 Highlight the importance of an "observational approach" and review the role of monitoring subsurface movements and pore water pressures at different locations in the region.

7   Refer to continuous real-time monitoring of selected sites including automatic
     transfer of data from the landslide sites to a computer server. Refer also to the
     display of processed information through a web-based interface.

11.2   REGIONAL PERSPECTIVE

The city of Wollongong is located approximately 70 km south of Sydney in the state
of New South Wales (NSW), Australia (Figure 11.1). The city is nestled on a narrow

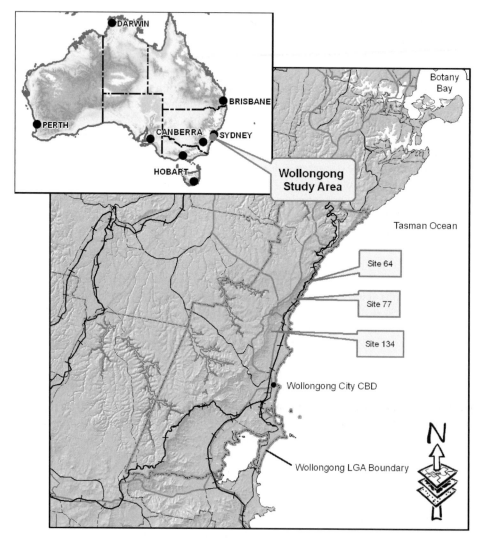

Figure 11.1 Location plan showing location of Wollongong, the escarpment and the location of three
          landslides discussed herein. (See colour plate section).

coastal plain and the adjacent slopes to the north, west and south are part of the spectacular Illawarra erosional escarpment, 300–500 m high, capped by near vertical cliffs of the Triassic aged Hawkesbury Sandstone The ground surface topography within the mid-slope section of the escarpment is characterised by moderate to steep slopes with intermediate gently sloping terraces. Over the last 150 years of settlement the population of the Wollongong area has increased to about 260,000 people. Many residential subdivisions have been developed in the lower to mid-slope areas over the last 50 years. Therefore, slope movements, even of relatively small magnitude, can have adverse, long-term economic consequences for residential houses, roads and railway lines and other associated infrastructure. The adverse consequences can be very high and even catastrophic when heavy and prolonged rainfall occurs. During such rainfall events widespread landsliding is triggered including some which are rapid and severely disruptive. Several such episodes have been observed in the region over the last 50 years.

The coastal plain is triangular in shape with a coastal length of 45 km. It is up to 17 km wide in the south and the width decreases steadily to the north. A few kilometres north of the suburb of Thirroul, the escarpment slopes reach the ocean as there is no coastal plain. However, even in these suburbs, a narrow ribbon of urban development does exist on the lower and mid-slopes of the escarpment and this includes the dual-electric South Coast railway line and a major urban road, the Lawrence Hargrave Drive.

As stated above, the escarpment consists of slopes with moderate to steep inclinations with several intermediate benches and cliff lines. The geological sequence encountered on the escarpment comprises an essentially flat-lying sequence of Late Permian to Mid Triassic interlayered sandstone, mudstone, claystone, shale and coal of the Illawarra Coal Measures, overlain by interbedded sandstones and mudstones/claystones of the Narrabeen Group. Spectacular cliffs of Hawkesbury Sandstone (quartz-cemented quartz sandstone of Middle Triassic age) cap the escarpment. A representative cross-section in the Northern suburbs is shown in Figure 11.2.

Over most of the slopes of the escarpment there is a mantle of colluvium of variable thickness (up to 30 m) and there is dense, temperate forest vegetation over most of the escarpment below the vertical cliffs. The composition of colluvium varies because of different source areas of contributing bedrock from which the colluvium is derived.

In particular, the clay content of colluvium, which has a significant influence on its shear strength, may differ widely from one site to the next. Indicative shear strength parameters may be determined by laboratory testing. Alternatively, shear strength may be estimated by performing stability analyses of failed slopes or landslides. However, such back-analyses enable only the estimation of the average shear strength operative over the slip surface of a failed slope.

The main road link to Sydney is the F6 Freeway that traverses the escarpment via Mount Ousley Road. There are several other road links from the coastal plain to the top of the escarpment and the freeway. At Bulli Pass the Princess Highway traverses the escarpment above the suburb of Thirroul to join the F6. To the north, the coastal road, Lawrence Hargrave Drive links the northern suburbs to the F6 via Clifton and the spectacular Seacliff Bridge. The South Coast railway line and the Unanderra to Moss Vale railway line also traverse the escarpment slopes and coastal plain; both

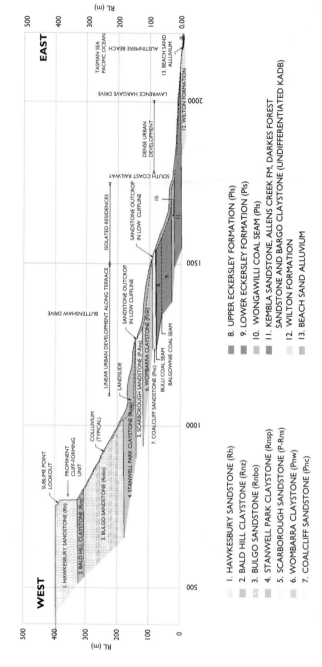

Figure 11.2 Representative escarpment cross-section in the northern suburbs region of Wollongong. (P. Flentje in association with GHD). (See colour plate section).

1. HAWKESBURY SANDSTONE (Rh)
2. BALD HILL CLAYSTONE (Rnz)
3. BULGO SANDSTONE (Rnbo)
4. STANWELL PARK CLAYSTONE (Rnsp)
5. SCARBOROUGH SANDSTONE (P-Rns)
6. WOMBARRA CLAYSTONE (Pnw)
7. COALCLIFF SANDSTONE (Pnc)

8. UPPER ECKERSLEY FORMATION (Pls)
9. LOWER ECKERSLEY FORMATION (Pls)
10. WONGAWILLI COAL SEAM (Pls)
11. KEMBLA SANDSTONE, ALLENS CREEK FM, DARKES FOREST SANDSTONE AND BARGO CLAYSTONE (UNDIFFERENTIATED KADB)
12. WILTON FORMATION
13. BEACH SAND ALLUVIUM

provide important freight and passenger services between Sydney, Wollongong and the surrounding areas.

Landsliding is a common occurrence along the Illawarra Escarpment. The University of Wollongong Landslide Inventory identifies 614 landslide sites within the Wollongong Local Government Area (WLGA). There are three main types of landslides, falls, flows and slides, although many are compound or complex landslides. Many of the slides have velocities in the very slow to extremely slow range (Cruden and Varnes 1996) characterised by intermittent stick-slip (episodically active) type of movements. Most of these documented landslides have occurred since 1950 and many of these are reactivations of old or ancient landslides. Whilst undated, most of these landslides would have developed within the Quaternary Period.

The processes and mechanisms of slope failure are controlled by factors such as stratigraphy, geotechnical strength parameters, hydrogeology, geomorphology, slope inclination and pore water pressure. Prolonged and/or intense rainfall typically causes pore water pressure rises which, in turn, initiate landsliding. There are many rainfall stations distributed throughout this region. On the other hand, pore water pressure data have been scarce until the last few decades where landslide monitoring has been introduced at some sites. Consequently, use of rainfall data for understanding and managing landslides has been quite helpful. The average annual rainfall for Wollongong varies from 1200 mm on the coastal plain near the city centre and up to 1600 mm along the top of the escarpment.

The University of Wollongong (UoW) Landslide Research Team has developed a web-site which summarises the research aims, scope and highlights of the research activities including monitoring. This web site can be found at: http://www.uow.edu.au/eng/research/landslide/index.html

11.3 LANDSLIDE INVENTORY

The Landslide Inventory, developed over the last fifteen years, comprises a relational MS Access and ESRI ArcGIS™ Geodatabase with 75 available fields of information for each landslide site (Chowdhury and Flentje 1998, Flentje and Chowdhury 2005a). Field mapping and compilation work have been carried out on GIS-based field maps at 1:4000 or larger scales. Each landslide is referenced by a three-digit key Site Reference Code (SRC). The Landslide Inventory currently contains 614 landslide locations with a total of almost 1000 landslide events (including first time occurrences and multiple recurrences at some sites). The number of recurrences or reactivations of each landslide are recorded. For example, Site 113 in Thirroul has 17 documented recurrences following its first recorded movement in March–April 1950.

The 614 landslides in the Landslide Inventory comprise 49 Falls, 43 Flows, 480 Slides and several others that have not been classified. A total of 426 Slide category landslides are located within a 188 km^2 area which has been chosen for modelling landslide susceptibility (Susceptibility Model Area). Landslide volumes have been estimated for 378 of these sites. The volumes range from less than 1 m^3 up to 720,000 m^3, with an average volume of 21,800 m^3. Figure 11.3 shows the temporal distribution of landsliding as reported in the Landslide Inventory. This shows that most of the landslide sites have been identified and recorded since 1950 with a marked increase

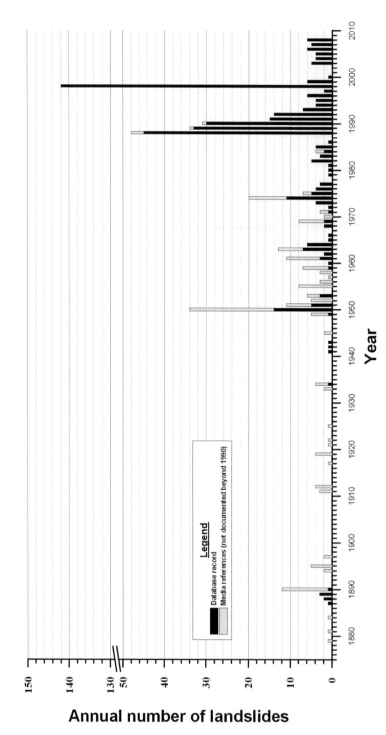

Figure 11.3 Temporal distribution of landslide events recorded in the UoW Landslide Inventory.

since 1988. Increased annual landslide occurrences have corresponded with relatively high-magnitude rainfall events.

Landslides are mapped showing the total affected area. No internal differentiation (i.e., head scarp, zone of depletion, source area, zone of accumulation, zone of deposition, main track, minor scarps etc.) have been identified within the inventory for individual landslides.

The slides are all considered to be episodically active, being activated by elevated pore water pressures resulting from periods of significant rainfall. Previous UoW research has led to the determination of regional rainfall thresholds for triggering landslides (Flentje and Chowdhury, 2006).

Landslide monitoring (ground survey, manual inclinometers, data logged in place inclinometers and extensometers) and other general field observations of landslides in the Wollongong region show that slide category landslide types typically move a few millimetres to a few tens of centimetres in response to a given rainfall event. It is rare for such a landslide to move a meter or more in one rainfall event. The velocities are in the range extremely slow to slow. Ongoing landslide monitoring will lead to a better understanding of the relationship between pore water pressure, antecedent rainfall magnitudes and rates of landslide movement.

In addition to the tabulated database, GIS-based maps of the known landslide locations have been developed for the region. GIS maps can be prepared at different scales and with different features displayed. For example, one set of 1:10,000 scale maps include a 10 m DEM (Digital Elevation Model) of the region as well as geology and cadastre. On each such map the locations of different landslides are superimposed and landslide types are distinguished by colour coding. Such geology and landslide inventory maps have been very useful reference documents. The Landslide Inventory, in combination with data-sets concerning the main influencing factors for slope stability has facilitated the modelling of landslide susceptibility and hazard in the region.

11.4 STABILITY ANALYSES OF THREE SITES

11.4.1 Introduction

In the following sections, three case studies of slope stability analyses are described. These sites are Site 64, Site 77 and Site 134 (Figure 11.1). The site reference codes correspond to the Landslide Inventory discussed above. By performing stability analyses, one may attempt to answer the following types of questions:

i   What is the estimated average shear strength of the colluvium along the slip surface at each site?

ii   Can both the peak and residual shear strength of the colluvium be estimated from back-analysis of these landslide sites?

iii   How can the analyses facilitate the planning and design of remedial measures?

iv   What factors contribute to the reliability of the results of back-analyses and the conclusions drawn from those results?

v   What is the role of monitoring in relation to stability-analysis?

vi   What are the similarities and differences amongst the sites for which analyses have been carried out?

Of course, it is unlikely that stability analyses can facilitate answers to all of the above questions for a particular case study without detailed knowledge of the area, careful consideration of data from detailed investigations, observation and subsurface monitoring. Moreover, there is an important role for expert judgment throughout the process of stability assessment.

11.4.2 Available information and assumptions

In order to answer the questions and to properly plan the analyses, the availability of information and data must be considered. Reasonable assumptions will have to be made where specific information is lacking. The topography of each site can be determined accurately at the time of investigation. For old landslides there may be no recorded information about the initial topography (before a first-time failure). It may, therefore, be difficult to assess the initial pre-failure conditions of the slope. Indeed, the dates of first time slope failures of many landslides in the region are unknown.

The general shape of the slip surface in each of the following cases has been interpreted from field investigations with a high degree of confidence. However, there may be some uncertainty regarding the exact location of the slip surface in each case. In some cases, there are reliable data concerning groundwater levels but there are relatively few cases in which accurate subsurface pore water pressures are known at the time of landslide occurrence. It is very rare to have accurate knowledge of the piezometric surface along the whole cross-section of a natural slope. Thus several analyses may be made, each corresponding to an assumed piezometric surface or an average pore pressure ratio. If a piezometric surface is assumed, the corresponding average pore pressure ratio may be estimated for convenience in comparing the results of analyses with different piezometric surfaces, the average pore pressure ratio being simply a label for the corresponding piezometric surface.

11.4.3 Failure mechanism

At each site, colluvium overlies bedrock and the slope movements are assumed to have occurred in the colluvial layer. Hence the behaviour of these slopes is likely to be similar or at least comparable to that of colluvial slopes in other regions with similar geology and climate. The known landslide reactivations, in each case, have occurred following significant rainfall in the region. Thus the mechanism of failure, in each case, is considered to be the decrease of shear strength associated with the development of high pore water pressure in response to preceding rainfall.

Due to intermittent slope movements, these landslides are often described as stick-slip landslides. Residual shear strength is considered to be operative over the slip surface at the time of failure of such a natural slope except during first-time landsliding. Past experience has shown that the effective residual cohesion is close to zero and that the effective angle of internal friction has a value reduced significantly from the peak to the residual value.

It is interesting to note that the slip surface is often located at or close to the colluvium-bedrock interface. Part of the slip surface may, in fact, be located in the highly weathered upper zone of the bedrock. The type and nature of bedrock may have a significant influence on stability of these colluvial slopes. In fact, significant differences in landslide susceptibility based on location and hence areas of geological subcrop have been noted in the Illawarra region.

11.4.4   Drainage conditions

Groundwater conditions and seepage have significant influence on the stability of natural slopes. Knowledge of regional and local ground water levels is, therefore, important for understanding slope processes and, in particular, the occurrence of landsliding. The change and rate of change in pore water pressure after significant rainfall will be controlled by a number of factors and, in particular, the permeability of a soil or rock mass. The permeability of a rock mass will, of course, be controlled by the number and orientation of discontinuities and how open or tight these are. Clayey soils and rocks with tight joints are characterised by poor subsurface drainage. On the other hand, granular soils and open-jointed rock masses can ensure very good subsurface drainage. With poor drainage, pore water pressures will increase quickly and dissipate slowly. On the other hand, pore water pressures will rise less quickly and dissipate relatively fast if natural drainage is good.

Within the Illawarra escarpment region, there is considerable spatial variability in the mass permeability and natural drainage of soil and rock masses. Consequently pore water pressures can vary significantly from one location to the next and the behaviour of individual slopes can be significantly different, even if other factors are similar.

Long-term behaviour of natural slopes can be understood only in terms of effective stress analyses. Therefore knowledge or reasonable assumptions concerning the pore water pressures along the slip surface of a slope is necessary for carrying out such analyses. Moreover, only effective stress shear strength parameters are relevant for such analyses.

Information from the landslide inventory may be useful in validating the results of stability analyses at particular sites or to supplement the outcomes and conclusions based on such analyses. Usually investigation of a site is limited to the potential sliding mass. It is obvious, however, that detailed knowledge of the underlying rocks and the surrounding areas can be very helpful. This is why it is so important to have previous experience of the area and regional knowledge. The comprehensive landslide inventory available for the Illawarra region is, therefore, a valuable resource.

11.4.5   Observed shapes of landslides and slip surfaces

Limit equilibrium analyses are often carried out on the basis of one-dimensional or two-dimensional geotechnical models. The overall three dimensional shape of a landslide surface is unknown. Moreover slip surfaces are assumed to have simple and regular shapes. The simplest and most useful example of a planar slip surface is the one-dimensional 'infinite slope' analysis. Curved surfaces approximating smooth circular or non-circular curves are often assumed for two-dimensional analysis. However, site investigations often reveal that the slip surfaces are not smooth but irregular and multi-planar. Moreover, shapes of the landslides in plan may differ greatly and this is evident in the three case studies presented in this chapter. It is very difficult, if not impossible, to predict the plan shape of a landslide area or the shape of a slip surface in advance. These aspects would be influenced by a number of factors such as local topography, geomorphology and the spatial variability in subsurface conditions including geological discontinuities and asperities along the bedrock-colluvium interface.

11.4.6 Software used for the Case Studies

For the three sites analysed in this chapter, the GeoStudio 2007 SLOPE/W software by GEO-SLOPE International Ltd. has been used. GEO-SLOPE International Ltd. can be found on the world wide web at the location: http://www.geo-slope.com/

The Morgenstern-Price method (one of the options in the SLOPE/W software) incorporating a half-sine interslice force function was used for all the analyses. The 'Piezometric Line Analysis' option was selected for all the analyses presented here.

11.5 CASE STUDY I – SITE 64 IN THE SUBURB OF SCARBOROUGH

11.5.1 Introduction

According to the classification system of Cruden and Varnes (1996), Site 64 is a slide-flow category landslide with an approximate surface area of 5000 m² and a volume of approximately 20,000 m³. It is ranked in the University of Wollongong Landslide Inventory as the 82nd largest landslide of a total of 553 landslides within the Wollongong Local Government Area (WLGA). The Narrabeen Group Wombarra Claystone bedrock subcrops below the landslide site. The Permian/Triassic boundary lies close to the top of the Wombarra Claystone. The head scarp and upper portion of the landslide area affects the alignment of the dual electrified South Coast Railway line between Sydney and Wollongong, whilst the remainder of the site extends across eight adjacent residential properties (Figure 11.4). The general direction of movement has been south-easterly towards Goodrich Street.

1.5.2 Background

This site has a moderately well documented history of movement dating from 1950s. The data concerning the site include that from inclinometer and survey monitoring since the late 1980s, which is still continuing (Figure 11.5).

Reducing rainfall-induced pore water pressures by surface and sub-surface drainage is considered to be the best way to manage the most important landslides in this region. Site 64 has had extensive subsurface engineering remedial works installed during the period from May to June 1992. These engineering works comprise an interconnected series of subsurface trench drains, excavated into the bedrock material, which feed downslope into the municipal storm water system (as shown in Figure 11.4). Following these subsurface works, extensive surface recontouring, including the construction of three retaining walls and fabriform lining of a surface drainage channel

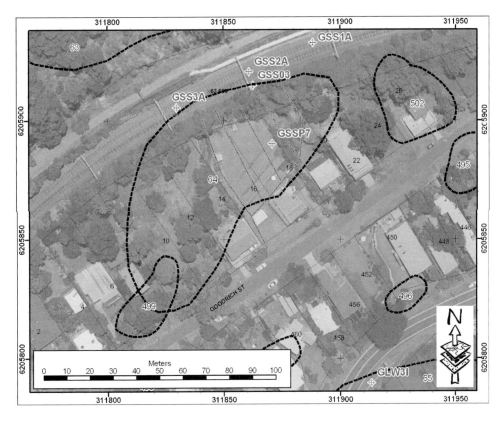

Figure 11.4 Plan highlighting the Site 64 landslide and showing extent of subsurface slot drains (marked in light blue lines). (See colour plate section).

were installed. These works were installed by the New South Wales Government State Rail Authority (currently known as RailCorp), partly on RailCorp land, but primarily on private residential land. Monitoring after the completion of construction work confirms that the remedial works have been quite successful in mitigating landsliding at this site. However, it is important to note that the cumulative rainfall levels which triggered instability at this site during the late 1980's have not been experienced since the remedial works were installed (see 30 and 90 day cumulative rainfall curves in Figure 11.5).

Standpipe water levels were monitored frequently during 1989 and 1990. On 21st of April 1990, the water levels in Boreholes 3 and 7 were 5.83 m and 1.24 m below ground level, respectively. With depths to the slide plane of 8 m in Borehole 3 and 2 m in Borehole 7, these piezometric levels on 21st of April 1990 correspond to piezometric lines with approximate r_u values of 0.15 and 0.21 respectively, or a simple average of 0.18. The highest piezometric levels for Borehole 3 (5.19 m on 17th of March 1989) and Borehole 7 (0.9 m on 12th of June 1990) correspond to r_u values of 0.19 and 0.3 respectively.

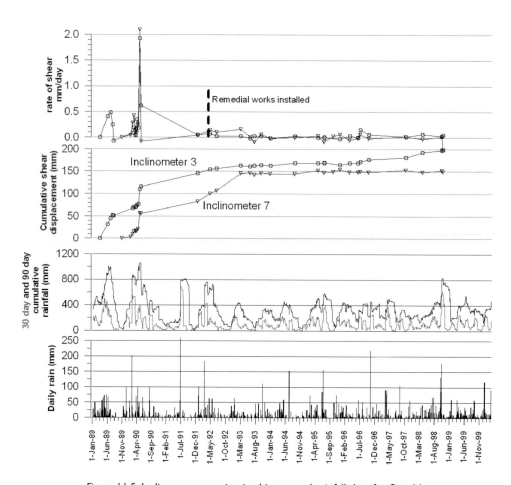

Figure 11.5 Inclinometer monitoring history and rainfall data for Site 64.

11.5.3   Geotechnical model for Site 64

At this site, a blast furnace waste ash layer, deposited as a fill, overlies a colluvium layer which, in turn, overlies bedrock. The geotechnical model employed for this analysis incorporates these aspects and the cross section of the slope is shown in Figure 11.6. The soil strength parameters used in the analyses are summarised in Table 11.1.

11.5.4   Pore water pressure assumptions

Four different piezometric lines (representing seepage in the slope occurring up to different levels) were assumed. For each of these assumed piezometric lines, average pore water pressure ratios were determined based on piezometric heights at different points along the slip surface (these r_u values are used only as a label in the following tables, since the option chosen in the software program was the direct use of a specified piezometric surface). The four piezometric lines represent the following average

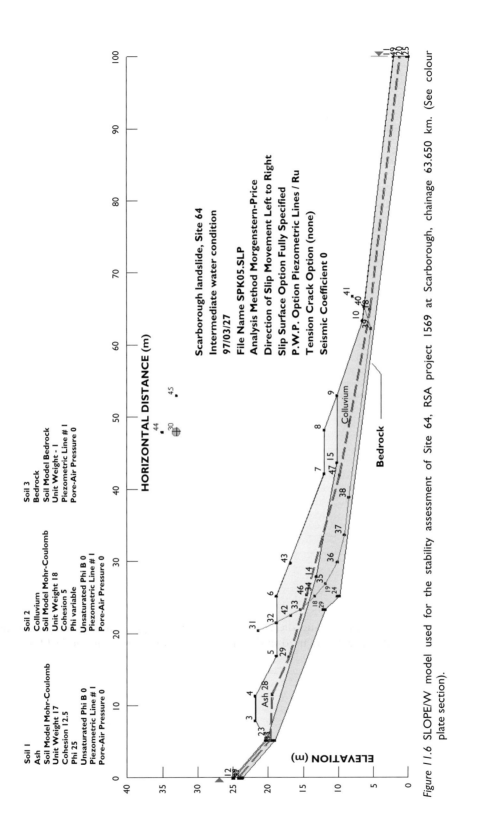

Figure 11.6 SLOPE/W model used for the stability assessment of Site 64, RSA project 1569 at Scarborough, chainage 63.650 km. (See colour plate section).

Table 11.1 Geotechnical data for the back-analysis of Site 64 using SLOPE/W.

Material	γ (kN/m³)	c' (kPa)	Ø (degrees)
Ash	17	7	20
Colluvium	18	0 and 5	13–20

Note: (i) For the ash layer, the values of γ, c' and Ø are known from testing. (ii) For the colluvium layer, γ is known. Two alternative values of c' and the range of Ø are shown.

Table 11.2 Factors of safety values compared using fully specified piezometric surfaces versus constant r_u values.

r_u =	0.18 surface	0.18 parameter	0.37 surface	0.37 parameter
Ø = 13°	1.01	1.02	0.81	0.84
Ø = 14°	1.06	1.08	0.85	0.88
Ø = 15°	1.11	1.13	0.89	0.92
Ø = 16°	1.17	1.19	0.93	0.97
Ø = 17°	1.22	1.24	0.97	1.01
Ø = 18°	1.28	1.30	1.01	1.05
Ø = 19°	1.33	1.35	1.05	1.10
Ø = 20°	1.39	1.41	1.09	1.14

Note: The above results correspond to a value of c' = 5 kPa for Colluvium.

r_u =	0.01	0.18	0.37	0.55
Ø = 15°	1.06	0.85	0.63	0.44
Ø = 17°	1.19	0.96	0.71	0.50
Ø = 18°	1.26	1.01	0.75	0.53
Ø = 19°	1.33	1.07	0.79	0.56
Ø = 20°	1.40	1.12	0.83	0.59
Ø = 22°	1.55	1.24	0.91	0.65

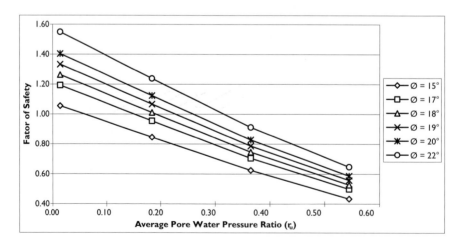

Figure 11.7 Site 64: calculated factors of safety (assuming c' = 0).

r_u values; 0.01, 0.18, 0.37, and 0.55. The piezometric surface with an average r_u value of 0.18 is shown in Figure 11.6.

In order to compare the use of a piezometric surface with the assumption of constant pore pressure ratio along the slip surface, some preliminary calculations were made which are shown in Table 11.2. This table shows that, in this example, use of an average r_u based on a piezometric surface gives a reduced F in comparison to the use of a constant r_u. In the table below, the third and fifth columns show results based on constant values of r_u.

While the differences in calculated F values are not significant for this geometry, all the analyses reported below are based on fully specified piezometric surfaces as represented by the corresponding average r_u values. The same approach has been used for the other two case studies in this chapter.

$r_u =$	0.01	0.18	0.37	0.55
$\emptyset = 12°$	1.12	0.96	0.77	0.62
$\emptyset = 13°$	1.19	1.01	0.81	0.65
$\emptyset = 14°$	1.25	1.06	0.85	0.68
$\emptyset = 15°$	1.32	1.12	0.89	0.70
$\emptyset = 16°$	1.39	1.17	0.92	0.73
$\emptyset = 17°$	1.45	1.22	0.96	0.76

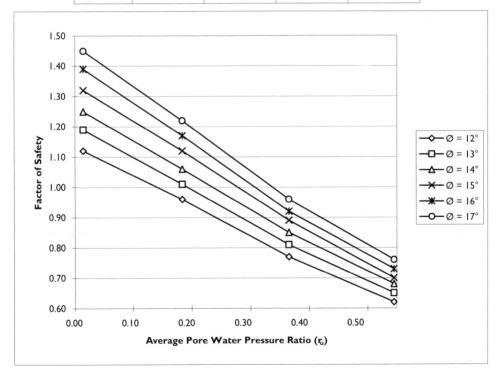

Figure 11.8 Site 64: calculated factors of safety (assuming $c' = 5$ kPa).

11.5.5   Results of analysis

Considering the history of landsliding at this site as discussed above, it was reasonable to assume that, during the 1989 and 1990 accelerated movement phases, residual shear strength conditions would have existed along the slip surface. The cohesion along the slide surface could have been reduced to a near-zero value. Two sets of analyses were made, one with a cohesion value of zero and the other with a cohesion value of 5 kPa. The results of these analyses are summarised in Figure 11.7 for the $c' = 0$ assumption and in Figure 11.8, for the $c' = 5$ kPa assumption for the four different piezometric conditions outlined above.

11.5.6   Shear strength at failure on the basis of the above analyses

The water levels recorded on the 21st April 1990 is considered indicative of an average $r_u = 0.18$. This would correspond to a residual friction angle $\varnothing'_r$ value at critical equilibrium ($F = 1$) in the range 17° to 18° for the $c' = 0$ assumption; and $\varnothing'_r$ value between 12° and 13° for $c' = 5$ kPa assumption. For a site such as this, which has been re-activated on numerous occasions, c' would be expected to be close to zero. Therefore, the value of $\varnothing'_r$ would be closer to the range 17° to 18° at this site.

It is instructive to study the variation of back calculated residual friction angle with the average pore pressure ratio as shown in Figure 11.9. Both curves in this figure

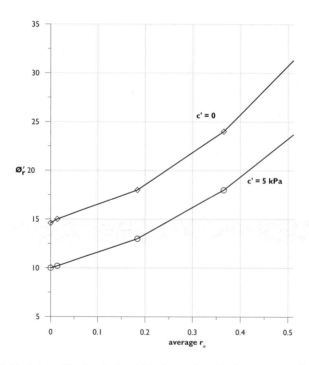

Figure 11.9 Site 64: Variation of back calculated friction angle with the average r_u (for $F = 1$) for $c' = 0$ and $c' = 5$ kPa.

reflect the relationship between the two parameters for $F = 1$. Such a graph would be a good aid to the design of effective remedial drainage works.

11.6 CASE STUDY 2 – SITE 77, MORRISON AVENUE, WOMBARRA

11.6.1 Introduction

The Morrison Avenue landslide has a plan area of approximately 46,600 m², a volume of approximately 233,000 m³. It is ranked in the Landslide Inventory as the 9th largest landslide within the WLGA. The site is in Wombarra, approximately 17 km north of Wollongong, and is located on a terrace on the mid-slopes of the escarpment between 80 m and 130 m above sea level. This area of the escarpment slopes gently to the south east. The terrace area itself has irregular hummocky slopes with ground slopes of 5°–15°. This gentle sloping terrace is bounded to the east and west by steeper slopes up to 30 m high. A site plan is shown in Figure 11.10 and the general direction

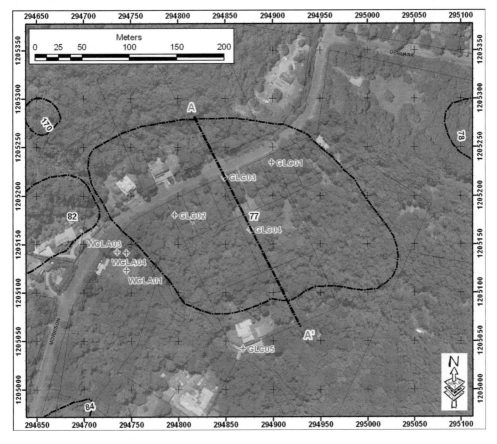

Figure 11.10 Site 77 landslide: Morrison Avenue, Wombarra. (See colour plate section).

of movement during landsliding is along the section line from A to A'. This is also the section shown in Figure 11.12.

The area contains some residential development including two houses within the landslide area, and several others in close proximity, one secondary urban road, one locally significant water course, and the associated urban services including water, electricity and telephone. Morrison Avenue is also an alternative route to the principal main thoroughfare, Lawrence Hargrave Drive. The landslide is situated between Denmark Street and Stockyard Creek. Periodic slope movement occur as a result of heavy and prolonged rainfall. The first visual evidence of failure from the road is often the cracking of the bitumen pavement of Morrison Avenue (Figure 11.11). However, residents may notice signs of ground movement on their properties even before cracking of pavements.

11.6.2 Background

A landslide occurred at this site in early 1974. The landslide occurred after a period of exceptional rainfall which resulted in increased pore water pressures within the colluvial soil mantling the slopes. While increased pore water pressure is considered to be the main cause of this landslide, there has been speculation concerning the possible effects of mine subsidence which is briefly outlined in a following paragraph.

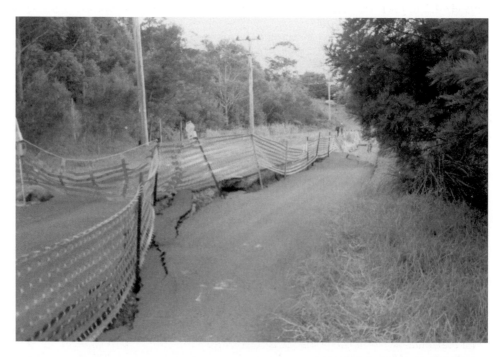

Figure 11.11 Damage to the pavement of Morrison Avenue within the Site 77. The rear main head-scarp of this landslide is approximately 40 m to the left and upslope of the road pavement. (See colour plate section).

However, the significance of mining subsidence as a contributing factor has never been confirmed by investigation and research.

As a result of this landslide seven residences were destroyed and/or subsequently abandoned. In the following two years the landslide extended laterally affecting land up to 100 m further to the south. This landslide was reactivated in April 1990. Subsequently, an extensive geotechnical investigation of site 77 was carried out by consultants for Wollongong City Council (WCC).

This landslide material is underlain primarily by Wombarra Claystone bedrock of the Narrabeen Group. Downslope of the terrace area, the landslide extends onto the area of steeper slopes, which is underlain by the Coalcliff Sandstone, the Bulli coal seam and the Upper Eckersley Formation.

The highest groundwater levels were recorded in June 1991. These levels correspond approximately to the piezometric line with an average $r_u = 0.22$. Following the resurfacing of Morrison Avenue by the end of 1990, no further cracking was observed during the 1991 wet period. Residual shear strength conditions would clearly have been reached by this time. It is, therefore, appropriate to assume that higher piezometric levels within the colluvium would have been required to initiate a first time movement of the landslide. The timing of a first time landslide occurrence at this site is not known. However, the geomorphology of the site and the surrounding area suggests that the site is an ancient landslide.

Underground mining within the Bulli Seam by the Bulli Main Colliery has occurred beneath and within areas adjoining this site. Boreholes show that the Bulli seam is approximately 1.2 m thick and occurs 25 m to 30 m below Morrison Avenue and has a local dip to the northwest of approximately 1.5°. The colliery opened in 1860 and mining was carried out by the conventional board and pillar methods. In preparation for abandoning the mine, full extraction is reported to have occurred in 1973, some 60 m to the north of this site. Ground surface subsidence within this area adjacent to the landslide site would have occurred following this extraction. Another interesting factor concerning the effect of mining is that mine drainage was required during mining operations. It is reasonable to assume that whilst the ground water was being pumped out during mining works, there would have been local reductions in groundwater pressures. This process of pore water pressure relief would have stopped when the mine was sealed on 1st June 1974, 3 months after the April 1974 landslide. The following stability analyses however, do not take into consideration the effect of mining or mine drainage.

11.6.3 Geotechnical model for Site 77

As in Case Study 1, colluvium overlies bedrock at Site 77. Based on investigation data, most of the slip surface below Morrison Avenue is interpreted to be located along or close to the base of this colluvium layer. No subsurface investigation data are available regarding the depth and shape of the part of slip surface upslope of Morrison Avenue. The cross section, as shown in Figure 11.12, is orientated approximately through the centre of the site along the alignment defined by A to A' in Figure 11.10. The rear main scarp of the landslide is located approximately 40 m to the northwest (upslope) of Morrison Avenue, as observed in the field in April 1990. The range of shear strength parameters used in the modelling were based on trial analyses and previous investigations.

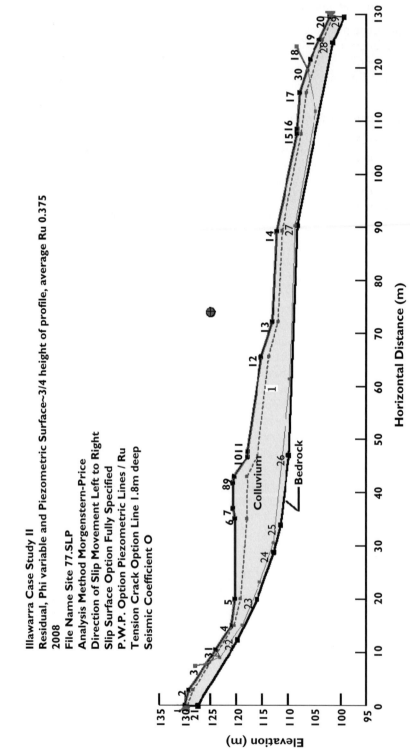

Illawarra Case Study II
Residual, Phi variable and Piezometric Surface~3/4 height of profile, average Ru 0.375
2008
File Name Site 77.SLP
Analysis Method Morgenstern-Price
Direction of Slip Movement Left to Right
Slip Surface Option Fully Specified
P.W.P. Option Piezometric Lines / Ru
Tension Crack Option Line 1.8m deep
Seismic Coefficient O

Colluvium

Bedrock

Horizontal Distance (m)

Elevation (m)

Figure 11.12 SLOPE/W model used for the stability assessment of Site 77, the Morrison Avenue landslide. (See colour plate section).

11.6.4 Pore water pressure assumptions

Four different piezometric lines (representative of the slope with seepage occurring up to different seepage levels) were assumed and these correspond to average pore pressure coefficient values of 0.09, 0.22, 0.38, and 0.55. As in Case Study-1, these piezometric lines have been fully specified in the model.

11.6.5 Results of analyses

Analyses of the slope were carried out by varying the values of cohesion, c'_r and the angle of internal friction, $\varnothing'_r$, and considering the four different piezometric surfaces mentioned above. Such analyses would allow estimation of the shear strength operative over the slip surface during reactivation of the landslide at this site. The results of analyses with an assumed $c'_r = 0$ are summarised in Figure 11.13 and, for an

$r_u =$	0.09	0.22	0.38	0.55
$\varnothing = 8°$	0.93	0.77	0.62	0.46
$\varnothing = 9°$	1.05	0.87	0.70	0.52
$\varnothing = 10°$	1.17	0.97	0.77	0.58
$\varnothing = 11°$	1.29	1.07	0.85	0.63
$\varnothing = 12°$	1.41	1.17	0.93	0.68
$\varnothing = 13°$	1.53	1.27	1.01	0.74
$\varnothing = 14°$	-	-	-	0.80
$\varnothing = 15°$	-	-	-	0.86
$\varnothing = 16°$	-	-	-	0.92
$\varnothing = 17°$	-	-	-	0.98

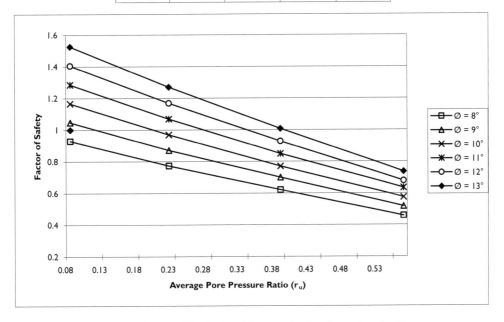

Figure 11.13 Site 77: calculated factors of safety (assuming $c'_r = 0$).

assumed $c'_r = 5$ kPa, the results are summarised in Figure 11.14. Considering $F = 1$, the relationship between pore pressure ratio and residual friction angle for both values of c'_r are shown in Figure 11.15.

11.6.6   Shear strength at failure based on results of analyses

Pore water pressures at the time of the disruptive slide failure in 1974 are unknown. Accurate pore water pressures during the April 1990 reactivation are also unknown. For this study, the approximate pore pressure ratio was assumed to be consistent with the highest monitored groundwater levels in 1991. This assumption correspond to an average pore water pressure ratio of $r_u = 0.22$. Based on the analyses presented above, the residual friction angle for $F = 1$ with $c'_r = 0$ and $r_u = 0.22$ would be in the range $10°–11°$. This relatively low shear strength is consistent with other reported investigations of slopes in which the slip surface is formed along a colluvium-bedrock interface within the Wombarra Claystone sequence.

$r_u =$	0.09	0.22	0.38	0.55
$\emptyset = 6°$	1.16	1.05	0.93	0.80
$\emptyset = 7°$	1.27	1.15	1.01	0.86
$\emptyset = 8°$	1.39	1.24	1.09	0.92
$\emptyset = 9°$	1.51	1.33	1.16	0.97
$\emptyset = 10°$	1.63	1.43	1.23	1.03
$\emptyset = 11°$	1.75	1.53	1.31	1.09
$\emptyset = 12°$	1.87	1.63	1.39	1.14

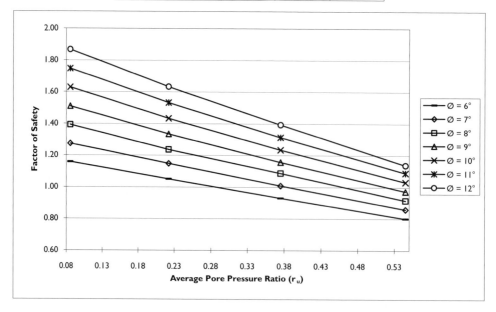

Figure 11.14 Site 77 calculated factors of safety (assuming $c'_r = 5$ kPa).

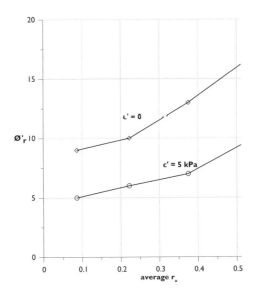

Figure 11.15 Site 77: Variation of back calculated friction angle with the average r_u (for $F = 1$) for $c' = 0$ and $c' = 5$ kPa.

11.7   CASE STUDY 3 – SITE 134, WOONONA HEIGHTS

11.7.1   Introduction

The Wonoona Heights Landslide has a plan area of approximately 20,500 m², a volume of approximately 225,000 m³ and is ranked in the land instability database as the 10th largest landslide within the subject area. The site is in the suburb of Woonona Heights, approximately 10 km north of Wollongong, and 700 m west of the Princess Highway. The landslide site is located within a densely developed urban area, extending from above Joanne Street, downslope through Joseph Street, to the cul-de-sac end of June Parade, as shown on Figure 11.16. The landslide is situated between the elevations of approximately 70 m and 110 m above sea level. A cross-section line through the landslide is shown between A and A′ (which is also the direction of movement) and this section is shown in Figure 11.17.

This area of the escarpment is situated at a relatively lower level than the geologically controlled and well developed terraces discussed in the two previous case studies. This level of the escarpment and, in particular, this area has been more heavily dissected by stream erosion. The landslide extends from the crest area of a broad shallow spur and trends obliquely from the spur line, downslope, towards a narrow and incised water course. The residential area is situated on a gentle south to southeast sloping area, with an inclination of less than 5° in the vicinity of Joanne Street, increasing up to 10° to 15° near the toe of the landslide close to the end of Joseph Street.

The landslide area is underlain by formations of the Illawarra Coal Measures. The Balgownie Coal Member is situated just metres above Joanne Street, and the

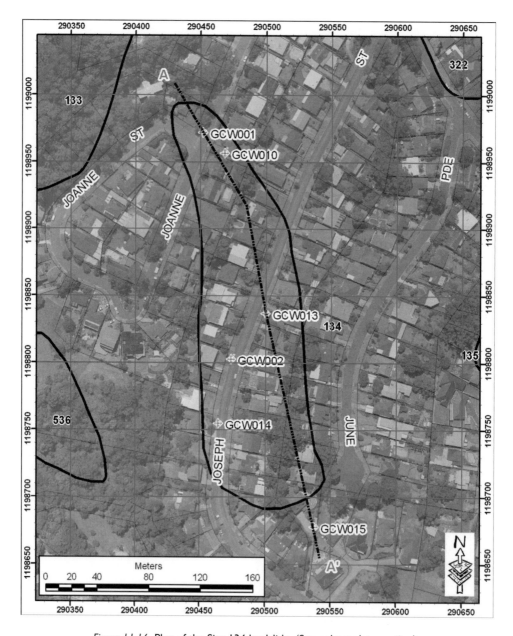

Figure 11.16 Plan of the Site 134 landslide. (See colour plate section).

Wongawilli Coal Seam is located just below the toe of the landslide. The bedrock subcropping below the landslide is, therefore, the Eckersley Formation, and contains at least one coal seam. Although several hundred metres away from the site, the water course south and west of the landslide provides an almost continuous bedrock exposure from the top of the Wongawilli Coal seam to the base of the Wombarra

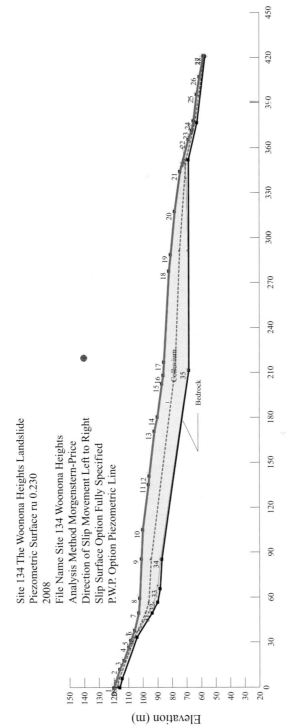

Site 134 The Woonona Heights Landslide
Piezometric Surface ru 0.230
2008
File Name Site 134 Woonona Heights
Analysis Method Morgenstern-Price
Direction of Slip Movement Left to Right
Slip Surface Option Fully Specified
P.W.P. Option Piezometric Line

Figure 11.17 SLOPE/W model used for the stability assessment of Site 134, the Woonona Heights landslide. (See colour plate section).

Claystone. This exposure, combined with the exposures of the Wongawilli Coal seam immediately to the southwest of Alanson Avenue, and borehole information from the geotechnical investigation of this site, have all helped to identify the geological sequence underlying this site.

Geotechnical investigation of this site has revealed that bedrock is located at up to 18.1 m below the ground surface, with the average thickness of the colluvial mantle over 15 boreholes in and around the landslide of 9.1 m. Some fill material of up to 4.4 m in thickness was encountered during the drilling. It is this colluvium and fill material and, at places, the upper few hundred millimetres of the residual bedrock material, that are being displaced by the landslide.

11.7.2 Background

The western (upslope) side of this landslide area, west of Joanne Street, comprises steeper slopes averaging 30° and up to 45 m in height. These steeper slopes also have a history of instability (for example, landslide Site 133 is seen in Figure 11.16). The south facing slope south of Joanne Street, which extends down to the water course, also has a history of instability.

The area contains up to 100 residential houses, 29 of which are situated within or straddling the margin of the landslide. Another 10 houses or so are located immediately adjacent to the margins of the landslide. One house in Joanne Street has been destroyed by ground movement, whilst at least 19 have required major repairs. The site also contains three local suburban roads, and the associated local services including water, sewer, electricity and telephone.

It is important to note that this landslide is a very subtle feature. Very little damage is visible from the streets unless it is being looked for. Road and kerb reconstruction have been carried out, and the one house that has been destroyed is now a vacant block of land.

Previous geotechnical investigations of this landslide refer to a 1948 aerial photograph which shows a gully traversing this area through a broad area of disturbed and hummocky ground. There is also reference to a 1952 plan related to a residential subdivision of the site which shows a spring located in the head area of the landslide and a creek bed along the alignment of the landslide. Local residents have also reported structural damage to houses since the 1960s. Following significant slope movements during 1977, Wollongong City Council had to reconstruct the road formations and kerbs. No damage had subsequently been recorded in the reconstructed pavement until the heavy rainfall event of 9th of April 1990. Following this rainfall event significant cracking was evident in the pavement and kerbing of the local streets. Minor cracking was evident in the bitumen surface of the June Parade cul-de-sac. It is of interest to note that Site 77 and Site 64 also experienced accelerated movement phases at this time.

The water levels are variable across the site. In the head area of the site, water levels are within 0.5 m of the surface. Near the centre of the landslide which encountered the deepest soil-bedrock interface at 18.4 m, water levels range between 1.0 m and 2.5 m below the ground surface. On the western side of the landslide, boreholes indicate that the water levels vary between 6.75 m and 10.9 m below ground level. Within the landslide on the western side near the toe, water levels of 4.2 m to 4.7 m below ground level have been recorded. Below the toe of the landslide, water levels between 0.05 m and 1.3 m below the ground surface have been recorded. All of these standpipes are slotted to allow the ingress of groundwater over the bedrock-colluvium interface. An approximate estimate is that the average pore pressure ratio for landslide reactivation would have been as high as 0.45.

11.7.3 Geotechnical model for Site 134

The geotechnical model is shown in Figure 11.17. Note that the cross section follows the approximate centre line of the landslide as shown in Figure 11.16. Some interpretation was involved in constructing the lower part of this cross section. No subsurface information is available near the centre-line of the landslide in this critical area of the site, although the section extends to one borehole 18 m beyond the toe of the landslide. The geotechnical model assumes that a massive body of colluvium is sliding over a shear surface fully developed within the colluvium itself. There is no evidence of sliding within the underlying bedrock. The location of the head-scarp and daylight-point of the toe are based on field observations and are consistent with the previous geotechnical investigations of the site.

In the upper half of the landslide, the slip surface dips at approximately 7.5° to the south-southeast. In the lower half of the landslide, the slide surface is approximately

r_u =	0.23	0.38	0.55
$\varnothing = 9°$	1.19	0.96	0.73
$\varnothing = 10°$	1.33	1.07	0.81
$\varnothing = 11°$	1.46	1.18	0.89
$\varnothing = 12°$	1.60	1.29	0.97
$\varnothing = 13°$	1.74	1.40	1.06
$\varnothing = 14°$	1.88	1.51	1.14

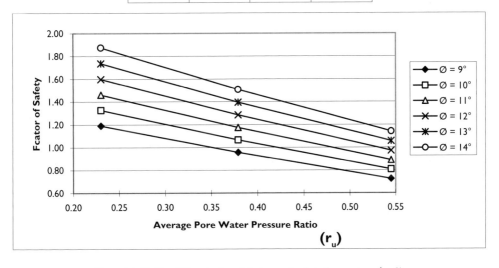

Figure 11.18 Site134: calculated factors of safety (assuming $c'_r = 0$).

horizontal. The depth to the sliding surface near the middle of the landslide is up to 18 m. Due to the documented history of landsliding at this site, it has been assumed, for the analyses reported here, that residual shear strength conditions would have existed along the slip surface.

11.7.4   Pore water pressure assumptions

Three different piezometric surfaces have been used for the analyses. As with the two other case studies, each piezometric surface was fully specified in the software package used for the analysis. These piezometric surfaces correspond to average pore pressure ratios of 0.23, 0.38 and 0.55.

11.7.5   Results of analyses

As stated above, shear strength parameters for the colluvium are expected to be at their residual values. On this basis, it was decided that the analyses need to be carried out for a value of $c'_r = 0$. The results for the analyses are shown in Figure 11.18.

For $F = 1$, the relationship between average pore pressure ratio and average friction angle is shown in Figure 11.19. The pore water pressures required for reactivation of movements during rainfall have been assumed to correspond to an average pore water pressure ratio of 0.45. On this basis, the residual friction angle is given by, $\varnothing'_r = 11°$.

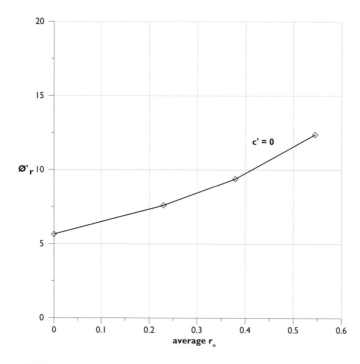

Figure 11.19 Site 134: Variation of back calculated friction angle with the average r_u (for $F = 1$) for $c' = 0$.

11.8 CONCLUDING REMARKS ON THE THREE CASE STUDIES

All the three landslides are relatively shallow (the depth to length ratio being relatively low). Consequently, parametric analyses have shown that the factor of safety is very sensitive to the value of cohesion. Even a small value of (assumed) cohesion has a significant effect on the factor of safety. In other words, the factor of safety will be overestimated if the value of cohesion is overestimated. Conversely, the back-calculated angle of internal friction for $F = 1$ will be underestimated if cohesion is assumed to have even a small value in cases where a zero value is appropriate.

Therefore, it was most important to arrive at the decision that residual shear strength parameters would be operative on the slip surfaces at these sites. It was also important to arrive at the decision that residual cohesion along the slip surfaces subject to continual sliding would have been very close to zero.

Movements and pore pressures at these three landslide sites have been monitored after the occurrence of the most significant reactivations. There are no accurate data concerning pore water pressures relevant to the time of occurrence of each landslide. The assumed data concerning triggering pore water pressures are, therefore, based on judgement after careful assessment of whatever data were available on groundwater levels. The accuracy of the conclusions reached would, therefore, be dependent on the above decisions and assumptions.

One may now attempt to answer the 'important questions' raised in the opening paragraphs of section 11.4:

i The factor of safety of a slope can be determined if the location of the slip surface is known along with the values of shear strength parameters and the location of the piezometric surface. For these case studies, the aim was to estimate the shear strength parameters. Since each of the slopes has been subjected to intermittent sliding movements over a number of years, the assumption of residual shear strength all along the slip surface is justified for each case. Zero or near-zero value of the residual cohesion is justified on the basis of previous research. Thus the value of the factor of safety depends only on the pore water pressures along the slip surface and the residual angle of internal friction. Assuming that a calculated factor of safety $F = 1$ corresponds to the condition of critical equilibrium, the angle of internal friction may be estimated for any known or assumed piezometric surface within the slope.

The relationship between average pore pressure ratio and residual angle of internal friction has been determined. From limited information concerning observed or inferred pore water pressure at the time of failure, the following estimates of residual internal friction angle have been estimated for each slope. A summary of these estimates are given below. (The corresponding pore pressure ratios are shown in parentheses).

Site 64: $\varnothing'_r = 17 - 18°$ $(r_u = 0.18)$
Site 77: $\varnothing'_r = 10 - 11°$ $(r_u = 0.22)$
Site 134: $\varnothing'_r = 11°$ $(r_u = 0.45)$

ii   For these slopes subjected to reactivation of landsliding over many years, the peak shear strength of the colluvium cannot be obtained from back analysis. This is because no information is available about the topography and pore water pressures prior to first-time landsliding. Indeed the date of the first time landsliding is unknown for each of these sites.

iii The analyses can be useful for planning or design of remedial measures such as installations for improved subsurface drainage. In particular, the curves showing the relationship between pore pressure ratio and residual friction angle for $F = 1$ can be very useful in this regard.

iv   The reliability of the results of back-analysis will depend primarily on the accuracy with which the main slip surface is determined and the accuracy of the pore water pressure distribution along the slip surface.

v   Monitoring of slopes can be very useful for stability analysis. If the slopes are instrumented with piezometers, pore pressures developed over time can be observed and the data used to validate the assumed values based on limited information.

vi   The three sites are all colluvial slopes in which intermittent movements are triggered by significant rainfall. Thus the failure mechanisms are basically the same. However, there are several differences amongst the sites due to differences in location and due to the spatial variability of geology, topography and drainage conditions within the region. Consequently, there are differences in the type of colluvium, the shape and size of each landslide and the shape of the slip surface. It is significant that the estimated average r_u at failure in each slope is different.

11.9   LANDSLIDE-TRIGGERING RAINFALL

11.9.1   Rainfall as triggering factor – threshold and variability

Rainfall is recognised internationally as a major triggering factor for the initiation of slope instability. Landslide movement triggered by rainfall may range from minor to catastrophic in terms of velocity and travel distance depending on the magnitude of pore water pressure increase and the rate at which this increase occurs. Extensive global research efforts have focused on the development of rainfall thresholds for the initiation of slope movements. Moreover, understanding the effects of rainfall is necessary for assessment of landslide hazard. An important source of uncertainty in hazard and risk assessment comes from both the spatial and temporal variation of rainfall (Chowdhury and Flentje, 2002). Therefore, it is important to study rainfall variability within a region and in particular the data concerning major rainstorms. Thus the spatial correlation of triggered landslides with the rainfall can be analysed in detail.

At the University of Wollongong, significant research has been directed to the analyses of rainfall and slope movements enabling estimation of such thresholds and the associated uncertainties. Initially the concept of Antecedent Rainfall Percentage Exceedance Time (ARPET) was proposed and a methodology was developed to use this concept for rainfall analysis and for the determination of landslide-triggering thresholds (Flentje and Chowdhury 1999, Chowdhury and Flentje, 2002). Subsequent work has been concerned with the study of spatial variability of rainfall and the relationship between rainfall duration and intensity.

11.9.2 Analyses of the 1998 rainstorm and associated landsliding

Wollongong experienced a major rainstorm event during the period 15th–19th of August, 1998. The intensity-frequency-duration curves derived from pluviometer rainfall monitoring stations around the city show that for intervals between 3 hours and 12 hours, some stations exceeded a 1 in 100 year event, and rainfall totals at one station for an 8 hour interval exceeded a 1 in 200 year event. However, many parts of the city experienced significantly less rainfalls over a wide range of durations equating to say a 1 in 20 year event for a 24 hour period.

The accumulated rainfall over the period 15th–19th of August 1998 was 745 mm recorded at Mount Ousley. The peak period of the rainstorm event was about three hours duration between the hours of 5 pm and 8 pm on August 17, the accumulated rainfall for the 24-hour period from 9 am August 17 to 9 am August 18 being 445 mm. Flash flooding, accompanied by shallow debris flows occurred during the peak rainfall period on the evening of August 17 with extensive damage to property and infrastructure and the loss of one life.

On the other hand, relatively deep-seated, slide-category landslides, occurred after August 18. (This refers to first-time landslides as well as to reactivations of existing landslide sites.)

Automatic rainfall pluviograph data showing the temporal pattern of rainfall distribution at 15-minute intervals is shown in Figure 11.20. According to an analysis of the rainfall event reported by Evans and Bewick (1999), return periods exceeding 1 in 100 years for durations between 30 minutes and 6 hours occurred along the top of the escarpment near Mount Ousley, Rixons Pass, Bulli and Beth Salem. These locations include parts of the urban Illawarra, which have historically had frequent landslide occurrences and where the adverse impact on residential property and infrastructure has been high.

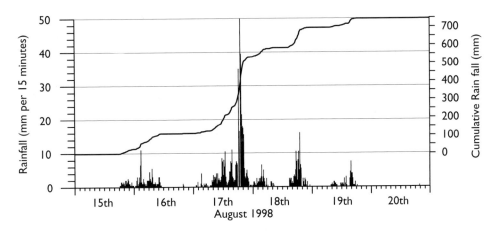

Figure 11.20 RTA Mount Ousley pluviograph rainfall data.

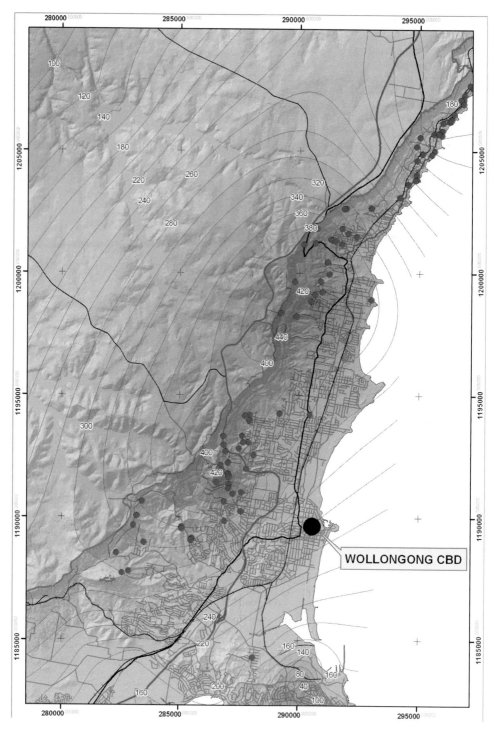

Figure 11.21 GIS based 24 hr rainfall distribution to 9 am on the 18th August 1998 (contours marked in mm rain) with observed landslides shown as dots. (See colour plate section).

The spatial distribution of the 24 hour rainfall totals to 9 am on the 18th of August and the known landslides that occurred during the event are shown in Figure 11.21. This figure clearly shows the spatial variability of the rainfall over this 24 hour period and also the good correlation between landslide locations and high rainfall intensity locations. Similar spatial variation exists for rainfall totals for other durations such as 4 hours and 12 hours. The full set of results has not been published but the results have facilitated the development of important relationships such as the one illustrated in Figure 11.22.

Figure 11.22 shows a rainfall intensity/duration graph with location-specific rainfall intensities for all landslide types (including debris flows) in the Illawarra during the August 1998 rain storm. For each duration, the rainfall intensities at each landslide is plotted, thereby creating clusters of points which appear as vertical lines. The lowest point plotted on of each such vertical line may, therefore, be regarded as the threshold intensity for that duration. For full details of rainfall analyses in the study area associated with 1998 rainstorm event, the reader may refer to Flentje and Chowdhury (1999, 2001), and Murray (2001).

A threshold relationship developed by Caine (1980) for internationally published rainfall intensity/duration and debris flow occurrence data on undisturbed slopes has been superimposed on the Wollongong data. An excellent correlation is found with the Wollongong data for debris flows associated with rainfall over a short duration. The Wollongong August 1998 series falls below the Caine threshold line for rainfall

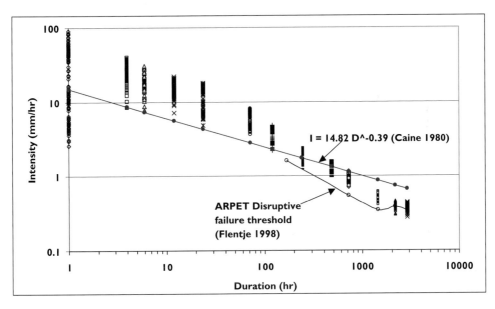

Figure 11.22 Rainfall intensity/duration thresholds for initiation of all landslide types (including debris flows) in the Illawarra during the August 1998 rainstorm event (vertical data series at various cumulative periods). Included is the Caine (1980) threshold line for internationally published rainfall intensity/duration and associated debris flow data on undisturbed slopes (Murray 2001). ARPET threshold line for disruptive failure involving deep-seated, slow-moving landslides (Flentje, 1998) is also included.

of longer durations. This would have been expected since the longer durations are clearly more relevant to deep seated landsliding. For this range of durations (240 hrs or 10 days up to 2280 hrs or 120 days), ARPET thresholds (Flentje, 1998) for deep seated slow moving landslides have been developed during previous research and are also shown on Figure 11.22.

11.10 LANDSLIDE SUSCEPTIBILITY AND HAZARD

11.10.1 Introduction and scope

Landslide susceptibility within a region varies due to differences in significant influencing factors which must be identified, carefully investigated and quantified as accurately as possible within local and financial constraints. Basic knowledge concerning topography, geology and drainage is essential. The location and distribution of known landslides in a region is very valuable for assessing future landslide susceptibility in the whole region. The development of a landslide inventory comprising all the available information on each landslide has already been discussed in the preceding sections of this chapter. The analysis of rainfall as a landslide triggering agent has also been discussed. Quantitative studies are facilitated by acquiring knowledge about geotechnical properties and pore water pressures from previous geotechnical reports, new geotechnical investigations and field monitoring. However, such data are available for only a limited number of locations and, therefore, regional studies of landslide susceptibility and hazard is usually based on data concerning the main influencing factors. The quality of assessment depends on the extent, quality and accuracy of the basic data and the type of methodology used for analysis and synthesis of different data sets. Modelling of landslide susceptibility and hazard in this study area has been discussed in detail by Flentje et al. (2007a, b). A brief outline of the important step in the modelling process is provided in sub-section 11.10.3 below.

11.10.2 Regional risk assessment outside the scope of this chapter

In chapter 10, a brief reference was made to the importance of qualitative and quantitative assessment of risk associated with the occurrence of landslides. In addition to hazard assessment, risk calculations require the assessment of elements at risk and the vulnerability of each such element. Simple examples of such calculations were presented in chapter 10. Integrated risk assessment covering several landslides of different type, size and frequency within an area requires a more comprehensive approach involving collection and analysis of considerable amount of additional data.

Similarly, quantitative assessment of risk in a regional context also requires considerable additional analysis beyond the landslide hazard zoning. The methodology for assessing regional landslide risk is, however, completely outside the scope of this book.

However, it is pertinent to mention a significant interdisciplinary study of landslide risk to human safety within the study area of this chapter. This risk study was concerned with the occurrence of landslides and rockfalls along a short section of

Lawrence Hargrave Drive, a coastal road located in the study area (Hendricks et al., 2005; Moon et al., 2005). Based on quantitative studies, the risk of fatality due to rockfalls and landsliding along this 1 km section of road was considered to be too high (unacceptable) in spite of remedial works carried out over a considerable period of time.

After consideration of several alternatives for reducing risk levels, a decision was taken to by-pass the particular short section of road with a bridge, the Seacliff Bridge, which has proved to be very effective. Photographs of this section of road before and after the completion of Seacliff Bridge were introduced in Chapter 1 (see also the book cover). Such case studies highlight the need for the development of strategic approaches for the management of risk in geomechanics (Chowdhury and Flentje, 2008).

11.10.3   Data-sets relevant to the study area

In addition to the GIS-based landslide inventory, other GIS-based data sets have been developed for this project including engineering geological mapping, data acquired through external agencies and data sets generated by the GIS software using the Digital Elevation Model (DEM). In total, ten GIS-based data sets have been compiled. The data sets include:

1   Geology (21 variables representing the mapped geological formations)
2   Vegetation (15 variables representing the mapped vegetation categories)
3   Slope Inclination (continuous floating point distribution)
4   Slope aspect (continuous floating point distribution)
5   Terrain Units (buffered water courses, spur lines and other intermediate slopes)
6   Curvature (continuous floating point distribution)
7   Profile Curvature (continuous floating point distribution)
8   Plan Curvature (continuous floating point distribution)
9   Flow Accumulation (continuous integer)
10 Wetness Index (continuous floating point distribution)

11.10.4   Knowledge based approach and Data Mining (DM) model

A knowledge-based approach has been used to assess landslide susceptibility based on analysis and synthesis of data concerning different influencing factors contained in the data-sets mentioned above. The specific approach used for this purpose is the Data Mining (DM) model or process.

The DM learning process is facilitated by the software "See 5" which is a well developed commercial application of earlier software "C 4.5" (Quinlan, 1993). Both of these have been applied to a variety of applications in diverse fields. Application to studies of landslide susceptibility and hazard has been developed for the first time in the context of landslide susceptibility and hazard modelling within the Wollongong Local Government Area (WLGA), the subject of this chapter.

The DM learning process extracts patterns from large databases related to the problem being studied. These patterns provide insight into aspects of the phenomena relevant to the associated natural and other processes. Moreover, the patterns can facilitate prediction and provide a useful basis for decision-making.

The process involves the use of known landslide areas as one half of the model training, the other half comprising randomly selected points from within the model area outside known landslide areas. Using a fully attributed data set representing all the above data sets, the DM analysis undertakes a process of pattern recognition and develops a rule-set which defines the data set. This process is automated by the DM software and is confined by several user defined parameters, such as the number of rules required and the number of occurrences required before a rule is generated. Each rule is assigned a numerical confidence value defined by well-defined parameters. Details concerning the rules and parameters such as the Laplace ratio have been discussed elsewhere (Flentje 2007a, b) and Flentje (2009).

Rules which relate to the presence of a landslide are assigned positive confidence values and rules which indicate non-presence of a landslide are assigned negative confidence values. The rule set is then re-applied within the GIS software using the ESRI Model Builder extension to produce the Susceptibility grid with floating decimal point values ranging from 1 to –1.

11.10.5   Analysis of DM results and landslide susceptibility zoning

To aid the post-DM analyses of the Susceptibility grid and particularly to aid the definition of credible Susceptibility Zone categories and zone boundaries, a script was written in Visual Basic code to produce the distributions shown in Figure 11.23. This code ranked the complete 1.88 million data points and also all the landslide pixels individually (29,480 points) according to decreasing order of model confidence and determined the cumulative percentage of each data represented in the ranked list. Figure 11.23 shows the distribution of DM model 'confidence' for the preferred final slide model. The graph displays two curves, the upper dashed curve shows the distribution of model confidence for the 'known landslide' pixels, and the lower dash-dot curve shows the distribution of model confidence for each pixel in the entire model (1.88 million points). Also shown in Figure 11.23 are the interpreted landslide Susceptibility zone boundaries. The confidence values used to define the Susceptibility zone boundaries are arbitrary. However, a simple logic has been followed whereby the maximum numbers of known landslides are incorporated into the highest Susceptibility zones, whilst at the same time keeping the extent of these highest susceptibility zones to a minimum.

Within the training area, the graph highlights the excellent performance of the modelling with approximately 70% of the known landslides being identified with a high model confidence. Considering the entire model area, a smaller but significant proportion of that area (approximately 10%) is predicted as being highly susceptible to landsliding with a relatively high confidence.

This quantitative 'review' validates the methodology to a significant extent, and ensures that the process of susceptibility zone classification is completely transparent and open for review. Field validation work has also been carried out and reported in published work.

For this phase of the project, the susceptibility zones were identified and classified as high susceptibility, moderate susceptibility, low susceptibility and very low

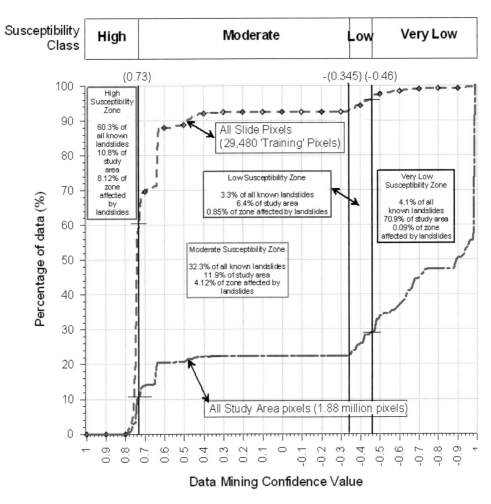

Figure 11.23 Classification of susceptibility zones using the distribution of the Data Mining model confidence for both the 'training data' and the complete model area.

susceptibility. The following findings relate to these zones: (a) high susceptibility (8.12%) of this area is subject to landslides and contains 60.3% of the known landslide population; (b) moderate susceptibility (4.12%) of this area is subject to landslides and contains 32.3% of known landslides; (c) low susceptibility (0.85%) of this area is subject to landslides and contains 3.3% of known landslides (d) very low susceptibility (0.09%) of the area is subject to landslides and contains (4.1%) of known landslides.

In terms of their area as a percentage of the total study area, the categories of susceptibility zones designated as 'high', 'moderate', 'low' and 'very low' comprise respectively 13.4, 9.2, 6.5 and 70.9 per cent. It is of interest to consider this in absolute terms. For example, the high landslide susceptibility zone identifies over 2,300 hectares of land, outside of known landslides, as being highly susceptible to landsliding.

Table 11.3 Summary of landslide hazard zoning: Relative annual likelihood and average landslide volume.

Hazard description	Map colour	% of zone affected by slides (S)	Zone area as % of study area	% of total slide population in hazard zone	Landslide annual average frequency (1950–2006)	Relative susceptibility of zone (S/Stotal) = Sr	Relative annual likelihood (Hazard) (Sr/T) where T = 126 years	Maximum landslide volume (m^3)	Average landslide volume (m^3)
Very low		0.10	70.86	4.1	1.65E-02	7.36E-03	5.84E-05	36,300	3,500
Low		0.85	6.47	3.7	1.72E-02	6.46E-02	5.13E-04	4,700	1,450
Moderate		4.12	9.23	35.1	2.21E-02	6.12E-01	2.48E-03	45,000	5,700
High		8.12	13.44	57.1	2.47E-02	6.16E-01	4.89E-03	720,000	28,700

Furthermore, the model also identifies over 13,000 hectares as having a very low susceptibility to landsliding.

11.10.6   Landslide hazard assessment and zoning

The spatial frequency of landsliding has been determined for each susceptibility zone as summarised in Table 11.3. Here, the percentage of each zone affected by landslides has been normalised and divided by the number of years represented by the period of coverage of the Landslide Inventory. In this case, the Wollongong landslide

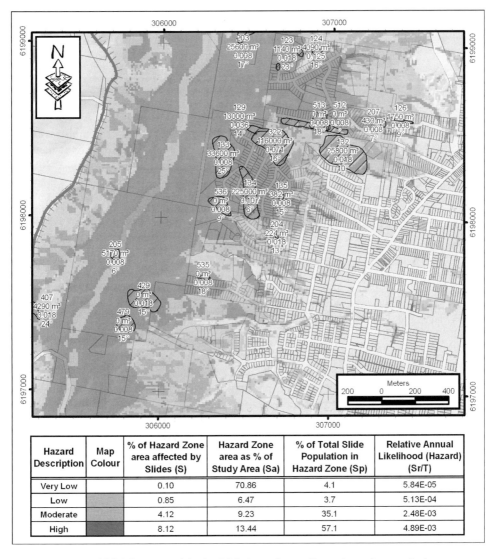

Hazard Description	Map Colour	% of Hazard Zone area affected by Slides (S)	Hazard Zone area as % of Study Area (Sa)	% of Total Slide Population in Hazard Zone (Sp)	Relative Annual Likelihood (Hazard) (Sr/T)
Very Low		0.10	70.86	4.1	5.84E-05
Low		0.85	6.47	3.7	5.13E-04
Moderate		4.12	9.23	35.1	2.48E-03
High		8.12	13.44	57.1	4.89E-03

Figure 11.24 Segment of the landslide hazard map. (See colour plate section).

Inventory covers a period of 126 years (1880–2006). Other techniques of assessing annual likelihoods of landsliding (i.e., process rates) are being investigated.

The landslide hazard zoning maps have been enhanced with additional detail regarding landslide volume, frequency of recurrence or reactivation of individual landslides and travel distance (Table 11.3 and Figure 11.24). This information appears as unique landslide site labels for each site and with text boxes appearing on the map sheet frames, outlining the distributions and averages of these values for each of the individual hazard zones.

On both the landslide Susceptibility and landslide Hazard maps, each landslide site is identified and labelled with its own unique Site Reference Code. On the Hazard maps, the label for each landslide also includes its volume (m^3) as the second label component. Landslide Frequency has been calculated from the total number of known recurrences at each landslide site as recorded in the Landslide Inventory. The specific landslide frequency for each landslide appears as the third label for each landslide.

11.11   OBSERVATIONAL APPROACH AND MONITORING

11.11.1   Introduction and definition

In this chapter, the term 'observational approach' is used to signify the monitoring of a number of locations within a study area and use of such observational data to assist with various aspects of landslide risk management such as the following:

- Estimating landslide-triggering rainfall thresholds.
- Estimating landslide-triggering pore water pressure thresholds.
- Assessing magnitudes and rates of landslide displacement with respect to triggering agents.
- Assessing landslide susceptibility, frequency, hazard and risk.
- Landslide risk management decision-making particularly during extreme rainfall events.
- Land management decision-making for medium to long term.
- Development of policies for land-use planning.

A landslide risk management strategy based on such an approach would involve a combination of both periodic (manual) and continuous (automated and real-time) monitoring of landslide displacement, pore water pressure and rainfall. Both types of monitoring are important. Continuous monitoring in real-time can facilitate the best understanding of increase in pore water pressures, initiation of landslide displacements, the occurrence of disruptive landsliding and the associated failure mechanisms. However, it must be pointed out that the traditional, periodic monitoring is also important. For example, data from periodic monitoring stations are important for designing continuous monitoring stations and, in particular, for selecting the depths at which shear movement and pore water pressure may be monitored continuously.

The definition of the 'observational approach' used here is different from that widely adopted in conventional geotechnical engineering practice. The conventional definition refers primarily to performance-based geotechnical design and construction in order to minimise over-conservatism and optimise safety. Moreover, that definition covers a wide range of geotechnical applications. Here, the term is used exclusively for slopes and landslides but in a more flexible way, to include a better understanding of slope performance based on observation under varying conditions coupled with the use of observed data in decision-making for risk management (Figures 11.25 and 11.26).

For landslide management, one may also extend the definition of the 'observational approach' even more broadly to include the whole process of landslide susceptibility,

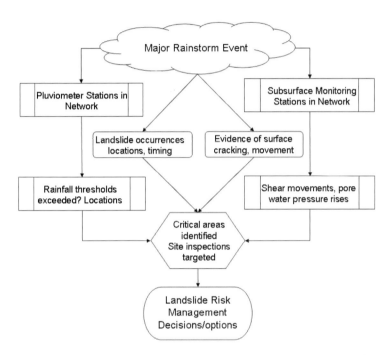

Figure 11.25 Overview of an 'Observational Approach' as applied during a major rainstorm event incorporating real-time information from a network of field stations (see Figure 11.26).

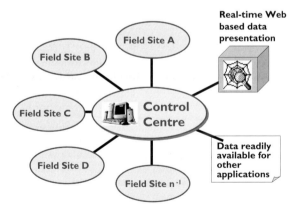

Figure 11.26 Continuous real-time monitoring landslide field stations, their automated linkage to a control centre and associated web-based data display.

hazard and risk assessment, including the development of a landslide inventory and the subsequent analyses and preparation of maps of landslide susceptibility. Moreover, data from monitoring may be used for emergency risk management in near-real-time during and in the immediate follow up response period of a significant rainstorm event.

This broad definition has been applied over the last decade by the landslide research team at the University of Wollongong. It is important to note that even the proper selection of sites for continuous monitoring cannot be done without knowledge concerning the location of existing landslides, their frequency of occurrence, and their severity. All of these aspects are greatly facilitated by observation and monitoring. The definition adopted here implies the establishment of a systematic monitoring regime within a region involving a network of continuous monitoring stations reporting data through a web-based interface (Figure 11.26).

The application of the 'observational approach' as defined here has less merit in the context of monitoring and managing a single landslide with the limited aim of designing remedial measures or validating a stability model.

11.11.2 Why an observational approach?

To answer this question, it is appropriate to consider how the role of observation and monitoring in slope stability is generally perceived by geotechnical engineers, engineering geologists and other professionals. One important role is as a tool for a detailed understanding of (a) slope performance at individual sites and (b) failure mechanisms in specific circumstances, so that assumed geotechnical models can be validated. In addition, a monitoring program at a site may have the specific purpose to help design the most appropriate remedial measures, and during the post construction stage, to determine the success of the works program. Another important use is as a research tool so that the relevance of important concepts can be verified such as the relationships between cumulative displacement, rate of displacement, pore water pressures and rainfall.

For landslide management in a regional context and, in particular, for urban landslide management, the widely accepted approach is to develop and use landslide susceptibility maps. In some instances, maps of landslide hazard or even of landslide risk may be used. The enormous usefulness of each of these types of maps is, of course, well known. The difficulty in preparing them is also well known. However it must be appreciated that such maps, however elaborate, are not predictive tools. During a significant landslide-triggering event such as a major rainstorm event, significant landslides and minor slope failures may occur at different locations. In addition, there will be subsurface shear movements which have not yet developed to the extent of being part of a recognizable landslide. The locations and timings of these effects are difficult, if not impossible to predict on the basis of susceptibility maps alone. Thus, there is considerable justification in advocating the use of observation and monitoring as key aspects of a more comprehensive approach for landslide management.

11.11.3 Example of landslide management based on monitoring

Landslide management during and after the August 1998 rainstorm event which affected the WLGA is a useful example of the role of an observational approach as defined in this paper. Previous research in the study area, which included observation and monitoring over many years, enabled predictions of widespread landsliding to be made and warnings to be issued. There was good information concerning preliminary rainfall thresholds, known pre-existing landslide locations and on subsurface shear movements at a number of locations. In fact, on this occasion, the rainfall was so intense (up to 750 mm in 5 days) that there was widespread professional and community recognition of the imminent danger of landsliding. Thus landslide management after the event was greatly facilitated. However, real-time management during and in the few days immediately following the rainstorm event was less successful, being more retro-active as there were no continuous monitoring stations and because 'an observational approach' had not been fully developed. All the monitoring that was carried out as a result of this event was manually undertaken and results were not available for days and weeks after the event.

An emergency geotechnical team of 3 experienced practitioners was assembled and carried out inspections at locations based on reports of damage and also at other sites of known previous instability within the urban area. This approach was successful and a range of geotechnical issues relating to approximately 150 landslides triggered during the rainfall event were addressed and expedited efficiently. However, the need for a fully developed 'observational approach' employing an automated network of Continuous Real-Time Monitoring (CRTM) Stations at selected representative landslide sites across the city of Wollongong (as conceptualised in Figure 11.26) was identified by the authors as a key requirement for enhancing the tools and capacity for landslide management within the region. Such a network of CRTM stations would be particularly useful during major rainstorm events. For more information about the development and significance of an approach based on continuous or real-time monitoring the reader may refer to Flentje et al. (2005), Flentje and Chowdhury (2006) and Chowdhury and Flentje (2007).

11.11.4 Field monitoring – periodic

In Wollongong, periodic inclinometer monitoring has been used extensively for over a decade. Among other benefits of such monitoring it is important to mention the estimation of preliminary landslide-triggering rainfall thresholds. A total of 50 inclinometer casings have been installed and monitored during the last decade across the Wollongong Local Government Area (WLGA). The University of Wollongong currently monitors nineteen of these inclinometers at ten different landslide sites. The manual monitoring has been carried out by the University since 1993 and by others since the early 1980's. As an example, landslide site 64 is a slide category landslide with an area of approximately 5000 m², a maximum depth of sliding of 7.5 m and an approximate volume of 18,000 m³. The crown of this landslide extends into the active track area of the dual electric railway line in the northern Wollongong suburb of Scarborough, and is located to the west of Site 355 (Figure 11.1). Subsurface remedial drainage slot drains, slope re-contouring and surface retaining structures were constructed during June 2002 by the State Rail Authority in a successful remediation strategy for the site. The manually monitored inclinometer profiles from borehole 3 near the crown of the landslide, for the period March 1989 to May 1996 are shown in Figure 11.27(a). The cumulative magnitude and rate of displacement indicated

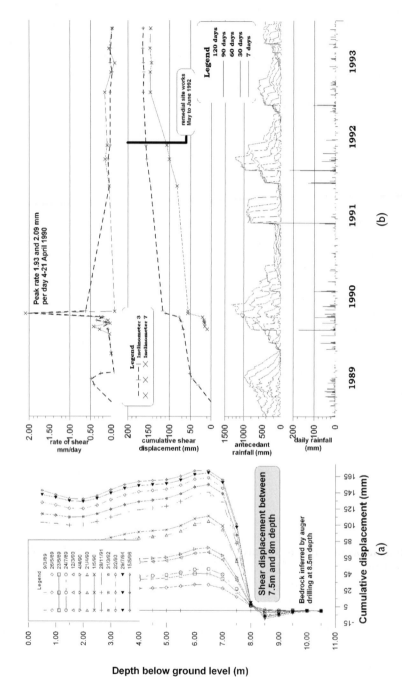

Figure 11.27 Manual monitoring record for Site 64 (a) Cumulative and rate of displacement graph for displacement at 6.5 m depth with daily and cumulative rainfall and (b) Manual inclinometer profiles.

by this record is shown as the dashed curve, together with daily rainfall and various antecedent rainfall curves in Figure 11.27(b). The remedial works appear to have substantially slowed subsurface shear movement at this site.

The daily rainfall station nearest to this site with data for this period is 650 m away at the Bureau of Meteorology Station 68223 at Reef Road Wombarra. A review of daily and cumulative rainfall data from this station, specifically for the period April 4–21, 1990, but also for the early April 1990 event and the April–May 1989 period, together with the rate of landslide displacement data has enabled the estimation of landslide triggering rainfall thresholds for this site. Geotechnical consultants for the railways have suggested that landslide movement at this site could be triggered by one month rainfall totals exceeding 350 mm and that movement would be maintained by subsequent monthly rainfall of 230 mm.

11.11.5 Field monitoring – continuous

11.11.5.1 Continuous Real-Time Monitoring (CRTM) stations – a summary

A CRTM Network of 23 landslide and weather field monitoring stations has been developed. Of these 23 stations, 15 are fully operational within the study area, whilst six are still being developed. Moreover, two stations within this network are installed at important landslide locations outside the state of New South Wales, one near Geelong in south-western Victoria and the other near the city of Hobart in Tasmania. Whilst the locations of the stations within this network are widely distributed, all the logged data are communicated to one computer server located at the University of Wollongong. Data from each of the CRTM stations are fed into individual databases on the server and accessed via a Graphical User Interface through an internet browser. Thus the landslide performance and weather data can be accessed and queried in a graphical form by an authorised user (network participant) via the internet.

The stations are all powered by 12 Volt batteries, some of which are charged by solar panels whilst others are charged by mains power. Tele-communications are performed by Internet Protocol (IP) broadband router devices. Data logging and on-site data management are carried out with Campbell Scientific Inc. CR10X and CR1000 data loggers and/or Data Taker dataloggers. Slope Indicator and Campbell Scientific have bundled these Campbell systems together and supplied them to the University of Wollongong. Slope Indicator and Campbell Scientific staff have completed the logger programming incorporating our research-based landslide triggering rainfall thresholds.

The instruments used so far in the Wollongong applications include In-Place-Inclinometers (IPI's) and Vibrating Wire Piezometers (VWP) installed at depth in boreholes. A discussion concerning the installation of inclinometer casing and vibrating wire piezometers is beyond the scope of this book. However, it is worth noting that the IPI instrument itself is approximately 44 cm from wheel to wheel centre and approximately 38.2 mm in diameter. These dimensions highlight two important points. Firstly, the 38.2 mm diameter of the IPI within the 58.5 mm ID of the standard 70 mm OD inclinometer casing allows for 20 mm of casing deflection before the IPI starts to get tight in the casing. Secondly, the length of the instrument can be extended by the addition of a length of stainless steel tubing to achieve whatever gauge length is

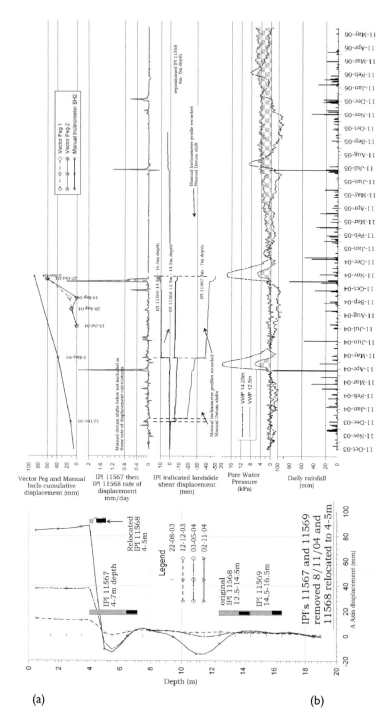

Figure 11.28 Site 355 monitoring history. (a) Continuous data–11th October 2003 to 30th September 2005. Rainfall, pore water pressure and landslide rate of shear and (b) Manual inclinometer profiles, Borehole 2 showing location of IPI instruments with gauge lengths.

required. Experience has shown that the gauge tubing easily bends, thereby masking actual shear displacement of the inclinometer casing. Therefore, ideally, the monitored IPI instrument length (instrument itself being 44 cm plus any additional gauge tubing) should be kept to a minimum. In Figure 11.28(a), IPI instrument and gauge lengths are indicated by black rectangles and hatched rectangles respectively.

Convergence monitors acting as Extensometers across ground surface landslide tension cracks have also been used in the Geelong application. GeoKon Long Range displacement meters have also been used in the study area. Rainfall pluviometers have been installed at all the field stations to record rainfall as it occurs (0.2 mm or 0.5 mm bucket tips).

11.11.5.2 CRTM field station example

Site 355 is a deep-seated slow moving 'slide' category landslide with a volume of approximately 35,000 m³. A limited geotechnical investigation of this landslide, carried out by the University of Wollongong, has shown that this landslide has the potential to move rapidly. Thus it could possibly adversely affect some of the houses that lie immediately upslope of and/or within the crown area of the landslide. The consequences of such landsliding at this site represent, as a worst case scenario, a high risk of loss of life for several specific adjacent residential dwellings. This assessment was an important factor that resulted in the construction of this continuous monitoring station in mid 2003. Three IPI's, two vibrating wire piezometers and one rainfall pluviometer were installed at the site. Following a review of past movement at this site, prior to continuous monitoring, it was determined that rainfall totalling 130 mm in 24 hours in combination with a 330 mm 60-day cumulative total would trigger landslide movement at this site. The manual and recent continuous monitoring at this site is facilitating more accurate estimation of landslide-triggering rainfall thresholds.

Manual inclinometer profiles recorded from Borehole 2 at the site, as shown in Figure 11.28(a), have confirmed that the depth of sliding in borehole 2 is between 4 and 5 m depth. The continuous monitoring record of Site 355 is shown as Figure 11.28(b).

The three original IPI's have been reduced to one and this instrument is now providing excellent data. The IPI 11567 rate of shear displacement curve in Figure 11.28 clearly displays two prominent spikes of accelerated displacement commencing on the 4th April and the 21st October 2004. The movement event, which commenced on the 4th April, continued for 5 days and peaked at 2.4 mm per day. This was triggered by rainfall of 110 mm and 106 mm on consecutive days.

The movement event commenced on the 21st of October 2004 lasted for 7 days and peaked at 2.5 mm per day on the second day. A maximum daily rainfall of 81.5 mm and several other days of 15 mm to 30 mm triggered this short duration of movement.

11.12 CONCLUDING REMARKS

A thorough understanding of factors which influence urban slope stability requires consideration of all the relevant influencing factors and the characteristics of triggering agents for landsliding. Historical information and data acquired from observational approaches form the basis for detailed assessments of landslide frequency, susceptibility and hazard. The quality of geotechnical slope analysis is dependent on the extent and quality of data obtained from field observations and geotechnical investigations. Both regional and site-specific analyses are important and the outcomes should be complementary.

Back-analyses for three landslide sites have been presented in this chapter and the results have served to highlight uncertainties concerning geotechnical parameters and, in particular, pore water pressures. Information has also been presented on the detailed analysis of rainfall data for an exceptional rainstorm event that occurred in August 1998 and triggered many landslides in the study area. Attention has been drawn to the monitoring of subsurface movements and pore water pressure related to landslide sites. Continuous or real-time monitoring offers considerable advantages over periodic monitoring and references have been made to recent work carried out in this regard for several sites in the study area.

An important goal of regional slope stability studies in an urban area is to model susceptibility of the terrain to landsliding. Recent work related to such modelling in the study area has been summarised in this chapter.

Chapter 12

Summing up

12.1 INTRODUCTION AND BRIEF OVERVIEW

Learning about geotechnical slope analysis requires that one should gain a good understanding of factors which control slope stability, the processes that lead to instability and the mechanisms of failure. Over many decades, theoretical development, experimental research, field studies and observational methods have led to good understanding of the basic causes and mechanisms of slope failure in many situations. Yet there may be uncertainties concerning many failures. Certain landslide events are still poorly understood and, in spite of many studies and analyses, there are serious gaps in the understanding of some catastrophic failures. Thus there is need for continued study, research and observation.

The development of geotechnical slope analysis has progressed as a consequence of improvement in the knowledge of basic geotechnical concepts and an understanding of the causes and processes associated with slope failures. Starting from simple and approximate methods based on a number of assumptions, advanced and relatively rigorous methods have been developed. Some of the latter are based on sophisticated models of geotechnical behaviour including non-linear, stress-dependent behaviour of soils. Advanced methods are versatile, enabling the analysis of a slope with complex geometry, formed in an anisotropic, non-homogeneous or reinforced earth mass. The history of slope formation can also be taken into consideration. Two-dimensional (2D) limit equilibrium analyses are, of course, the most widely used. However, considerable progress has been made in the development and use of three-dimensional (3D) analyses. Limit equilibrium methods can be easily extended to reinforced slopes by the inclusion of the additional forces due to reinforcing elements in the equilibrium equations.

The use of stress-deformation analysis is essential when the estimation of strains and deformations within a slope is required. In most cases, two-dimensional (2D) stress-deformation analyses would suffice. However, there are significant problems which need to be modelled and analysed in three-dimensions. Methods appropriate for 3D stress-deformation analysis have been developed and used successfully.

Dealing with seismic slope stability requires consideration of slope behaviour during earthquake shaking and thus soil properties under dynamic or cyclic loading can be important. Thus methods of analysis must be modified accordingly, and a full chapter has been devoted in this book to this important and vast subject.

Rainfall-induced slope failures occur generally, but not always, in saturated soils. Such failures are caused by increase of pore water pressures to critical values. Limit equilibrium methods are well suited to the analysis of saturated soils under conditions of seepage including rainfall infiltration. Moreover, special cases such as short-term, undrained behaviour and draw-down can also be dealt with. Back-analyses of rainfall-induced slope failures enable the estimation of critical pore water pressures.

Most of the widely used methods of analysis can be extended to slopes in unsaturated soils provided the relevant shear strength equation (different from that applicable to saturated soils) is used. Thus additional shear strength parameters must be determined and the distribution of suctions (negative pore pressures) within the soil mass estimated. Studying the change in stability during rainfall infiltration requires modelling of the change in suctions.

Increasing appreciation of the importance of geotechnical parameter variability (e.g., variability of shear strength parameters and pore water pressures), spatial and temporal, has led to the development of probabilistic approaches. There are, of course, other uncertainties which may require to be included in a probabilistic analysis such as statistical uncertainty, bias, and geotechnical model uncertainty. Although the adoption of a probabilistic approach by the geotechnical profession was initially a slow process, the considerable benefits in doing so are now increasingly recognised. In this book, attention is drawn to the vast scope offered by adopting a probabilistic perspective. Thus replacement of performance indicator from factor of safety to probability of failure or to reliability index is just one of the many benefits that accrue from consideration of slope analysis within a probabilistic framework. Thus it was considered desirable to introduce the basic probability concepts at an early stage of this book (Chapter 3). A full chapter, Chapter 10, is then devoted to the scope of probabilistic slope analysis, the methods and techniques that are widely used, and relevant examples and case studies including special analyses.

Understanding of the regional context of a site in terms of topography, geology, groundwater flow and geomorphology is important. Knowledge about the location, character, types and behaviour of regional landslides can be very valuable. It is important to study the occurrence and spatial distribution of first-time slope failures as well as reactivated landslides. Accordingly, in this book, reference has been made to the development of a comprehensive data base such as a landslide inventory and the modelling of landslide susceptibility and hazard.

It has also been necessary to refer to the importance of observation and, in particular, the monitoring of slope movement and subsurface pore water pressures. Monitoring of slope performance is often part and parcel of an important geotechnical project such as an earth dam or a reinforced embankment or major excavation. However, it is also desirable to monitor the performance of natural slopes in urban areas because of the consequences of failure to human safety in addition to the economic consequences. Moreover, analysis of data from such monitoring can help validate concepts concerning causes and mechanisms of landsliding, contribute to decisions concerning method of improving slope stability, and help design warning systems.

12.2   SEEKING EMERGING THEMES

This book started with an overview of recent developments, perspectives and trends before outlining the aims of geotechnical slope analysis. The importance of an interdisciplinary approach was highlighted and it was suggested that regional and site-specific analyses should complement each other. The book is primarily about the analysis of individual slopes or site-specific studies and detailed coverage of regional studies is outside its scope. Yet it has been useful to include some regional perspectives in chapters 9, 10 and 11. This coverage, although very limited, serves as a reminder to the reader that the era of exclusivity is over and that it can be very beneficial to consider geotechnical analysis in a regional context. In some instances, it is vitally important to do so. By increasingly working in interdisciplinary teams on important or complex projects, geotechnical engineers are learning about such benefits. This is particularly evident in projects concerned with urban slope stability.

The reader may identify important themes or lessons that have emerged as a result of studying this book. One way to do so is to pose specific questions and then try to answer them. These questions could include the following:

- How important is it to consider geotechnical slope analysis, focussed on individual slopes and on specific performance indicators, in a regional context and why?
- How well can one balance the use of simpler methods of analysis requiring limited input data and computational effort, in comparison to the use of sophisticated methods of analysis, given the availability of increasing power of computing and appropriate geotechnical software?
- Are complex or sophisticated geotechnical models necessary in order to account for mechanisms or phenomena such as stress redistribution and progressive failure?
- Is probabilistic analysis superior to deterministic analysis in some situations and why?
- What is the role of an observational approach in relation to slope analysis and why should its scope be different from that of a traditional 'observational method' in geotechnical engineering?
- Should the goal of slope analysis be performance prediction or simply the assessment of a measure of stability? Alternatively, should slope analysis be considered simply as a component of the assessment of hazard and risk?
- In meeting the emerging and future challenges facing geotechnical engineers, amongst many others, how good are the available methods as tools of geotechnical slope analysis?

12.3   GEOTECHNICAL SLOPE ANALYSIS IN A REGIONAL CONTEXT

The strategies, methods and techniques for regional slope analysis involve collection, assessment, analysis and synthesis of a wide range of data concerning influencing factors for slope stability as well as observational data. Regional analysis may range from qualitative to quantitative. The latter requires the development and use of appropriate models to extrapolate from existing information about the occurrence of slope failures in a region. Even the results of quantitative analysis are generally expressed in qualitative terms as in landslide susceptibility zoning. In contrast, geotechnical slope analysis is invariably quantitative and the results are always expressed in quantitative terms. However, the two types of analysis, regional and site-specific are inextricably linked as follows. For example, one or more of the following factors may have a very strong influence on how modelling and analysis methods are developed. Such factors would also influence the outcomes of both types of analysis.

- Understanding of geology, geomorphology and groundwater flow is of key importance. As Peck (1973) observed "We deal with geological materials, yet geological techniques, geological reasoning, and the implications of geology are rarely utilised to maximum advantage ... many a deposit considered to be of unpredictable variability and depth has turned out to be exactly what should have been expected on the basis of the patterns of jointing, shearing, folding and faulting that could be worked out by geological methods; ... geology enables us to establish what constraints may exist on the shape and depth of the surface of sliding when we consider the stability of natural slopes ..."
- There are known uncertainties which will influence the results of analysis or assessment and which must therefore be identified and, if possible, quantified. Again there may be unknown uncertainties which will limit the accuracy of analyses and of any predictions based on them.
- Variability of ground conditions, spatial and temporal, is important in both regional and site-specific analysis.
- Probability concepts are very useful in both cases although they may be applied in quite different ways.
- Spatial and temporal variability of triggering factors such as rainfall influence the occurrence and distribution of landslides in a region. This context is important for understanding of uncertainties concerning development of critical pore water pressures. Consequently, it helps in the estimation of rainfall threshold for on-set of landsliding. Regional and local factors both would have a strong influence on the combinations of rainfall magnitude and duration leading to critical conditions.

Considering the regional context of an individual slope at a given site will thus provide access to a wealth of information which otherwise would be considered irrelevant to that site. Consequently, information and data from a regional study will improve the capacity to learn about the performance of an individual slope and the capacity for proper selection and use of a specific method of geotechnical slope analysis.

12.4   CHOICE BETWEEN CONVENTIONAL AND ADVANCED METHODS OF ANALYSIS

There is considerable choice amongst limit equilibrium methods and choice amongst these depends on the type of slope (e.g., soil, rock), shape of slip surface (e.g., planar, multi-planar, circular, non-circular) and other aspects. Even so, more than one method may be suitable and many available software packages do include several alternative methods and options. Similarly there are several sophisticated methods of analysis for determining stresses and deformations and there is a corresponding choice of software packages.

The use of one or more limit equilibrium methods is sufficient in most slope problems where the aim is to determine values of factor of safety F as the main performance indicator. Moreover, one of these methods can serve as a useful geotechnical basis for probabilistic modelling and analysis. On the other hand, if slope deformations need to be calculated and if detailed knowledge of stress and strain distributions is important, the use of advanced stress-deformation methods is desirable and, in fact, may be necessary. However, the required input data must be available and in fact deformations measured in the field would be desirable in order to validate the results based on the input data. Using a finite element solution simply to calculate the factor of safety offers little or no advantage over a limit equilibrium approach.

Writing under the heading, "Simple calculations based on a range of variables are better than elaborate ones based on limited input", Peck (1973) acknowledged that advanced techniques like the finite element method are valuable for solving problems which formerly could only be tackled by crude methods. However, he warned about inappropriate use of such methods as follows:

"All too often those skilled in such techniques are unskilled in selecting the appropriate physical properties for inclusion in the analysis or in appreciating the physical constraints on the problem".

He went on to say

"We should be on guard not to ascribe to elaborate analytical routines a reliability they do not possess".

More than three decades later, the wisdom of these comments is still borne out by trends in geotechnical practice.

There may be complex projects in which limit equilibrium approach requires to be supplemented by advanced methods. Certainly there are known, well-documented failures of slopes and dams in which the conventional limit equilibrium approach has not provided all the answers. In some of those cases, stress-deformation analyses have also proved to be of limited value. This is because knowledge gaps concerning geotechnical parameters and failure mechanisms would be more important in those cases than limitations in the method of analysis.

12.5   UNDERSTANDING AND MODELLING IMPORTANT PHENOMENA

Throughout this book the reader would have noted references to important concepts and phenomena such as non-uniform stress and strain distributions, progressive failure, initial stresses and slip surface development and propagation. Research and observation have contributed to an understanding of such concepts and to the development of relevant methods of analysis. However, much more remains to be done. Basic concepts of progressive failure were considered in Chapter 2 and followed up in several other chapters. During the early stages of the development of soil mechanics, the focus was primarily on non-uniform stress and strain redistributions within an earth mass. However, manifestations of progressive failure can be different in different types of soil and may also depend on other factors and conditions and, in particular, on site-specific factors. Initial stress concepts and analyses based on them were considered primarily in chapter 7. Modelling of slip surface propagation was also considered in the same chapter.

While analysis has an important role in understanding these effects, the outcomes and results must be combined with lessons learnt from observation and monitoring.

Increasingly sophisticated stress deformation methods have been developed in order to model these phenomena or effects based on them. The requirements in the form of input data are often forbidding. Yet these methods have an important role to play in large projects where the time and expense required to obtain the relevant data can be easily justified. However, success in modelling complex phenomena cannot be assured simply because a sophisticated method is available. Continued research is thus important. In particular; success in tackling difficult problems may depend on the development of new concepts and ways of modelling which reflect observed phenomena more closely.

Meanwhile, it is always prudent to consider suitable modifications of proven conventional method of analysis. In their basic form, convention methods of limit equilibrium analysis have severe limitations. However, relatively simple modifications and adaptations may be made to simulate strain-softening and stress redistribution. In chapter 5, it was shown that the influence of strain-softening on the factor of safety could be estimated reliably by using such modified methods. More importantly, there are no requirements of additional input data such as detailed stress-strain properties.

12.6   APPROPRIATE USE OF PROBABILISTIC ANALYSIS

The importance of a probabilistic perspective has been emphasised in this book and is evidenced by increasing number of papers published in professional journals and those presented at international conferences. A recent paper, Silva et al. (2008) is the latest manifestation of continuing interest by practising engineers and this paper will be discussed further below. Probabilistic analysis should be considered as complementary to deterministic analysis; the latter is not to be considered as superior to the former. Indeed any type of analysis is useful only if the geotechnical model is sound and, in turn, that depends on a proper understanding and interpretation of site conditions including geology. Improper use of probability will prove to be counterproductive.

At a time when probabilistic geomechanics was in its early stages of development Peck (1973) observed "... The statistical methods are sometimes remarkably refined. Yet they are frequently entirely inappropriate because randomness is assumed to be a characteristic of the deposits. Nature, however, did not create deposits by random processes but in accordance with strict physical laws such as those of hydraulics and sediment transport. Alluvial deposits are likely to consist of a multiplicity of lenses, each of which might be called a sedimentation unit; each laid down under remarkably uniform conditions but each differing from its neighbours ...".

Contrast this with the following comment made about a decade later: "The literature also has been directed to probability-based assessment of strengths to be used in stability analyses. When strengths can be considered a random variable, as in a compacted embankment, this approach can be certainly defended ..." (Peck, 1982).

In the same paper, it is argued that assessing the likelihood of a dam failure by piping would require a working knowledge of geology, as well as a theoretical and practical knowledge of seepage and asks "How many such people would be equally experienced in the techniques of formal risk analysis? The important requirements for safety require understanding of field conditions, good dam design in accordance with those conditions, adequate safety measures against piping failure, such as filter blankets, filter wells and weight berms, and a provision for adequate surveillance. Peck (1982) concludes by saying that, when all these relevant factors can be taken into consideration in a risk analysis, "... I shall become an enthusiastic supporter. I think that this may be possible, and I endorse efforts to that end ... I don't believe the implications of these factors can be quantified by asking the most qualified of experts to choose a number between 1 and 10." The last comment shows that Peck rejected subjective probability assessment as it was projected in 1982.

Three decades have passed since the above comments were made. Probability-based risk analysis has indeed progressed significantly during this period both for slope stability and dam safety. Yet, in order to avoid inappropriate use of probabilistic analysis, the need for scepticism and caution is as important today as it was then.

One may ask:

"What is the status today of the subject 'probability assessment based on expert judgement'?"

In this regard it is pertinent to refer to a recent paper (Silva et al., 2008) where the development of empirical non-linear relationships between the factor of safety F and annual probability of failure p_f is outlined. Slope stability problems are classified into one of four types, category I to category IV, depending on a number of factors such as the extent of investigation, the reliability of shear strength data and the quality of engineering including construction supervision. Category I projects are the best and category IV the worst in terms of the level of engineering based on criteria outlined in detail by the authors. Level of engineering is established by considering the practices followed in design, investigation, testing, analysis and documentation, construction, operation and monitoring.

Each category is represented by one nonlinear curve of F vs. p_f showing how the probability of failure decreases as the value of F increases. Each curve is developed from experience backed by relevant case studies along with a consideration of published results of probabilistic analyses concerning slopes and earth dams. For factor of safety below 1, each curve approaches $p_f = 1$ asymptotically and the curves flatten out for factor of safety greater than 2, which reflects "... diminishing returns obtained from overbuilding a constructed facility".

It is difficult to compare empirical curves to theoretical curves such as a family of curves of mean F vs. p_f, each representing a different standard deviation or coefficient of variation of F. However, the authors claim that the general shapes of the proposed curves compare reasonably with relationships based entirely on probability calculations.

For using their empirical curves, the authors (Silva et al., 2008) detail a number of conditions that must be satisfied for a problem to be classified into one of the four different categories. Once a problem is categorised, the probability of failure for a given value of factor of safety F may be read from the corresponding curve.

For example, for $F = 1.5$, the approximate pf values read from their curves are: 0.1 for category IV (poorest engineering), 0.01 for category III, 0.0001 for Category II and 0.000001 for Category I (best engineering). Before using the curves, conventional

F would have to be estimated. Considerable uncertainty would exist regarding the method of assessing F, especially for categories III and IV where minimal data concerning geotechnical parameters are available. This aspect is not discussed in the paper.

In evaluating this proposed approach, let us consider both the merits and the limitations. This approach offers a good guide to the considered and thoughtful estimation of failure probabilities for practical slope problems. A considerable amount of study, thought and effort has led to the development of these guidelines. To quote the authors "We have concluded that quantified expert judgement places at our disposal an underutilised tool for making better engineering and management decisions." With increasing use for number of cases, the context and scope for the best use of such an approach will become clearer. At this time, it can be said that this approach significantly upgrades subjective probability assessment by including detailed information on the level of engineering. In that sense it is a sophisticated subjective approach in comparison to the way that subjective judgement was used in the past.

On the other hand, adopting such an approach discourages the consideration of each problem as unique and inhibits an understanding of the components of uncertainty and their relative influence on the results. For example, consider problems of natural slope stability in which the variability of pore water pressure, spatial and temporal, is often a significant source of uncertainty. Clearly, in such cases, relying on empirical curves may be misleading. Region-specific and site-specific factors based on observational data would have to be considered to assess the uncertainty and formal analysis would be required to determine its influence on the annual failure probability.

The authors refer to past practice and mention "The difficulty and expense associated with determining probability of failure by rigorous mathematical means …". Over the last few decades, these difficulties have already been overcome and simpler methods of probabilistic analysis have also been made available. One would expect present and future generations of geotechnical engineers to be familiar with the basic concepts of probability and with probabilistic geotechnical analysis.

One must be reminded that estimation of a value of p_F for individual slopes is a limited aim. The broader aim is to adopt a probabilistic perspective in order to further advance the understanding of important phenomena related to stability and safety. For instance, formal probabilistic analysis is required to consider multiple failure modes and, more generally, the probability of failure of a geotechnical system. Similarly, formal analysis is required to consider the probability of progressive failure. Finally, one must be prepared to deal with future challenges. New problems will arise for which there is no previous experience available, requiring careful consideration of their unique features and how those features may be incorporated in modelling and analysis.

12.7　OBSERVATIONAL APPROACH

Throughout this book, it has become clear that slope analysis cannot be considered in isolation. Having access to equations, formulae and computer programs is not enough. Understanding site conditions and field performance is essential. While this book is primarily about geotechnical slope analysis, observation and monitoring are very important for understanding all aspects of slope performance from increases in pore water pressures to the evidence of minor deformations, and from the development of tension cracks and small shear movements to progressive failure and the development of a complete landslide including post-failure movement.

Observation and monitoring also facilitate an understanding of the occurrence of multiple slope failures within a region after a significant triggering event such as a rainfall event or an earthquake. Most importantly, observational approach helps in the back analyses of slope failures and landslides. From the beginning of soil mechanics as a discipline, back analyses have been very useful in understanding the mobilisation of shear strength, the development of stresses and deformations and several other aspects of slope behaviour. Whether considering new or existing slopes or the strengthening of slopes, a well designed program of observation and monitoring can be useful for validating geotechnical analyses. Moreover, data for slope analysis, such as pore water pressure and shear strength can be updated as more observational data become available. Observation and monitoring of natural slopes including real-time monitoring has been discussed in Chapter 11. The availability of real-time data will contribute to more accurate assessments and to more accurate back-analyses. Consequently, real-time monitoring will lead to further advancement in the understanding of slope behaviour.

12.8   MEETING EMERGING CHALLENGES

First and foremost we must consider the challenge concerning increasing number of slope failures and their increasingly adverse consequences. These trends have developed in spite of significant progress in our understanding of natural processes and in spite of the successful development of experimental, analytical and design tools. Attention was drawn in Chapter 1 to the increasing frequency of catastrophic slope failures and landslides all over the world and especially in the less developed parts of the world.

Often catastrophic landslides are caused by high magnitude natural events such as rainstorms and earthquakes. It is also important to consider the contribution of human activities such as indiscriminate deforestation and rapid urbanisation to landslide hazard. There is an increasing realisation that poor planning of land and infrastructure development has increased the potential for slope instability in many regions of the world.

Adverse consequences are a product of hazard and vulnerability and there is considerable evidence that vulnerability of infrastructure and human safety is increasing. Consequently, human costs in terms of lives lost and injuries suffered are increasing and so are the adverse economic and environmental consequences.

Issues concerned with increasing hazard and vulnerability are very complex and cannot be tackled by geotechnical engineers alone. Therefore, the importance of working in interdisciplinary teams must again be emphasised. In educating geotechnical engineers, greater attention needs to be given to the reasons for the increasing occurrence of slope failures and the role of both natural and human factors. Greater emphasis also needs to be given to understanding long-term slope performance. In a modern educational curriculum for civil and geotechnical engineers, the traditional emphasis on good engineering design is important but not sufficient.

Developing better method of hazard and risk assessment will continue to be important. This can be done rationally within a probabilistic framework. Thus the emphasis on probabilistic perspectives is important for meeting the challenges of the future. Existing methods of landslide risk management may be developed further and more innovative methods need to be developed.

At the level of analysis methods and techniques, one of the important challenges is to use slope deformation as a performance indicator rather than the conventional factor of safety. More needs to be learnt about what level of slope deformation is critical for each type of slope considering different applications such as embankments and cut slopes for roads, railways and natural slopes in urban areas. Increased knowledge based on research and observation can then be used to develop better methods of deterministic and probabilistic analysis. Also at the level of analysis, attention needs to be given to better description of uncertainties related to construction of slopes including the quality of supervision.

So far the focus has been on uncertainties in geotechnical parameters and, in particular, on shear strength data. Attention has also been drawn in this book to the variability of triggering factors such as rainfall. This contributes to a different type of uncertainty which deserves more attention.

With projected changes in climate and weather, variability of influencing factor like rainfall will increase and, therefore, geotechnical engineers need to be equipped with better tools for dealing with variability and uncertainty. There may also be other changes in the rate at which natural processes like weathering and erosion occur. Sea level rise is another important projected consequence of global warming and climate change and it would have adverse effects on the stability of coastal slopes. While one can expect changes in rainfall patterns and pore pressures, and changes in sea levels, there is significant uncertainty in the occurrence, magnitude and rate of these changes. Based on whatever limited data become available, modelling of future scenarios is necessary and this can only be done by interdisciplinary teams. Once certain scenarios are accepted as a basis for assessment and analysis, objectives and goals must be defined. Once that has been done, regional and site-specific assessments can be carried out in that context.

12.9 CONCLUDING REMARKS

As evidenced by the material and discussions in this book, a wide range of methods is available for analysis of geotechnical slopes, from the simplest to the most sophisticated. Similarly there is a wide range of aids ranging from slope stability graphs, charts and tables to computer programs and comprehensive softwares. Discussion of the merits and limitations of geotechnical software is outside the scope of this book. However, the use of such softwares is frequently required and this trend will grow. Consequently, the assumptions made in developing the software must be explored and the validity of these assumptions assessed. This is an important responsibility of geotechnical engineers since they must ensure that the choice and use of computer software is appropriate for the problems being analysed. Exploration of such issues will be facilitated by a proper understanding of the basic concepts of geotechnical slope analysis and the fundamental principles on which the available methods of analysis are based. These concepts and principles are covered extensively in this book.

Shear strength parameters of residual soils, weathered rocks and related minerals

The following tables of shear strength parameters for residual soils, weathered rocks and related minerals were compiled by Deere and Patton (1971) from a number of sources. The following symbols and units are used:

ϕ' = effective angle of shearing resistance in degrees
ϕ_r = residual angle of shearing resistance (usually drained) in degrees
ϕ = angle of shearing resistance in degrees
c = cohesion (kg/cm^2)
c' = effective cohesion (kg/cm^2)

Table I.I Metamorphic rocks. With permission, see page 714, No 37.

Rock type	Degree of weathering	Strength kg/cm^2	Parameters Degrees	Remarks
Gneiss (micaceous)	muram (zone IB) decomposed rock	$c = 0.6$ $c = 0.3$	$\phi = 23°$ $\phi = 37°$	direct shear tests
Gneiss	decompressed (zone IC)	–	$\phi = 18.5°$	consol. undrained tests
Gneiss	decompressed (fault zone)	$c = 1.5$	$\phi = 27°$	direct shear tests on concrete rock surfaces
	much decomposed	$c = 4.0$	$\phi = 29°$	
	medium composed	$c = 8.5$	$\phi = 35°$	
	unweathered	$c = 12.5$	$\phi = 60°$	
Schist	weathered (mica-schist soil)	–	$\phi = 24.5°$	both from analysis of slides perpendicular to schistocity
	Partly weathered (mica-schists and phyllites) (highly fractured)	$c = 0.7$	$\phi = 35°$	
Schist	weathered – intermediate (zone IC)	$c' = 0.5$ $c' = 0.7$	$\phi = 15°$ $\phi' = 15°$ $\phi = 18°$ $\phi' = 21°$	50% saturated consol 100% saturated undrained tests

(Continued)

Table I.I (Continued).

Rock type	Degree of weathering	Strength kg/cm²	Parameters Degrees	Remarks
Schist	weathered	–	$\phi = 26°{-}30°$	compacted rock fill field direct shear tests
Phyllite	residual soil (zone IC)	$c = 0$	$\phi = 24°$	perpendicular to schistosity
		$c = 0$	$\phi = 18°$	parallel of schistosity (both from analysis of slides)

Table I.2 Igneous rocks. With permission, see page 714, No 37.

Rock type	Degree of weathering	Strength kg/cm²	Parameters Degrees	Remarks
Granite	decomposed granite	$c = 0$	$\phi = 27°{-}31°$ ϕ average = 29°	500 tests Cherry Valley Dam
Granite	quality index, i 15 10 7 5 3	c 1 2 3 5 6–13	ϕ 41° 45°–46° 49°–50° 57° 62°–63°	In-situ direct shear tests Alto Rabagao
Granite	weathered (zone IIB) i/7+ partly weathered (zone IIB) 3+ relatively sound (zone III) 1–2		 $\phi_r = 26°{-}33°$ $\phi_r = 27°{-}31°$ $\phi_r = 29°{-}32°$	lab direct shear tests Alto Lindoso
Granite	Red earth (zone IB) decompo-sed granite (zone IC)		$\phi' = 28°$ ϕ' average = 35°	
Granite	decomposed (fine grained) decomposed (coarse rained) decomposed, remoulded	$c = 0$ if saturated	$\phi = 25.5°{-}34°$ $\phi = 36°{-}38°$ $\phi = 22°{-}40°$	
Quartz Diorite	sandy, silt decomposed rock	$c = 0.1$	$\phi = 30°{+}$	lab tests, undisturbed samples
Diorite	weathered	$c = 0.3$	$\phi = 22°$	consol. Undrained tests
Rhyolite	decomposed		$\phi' = 30°$	

The manner in which weathering influences the shear strength of rocks is shown in Figs. 17 and 18 of Deere and Patton (1971). The reader may also refer to:

Hamrol, A. (1961). A quantitative classification of the weathering and weatherability of rocks, Proc. 5th Int. Conf. Soil Mech. Found. Engg., Paris, 2; 771–774.

Table I.3 Sedimentary rocks, joint filling and minerals common in soils and weathered rocks. With permission, see page 714, No 37.

Rock type	Degree of weathering	Strength kg/cm^2	Parameters Degrees		Remarks
Keuper Marl	highly weathered	$c' \leq 0.1$	$\phi' = 25\text{--}32°$	$\phi_r = 18\text{--}24°$	2% carbonates
	intermediately weathered	$c' \leq 0.1$	$\phi' = 32\text{--}42°$	$\phi_r = 22\text{--}29°$	14% carbonates
	unweathered	$c' \leq 0.3$	$\phi' > 40°$	$\phi_r = 23\text{--}32°$	20% carbonates all triaxial tests drained and consol. undrained and cut plane triaxial tests
London Clay	weathered (brown)	$c' = 1.2$	$\phi' = 19\text{--}22°$	$\phi_r = 14°$	
	unweathered	$c' = 0.9\text{--}1.8$	$\phi' = 23\text{--}30°$	$\phi_r = 15°$	
"Black seams"	in zone IC			$\phi_r = 10.5°$	seam with slickensides
Joint filling				$\phi_r = 14.5°$	seam without slickensides
Quartz Sand				$\phi_r = 30°$ $\phi_r = 35°$	dune sand crushed sand
Kaolinite				$\phi_r = 22°$	Remolded Kaolinite-limited displacement
	minerals common in			$\phi_r = 12°$	Remolded Kaolinite-limestone
	residual			$\phi_r = 12°$	Intact Kaolinite-precut surface
Illite	soil			$\phi_r = 6.5°$	Remolded Illite-limestone
	and			$\phi_r = 11.5°$	Remolded Illite
Montmor- illonite	rocks			$\phi_r = 4\text{--}11°$	
Muscovite				$\phi_r = 17\text{--}24°$	
Hydrous mica				$\phi_r = 16\text{--}26°$	

The reader may like to compare the information given in the tables to the information included in chapter 1. It is also of interest to note for comparison that for overconsolidated clays values of c' ranging from 100 to 500 Ibs/ft^2 are often used (Lambe and Whitman, 1969). According to Lambe and Whitman, large 'measured' c' values frequently result from running CD tests too rapidly so that pore pressures develop. Therefore extreme caution must be exercised when a value of c' has to be adopted for practical purposes. For normally consolidated soils the value of c' is generally considered to be negligible.

The value of ϕ' for normally consolidated clays decreases in a general way with increasing plasticity-index. For extremely plastic clays e.g., those containing a large percentage of montmorillonite, the dissipation of excess pore pressure during a shear test takes an extremely long time. Therefore, according to Lambe and Whitman

(1969) the magnitude of ϕ' for very plastic clays is uncertain. For oversonsolidated clays with low overconsolidation ratio (OCR), ϕ' is slightly less than for the same clay in its normally consolidated state and c' depends on the magnitude of the pre-consolidation stress or on void ratio. For overconsolidated clays with high OCR, c' is relatively small and ϕ' depends on the magnitude of the preconsolidation stress or void ratio. These differences arise because the envelope of shear strength for overcon-solidated clays is generally curved and the values of c' and ϕ' for a given soil depend on the stress range over which a straight line fit is made to the curved envelope. The magnitude of strength parameters may also depend on how long the clay has been under preconsolidation stress. In compacted soils the compaction effort supplies the preconsolidation and both c' and ϕ' increase with compaction effort.

Slope stability charts and their use for different conditions including rapid draw down

AII.1 CHART FOR PARAMETER m_α IN BISHOP SIMPLIFIED METHOD (ALSO JANBU'S METHOD)

In Chapter 5, Equation (5.10) gives the factor of safety which must be calculated by iteration since m_α appearing on the right hand side contains F as shown in Equation (5.10a). A trial value of F is first used to evaluate the right hand side of (5.10). This gives a new value of F which is then used in the next calculation. Convergence is usually rapid and only a few iterations are required to get the correct value of F. The following chart, Figure II.1 is used for rapid determination of the term m_α. Note that α may have both positive and negative values as shown.

This chart may also be used for analysis by Janbu's Method (rigorous or simplified). Note that the denominator of (5.14a) on page (Ch. 5.21) is (m_α sec α). There-

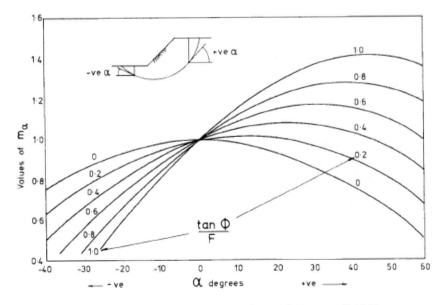

Figure II.1 Chart for evaluating m_α [refer to chapter 5, Equation (5.10a)].

fore this denominator can be calculated rapidly by using the chart Figure II.1. Once s has been evaluated from (5.14a) *F* may be obtained from (5.14). See also pages 264 and 265 for Janbu's simplified method including Equations (5.14b) and (5.14c). For the most detailed discussion concerning the use of Janbu's method the reader may refer to Janbu (1973) in Hirschfeld and Poulos (1973). It is of interest to note that a large number of vertical slices *should not* be used in Janbu's method. Typically about 15 slices may be sufficient. The ratio between width *dx* and height *z* of each slice must lie within reasonable limits so that terms of second order are truly negligible (finite difference approximation is used in developing the equations). The following criterion may be used as a rough guide:

$$1.5z > dx > 0.4z$$

This information is provided by K. Karal in a discussion of Workshop session 9, Analysis and Design in Geotechnical Engineering, Vol. 2, pages 150–153. (Am. Soc. Civ. Engrs. 1974.)

AII.2   INTRODUCTION TO SLOPE STABILITY CHARTS

Most slope stability charts have been devised on the following assumptions:

1   Two-dimensional limit equilibrium analysis
2   Simple homogeneous slopes
3   Slip surfaces of circular shape only

A user of charts must always bear these and any other assumptions in mind. In some cases charts have been devised on the basis of assumptions different from those noted above. For example Hoek (1970) devised charts for plane slip surfaces in rock. Hoek and Bray (1974, 1977) have also given some charts for plane surfaces in rock which are different from those in Hoek (1970). The charts in Hoek (1970) are not accurate over a wide range of the values of the slope parameters and plane failure charts in the book by Hoek and Bray (1974, 1977) are in fact preferable (E. Hoek pers. comm. 1978). In their book Hoek and Bray gave charts for failure along circular slip surfaces as well. These charts consider tension cracks as well as specific seepage conditions. Some charts and tables for non-uniform slopes and non-homogeneous soils based on the limit analysis technique of plasticity have been given by Chen (1975). The reader may recall from the text (chapter 8) that the results of limit equilibrium and limit analysis (upper bound technique) solutions are in very good agreement for uniform homo-geneous soils whether the shear strength is isotropic or anisotropic. Therefore Chen's results may be adopted for practice with the same confidence which is placed on limit equilibrium solutions.

The first slope stability charts were devised by Taylor (1937, 1948). These are the most well known charts and are strictly applicable for analysis in terms of 'total stress' approach only. (Note that pore pressure *u* or pore pressure ratio r_u are not considered in these charts). Taylor used the friction circle method. The same method has now been used by Cousins (1977) to prepare charts in terms of effective stress so that parameter r_u is included. Cousins' charts are discussed separately in sections AII.4 and AII.5 of this Appendix.

AII.3   TAYLOR'S CHARTS AND THEIR USE

Figure II.2 shows Taylor's chart for $\phi = 0$ analysis. The $\phi = 0$ concept has already been discussed in chapter 2 and the user must carefully consider the site conditions before using a $\phi = 0$ approach. Note from the chart that a minimum factor of safety may correspond to different depth factors D for different slope angles. For slope angles less

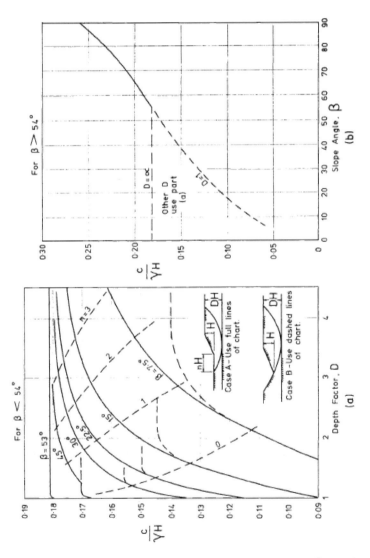

Figure II.2 Taylor's chart for $\phi = 0$ conditions for slope angles (a) less than 54° and (b) greater than 54°, (after Taylor, 1948).

than 54°, chart (a) is applicable and values of n can be read to locate the critical slip circle which is tangent to the assumed hard stratum at depth DH. For values of slope angle greater than 54°, chart (b) is applicable and critical slip circle passes through the toe i.e., $D = 1$. (For slope angles less than 54° when there is no hard stratum, i.e. $D = \alpha$, the horizontal dashed line in curve (b) is relevant).

The value of c obtained from the chart for given values of D, B, γ and H is the unit cohesion required for stability c_m (also called mobilised cohesion). The factors of safety may be defined as the ratio of available cohesion c_a to mobilised cohesion c_m i.e., $F = c_a/c_m$.

Figure II.3 shows the chart for locating the centre of the critical toe circle. Information about the location of critical slip surfaces is always useful. For instance a comparison can be made between observed locations of slip surfaces on the one hand and theoretical locations on the other hand.

Figure II.4 shows Taylor's chart for $\phi \neq 0$ as redrawn by Terzaghi and Peck (1967). Note that in this replotted version $\gamma H/c$ is plotted as a dimensionless parameter instead of its inverse $c/\gamma H$ plotted in Figure II.2. The use of such a chart has already been explained in the text and is repeated here for convenience of the user.

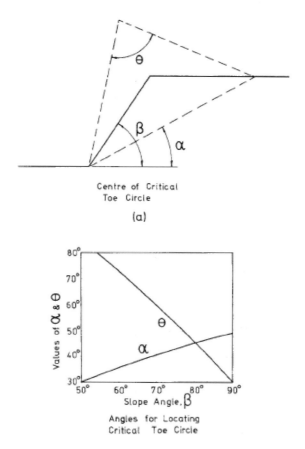

Figure II.3 Location of critical toe circle for simple homogeneous slope
(a) geometry of slope (b) chart for locating centre of critical circle.

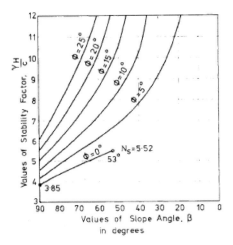

Figure II.4 Taylor's charts for the case when both c and φ are non-zero, (after Terzaghi and Peck, 1967). Permission requested, see page 714, No 44.

- Suppose it is desired to have the same factor of safety with respect to both c and φ. Assume a value $F = F_1$. From available value of $\phi = \phi_a$ obtain ϕ_m from $\tan \phi_m = \tan \phi_a / F_1$. Read $c = c_m$ from the chart corresponding to ϕ_m, γ, H and β. Then check the ratio of available to mobilised cohesion $F_2 = c_a / c_m$. If F_2 is equal to or very close to F_1, then the required $F = F_1$ or F_2. Otherwise use F_2 to get a new value of ϕ_m and use the chart again to get a new value $F_3 = c_a / c_m$. The correct F is usually found in just a few iterations.
- Alternatively, F_ϕ may be specified so that $\tan \phi_m = \tan \phi_a / F_\phi$ is fixed i.e., ϕ_m is fixed. Then F_c is obtained from c_m (which is read from the chart) as $F_c = c_a / c_m$. When $\phi_m = \phi$, $F_c = F_H$ is known as factor of safety with respect to height.

(c) Suppose neither (a) nor (b) above are specified. It may then be useful to assume different values of F_ϕ and obtain corresponding values of F_c. This information could be useful for the designer.

AII.3.1   Special conditions considered by Taylor (1948)

AII.3.1.1   *Submerged slope*

If a slope is fully submerged use Taylor's charts with $\gamma = \gamma'$, given values of φ, c, H etc. (Note $\gamma' = \gamma - \gamma_w$ is the submerged unit of the slope material).

AII.3.1.2   *Rapid or sudden draw down*

Suppose a slope suffers a complete rapid draw down (as may happen for earth dams) and the material of the slope is considered to be impermeable so that no increase of strength can be assumed during rapid draw down. The factor of safety for this condition is obtained by using Taylor's charts with a modified or weighted friction angle ϕ_w:

$$\phi_w = \frac{\gamma'}{\gamma} \phi_m$$

ϕ_w, γ (total unit weight of saturated material), H and β are then used to get the value of c_m from Taylor's chart in the ordinary way. Again, iterations will be required if it is required that $F = F_c = F_\phi$.

Effective stress approach to this draw down case is explained in section AII.6 of this Appendix. Note that values of c and ϕ corresponding to total stress approach are applicable for Taylor's charts. (See item 4 of Table 5.5 in text, chapter 5, for suggested refinements).

AII.3.1.3   Steady seepage case

Taylor's chart cannot be used for an arbitrary pore pressure condition such as long-term condition of steady seepage.

AII.3.1.4   Zero boundary neutral force

This was another condition considered by Taylor which may more accurately be described as a long-term condition when pore pressure is zero or negligible. For such a case use total unit weight γ, and effective stress values of c and ϕ in Taylor's chart. Note that in the example solved by Taylor on page 471–473 of his book, undrained values of c and ϕ are used for this case even though the problem states, "… eventually the water table may recede to an average level below the toe of the slope … values of present and eventual factors of safety are also desired … . Laboratory tests on specimens in which no drainage is permitted furnish the following average soil characteristics…". It is now accepted practice that 'eventual' or long-term conditions must be analysed using effective stress parameters. However, Taylor's chart can be used as the pore pressures are considered zero in this case.

AII.4   COUSINS' (1977) CHARTS – STUDIES IN TERMS OF EFFECTIVE STRESS

Several types of slope stability charts have been devised from time to time for effective stress analysis. In order to account for pore pressure on assumed or actual slip surfaces the parameter r_u indicating a uniform pore pressure ratio is used in most of these charts. The actual pore pressure ratio is generally non-uniform and care is required in selecting an average value for use in the charts. The location of the critical slip circle must be known or assumed before an average value of r_u can be estimated.

There are usually some limitations restricting the use of a given set of charts. For instance the charts prepared by Bishop and Morgenstern (1960) are for a slope angle range of (11°–27°) only and considerable interpolation and extrapolation may be required to determine the value of the factor of safety. Also no information is given concerning the location of the critical slip circles. The charts prepared by Spencer (1967) cover a slope angle range upto 34°. These charts are for toe circles only and an iterative procedure is required to determine the factor of safety for a given slope. Charts prepared by Janbu* (1967) are also for toe circles only. One good feature of his charts is that all the information has been packed in a relatively small number of charts. This is achieved by plotting the stability number $N_F = F\gamma H/c'$ against the slope angle α for a series of values of the dimensionless parameter $\lambda_{c\phi} = (1 - r_u)\, \gamma H \tan \phi'/c'$.

Cousins (1977) used Taylor's (1937, 1948) friction circle method to devise charts in terms of effective stresses. (Different analytical procedures have been used by others referred to above). He used the parameter $\lambda_{c\phi} = \gamma H \tan \phi'/c'$ proposed by Janbu and also investigated the usefulness of the modified parameter $\lambda_{c\phi} = (1 - r_u)\, \lambda c\phi$ also proposed by Janbu. Cousins' charts have the following desirable features:

(1) Critical toe circles are considered and in addition critical circles are also considered for given depth factors D of 1, 1.25, 1.50. The depth factor is defined as the ratio:

$$\frac{\text{Vertical distance between top of slope and lowest point on the slip circle}}{\text{Height of Slope}} = \frac{DH}{H}.$$

Even toe circles may have a depth factor greater than 1. In fact values of $D \geq 1$ for toe circles are shown on the corresponding charts. Charts which refer to specific values of D greater than 1 may or may not indicate base failure. Depending on relevant slope parameters, the lower end of the critical circle may intersect the slope either above or below the toe even when D is greater than 1. In terms of effective stress, critical circles are not always toe circles for values of ϕ greater than approximately 3° as is generally believed (e.g., Terzaghi and Peck, 1967, p. 242).

In chapter 5 of the text a statement was repeated after Terzaghi and Peck to the following effect: "If a typical base failure has occurred in fairly homogeneous soil in the field, it can be concluded that with respect to total stresses the value of ϕ for the soil at the time of the failure was close to zero." This statement is based on interpretation in terms of 'total stress'. However, there are many problems in which a 'total stress' approach may not be applicable at all and this point has been emphasised in the text at several places. For example the long-term stability of a cutting or a natural slope cannot be assessed in terms of 'total stress' analysis when non-zero pore pressures are considered. Therefore, the above statement must be restricted to slides or failures in which a 'total stress' analysis is valid.

(2) Cousins' charts cover a wide range of slope angles upto 45° and pore pressure ratios $r_u = 0$, 0.25 and 0.5.

(3) The necessity for interpolation, extrapolation and iteration has been reduced to a minimum by good choice of dimensionless parameters as suggested by Janbu. In contrast to other types of charts the value of $F = F_c = F_\phi$ is directly obtained. (If it is desired to have F_c different from F_ϕ the charts are still useful although a couple of iterations may be required.)

---

* Janbu, N. (1967). Discussion of paper, 'Dimensionless parameters for homogeneous slopes by J.M. Bell, J. Soil Mech. Found. Div., ASCE, 93, SM6, 367–374.

(4) Information is provided about the location of the critical circles. This information is useful in many ways e.g., comparing actual slip surface locations to theoretical slip surface locations, estimating average pore pressure ratio r_u for use in analysis etc.

In view of all these features, the entrie set of chartis included here.

Figures II.5, II.6 and II.7 are for critical toe circles with different values of r_u. Figures II.8, II.9 and II.10 each cover depth factors of 1, 1.25 and 1.5 and different values of r_u. Figures II.11 to II.13 give the co-ordinates of centre of critical toe circles for the three values of r_u chosen for the charts. Figures II.14 to II.16 give the co-ordinates

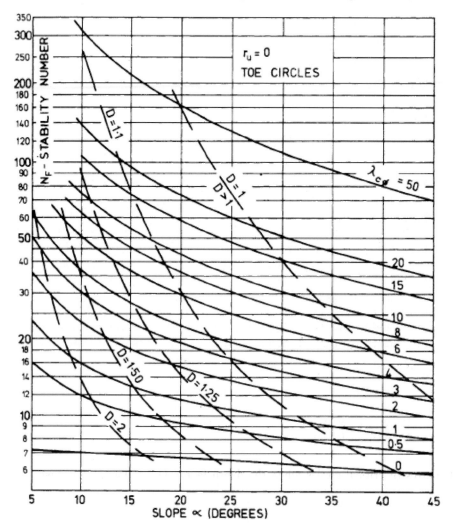

Figure II.5 Stability number N_F considering critical toe circles when $r_u = 0$. With permission, see page 714, No 38.

Note: Charts AII.5 to AII.18 are taken from Cousins (1977) a shortened version of which has been published as the following paper. Cousins, B.F. (1978). Stability charts for simple earth slopes, journal of Geotechnical Engineering Division, ASCE, 104, February, 1978.

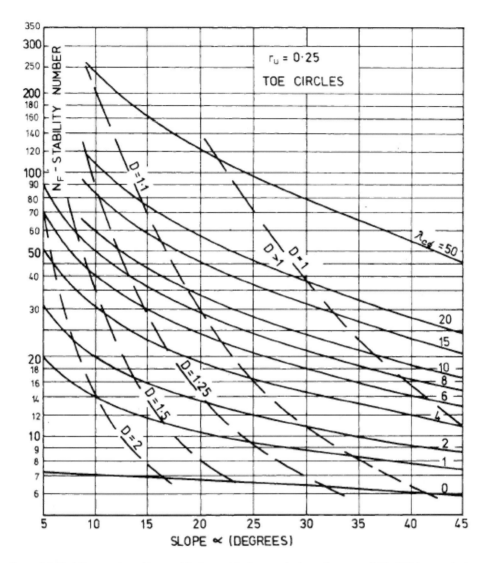

Figure II.6 Stability number N_F considering critical toe circles when $r_u = 0.25$. With permission, see page 714, No 38.

of centres of critical circles when the depth factor $D = 1$. Figure II.17 gives the co-ordinates of the centre of the critical circle for $D = 1.25$ and $r_u = 0$ and Figure II.18 for $D = 1.5$ and $r_u = 0$. Note that in all these charts for critical slip surface location the co-ordinates X and Y of the centre are defined with respect to the origin at the toe of a simple homogeneous slope. (X positive into the slope, Y positive upward).

Before considering an example concerning the use of these charts, let us give some attention to the usefulness of the parameter $\lambda'_{c\phi} = (1 - r_u)\lambda_{c\phi}$. Cousins investigated the possibility of allowing for pore pressure by using such a parameter. If such a procedure were correct the number of charts could be considerably reduced.

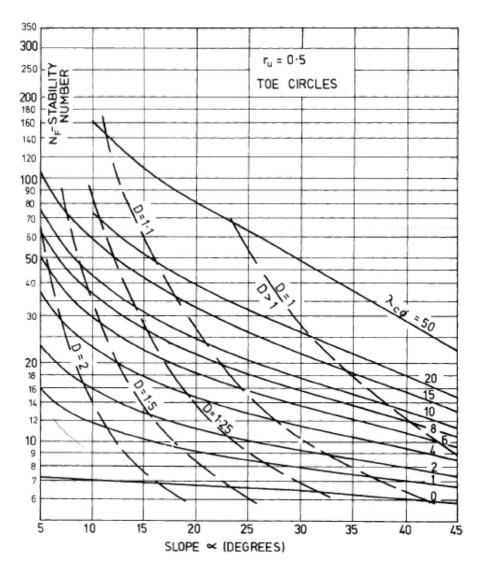

Figure II.7 Stability number N_F considering critical toe circles when $r_u = 0.5$. With permission, see page 714, No 38.

One chart (for $r_u = 0$) would be sufficient instead of different charts for different values of r_u, other conditions remaining the same. For example in Figure II.6 curves for $\lambda_{c\phi} = 20,8,4$ for $r_u = 0.25$ would be identical to curves for $\lambda_{c\phi} = 15,6,3$ in Figure II.5 for $r_u = 0$. However, general agreement was not found and care is required if $\lambda_{c\phi}'$ is to be used as a parameter. There is reasonable agreement for low values of (1) slope angle α, (2) pore pressure ratio r_u and, (3) parameter $\lambda_{c\phi}$. As the values of these parameters increase the inaccuracy in F calculated by using $\lambda_{c\phi}'$ (and the chart for $r_u = 0$) also increases. The loss of accuracy is very high for extreme cases. For example, if $\alpha = 45°$, $r_u = 0.5$ and $\lambda_{c\phi} = 20$, use of $\lambda_{c\phi}'$ gives F value 50% higher than

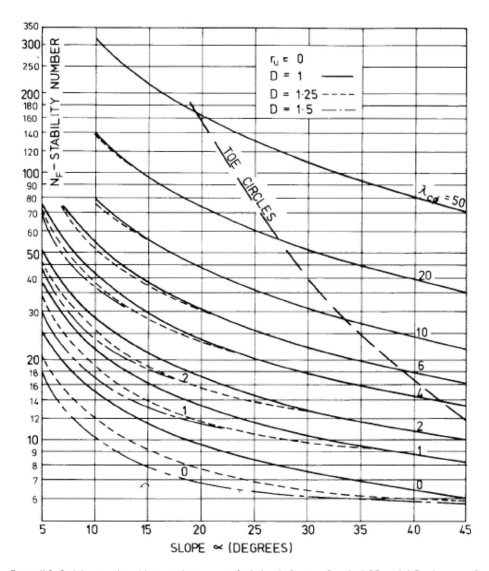

Figure II.8 Stability number N_F considering specified depth factors $D = 1$, 1.25 and 1.5 when $r_u = 0$. With permission, see page 714, No 38.

the value of F given by use of $\lambda_{c\phi}$ and the correct chart for $r_u = 0.5$. The error is always on the unsafe side. In order to restrict the error to about 5%, Cousins provides the following guidelines:

1   Slope angle α should be less than 17.5°, while r_u and $\lambda_{c\phi}$ may have any values. Alternatively,

2   Slope angle α should be less than 25°, r_u should be less than 0.25 and $\lambda_{c\phi}$ may have any value.

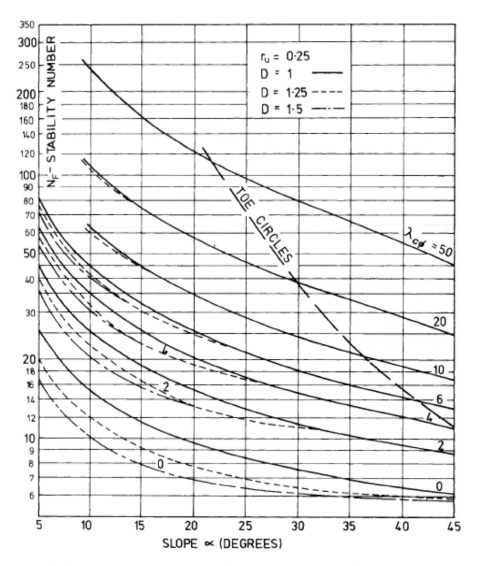

Figure II.9 Stability number N_F considering specified depth factors $D = 1$, 1.25 and 1.5 when $r_u = 0.25$. With permission, see page 714, No 38.

If either of these conditions is met $\lambda'_{c\phi}$ and chart for $r_u = 0$ may be used with confidence since an error of about 5% is generally considered acceptable.

As a final comment, Cousins' charts give results which are in good agreement with the results obtained by methods used by Bishop and Morgenstern (1960), Spencer (1967) and Taylor (1937, 1948) for the range of values of parameters for which respective charts can be used. However, Cousins found that Janbu's (1967) charts give F values (for the case when $r_u = 0$) which are low in comparison with values from other charts. The use of Cousins' charts is explained below in section AII.5.

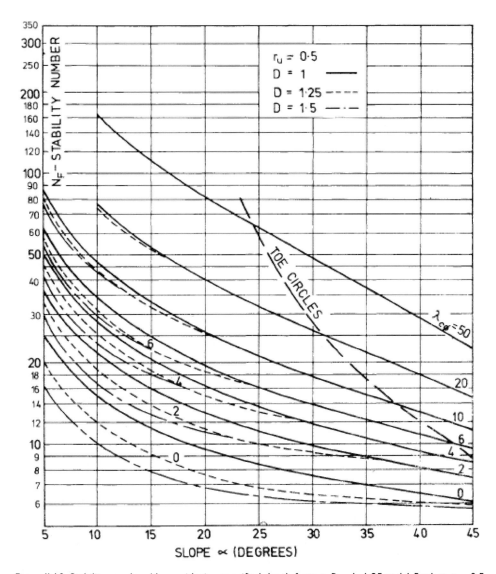

Figure II.10 Stability number N_F considering specified depth factors $D = 1$, 1.25 and 1.5 when $r_u = 0.5$. With permission, see page 714, No 38.

Cousins, B.F. (1978). Stability charts for simple earth slopes, Journal of Geotechnical Engineering Division, ASCE, 104, February, 1978.

AII.5 EXAMPLE CONCERNING USE OF COUSINS' CHARTS

Problem: Find the factor of safety of a slope for the following parameters: $\alpha = 20°$, $H = 20$ m, $c' = 23.8$ kN/m² (kpa), $\phi' = 20°$, $\gamma = 19.6$ kN/m³. Consider that the analysis

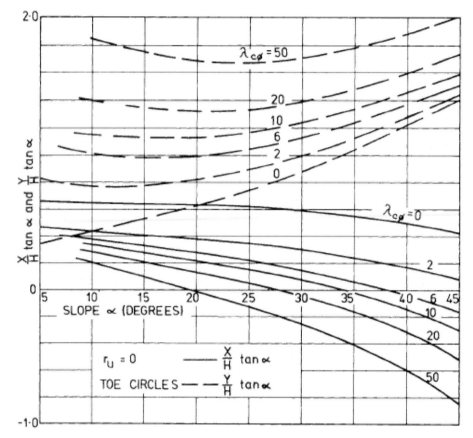

Figure II.11 Co-ordinates (*X* horizontal, *Y* vertical, measured from toe of slope) of centre of critical toe circle when $r_u = 0$. With permission, see page 714, No 38.

Note: *X* is positive into slope and *Y* positive upwards.

is to be made for the steady seepage condition and that pore pressures at each point can be determined readily from a known flow net for the relevant seepage condition. (Note that the accurate determination of pore pressures during steady seepage requires construction of a good flow net. Approximately the pore pressure at any point at depth z below the phreatic surface may be obtained by considering $u = \gamma_w z$. Some idea of the approximation may be had by recalling from chapter 4 that when the phreatic surface is a straight line of inclination β, the pore pressure is given by $u = \gamma_w z \cos^2\beta$).

The solution of the problem requires the following steps.

Step 1   Construct contours of $r_u = u/\gamma z$ by Joining points with equal r_u values 0.1, 0.2, 0.3, 0.4 etc. (See Figure II.E1)

Step 2   Calculate dimensionless parameters. In this case $c'/\gamma H = 0.0607$, $\lambda_{c\phi} = 6.00$.

Step 3   Examine Figures II.8 to II.10 to find critical depth factor using $\alpha = 20°$ and $\lambda_{c\phi} = 6$.

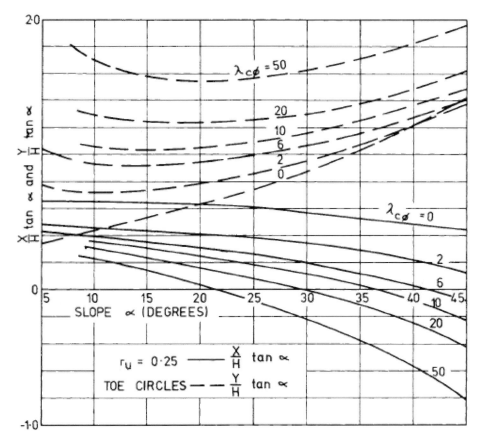

Figure II.12 Co-ordinates (*X* horizontal, *Y* vertical, measured from toe of slope) of centre of critical toe circle when $r_u = 0.25$. With permission, see page 714, No 38.

Note: *X* is positive into slope and *Y* positive upwards.

With $r_u = 0$, $N_F = 30.5$ for both $D = 1$ and 1.25; with $r_u = 0.25$, $N_F = 25$ for $D = 1$ and $N_F = 24.5$ for $D = 1.25$. $D = 1.50$ is not critical even for $r_u = 0.5$. Thus $D = 1.25$ gives the lowest N_F i.e. the lowest factor of safety.

Step 4   Locate critical circle ($D = 1.25$) from Figure II.17.

For $r_u = 0$, co-ordinates of centre are $X = 16.5$ m and $Y = 45.65$ m. For $r_u = 0.25$, use $\lambda'_{c\phi} = (1 - r_u)\lambda_{c\phi} = 4.5$ and Figure II.17 again. The co-ordinates are $X = 18.2$ m, $Y = 46.2$ m.

The co-ordinates of centres as well as the slip surfaces are shown in Figure II.E1.

Step 5   In order to estimate the average value of r_u applicable to each critical circle these circles are plotted on the same diagram on which contours of actual r_u have already been drawn. Suppose that the position of the alternative slip circles considered in step 4 with respect to r_u contours is such that a value of $r_u = 0.2$ *appears reasonable and conservative as an average*. Obviously this requires some judgement which can develop with a bit of experience.

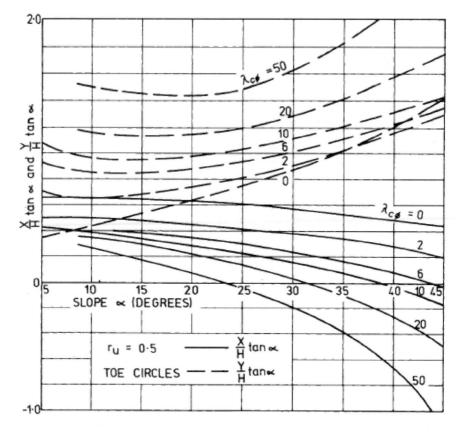

Figure II.13 Co-ordinates (*X* horizontal, *Y* vertical, measured from toe of slope) of centre of critical toe circle when $r_u = 0.5$. With permission, see page 714, No 38.

Note: *X* is positive into slope and *Y* positive upwards.

The value $r_u = 0.2$ may now be adopted for calculation. N_F for $r_u = 0.2$ by interpolation between $r_u = 0$ and $r_u = 0.25$ is given by:

$$NF = 30.5 - (30.5 - 24.5) \times 0.20/0.25 = 25.7$$

$$F = N_F \times \frac{c'}{\gamma H} = 25.7 \times .0607 = 1.56 \, (\text{for } D = 1.25)$$

Alternatively
Instead of interpolation make use of $\lambda'_{c\phi}$ and use Figure II.8 directly.

$$\lambda'_{c\phi} = (1 - r_u)\lambda_{c\phi} = (1 - 0.2)6 = 4.8$$
$$\therefore N_F = 2.6 \text{ from Figure II.8}$$
$$\therefore F = 1.58 \, (\text{for } D = 1.25)$$

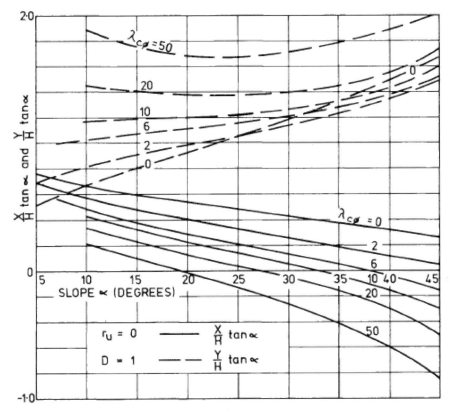

Figure II.14 Co-ordinates (X horizontal, Y vertical, measured from toe of slope) of centre of critical circle with specified depth factor D = 1 when r_u = 0. With permission, see page 714, No 38.

Note: X is positive into slope and Y positive upwards.

In a similar manner charts for toe circles may be used. Note that the value of average r_u with respect to critical toe circle will be different. For this case average value of r_u will be less because the toe circle is located higher than the base circle with D = 1.25. To get the values of D for critical toe circles, refer to the relevant charts II.5 and II.6. Then draw these circles on the same diagram on which contours of actual r_u have been drawn. Suppose that the location of the circles with respect to these contours is such that r_u = 0.15 *appears a reasonable and conservative value as an average*.

With r_u = 0, N_F = 29.5 (Figure II.5)
With r_u = 0.25, N_F = 24 (Figure II.6)
$\therefore N_F$ for r_u = 0.15 by interpolation is given as:
N_F = 29.5–(29.5–24) × 0.15/0.20 = 26.2
$\therefore F$ = 26.2 × 0.0607 = 1.59

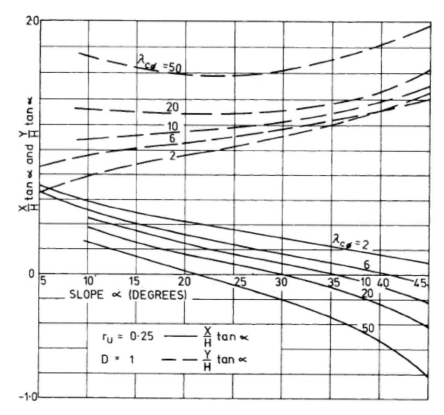

Figure II.15 Co-ordinates (*X* horizontal, *Y* vertical, measured from toe of slope) of centre of critical circle with specified depth factor *D* = 1 when r_u = 0.25. With permission, see page 714, No 38.

Note: *X* is positive into slope and *Y* is positive upwards.

Alternatively

Instead of interpolation use $\lambda'_{c\phi} = 0.85 \times 6 = 5.10$. This gives $N_F = 26.5$ and $F = 1.61$ (using Figure II.5). Note that the values of the factor of the safety obtained in this example are such that $F = F_c = F_\phi$. This is a useful feature of Cousins' charts.

AII.6   CHARTS BY HOEK (1970) AND HOEK AND BRAY (1974, 1977)

Reference has already been made in chapter 5 to stability charts prepared by Hoek (1970). A typical chart for circular failure is shown in Figure II.19. The slope height function $Y = \gamma H/c$ is plotted against slope angle function *X*. The slope angle function is calculated for different positions of phreatic surface and by making different assumptions with respect to tension crack depth, depth of water in tension cracks. One case is shown in Figure II.19 (the phreatic surface is assumed to be horizontal and there is no tension crack). Different equations for slope angle function *X* are given

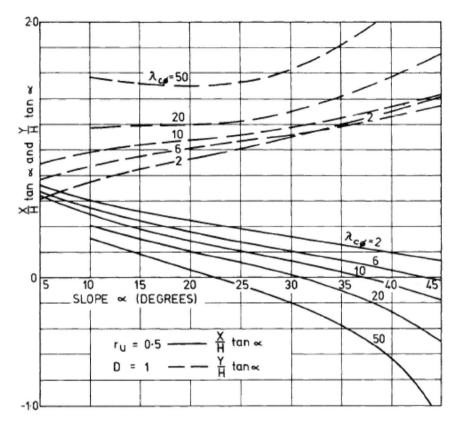

Figure II.16 Co-ordinates (X horizontal and Y vertical, measured from toe of slope) of centre of critical circle with specified depth factor $D = 1$ when $r_u = 0.5$. With permission, see page 714, No 38.

Note: X is positive into slope and Y is positive upwards.

by Hoek (1970) for other cases. This type of stability chart may lead to inaccuracies which become unacceptable for extreme values of slope parameters (E. Hoek, pers. comm. 1978). Therefore Hoek and Bray (1974, 1977) used a different approach to devise improved stability charts. As their charts are widely available, they are not reproduced here. Their charts are based on specific positions of the phreatic surface and, therefore, do not require estimation of an average $\bar{r}_u$. However, the charts can be used only for the four specific seepage conditions to which they correspond. For any other seepage or pore pressure condition, the charts are not directly applicable. Hoek and Bray also assumed a tension crack at any arbitrary position in devising their charts. To give the reader an idea of their approach, Figures II.20 and II.21 are included here. Figure II.20 shows a drained slope (with zero pore water pressure and charts are given to locate the centre of the critical toe circle and the critical position of a tension crack for different slope angles and different values of ϕ. Figure II.21 shows a specific groundwater surface and again charts are given for location of the centre of the critical toe circle and critical position of the tension crack. It is obvious that the

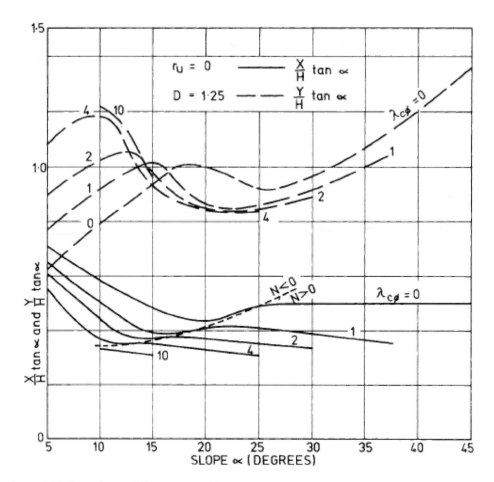

Figure II.17 Co-ordinates (*X* horizontal and *Y* vertical, measured from toe of slope) of centre of critical circle with specified depth factor *D* = 1.25 when r_u = 0. With permission, see page 714, No 38.

pressure of ground water has a significant influence on these critical positions. These two seepage conditions correspond to two of their stability charts.

AII.7 RAPID DRAW DOWN-EFFECTIVE STRESS APPROACH (AFTER BISHOP, 1954 AND SKEMPTON, 1954)

The pore pressure changes occurring during rapid draw down may be estimated if the values of pore pressure parameters *A* and *B* (Skempton, 1954) are known.

Following Bishop (1954) the following equations are relevant:

Initial pore pressure in an element of soil beneath the upstream slope of an earth dam is given by (Figure II.22) u_0:

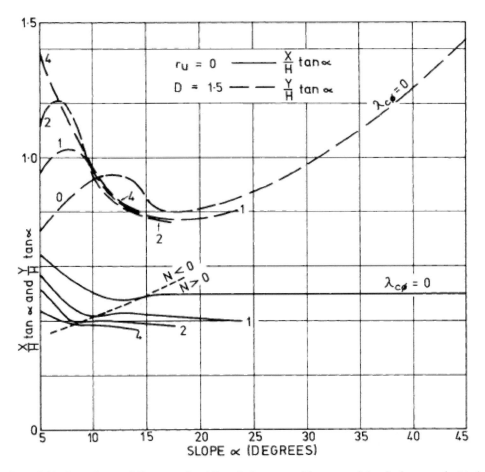

Figure II.18 Co-ordinates (X horizontal and Y vertical, measured from toe of slope) of centre of critical circle with specified depth factor $D = 1.5$ and $r_u = 0$. With permission, see page 714, No 38.

$$u_0 = \gamma_w(h_c + h_r + h_w - h')$$ (AII.1)

After rapid draw down the pore pressure is u where:

$$u = u_0 + \Delta u$$ (AII.2)

Δu is the excess pore pressure (or pore pressure increment) resulting from change of total stresses during draw down and in terms of parameters A and B:

$$\Delta u = B[\Delta\sigma_3 + A(\Delta\sigma_1 - \Delta\sigma_3)]$$ (AII.3)

The pore pressure increment may be expressed as a ratio of the major principal stress increment as follows: (Skempton, 1954)

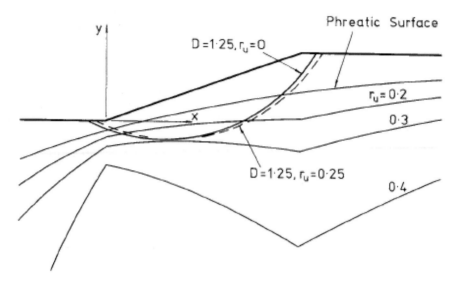

Figure II.E1 Procedure for plot of contours of r_u to estimate $\bar{r}_u$ for different critical slip surfaces. Co-ordinates of critical slip surfaces are shown for two values of depth factor D and r_u.

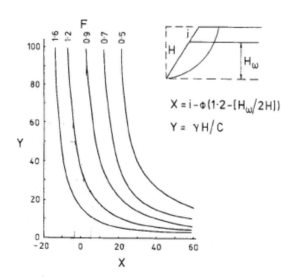

Figure II.19 Chart for approximate calculation of F considering different seepage conditions from which slope angle function is calculated (after Hoek, 1970). For extreme values of slope parameters the accuracy of F from this type of chart may be in doubt (E. Hoek, pers. comm. 1978). With permission, see page 714, No 40.

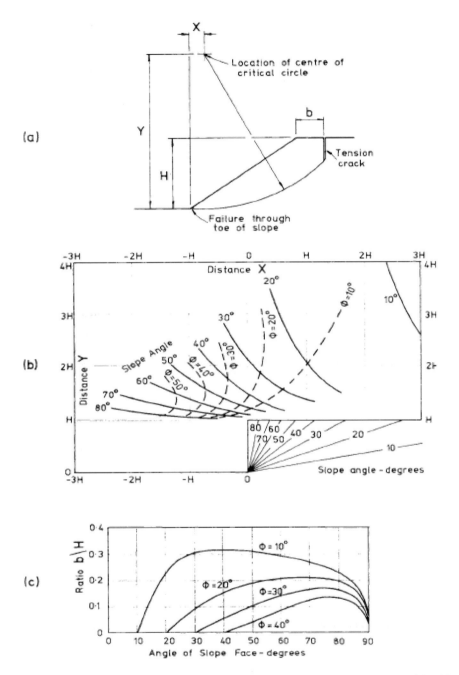

Figure II.20 Location of critical failure surface and critical tension crack for drained slopes, (after Hoek and Bray, 1977). With permission, see page 714, No 39 & 40.

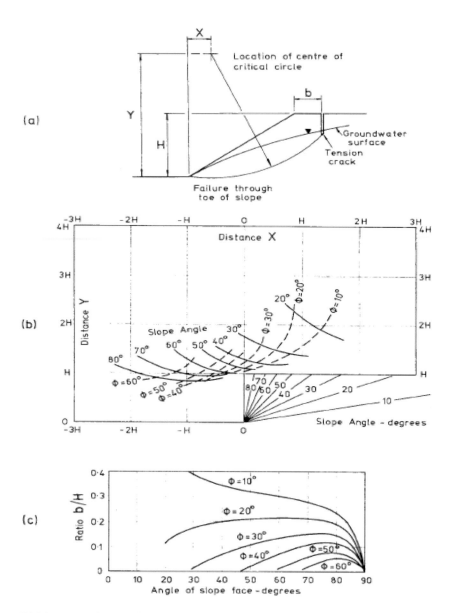

Figure II.21 Location of critical failure surface and critical tension crack for slopes with groundwater present, (after Hoek and Bray, 1977). With permission, see page 714, No 39 & 40.

$$\frac{\Delta u}{\Delta \sigma_1} = \bar{B} = B \left\{ 1 - (1 - A) \left(1 - \frac{\Delta \sigma_3}{\Delta \sigma_1} \right) \right\} \tag{AII.4}$$

Thus $\bar{B}$ is an overall pore pressure co-efficient so that:

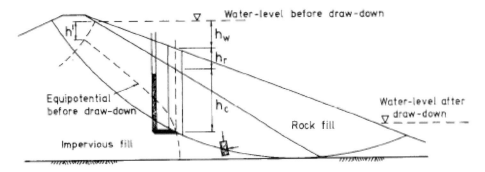

Figure II.22 Diagram. explaining effective stress approach using pore pressure parameters for rapid draw down, (after Bishop, 1954).

$$\Delta u = \bar{B}\Delta\sigma_1 \tag{AII.4a}$$

From equation (AII.3) we now have

$$u = u_0 + \bar{B}\Delta\sigma_1 \tag{AII.5}$$

The magnitude and direction of the major principal stress varies from point to point. But as an approximation the magnitude of the major principal stress at any point in an embankment may be considered as equal to the vertical head of soil above that point. Therefore we have:

$$\text{Before draw down } (\sigma_1)_0 = \gamma_c h_c + \gamma_r h_r + \gamma_w h_w \tag{AII.6}$$

$$\text{After draw down } \sigma_1 = \gamma_c h_c + \gamma_{rd} h_r \tag{AII.7}$$

where γ_c is saturated unit weight of clay fill or clay core, γ_r is saturated unit weight of rock fill, γ_{rd} is drained unit weight of rockfill. Thus

$$\Delta\sigma_1 = \sigma_1 - (\sigma_1)_0 = -\{(\gamma_r - \gamma_{rd})h_r + \gamma_w h_w\} \tag{AII.8}$$

Assuming the free-draining rockfill to have a specific porosity n

$$\gamma_{rd} = \gamma_r - n\gamma_w \quad \text{and} \quad \Delta\sigma_1 = -\gamma_w(nh_r + h_w) \tag{AII.9}$$

From Equations (AII.1), (AII.4a) and (AII.9)

$$u = \gamma_w\{h_c + h_r\,(1 - \bar{B}n) + h_w(1 - \bar{B}) - h'\} \tag{AII.10}$$

From Equation (AII.10) it follows that the residual pore pressure u increases as $\bar{B}$ decreases. Bishop (1954) concluded that as a safe working rule $\bar{B}$ may be taken as unity. (For saturated soils $B = 1$ and upper limit of A in practice is also 1. During draw down total major principal stress is decreased and total minor principal stress is decreased by an even greater extent. Thus $\bar{B}$ is likely to be greater than 1. Therefore $\bar{B} = 1$ giving greater u is a conservative assumption.) With $\bar{B} = 1$, Equation (AII.10) becomes:

$$u = \gamma_w \{h_c + h_r (1-n) - h'\} \tag{AII.11}$$

According to Bishop (1954) this has been found to give satisfactory agreement with field measurements.

Full saturation may not occur in practice so that B is less than 1. However, the magnitudes of A and B measured in a conventional undrained test are not applicable. The recommended test procedure is:

1   Allow the sample to come to equilibrium under total principal stresses and pore pressure corresponding to a particular element of soil during steady seepage. Maintain flow of water to reproduce a representative degree of saturation.
2   Reduce principal stresses under undrained conditions to reproduce decrease in major principal stress and increase in shear stress after draw down. The shear stresses may be deduced from a typical slip surface passing through the element under consideration.
3   Measure pore pressure changes.

The reduction in stress is best carried out in two stages – i.e., (a) equal reduction in σ_1 and σ_3 so that B can be obtained. B gives an indication of the degree of saturation and (b) further reduction in σ_3 to give additional shear stress, enabling value of $\bar{B}$ to be determined.

For a moraine and a clay-gravel (boulder clay) Bishop found $\bar{B}$ between 1.1 and 1.4. In one case $\bar{B}$ was 1.14 but B was 0.57 and A was -1.0. These values show the marked influence of change in shear stress on pore pressure.

Once values of pore pressure immediately after draw down have been calculated for saturated or partially saturated soil by the above procedure, an effective stress analysis may be carried out for stability. For circular slip surfaces charts such as these of Cousins (1977) included here may be used.

Pore pressures after draw down must be expressed in terms of ratio r_u to use the charts.

AII.8   CONSTRUCTION PORE PRESSURES IN IMPERVIOUS FILL OF EARTH DAM (AFTER BISHOP, 1954)

Equation (AII.4a) may be expressed in terms of effective stress ratio K as follows:

$$K = \frac{\Delta\sigma_3'}{\Delta\sigma_1'} = \frac{\Delta\sigma_3 - u}{\Delta\sigma_1 - u} = \frac{\Delta\sigma_3 - \bar{B}\Delta\sigma_1}{\Delta\sigma_1 - \bar{B}\Delta\sigma_1} \tag{AII.12}$$

giving

$$\bar{B} = B \frac{1-(1-A)(1-K)}{1-B(1-A)(1-K)} \tag{AII.12a}$$

For a sandy gravel with value of K ranging from 0.5 (at rest) to 0.3 (failure) and with $A = 0.5$ and $B = 0.8$, $\bar{B}$ lies between 0.75 and 0.72. For a clay-gravel with K ranging from 0.4 (at rest) to 0.25 (failure) and with $A = 0$ and $B = 0.8$, $\bar{B}$ lies between 0.6 and 0.5.

For a more accurate estimate attention should be given to factors such as:

1   Variation of A and B with magnitude of stresses
2   Variation of A with principle stress ratio.

Once (A and B) or $\bar{B}$ are known, Δu can be calculated from Equations (AII.3) or (AII.4a).

To get values of A and B accurately follow the same stress paths or loading sequence as occurs during construction with respect to element of soil under consideration.

Morgenstern and Price approach – some additional particulars

AIII.1 SIDE FORCE ASSUMPTIONS

In the Morgenstern and Price method of limit equilibrium stability analysis, an assumption is made about the relationship between horizontal or normal components E and vertical or tangential components T of the force acting on any boundary between two vertical slices. (The potential sliding mass is divided into a number of vertical slices in all variants of the method of slices). The assumption may take either of the following forms corresponding respectively to total stress normal force E or effective stress normal force $\bar{E}$:

$$T = \lambda f(x)E \tag{AIII.1}$$

or

$$T = \lambda f(x)\bar{E} \tag{AIII.2}$$

Several types of functions $f(x)$ may be assumed to represent the manner in which the relationship between T and E (or $\bar{E}$) forces changes from one end of a sliding mass to the other (e.g. see Bailey, 1966; Hamel, 1968). Figure III.1 shows the following assumptions:

No. 1. Constant side force assumption $f(x) = $ constant. This implies parallel inter-slice forces

No. 2. $f(x) = $ half sine curve

No. 3. $f(x) = $ half sine curve of amplitude 2 clipped at value greater than 1

No. 4. $f(x) = $ half sine wave added to a trapezoid. Here a and b are specified by the use of a computer program

No. 5. $f(x) = $ full sine wave adjusted as shown

No. 6. $f(x) = $ full sine wave of amplitude 2 but clipped at values greater than 1

No. 7. $f(x) = $ full sine wave added to trapezoid

No. 8. $f(x) = $ arbitrary.

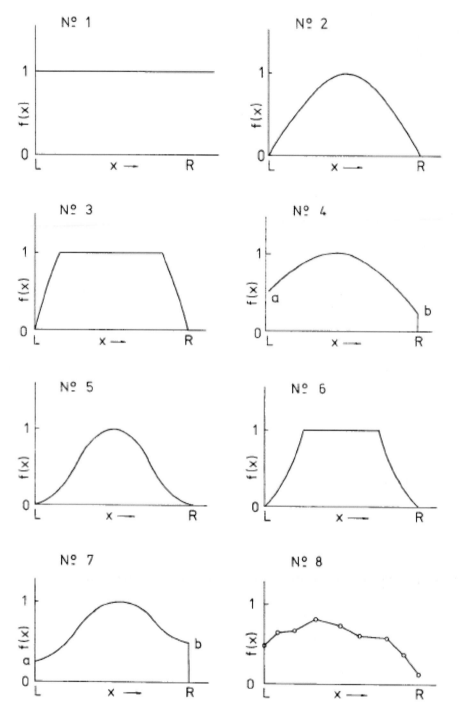

Figure III.1 Some side force assumptions that may be made when using the Morgenstern and Price Method (after Hamel, 1968). With permission from Dr. James V. Hamel, see page 714, No 41.

Any one of the side force assumptions listed above or other curvilinear assumptions may be used in a program. However, the chosen side force assumption may not lead to acceptable results (acceptability criteria are discussed separately below). Therefore, provision is made for several side force assumptions in a computer program and results are computed using all these alternative assumptions unless experience has demonstrated the use of a particular side force assumption produces the best results for a given type of problem.

The first assumption $f(x)$ – constant, which implies parallel inter-slice forces, is usually a satisfactory one and should be used as a first trial. Hamel (1968) found that this assumption leads to admissible solutions in a wide range of problems involving soil and rock slopes. Chowdhury and Bertoldi[*] (1977a) found that results given by Morgenstern Price Method compared well with results of other methods if $f(x) =$ constant assumption was made. On the other hand, significant errors could arise if the other alternative assumptions were made. However, this conclusion applied only to some specific problems. There may well be cases in which a constant side force assumption does not prove satisfactory and several alternative assumptions have to be tried before a satisfactory result is obtained. For example Hamel (1968) found that $f(x) =$ constant does not give a solution satisfying the criteria for the heights of the points of application of the effective normal side forces where the toe of the potential failure mass is acted upon by high water pressures e.g., a submerged toe (the points of application of the effective normal side forces $\bar{E}$ frequently fall above the tops of the slices in the toe region). In these cases admissible solutions were obtained with $f(x) =$ a parabola or $f(x) =$ a half sine wave. Such a curve should have a zero amplitude at the toe of the failure mass but its amplitude across the rest of the mass must be adjusted to give an admissible solution.

In practice it is necessary to gain some experience with different types of problems before a user can know in advance what side force distribution to use for best results.

AIII.2   ADMISSIBILITY CRITERIA FOR MORGENSTERN AND PRICE SOLUTION

It is generally agreed that to be admissible a limit equilibrium solution must give a reasonable distribution of normal stresses on the assumed failure surface. The general limit equilibrium slope stability problem is statically indeterminate and there is no unique normal stress distribution for a given failure surface. In the Morgenstern and Price method a set of assumptions is made to render the problem statically determinate and each set of assumptions leads to a corresponding normal stress distribution and value of factor of safety F. A reasonable normal stress distribution may be defined as one which is consistent with the assumed physical or mechanical behaviour of the sliding mass. It is usual to examine not only the stresses on the failure surface but also on the vertical slice boundaries between slices. The following criteria for the admissibility of limit equilibrium solutions to soil slope stability problems have

* Chowdhury, R.N. and Bertoldi, C. (1977a). Unpublished work concerning Progressive Failure Studies by Limit Equilibrium Using Morgenstern and Price Method.

been proposed (e.g., Morgenstern and Price, 1965; Bailey, 1966; Whitman and Bailey, 1967):

1 There must be no effective tensile stresses on inter-slice boundaries
2 The shear stresses acting on any inter-slice boundary must be less than those required for local critical equilibrium. In other words, the assumed shear strength criterion or failure criterion must not be violated within a failure mass.

In practice a computer program usually calculates the total and effective forces on vertical inter-slice boundaries rather than stresses. The line of thrust (locus of points of application of the inter-slice or side wall forces) may be plotted for either 'total stress' side forces or 'effective stress' side forces. The latter is useful in assessing admissibility criteria in terms of stresses stated above.

Hamel (1968) proposed specific criteria for evaluating Morgenstern and Price solutions which are useful in practice. These criteria are in terms of calculated forces on slice boundaries rather than stresses. He gave separate criteria for soil slopes and rock slopes as shown below:

Table III.1 Admissibility criteria for evaluating Morgenstern and Price solution for soil and rock slope stability problems, (after Hamel, 1968).

Soil slope problems
Criteria
1 The effective normal forces on the sides and bases of slices should be compressive.
2 The height of the point of application of each of the effective normal side forces should be between 0.25 H and 0.65 H, where H is the height of any inter-slice boundary.
3 The average friction angle required (or mobilised) on the sides of any slice (when cohesion is considered fully mobilised) should be less than 80% of the average available friction angle along that surface.

Rock slope problem
Criteria
1 The effective normal forces on the sides and bases of slices should be compressive.
2 The height of the point of application of each effective side force should be between 0.15 H and 0.75 H where H is the height of any inter-slice boundary.
3 The average friction angle required or mobilised on the side of each slice (when cohesion is considered to be fully mobilised) should be equal to or less than the average available friction angle.

Notes: 1 The criteria for rock slope problems are somewhat less conservative than those for soil slope problems.
2 The criteria may be modified at the discretion of the geotechnical engineering expert on the basis of experience.
3 In general it is difficult to satisfy the criteria simultaneously for all slices. Therefore the criteria may be relaxed somewhat near the crest because theoretical and experimental investigations have shown that tensile stresses generally exist in the region.
4 The criteria may also be relaxed for slopes which are failing progressively.
5 While different solutions (based on different side force assumptions) lead to different factors of safety, the difference is not significant if the above admissibility criteria are satisfied in each solution. The difference in F seldom exceeds 0.05 for soil slopes or 0.08 for rock slopes.

AIII.3   TYPICAL COMPARISONS

AIII.3.1   Brilliant cut slide

Factor of safety F from an Admissible Morgenstern and Price Solution compared to F from other methods, (after Hamel, 1969).*

Method of analysis		Factor of safety
1 Morgenstern and Price		1.02
2 Sliding block		
inclination of	$\alpha = 0°$	0.77
inter-block	$\alpha = 30°$	0.87
forces	$\alpha = 45°$	1.00
3 Fellenius		0.97
4 Bishop		1.09

Notes: The failure surface had a 100 ft. deep water filled tension crack at the rear and passed mostly through rock with $c = 1.8$ kips/ft^2 and $\phi = 23°$. The existence of large horizontal thrust due to water pressure as the main disturbing force perhaps explains why Fellenius' approach is not very inaccurate here.

*Hamel, J.V. (1969). Stability of Slopes in Soft, Altered Rocks, Ph.D. Thesis, Univ. of Pittsburgh – chapter 6.

AIII.3.2   Navdocks example problem

Factor of safety with different side force assumptions. (Solutions satisfy acceptability criteria to different degrees, (after Hamel, 1968).

Solution and assumption	Factor of safety F	Computed λ
Earth pressure sliding block approach	1.08	
Morgenstern and Price with $f(x)$		
• constant side force	1.53	–0.15
• half sine wave	1.43	–0.21
• clipped half sine wave	1.47	–0.17
• bell shape	1.36	–0.26
• clipped bell shape	1.41	–0.20

AIII.4   CONCLUSIONS

1   The Morgenstern and Price Method requires a computer solution and hand calculations are totally impracticable. It requires the entire potential sliding mass to be in complete statical equilibrium.

2   Assumptions must be made with regard to inter-slice forces. Different side force assumptions may lead to quite different values of the factor of safety in some situations.

3   Acceptability or admissibility criteria must be adopted before the results are evaluated. These criteria must depend on the type of stability problem being solved.

4   The Morgenstern and Price Method can handle a failure surface of irregular shape and is suitable for both soil and rock slopes.

5   The method is suitable only for two-dimensional problems and should not be relied upon when three-dimensional effects are important in a slope stability problem.

6   It is useful to compare the results with results obtained by other methods based on limit equilibrium.

7   It is desirable to make comparisons with stress analysis solutions. These comparisons may prove useful for interpretation of results.

8   Results of field observations of actual slope failures, back analyses etc. are useful in evaluating the usefulness of limit equilibrium methods under a wide range of conditions.

9   Improved criteria for admissible solutions must be found. These must be based on a better understanding of the behaviour of soil and rock masses in the field. Such an understanding can only be gained by observation of failures and research into the behaviour of slopes and slope forming materials.

References

Aas, G., 1976. Soil properties, their determination and use in stability analysis of clays, NIF Course, Gol 1976, Five lectures in Norwegian Geotechnical Society, 69 pp.

Abdelhamid, M.S. and Krizek, R.J., 1976. At-rest lateral earth pressure of a consolidating clay, J. Geotech. Engg. Div., ASCE, 102, GT7; 712–738.

Abramento, M. and Carvalho, C.S., 1989. Geotechnical parameters for the study of natural slopes instabilisation at "Serra do Mar", Brazil, proc. 12th int. Conf. on Soil Mech. and Found. Engg., Rio de Janeiro, 3, 1599–1602.

AGS, 2000. Landslide Risk Management Concepts and Guidelines, Australian Geomechanics, Vol. 35, 49–92.

Aleotti, P., 2004. A warning system for rainfall-induced shallow slides, Engineering Geology, 73(3–4); 247–265.

Aleotti, P. and Chowdhury, R. 1999. Landslide hazard assessment: summary review and new perspectives. Bulletin of Engineering Geology and the Environment, 58, 21–44.

Ambraseys, N.N., 1960. The seismic stability of earth dams, Proc. Second World Conference on Earthquake Engineering, 2, Japan.

Ambraseys, N.N. and Menu, J., 1988. Earthquake-induced ground displacements, Earthquake Engineering and Structural Dynamics, Vol. 16, 985–1006.

Ambraseys, N.N. and Sarma, S.K., 1967. The response of earth dams to strong earthquakes, Geotechnique, 17, 3; 181–213.

Ambraseys, N.N. and Srbulov, M., 1995. Earthquake induced displacement of slopes, Soil Dynamics and Earthquake Engineering, 14, 59–71.

American Society of Civil Engineers, 1974. Analysis and Design in Geotechnical Engineering, Vol. 1, p. 327, Vol. 2, 179 pp.

ANCOLD, 1994. Guidelines on Risk Assessment, Australian National Committee on Large Dams, Sydney, 116 pp.

Anderson, D.L., 1985. Static slope analysis method used for the Vaiont Slide analyses (Appendix B), Calculation of slide velocities (Appendix E), and Heat generated pore pressure mechanisms (Appendix F), all three in the Report of Hendron and Patton, Vol. II.

Ang, A.H-.S. and Cornell, C.A., 1974. Reliability bases of structural safety and design, Journal of the Structural Division, ASCE, 100, ST9; 1755–1769.

Ang, A.H-S and Tang, W.H., 1975. Probability Concepts in Engineering Planning and Design, Vol. 1 – Basic Principles, John Wiley & Sons, 409 pp.

Ang, A.H-S. and Tang, W.H., 1984. Probability Concepts in Engineering Planning and Design, Vol. II – Decision, Risk and Reliability, John Wiley & Sons, Inc, 562 pp.

Ang, A.H-S. and Tang, W.H., 2007. Probability Concepts In Engineering, Emphasis on applications to Civil and Environmental Engineering, (2nd edition of Probability Concepts in Engineering Planning and Design, Vol. I, Basic Principles, 1975), John Wiley & Sons, Inc, 406 pp.

Arai, K. and Tagyo, K., 1985. Determination of non-circular slip surface giving the minimum factor of safety in slope stability analysis, Soils and Foundations, 25(1); 43–51.

Araya, R and Saragoni, R., 1984. Earthquake accelerogram destructiveness potential factor, Proc 8thWCEE, San Francisco, 2, 835–841.

Ashford, S.A. and Sitar, N., 1997. Analysis of topographic amplification of inclined shear waves in a steep coastal bluff, Bulletin of the Seismological Society of America, 87(3); 1997, 692–700.

Ashford, S.A. and Sitar, N., 1998. Topographic amplification in the 1994 Northbridge earthquake: analysis of observations, Proc 6th US National Conference on Earthquake Engineering, Seattle, 9.

Ashford, S.A., Sitar, N., Lysmer, J. and Deng, N., 1997. Topographic effects on the seismic response of steel slopes, Bulletin of the Seismological Society of America, 48(3); 701–709.

Attewell, P.B. and Farmer, I.W., 1976. Principles of Engineering Geology. Chapman and Hall, London, 1045 pp.

Babu, G.L.S. and Murthy, D.S.N., 2005. Reliability analysis of unsaturated soil slopes, Technical Note, Journal of Geotechnical and Geoenvironmental Engineering Division, ASCE, Vol. 131, No. 11, 1423–1428.

Baecher, G.B. and Christian, J.T., 2003. Reliability and Statistics in Geotechnical Engineering, John Wiley & Sons Ltd., 605 pp.

Bagnold, R.A., 1954. Experiments on a gravity-free dispersion of large solid spheres in a Newton fluid under shear. Proc. Royal Soc. Lond., Ser. A, 225: 49–63.

Bagnold, R.A., 1956. The flow of cohesionless grains in fluids, Proc. Royal Soc. Lond., Ser. A, 249: 235–297.

Baguelin, F., Jezequel, J., Lemeeg, E. and Mehaute, A. Le., 1972. Expansion of cylindrical probes in cohesive soils, J. Soil Mech. Found. Div., ASCE, 98, SM11; 1129–1142.

Bailey, W.A., 1966. Stability Analysis by Limiting Equilibrium, C.E. Thesis, Massachusetts Institute of Technology, U.S.A.

Baker, B., 1881. The actual lateral pressure of earthwork, Min. Proc. Ins. Civ. Eng., 65: 140–186.

Baker, R., 1980. Determination of critical slip surface in slope stability computations, Int. J. Numerical and Analytical Methods in Geomechanics, 4: 33–359.

Baker, R. and Garber, M., 1977. Variational approach to slope stability, Proc. 9th Int. Conf. Soil Mech. Found. Eng., 2: 9–13.

Baker, R., Shukha, R. and Leshchinsky, D., 2005. Stability of cohesionless partially submerged slopes, International Journal for Numerical and Analytical Methods in Geomechanics. 29(12); pp. 1157–1170.

Baligh, M.M. and Azzouz, A.S., 1975. End effects on stability of cohesive soils, J. Geotech. Eng. Div., ASCE, 101, GT11; 1105–1117.

Banks, D.C., 1975. Study of clay shale slopes along the Panama Canal; Engineering analyses of slides and strength properties of clay shales along the Gaillard Cut, U.S. Army Engineers Waterways Expt. Station, Tech. Rep. S-70-9, Report 3, Vicksburg, U.S.A.

Banks, D.C. and MacIver, B.N., 1969. Variation in angle of internal friction with confining pressure, U.S. Army Engineers Waterways Experiment Station, Paper S-169-12, Vicksburg, U.S.A.

Banks, D.C. and Strohm, W.F., 1974. Calculation of rock slide velocities, Proc. 3rd Int. Cong. Rock Mech., Denver, 2, B; 839–847.

Barton, N., 1971. A model study of the behaviour of excavated slopes, Ph.D. Thesis, University of London, Imperia College of Science and Technology, 520 pp.

Barton, N., 1972. Progressive failure of excavated rock slopes, 13th Symp. Rock Mech., Urbana (Illinois), Ed. E.J. Cording, ASCE; 139–171.

Barton, N., 1973. Review of new shear strength criterion for rock joints, Engineering Geology, 7: 287–332.

Barton, N., 1974. A review of the shear strength of filled discontinuities in rock, Norwegian Geotechnical Institute, Publication No. 105, 38 pp.

Barton, N., 1976. The shear strength of rock and rock joints, Int. Jour. Rock Mech. and Min. Sci. and Geomech. Abs., 13: 255–279.

Basudhar, P.K., 1976. Some Applications of Mathematical Programming Techniques to Slope Stability Problems in Geotechnical Engineering,, Ph.D. Thesis, Indian Institute of Technology, Kanpur, India.

Basudhar, P.K. and Bhattacharya, G., 2008. Predicted Versus Observed Failure Surface: A Case Study. Proc of the 6th Int. Conf. on Case Histories in Geotechnical Engineering (6ICCHGE), Arlington (VA), USA, during, August 11–16, 2008.

Bell, J.M., 1968. General slope stability analysis, J. Soil. Mech. Found. Div., ASCE, 94, SM6; 1253–1270.

Benjamin, J.R. and Cornell, C.A., 1970. Probability, Statistics and Decisions for Civil Engineers, McGraw-Hill.

Berg, P.N., 1962. Calculus of variations, Handbook of Engineering Mechanics, Ed. W. Flugge, McGraw-Hill.

Bhattacharya, G., 1990. Sequential Unconstrained Minimization Technique in Slope Stability Analysis. Ph.D. Thesis, Indian Institute of Technology, Kanpur, India.

Bhattacharya, G. and Basudhar, P.K., 1996. A note on the back analysis of slope failures, Technical Note, Indian Geotech. J., 26(4); 430–441.

Bhattacharya, G. and Basudhar, P.K., 2001. A new procedure for finding critical slip surfaces in slope stability analysis, Indian Geotech. J., 31(1); 149–172.

Bhattacharya, G., Ojha, S., Jana, D. and Chakraborty, S.K., 2003. Direct search for minimum reliability index of earth slopes. Computers and geotechnics, Elsevier Science Ltd., Vol. 30, No. 6, pp. 455–462.

Bieniawski, Z.T., 1974. Estimating the strength of rock materials, J. South African Inst. of Min. & Met., 749, 312–320.

Bishop, A.W., 1952. The stability of earth dams, Ph.D. Thesis, University of London.

Bishop, A.W., 1954. The use of pore pressure co-efficients in practice, Geotechnique, 4: 148–152.

Bishop, A.W., 1955. The use of the slip circle in the stability analysis of slopes, Geotechniqiie, 5: 7–17.

Bishop, A.W., 1958. Test requirements for measuring the co-efficient of earth pressure at rest. Proc. Conf. on Earth Pressure Problems, Brussels, 1: 2–14.

Bishop, A.W., 1960. The principle of effective stress, Norwegian Geotechnical Institute Publication No. 32: 1–15.

Bishop, A.W., 1966. The strength of soils as engineering materialst 6th Rankine Lecture, Geotechnique, 16, 2.

Bishop, A.W., 1967. Progressive failure with special reference to the mechanism causing itv Proc. Geotech. Conf., Oslo, 2: 142–154.

Bishop, A.W., 1971. The influence of progressive failure on the method of stability analysist Geotechnique, 21: 168–172.

Bishop, A.W., 1973. The stability of tips and spoil heaps Quart. J. Eng. Geol., 6(3–4); 335–377.

Bishop, A.W. and Bjerrum, L., 1960. The relevance of the triaxial test to the solution of stability problems, ASCE Research Conference on Shear Strength of Cohesive Soils, Boulder (Colorado); 437–501.

Bishop, A.W., Green, G.E., Garga, V.K., Anderson, A. and Brown, G.D., 1971. A new ring shear apparatus and its application to the measurement of residual shear strength, Geotechnique, 21: 273–328.

Bishop, A.W. and Henkel, D.J., 1962. The measurement of soil properties in the triaxial test, Second Edition, Edwin Arnold, London, 225 pp.

Bishop, A.W. and Morgenstern, N.R., 1960. Stability coefficients for earth slopes, Geotechnique, 10: 129–150.

Bishop, A.W., Webb, D.L. and Lewin, P.J., 1965. Undisturbed samples of London Clay from the Ashford Common Shaft: strength-effective stress relationships, Geotechnique, 15, 1: 1–34.

Bjerrum, L., 1967. Progressive failure in slopes in overconsolidated plastic clays and clay-shale, Terzaghi Lecture, J. Soil Mech. Found. Div., ASCE, 93, SM5; 3–49.

Bjerrum, L., 1972. Embankments on soft ground, ASCE Conf. on Performance of Earth and Earth supported Structures, Purdue Univ., 2: 1–54.

Bjerrum, L., 1973. Problem of soil mechanics and construction on soft clays and structurally unstable soils (collapsible, expansive and others), Proc. 8th Int. Conf. Soil Mech. Found. Eng., Moscow, 3: 111–159.

Bjerrum, L. and Anderson, K.H., 1972. In situ measurement of lateral pressures in clay, Proc. 5th European Conf. Soil Mech. Found. Eng., 1: 11–20.

Bjerrm, L. and Jorstad, F.A., 1968. Stability of rock slopes in Norway, Norwegian Geotechnical Institute, Publication No. 79.

Bjerrum, L. and Kjaernsli, B., 1957. Analysis of the stability of some Norwegian natural clay slopes, Geotechnique, 7: 1–16.

Bjerrum, L., Nash, J.K.T.L., Kennard, R.M. and Gibson, R.E., 1972. Hydraulic fracturing in field permeability testing, Geotechniqiie, 22(2); 319–322.

Blackwood, R.L., Hargraves, A.J. and Mackay, J., 1976. Absolute stress investigation in coal at Appin Colliery, New South Wales, preprint Int. Soc. Rock Mech. Symposium, Sydney; 1–7.

Blight, G.E., 1967. Horizontal stresses in stiff and fissured lacustrine clays, Proc. 4th Regional Conference Soil Mech. Found. Eng., Africa, 1: 95–99.

Blight, G.E., 1977. General report on slopes in mining and industrial wastes and on slopes in residual soils, Proc. 9th Int. Conf. Soil Mech. Found. Eng., Tokyo, 2: 600–604 and 582–590.

Blyth, F.G.R. and de Freitas, M.H., 1974. A Geology for Engineers, 6th Edition, Edwin Arnold, London, 557 pp.

Booker, J.R. and Davis, E.H., 1972. A note on a plasticity solution to the stability of slopes in inhomogeneoiis clays, Geotechnique, 22(3); 509–513.

Borges, J.F. and Castenheta, M., 1971. Structural Safety, Laboratorio Nacional de Engeriharia Civil, Lisbon, Portugal.

Bowles, J.E., 1977. Foundation Analysis and Design, McGraw-Hill, New York., 750 pp.

Brace, W.F. and Byerlee, D., 1966. Recent experimental studies of brittle fracture of rocks, M.I.T. Report, published in Proc. 8th Symp. Rock Mech., Univ. of Minnesota, 1967; 58–81.

Brandon, T.L., Wright, S.G. and Duncan, J.M., 2008. Analysis of i-walls with gaps between the i-wall and the level fill, Journal of Geotechnical and Geoenvironmental Engineering,, ASCE, Vol. 134, No. 5, pp. 692–717.

Briaud, J.L., 2008. Case histories of soil and rock erosion: woodrow wilson bridge, brazos river meander, normandy cliffs and new orleans levees, Journal of Geotech and Geoenvironmental Engineering, Vol. 134, No. 10, 1425–1447.

Broadbent, C.D. and Ko, K.C., 1972. Rheological aspects of rock slope failures, stability of rock slopes, 13th Symposium on Rock Mechanics, Ed. by E.J. Cording, ASCE, New York; 573–595.

Broch, E. and Franklin, J.A., 1972. The point load strength test, Int. J. Rock Mech. and Min. Sci., 9: 669–697.

Broili, L., 1967. New Knowledge on the geomorphology of the Vajont slide slip surface, Rock. Mech. Eng. Geol., 5, 1.

Bromhead, E.N. and Dixon, N., 1986. The field residual strength of London Clay and its correlation with laboratory measurements, especially the ring shear tests, Geotechnique, 36, (3); 449–452.

Brooker, E.W. and Ireland, H.O., 1965. Earth pressures at rest related to stress history, Canadian Geotechnical Journal, 2(1); 1–15.

Broscoe, A.J. and Thompson, S., 1967. The Devon Road landslide, Assoc. of Eng. Geol. Meeting, Dallas, Texas.

Brown, C.B. and Goodman, L.E., 1963. Gravitational stresses in acereted bodies, Proc. Royal Society, Series A, 276.

Brown, C.B. and King, I.P., 1966. Automatic embankment analysis; equilibrium and instability conditions, Geotechnique, 16: 209–219.

Brown, E.T., 1970. Strength of models of rock with intermittent joints, J. Soil Mech. Found. Div., ASCE, 96, sm6; 1917–1934.

Brunsden, D., Doornkamp, J.C., Fookes, P.G., Jones, D.K.C. and Kelly, J.M.H., 1975. Large scale geomorphological mapping and highway engineering design, Qnart. J. Eng. Geol., 8(4); 227–255.

Bruückl, E. and Scheidegger, A.E., 1973. Application of the theory of plasticity to slow mudflows, Geotechnique, 23: 101–107.

Bryant, E.A., Head, L. and Morrison, R.J., 2005. Planning for natural hazards-how can we mitigate the impacts, Proceedings of a symposium with the same title, Eds., R.J. Morrison, Sandra Quin and E.A. Bryant, GeoQuEST Research Centre and School of Earth and Environmental Sciences, University of Wollongong, February 2005, pp. 1–21.

Bunce, C.M., 2008. Risk estimation for railways exposed to landslides, Ph D Thesis, University of Alberta, Alberta, Canada, 417 pp.

Burland, J.B., 1973. Discussion of paper entitled 'Initiation and Growth of Shear Bands' by J.H. Rice, Proc. Symp. on Plasticity and Soil Mechanics, Ed., by A.C. Palmer, Cambridge Univ. Eng. Dept., England.

Burland, J.B., Longworth, T.I. and Moore, J.F.A., 1977. A study of ground movement and progressive failure caused by a deep excavation in Oxford clay, Geotechniqiie, 27, 4t 557–593.

Byerlee, J.D., 1967. Theory of friction based on brittle fracture, J. Appl. Phys., 38: 2928–2934.

Byrne, P.M., 1994. A model for predicting liquefaction induced displacements, Soil Mechanics Series No. 147, Department of Civil Engineering, UBC, Vancouver, Canada, 1–34.

Caine, N., 1980. The Rainfall Intensity – Duration Control of Shallow landslides and Debris Flows, Geografiska Annaler, Vol. 62, A 1–2, pp. 23–27.

Carrara, A. and Guzzetti, F., (Editors) 1995. Geographical Information Systems in Assessing Natural Hazards, Advances in Natural and Technological Hazards Research, Vol. 5, Kluwer Academic Publishers.

Carson, M.A. and Kirkby, M.J., 1972. Hillslope Form and Process, Cambridge University Press, England, 475 pp.

Carter, J.P., Desai, C.S., Potts, D.M., Schweiger, H.F. and Sloan, S.W., (2000) Computing and computer modeling in geotechnical engineering, GeoEng 2000, 19–24 November, Melbourne, Australia, Volume-1: Invited papers, 1157–1252.

Casagrande, A., 1950. Notes on the design of earth dams, Proc. Boston Soc. Civil Eng., 37(4); 405–429.

Casagrande, A. and Carrillo, N., 1944. Shear failure of anisotropic materials, J. Boston Soc. Civil Eng., 31(2); 74–87.

Cavounidis, S., 1987 On the ratio of factors of safety in slope stability problems, Geotechnique, 37(2); 207–210.

Cedergren, H.R., 1967. Seepage, Drainage and Flow Nets, John Wiley, New York.

Celestino, T.B. and Duncan, J.M. 1981. Simplified search for non-circular slip surfaces, Proc. 10th Int. Conf. S.M.F.E., Stockholm, Sweden, 391–394.

Chandler, R.J., 1969. The effect of weathering on the shear strength properties of Keuper marl, Geotechnique, 19: 321–334.

Chandler, R.J., 1972. Lias clay, weathering processes and their effect on shear strength, Geotechnique, 22: 403–431.

Chandler, R.J., 1974. Lias clay, the long-term stability of cutting slopes, Geotechnique, 24: 24–38.

Chang, C.Y. and Duncan, J.M., 1970. Analysis of soil movements around a deep excavation, J. Soil Mech. Found. Div., ASCE, SM5; 1655–1681.

Charles, J.A. and Bromhead, E.N., 2008. Contributions to Geotechnique 1948–2008: Slope stability and embankment dams,Geotechnique, Vol. 58, No. 5, 385–389.

Chen, H., Lee, C.F. and Law, K.T. 2004 Causative mechanisms of rainfall-induced fill slope failures, Journal of Geotechnical and Geoenvironmental Engineering, ASCE, 130, No. 6, June, 593–602.

Chen, R.H. and Chameau, J.L., 1982. Three-dimensional slope stability analysis, Proc. 4th Int. Conf on Numerical Methods in Geomechanics, Edmonton 2: 671–677.

Chen, W.F., 1975. Limit Analysis and Soil Plasticity, Elsevier, Amsterdam, 638 pp.

Chen, W.F. and Giger, M.W., 1971. Limit analysis of stability of slopes, J. Soil Mech. Found. Div., ASCE, 97, SM6; 19–26.

Chien-Yuan, C., Tien-Chien, C., Fan-Chieh, Y., Wen-Hui, Y. and Chun-Chieh, T., 2005. Rainfall duration and debris flow initiated studies for real- time monitoring, Environmental Geology, 47: 715–724.

Chlimintzas, G.O., 2003. Seismic displacements of slopes using multi-block sliding model. Ph.D. Thesis, Imperial College London, 2003.

Chopra, A.K., 1967. Earthquake response of earth dams, J. Soil Mech. Found. Div., ASCE, 93, SM2; 65–82.

Chowdhury, R.N., 1970a. The Application of the Finite Element Method to Stress Deformation and Seepage Problems in Soil Mechancis, Ph.D. Thesis, University of Liverpool, England.

Chowdhury, R.N., 1970b. Discussion on paper 'Stiff-fissured clays and shales', J. Soil Mech. Found. Div., ASCE, 96, SM1; 336–338. (See also 97, SM4, 1971).

Chowdhury, R.N., 1972. Deformation problems in anisotropic soil – application of the finite element method, Finite Element Methods in Civil Engineering, Ed. by Mirza et al., Montreal. 5: 653–675.

Chowdhury, R.N., 1975. Comparison of simplified and rigorous analyses for natural slopes, Proc. Baltic Conf. Soil Mech. Found. Eng., Poland, 3(4); 347–357.

Chowdhury, R.N., 1976. Initial stresses in natural slope analysis, Rock Engineering for Foundations and Slopes, ASCE, Geotech. Eng. Specialty Conf., Boulder (Colorado), 1: 404–415.

Chowdhury, R.N., 1977a. A new approach to slope stability studies, Research Report, Dept. of Civil Eng., University of Wollongong, (New South Wales), Australia.

Chowdhury, R.N., 1977b. Understanding landslides in relation to initial ground stresses, Proc. 2nd Int. Symp. on Landslides and their Control, Japan Soc. of landslides and Public Works Research Institute, Tokyo, Japan.

Chowdhury, R.N., 1977c. Propagation of failure surfaces in natural slopes, Research Report, Dept. of Civil Eng., University of Wollongong (New South Wales), Australia.

Chowdhury, R.N., 1978a. Analysis of the Vajont slide – New Approach, Rock Mechanics and Rock Engineering, Vol. 11, 29–38.

Chowdhury, R.N., 1978b. Propagation of failure surfaces in natural slopes, Journal of Geophysical Research, Vol. 83, No. B12, December, 5983–5988.

Chowdhury, R., 1980. Landslides as natural hazards – mechanisms and uncertainties, Geotechnical Engineering, Vol. 11, 135–180.

Chowdhury, R., 1984. Recent Developments in Landslide Studies-Probabilistic Methods, State of the Art Report, Proc. International Symposium on Landslides, Toronto, Vol. 1, 209–229.

Chowdhury, R., 1985. Successive Failures-A Probabilistic Approach, Proc. of the Eleventh International Conference on Soil Mechanics and Foundation Engineering, San Francisco, 1C5, 819–824.

Chowdhury, R., 1986. Geomechanics risk model for multiple failures along discontinuities, Int. J. Roc Mech. Min. Sci & Geomech. Abstr. Vol. 23, No. 5, 337–346.

Chowdhury, R., 1987a. Risk of Slip Along Discontinuities in a Heterogeneous Medium, Minig Science and Technology, Vol. 4, 241–255.

Chowdhury, R., 1987b. Retrospective comments-Aspects of the Vajont Slide, Engineering Geology, 24 (1987), 533–540, also Proc. Int. Coinf. on Dam Failures, Purdue University, Lafayette, Indiana, USA, August 5–8, 1985.

Chowdhury, R., 1988. Special Lecture: Analysis Methods For Assessing Landslide Risk-Recent Developments, Proc. Fifth International Symposium on Landslides, Laussane, 515–524.

Chowdhury, R., 1992. Simulation of Risk of Progressive Slope Failure, Canadian Geotechnical Journal, Vol. 29, No. 1, 94–102.

Chowdhury, R., 1995. Assessing embankment safety during an earthquake, proceedings Pacific Conference on Earthquake Engineering, 22–25, Paper 201, 67–75.

Chowdhury, R., 1996. Evaluation of the seismic performance of earth structures, Proceedings of the Eleventh World Conference on Earthquake Engineering, Acupulco, Mexico, Paper No. 549, ISBN 0-080-42822.

Chowdhury, R., 2001. Contribution to discussion on "Earthquake destructiveness potential factor and slope stability (Cresspellani et al., (1998)", including reply by the authors, Geotechnique, 51(3); 281–284.

Chowdhury, R. and A-Grivas, D., 1982. Probabilistic Model Of Progressive Failure Of Slopes, Journal of Geotechnical Engineering Division, ASCE, 108, GT6; 803–819.

Chowdhury, R.N. and Bertoldi, C., 1977. Residual shear strength of soil from two natural slopes, Australian Geomechanies Journal, G7; 1–9.

Chowdhury, R. and Flentje, P., 1998. A Landslide Database for Landslide Hazard Assessment, Proceedings of the Second International Conference on Environmental Management, (ICEM2), Elsevier (Oxford), Vol. 2, 1229–1238.

Chowdhury, R. and Flentje, P., 2002. Uncertainties in Rainfall-Induced Landslide Hazard. Quarterly Journal of Engineering Geology and Hydrogeology. Symposium in Print on Landslides. London (UK), Volume 35 Part 1, February 2002, pp. 61–70.

Chowdhury, R. and Flentje, P., 2003 Role of Slope Reliability Analysis in Landslide Risk Management, Bulletin of Engineering Geology and the Environment, Vol. 62, 41–46.

Chowdhury, R. and Flentje, P., 2007. Perspectives For The Future of Geotechnical Engineering, Keynote Paper, Proceedings of the International Conference on Civil Engineering in the New Millennium: Opportunity and Challenges (CENeM-2007), 150 – year anniversary conference at Bengal Engineering and Science University, Shibpur, India, January 11–14, 2007, Vol. III, pp. 1291–1312.

Chowdhury, R. and Flentje, P., 2008. Strategic Approaches for the Management of Risk in Geomechanics, Theme Paper, Proc. 12 IACMAG conference, Goa, India, CD-ROM, 3031–3042.

Chowdhury, R.N. and Gray, P.A., 1976. Finite elements in natural slope analysis, Finite Element Methods in Engineering, Ed. by Y.K. Cheung et al., Adelaide, 13: 1–15.

Chowdhury, R.N. and King, G.J.W., 1972. Stresses due to strip loads on saturated soil, J. Soil Mech. Found. Div., ASCE, SM12; 1433–1438.

Chowdhury, R. and Tabesh, A., 1998. Seismic response of coastal escarpments, Proc Sixth US National Conference on Earthquake Engineering, Seattle, Washington, USA, May 31–June 4, 1998, CD Rom, 8.

Chowdhury, R. Tang, W.H. and Sidi, I., 1987. Reliability Model of Progressive Slope Failure, Geotechnique, 37: 467–481.

Chowdhury, R. and Xu, D.W., 1992. Reliability Index for Slope Stability Assessment – Two Methods Compared, Reliability Engineering and System safety, 37: 99–108.

Chowdhury, R. and Xu, D.W., 1994. Slope System Reliability with General Slip Surfaces, Soils And Foundations, Vol. 34, No. 3, 99–105.

Chowdhury, R. and Xu, D.W., 1995. Geotechnical System Reliability of Slopes, Reliability Engineering and System Safety, 47: 141–151.

Chowdhury, R. and Zhang, S., 1989. Updating Open Pit Slope Stability Based On Bayesian Approach, Second Large Open Pit Mining Conference, April 1989, 9–12.

Chowdhury, R. and Zhang, S., 1990. Convergence aspect of limit equilibrium method for slopes, Can. Geotech. J., 27: 145–151.

Chowdhury, R. and Zhang, S., 1993. Modelling the Risk of Progressive Slope Failure: A New Approach, Reliability Engineering and System Safety, 40: 17–30.

Chowdhury R; Zhang, S and Flentje, P., 2004. Reliability Updating and Geotechnical Back-analysis, Advances in Geotechnical engineering, Proc of the Skempton Conference, Institution of Civil Engineers, Thomas Telford, London, Vol. 2, 815–821.

Christian, J.T., 1968. Undrained stress distribution by numerical methods, J. Soil Mech. Found. Div., ASCE, 94, SM6; 1333–1345.

Christian, J.T., 2004. Geotechnical Engineering Reliability "How well do we know what we are doing?", The 39th Terzaghi Lecture, Journal of Geotechnical and Geoenvironmental Engineering, ASCE, Vol. 130, No. 10, 985–1003 C163.

Christian, J.T. and Baecher, G.B., 2001. Discussion on "Factors of Safety and Reliability in Geotechnical Engineering" by JM Duncan, Journal of Geotechnical and Geoenvironmental Engineering, ASCE, Vol. 127, No. 8, 700–703 (see also rest of discussion, pp. 703–716 and closure by the author on pp. 717–721).

Christian, J.T., Ladd, C.C. and Baecher, G.B., 1992. Reliability and Probability in Stability Analysis, Invited Lecture, Stability and Performance of Slopes and Embankments-II, A 25 year perspective, ASCE Geotechnical Special Publication No. 31,Vol. 2, 1071–1111.

Christian, J.T., Ladd, C.C. and Baecher, G.B., 1994. Reliability Applied to Slope Stability Analysis, Journal of Geotechnical and Geoenvironmental Engineering, ASCE, Vol. 120, No. 12, 2187–2207.

Christian, J.T. and Urzua, A., 1999. "Probabilistic Evaluation of Earthquake-Induced Slope Failure", Journal of Geotechnical and Geoenvironmental Engineering, ASCE, Vol. 124, No. 11, Nov. 1998, pp. 1140–1143.

Christian, J.T. and Whitman, R.V., 1969. A one-dimensional model for progressive failure, Proc. 7th Int. Conf. Soil Mech. Found. Eng., 2: 541–545.

Cleary, M.P. and Rice, J.R., 1974. Some elementary models for the growth of slip surfaces in progressive failure, Report M.R.L.E.-91, Div. of Eng., Brown University, U.S.A., 1–65.

Close, U. and McCormick, E., 1922. Where the mountains walked, National Geographic, Vol. 41, No. 5, 445–464.

Clough, G.W. and Duncan, J.M., 1971. Finite element analysis of retaining wall behaviour, J. Soil Mech. Found. Eng., ASCE, 97, SM12; 1657–1673.

Clough, R.W. and Chopra, A.K., 1966. Earthquake stress analysis of earth dams, J. Eng. Mech. Div., ASCE, 2, EM2; 197–212.

Clough, R.W. and Woodward, R.J., 1967. Analysis of embankment stresses and deformations, J. Soil Mech. Found. Div., ASCE, 93, SM4; 529–549.

Collins, B.D. and Znidarcic, D. 2004. Stability analyses of rainfall induced landslides, Journal of the Geotechnical and Geoenvironmental Engineering, ASCE, 130, No. 4, April, 362–372.

Cooke, R.U. and Doornkamp, J.C., 1974. Geomorphology in environmental management, Clarenden Press, Oxford, 413 pp.

Cooper, M.R., 1988. A displacement based analysis of progressive failure by the reserve capacity method, Vth Int. Symp. on Landslides (ISL 1988), Laussane, 1, 387–392.

Cooper, M.R., Bromhead, E.N., Petley, J. and Grant, D.I., 1998. The Selborne cutting stability experiment", Geotechnique, 48, No. 1: 83–101.

Cording, E.J., 1972. (Editor) Stability of Rock Slopes, 13th Symp. Rock Mechanics, Urbana (Illinois), ASCE, New York, 912 pp.

Cornell, C.A., 1969. A Probability based structural Code, Journal of ACI, Vol. 66, No. 12, pp. 974–985.

Cornforth, D.H., 2005. Landslides in Practice, Investigation, analysis and remedial/prevention options in soils, John Wiley & sons Inc., 596 pp.

Cornforth, D.H., 2007. Seven deadly sins of landslide investigation, analysis and design, in A K Turner and R L Schuster(Editors) Landslides and Socirty, AEG Special Publication No. 22, 1st North American Landslide Conference, Vail Colorado, June, 149–178.

Cousins, B.F., 1977. Stability charts for simple earth slopes, Research Report, CM-77/2, Univ. of Tasmania, Hobart (Tasmania) Australia, 45 pp.

Couture, R., Evans, S.G., Locat, J., Hadjigeorgiou, J. and Antoine, J.P., 1999. A methodology for rock avalanche analysis, Proc. Int. Symp. On slope stability engineering, Matsuyama, Japan, November, Vol. 2, 1369–1378.

Crawford, C.B. and Eden, W.J., 1967. Stability of natural slopes in sensitive clay, J. Soil Mech. Found. Div., ASCE, 93, SM4; 419–436.

Crespellani, T., Madiai, C. and Vannucchi, G., 1998. Earthquake destructiveness potential factor and slope stability, Geotechnique, 48(3); 411–419.

Crozier, M.J., 1973. Technique for morphometric analysis of landslips, Zeit fur Geom., 17: 78–101.

Cruden, D.M., 1976. Major rock slides of the Rockies, Canadian Geotech Journal, 13: 8–20.

Cruden, D.M, and Varnes, D.J., 1996. Landslide Types and Processes. In Turner and Schuster, 1996. In Turner, A.K. and Schuster, R.L., 1996. Landslides, Investigation and Mitigation. Special Report 247. Transportation Research Board, National Research Council. National Academy Press Washington DC.

D'Appolonia, D.J., Lambe, T.W. and Poulos, H.G., 1971. Evaluation of pore pressures beneath an embankment, J. Soil Mech. Found. Eng., ASCE, 97, sm6; 881–898.

D'elia, B., Esu, F., Pelliegrino, A., and Pescatore, T.S., (1985) Some effects on natural slope stability induced by the 1980 Italian earthquake, Proc XI International Conference Soil Mechanics and Foundation Engineering, San Francisco, Vol. 4, 1985, 1943–1949.

Dai, F.C. and Lee, C.F., 2003. A spatiotemporal probabilistic modeling of storm-induced shallow landsliding using aerial photographs and logistic regression, Earth Surface Processes and Landforms, 28: 527–545.

Dai, S.H. and Wang, M.O., 1992. Reliability Analysis in Engineering Applications, Van Nostrnad Reinhold, New York.

Davies, W.N. and Christie, D.H., 1996. The Coledale Mudslide, New South Wales, Australia-A lesson for geotechnical engineers, Proc. Seventh International Symposium on Landslides, Trondheim, Norway, Senneset K (ed.) Vol. 2, 701–706.

Davis, E.H. and Booker, J.R., 1973. Some applications of classical plasticity theory for soil stability problems, Proc. Symp. on Plasticity and Soil Mechanics, Cambridge Univ. Eng. Dept., England.

Davis, E.H. and Poulos, H.G., 1963. Triaxial testing and three-dimensional settlement analysis, 4th Aust.-New Zealand Conf. Soil Mech. Found. Eng., Adelaide, 233–243.

Dawei, X., 1994. Ph.D. Thesis, University of Wollongong.

Dawson, E.M., Roth, W.H. and Drescher, A., 1999. Slope stability analysis by strength reduction. Geotechnique, 49, No. 6, 835–840.

De Natale, J.S., 1991. Rapid identification of critical slip surface Structure. J. Geotech Engrg., ASCE, 117(10); 1568–1589.

Deere, D.U., 1963. Technical description of rock cores for engineering purposes, Rock Mech. Eng. Geol., 1: 18–22.

Deere, D.U. and Patton, F.D., 1971. Slope stability in residual soils, Proc. 4th Pan. Am. Conf. on Soil Mech. Found. Eng., State of the Art Report, 1: 88–171.

DeLory, F.A., 1957. Long-term stability of slopes in overconsolidated clays, Ph.D. Thesis, University of London.

De Mello, V.F.B., 1977. Reflections on design decisions of practical significance to embankment dams, Rankine Lecture, Geotechnique, 27(3); 279–355.

Desai, C.S., 1971. Non-linear analysis using spline functions, J. Soil Mech. Found. Div., ASCE, SM10; 1461–1480.

Desai, C.S., 1972. (Editor) Proe. Symp. Appl. of Finite Element Method in Geotechnical Engineering, U.S. Waterways Experiment Station, Vicksburg, 1227 pp.

Desai, C.S., 1976. (Editor) Numerical Methods in Geomechanies, 3 Vols., Proc. Int. Conf. on Numerical Methods in Geomechanics, Blacksburg (Virginia), ASCE, 1273 pp.

Desai, C.S. and Abel, J.P., 1972. Introduction to Finite Element Method, Van Nostrand, Reinhold, New York.

Desai, C.S. and Wu, T.H., 1976. A general function for stress-strain curves, Numerical Methods in Geomechanics, Ed. by C.S. Desai, 1: 306–319.

Dodd, J.S. and Anderson, H.W., 1972. Tectonic stresses and rock slope stability, Stability of Rock Slopes, Thirteenth Symp. Rock Mechanics, Ed. by E.J. Cording, ASCE; 171–182.

Donald, I.B. and Giam, S.K., 1988. Application of the nodal displacement method to slope stability analysis, Proc 5th Australia New Zealand Conference on Geomechanics, Sydney, 456–460.

Dounias, G.T., Potts, D.M. and Vaughan, P.R., 1996. Analysis of progressive failure and cracking in old British dams, Geotechnique, 46, No. 4, 621–641.

Drucker, D.C., 1953. Limit analysis of two and three-dimensional problems, J. Mech. Phys. Solids, 1: 217–226.

Drucker, D.C., Gibson, R.E. and Henkel, D.J., 1957. Soil mechanics and work hardening theories of plasticity, Transactions, ASCE, 122: 338–346.

Drucker, D.C. and Prager, W., 1952. Soil Mechanics and plastic analysis or limit design, Quart. App. Meth., 10: 157–165.

Duncan, J.M., 1992. State-of-the-Art: Static stability and deformation analysis, Invited lecture, Stability and Performance of slopes and Embankments II, Geotechnical Special Publication No. 31, ASCE, Vol. 1, 222–266.

Duncan, J.M., 2000. Factors of Safety and Reliability in Geotechnical Engineering, Journal of Geotechnical and Geoenvironmental Engineering, ASCE, Vol. 126, No. 4, 307–316 (See also discussion of this paper by various writers including reply by author in Vol. 127, No. 8, pp. 700–721).

Duncan, J.M., 2001. Closure to the discussion on "Factors of Safety and Reliability in Geotechnical Engineering" by J.M. Duncan, Journal of Geotechnical and Geoenvironmental Engineering, ASCE, Vol. 127, No. 8, 717–721 (discussion pp. 700–717).

Duncan, J.M. and Chang, C.Y., 1970. Non linear analysis of stress and strain in soils7 J. Soil Mech. Found. Div., ASCE, sm5; 1629–1653.

Duncan, J.M. and Dunlop, P., 1969. Slopes in stiff-fissured clays and shales, J. Soil Mech. Found. Div., ASCE, 95, SM2; 467–491.

Duncan, J.M. and Goodman, R.E., 1968. Finite element analysis of slopes in jointed rock, Contract Report S-68-3, U.S. Army Engineers Waterways Experiment Station, Vicksburg.

Duncan, J.M. and Seed, H.B., 1966a. Anisotropy and stress reorientation in clay, J. Soil Mech. Found. Div., ASCE, 92, SM5; 21–50.

Duncan, J.M. and Seed, H.B., 1966b. Strength variation along failure surfaces in clay, J. Soil Mech. Found. Div., ASCE, 92, sm6; 81–104.

Duncan, J.M. and Wright, S.G., 2005. Soil strength slope stability, John Wiley & Sons.

Duncan, J.M., Brandan, T.L., Wright, S.G. and Vraman, N., 2008. Stability of I-walls in New Orleans during Hurricana Katrina, J. of Geotech & Geoenvironmental Engineering, ASCE, Vol. 134, No. 5, 681–691.

Dunlop, P. and Duncan, J.M., 1970. Development of failure in excavated slopes, J. Soil Mech. Found. Div., ASCE, 96, SM2; 471–495.

Durney, D.W., 1972. Solution-transfer, an important geological deformation mechanism, Nature, 235(5337); 315–317.

E.T.B., 1977. Review of book 'Principles of Engineering Geology' in Int. J. Rock Mech. & Min. Sci. & Geomech. Abs., Pergamon Press, 14: 161–162.

Early, K.R. and Skempton, A.W., 1972. Investigation of the landslide at Waltonts Wood, Staffordshire~ Quart. J. Eng. Geol., 5: 19–42.

Eckel, E.B., 1958. (Editor) Landslides and Engineering Practice, Highway Research Board, Special Report 29, Washington, 232 pp.

Eigenbrod, K.D., 1975. Analysis of the pore pressure changes following the excavation of a slope, Canadian Geotechnical Journal, 12: 429–440.

Eigenbrod, K.D. and Morgenstern, N.R., 1972. A slide in Cretaceous bedrock at Devon, Alberta, Geotechnical Practice for Stability in Open Pit Mining, Ed. by C.O. Brawner and V. Milligan, AIME, New York, 223–238.

Einstein, H.H. and Hirschfeld, R.C., 1973. Model studies on mechanics of jointed rock, J. Soil Mech. Found. Div., ASCE, 99, SM3; 229–248.

Endersbee, L.A., 1969. Application of Rock Mechanics in Hydro-Electric Development in Tasmania, Hydro-Electric Commission, Tasmania, Australia.

Evans, J. and Bewick, B., 1999. The Wollongong Flash Flood Event, 17 August 1998,Proceedings of symposium on "August 1998 Wollongong Storms" organised by The Institution of Engineers, Australia, Sydney Division, Water Engineering Panel, held on 23 February 1999 at the University of Wollongong, Wollongong, Australia: 30 pages, The Institution of Engineers, Australia.

Evans, S.G, and DeGraff, J.V., 2002. eds., Catastrophic Landslides: Effects, Occurrence and Mechanisms, Reviews in Engineering Geology XV, The Geological Society of America, 411 pp.

Fairhurst, C., 1964. Measurement of in situ rock stresses with particular reference to hydraulic fracturing, Rock. Mech. Eng. Geol., 2, 129.

Fan, K., Fredlund, D.G., and Wilson, G.W., 1986. An interslice force function for limit equilibrium slope stability analysis, Can. Geotech. J., 23: 287–296.

Fell, R. and Hartford, D., 1997. Landslide risk management, In, Landslide Risk Assessment, edited by:- D. Cruden and R. Fell, Balkema, Rotterdam, 51–109.

Fellenius, W., 1927. Erdstatische Berechnungen mit Reibung and Kohaesion, Ernst, Berlin.

Fellenius, W., 1936. Calculation of stability of earth dams, Transactions, 2nd Congress Large Dams, 4: 445.

Ferguson, H.E., 1967. Valley stress relief in the Allegheny Plateau, Bulletin Assoc. of Eng. Geol., 14(1); 63–71.

Ferguson, H.E., 1974. Geologic observations and geotechnical effects of valley stress relief in Allegheny Plateau, preprint of paper presented to ASCE National Meeting on Water Resources Engineering, Los Angeles, California, 31 pp.

FHWA., 2000. Mechanically Stabilised Earth Walls and Reinforced Soil Slopes: Design and Construction Guidelines, Report FHWA-NHI-oo-043,FHA, US Dept. of Transportation.

Finn, W.D.L. and Khanna, J., 1966. Dynamic response of earth dams, Pro. 3rd Earthquake Symposium, Roorkee (U.P.) India.

Flentje, P., 1998. Computer Based Landslide Hazard and Risk Assessment. Ph.D. Thesis, University of Wollongong, Australia.

Flentje, P., 2009. Landslide Inventory Development and Landslide Susceptibility Zoning in the Wollongong City Council Local Government Area, Unpublished report to Industry Partners – Wollongong City Council, RailCorp and the Roads and Traffic Authroity, University of Wollongong, Australia, 73 pp.

Flentje, P. and Chowdhury, R., 1999. Geotechnical Assessment and Management of 148 Landslides Triggered by a Major Storm Event in Wollongong, Australia. Proceedings of the Australian Disaster Conference 1999. 1–3 November, Canberra, Australian Capital Territory, Australia. pp. 269–274.

Flentje, P. and Chowdhury, R., 2001. Aspects of Risk Management for Rainfall – Triggered Landsliding. Proceedings of the Engineering and Development in Hazardous Terrain

Symposium, New Zealand Geotechnical Society Inc. University of Canterbury, Christchurch, New Zealand. The Institution of Professional Engineers New Zealand, August 24–25, pp. 143–150.

Flentje, P. and Chowdhury, R., 2002. Frequency of landsliding as part of risk assessment, Australian Geomechanics, 37(2); 157–167.

Flentje, P. and Chowdhury, R. 2005a. Managing landslide hazards on the Illawarra escarpment. Proceedings of the GeoQuest Symposium entitled 'Planning for Natural Hazards – How can we mitigate the impacts?' Editor: Associate Professor John Morrison. University of Wollongong, 2–5 February 2005. Published by GeoQuest Research Centre, University of Wollongong 2005, pp. 65–78.

Flentje, P. and Chowdhury, R., 2005b Towards real-time landslide risk management in an urban area., Proc. of Conference on Landslide Risk Management, Vancouver May 31–June 3, Hungr, Fell, Couture & Eberhardt (eds), Taylor and Francis Group, London, 741–751.

Flentje, P. and Chowdhury, R., 2006. Observational Approach for Urban Landslide Management, Engineering geology for tomorrow's cities. The 10th International Association of Engineering Geology and the Environment (IAEG) Congress, Nottingham, United Kingdom, 6–10 September 2006.

Flentje, P. Chowdhury, R., Tobin, P. and Brizga, V., 2005. Towards real-time landslide risk management in an urban area. Landslide Risk Management, Editors Hungr, O., Fell, R., Couture, R. and Eberhardt, E. Vancouver. Joint Technical Committee on Landslides and Engineered Slopes, JTC-1, in association with Vancouver Geotechnical Society. Proceedings of the International Conference on Landslide Risk Management/18th Annual Vancouver Geotechnical Society Symposium, May 31 to June 4, pp. 741–751.

Flentje, P., Stirling, D. and Chowdhury, R., 2007a. Landslide Susceptibility and Hazard derived from a Landslide Inventory using Data Mining – An Australian Case Study. Proceedings of the First North American Landslide Conference, Landslides and Society: Integrated Science, Engineering, Management, and Mitigation. Vail, Colorado June 3–8, 2007. CD, Paper number 17823–024, 10 pp.

Flentje, P., Stirling, D., Palamara, D. and Chowdhury, R., 2007b. Landslide susceptibility and landslide hazard zoning in Wollongong, Common Ground, Proc. 10th Australia New Zealand Conference on Geomechanics, Brisbane, October 21–24, Vol. 2, 392–397 Australian Geomechanics Society, printed by Carillon Conference Management Pty Ltd.

Fookes, P.G., Dearman, W.R. and Franklin, J.A., 1971. Some engineering aspects of rock weathering with field examples from Dartmoor and elsewhere, Quart. J. Eng. Geol., 4: 139–185.

Fookes, P.G., Lee, E.M. and Milligan, G., 2005. eds., Geomorphology for Engineers, Whittles Publishing, CRC Press, 851 pp.

Fookes, P.G., Lee, E.M. and Griffiths, J.S., 2007. Engineering Geomorphology, theory and practice, Whittles Publishing, CRC Press LLC, 279 pp.

Foott, R. and Ladd, C.C., 1977. Behaviour of Atchafalaya Levees during construction, Geotechnique, 27(2); 137–161.

Fox, R.L. 1971. Optimization Methods for Engineering Design, Addison-Wesley, Reading Mass.

Franklin, J.A. and Chandra, A., 1972. The slake durability test, Int. J. Rock Mech. & Min. Sci., 9: 325–341.

Fredlund, D.G. and Barbour, S.L., 1992. Integrated seepage modelling and slope stability analyses: a generalised approach for saturated/unsaturated soils, chapter in the book, Geomechanics and Water Engineering in Environmental Management, (Edited R. Chowdhury), Balkema, 1992, pp. 3–35.

Fredlund, D.G. and Rohardjo, H., 1993. Soil Mechanics for Unsaturated Soils, John Wiley & Sons Inc., 517 pp.

Fredlund, D.G. and Scoular, R.E.G., 1999. Using limit equilibrium concepts in finite element slope stability analysis, Proc. Int. Symp. on slope stability engineering, Matsuyama, Japan, November, Vol. 1, 31–48.

Frydman, S. and Beasely, D.H., 1976. Centrifugal modelling of riverbank failure, J. Geotech. Eng. Div., ASCE, 102, GT5; 395–409.

Gibson, R.E. and Morgenstern, N.R., 1962. A note on the stability of cuttings in normally consolidated clays, Geotechnique, 12, 212–216.

Gilboy, G., 1934. Mechanics of hydraulic fill dams, J. Boston Society of Civil Engineers, Reprinted in Boston Society of Civil Engineers: Contributions to Soil Mechanics, 1925–1940.

Girijivallabhan, C.V. and Reese, L.C., 1968. Finite element method for problems in soil mechanics, J. Soil Mech. Found. Div., ASCE, 94, SM2; 473–495.

Goguel, J., 1978. Scale-dependant rockslide mechanisms with emphasis on the role of porefluid vaporisation, Chapter 20, pp. 693–705, in: Rockslides and Avalanches, 1, Natural Phenomena, Barry Voight, ed., Elsevier.

Goh, A.T.C., Kulhawy, F.H. and Wong, K.S., 2008. Reliability Assessment of Basal-Heave Stability for Braced Excavations in Clay, Journal of Geotechnical and Geoenvironmental Engineering, ASCE, Vol. 134, No. 2, 145–153.

Goodman, L.E. and Brown, C.B., 1963. Dead load stresses and the Instability of slopes, J. Soil Mech. Found. Div., ASCE, 89, SM3; 103–137.

Goodman, R.E., 1970. The deformability of joints, Determination of In-situ Modulus of Deformation of Rocks, ASTM, Special Technical Publication, 477: 174–196.

Goodman, R.E., 1976. Methods of Geological Engineering in Discontinuous Rocks, West Publishing Co., St. Paul, Minn.

Goodman, R.E. and Dubois, J., 1972. Duplication of dilatancy in analysis of jointed rocks, J. Soil Mech. Found. Div., ASCE, 98, SM4; 399–422.

Goodman, R.E. and Taylor, R.L., 1967. Methods of analysis for rock slopes and abutments, Proc. 8th Symp. Rock Mech., Minneapolis, 9: 303–320.

Goodman, R.E., Taylor, R.L. and Brekke, T.L., 1968. A model for the mechanics of jointed rock, J. Soil Mech. Found. Div., ASCE, 94, SM3; 637–659.

Govt. of Hong Kong, 1977. Report on the slope failures at Sau Mau Ping, Reports of (a) Independent Review Panel and (b) Binnie and Partners, P.W.D., Hong Kong, 104 pp.

Greco, V.R., 1988. Numerical Methods for Locating the Critical Slip Surface in Slope Stability Analysis, Proc. of the Sixth Int. Conf. on Numerical methods in Geomechanics, Innsbruck, 1219–1223.

Greco, V.R., 1996. Efficient Monte Carlo technique for locating critical slip surface, J. Geotech Engg., ASCE, 122(7); 517–525.

Greco, V.R., and Gulla, G., 1985. Slip surface search in slope-stability analysis, Rivista Indiana di Geotecnica, 19(4); 189–198.

Griffith, A.A., 1921. The phenomena of rupture and flow in solids, Phil. Trans., Royal Soc. London, Series A, 221: 163–198.

Griffith, A.A., 1924. Theory of rupture, lst Conf. App. Mech., Delft; 55–63.

Griffiths, D.V. and Lane, P.A., 1999. Slope stability analysis by finite elements, Geotechnique, 49(3); C55, 387–403.

Guzzetti, F., Peruccacci, S., Rossi, M., and Stark, C.P., 2007. Rainfall thresholds for the initiation of landslides in central and southern Europe, Meteorology and Atmospheric physics, DOI 10.1007/s00703-007-0262-7.

Habib, P., 1976. Production of gaseous pore pressure during rockslides, Rock Mechanics, 7: 193–197.

Haimson, B., 1968. Hydraulic fracturing in porous and non-porous rock and its potential for determining in situ stresses at great depth, U.S. Army Engineers, Missouri River Division, Tech. Report; 4–68.

Hamel, J.V., 1968. Morgenstern and Price Method of Slope Stability Analysis, Report by Dept. Civil Eng., Univ. of Pittsburgh to U.S. Bureau of Mines, 149 pp.

Hamel, J.V., 1971. Kimbley pit slope failure, Proc. 4th Pan Am. Conf. Soil Mech. Found. Eng., San Juan, Puerto Rico; 2: 117–127.

Hamel, J.V., 1972. The slide at Brilliant Cut, Proc. 13th Symp. Rock Mech., Urbana (Illinois), Ed. by E.J. Cording, ASCE; 487–570.

Hamel, J.V., 1973a. Rock strength from failure cases: Powerhouse slope stability study, Fort Peck Dam, Montana, Report MRD-l-73, Missouri River Division, U.S. Army Corps of Engineers, Omaha, Nebraska, U.S.A.

Hamel, J.V., 1973b. Large scale laboratory direct shear tests on desert alluvium, Proc. 15th Symp. rock mechanics, South Dakota, Ed. by E.R. Hoskins; 385–414.

Hamel, J.V., 1974. Rock strength from failure cases, Left bank slope stability study, Libby Dam and Lake Koocanusa, Montana, MRD-1-74, Missouri River Division, Corps of Engineers, Omaha, Nebraska, U.S.A.

Hamel, J.V., 1976. Libby Dam left abutment rock wedge stability, Rock Engineering for Foundation and Slopes, Proe. ASCE, GeotecE. Eng. Div. Specialty Conf. Boulder (Colorado), 1: 361–385.

Hamel, J.V., 1977. Personal Communication.

Hamel, J.V. and Flint, N.K., 1972. Failure of colluvial slope, J. Soil Mech. Found. Div., ASCE, 98, SM2; 167–180.

Hamel, J.V., Long, S.B. and Ferguson, H.P., 1976. Mahoning dam foundation reevaluation, Rock Engineering for Foundations and Slopes, Proc. ASCE, Geotech. Eng. Div. Specialty Conf. Boulder (Colorado), 1: 217–243.

Hamrol, A., 1961. A quantitative classification of the weathering and weather-ability of rocks, Proc. 5th Int. Conf. Soil Mech. Found. Eng., Paris, 2: 771–774.

Hand, D., 2000. Report of the inquesy into the deaths arising from the Thredbo landslide, Inquiry by the NSW Coroner, 29 June 2000, p. 212 plus attached maps and several technical reports available separately.

Hansen, J.B., 1952. A general plasticity theory for clay, Geotechnique, 3(4); 154–164.

Hansen, J.B. and Gibson, R.E., 1949. Undrained shear strengths of anisotropically consolidated clays, Geotechnique, 1(3); 189–204.

Harr, M.E., 1962. Groundwater and Seepage, McGraw-Hill, New York.

Harr, M.E., 1966. Foundations of Theoretical Soil Mechanics, McGraw-Hill, New York, 381 pp.

Harr, M.E., 1977. Mechanics of particulate media-a probabilistic approach, McGraw-Hill, New York, 543 pp.

Harr, M.E., 1987. Reliability-Based Design in Civil Engineering, McGraw-Hill, New York, 290 pp.

Hasofer, A.M. and Lind, N.C., 1974. A extract and Irvariant First Order Reliability Format, Journal of Engg. Mech., ASCE, Vol. 100, EM-1, pp. 111–121.

Hassan, A.M. and Wolff, T.F., 1999. Search Algorithm for Minimum Reliability Index of Earth Slopes, J. Geotechnical and Geoenviormental Engrg. 125(4); 301–308.

Hast, N., 1958. The measurement of rock pressure in mines, Sveriges Geologiska Undersokningg Stockholm, Ser. C, 52; 560.

Hast, N., 1967. The state of stress in the upper part of the earth's crust, Engineering Geology, 2(1); 5–17.

Hatzor, H. and Goodman, R.E., 1997. Three-dimensional back analyses of saturated rock slopes in discontinuous rock-a case study, Geotechnique, 47, No. 4, 817–839.

Heard, H.C., 1960. Transition from brittle fracture to ductile flow in Solenhofen limestone as a function of temperature, confining pressure and interstitial fluid pressure, Geol. Soc. Am. Mem., 79.

Heim, A., 1932. Bergsturz und Menschenleben, Fertz and Wasmuth, Zurich, 218 pp.

Heins, D.M., 1986. Slope Stability and Progressive Failure, Final Year Undergraduate Thesis, Department of Civil, Mining and Environmental Engineering, University of Wollongong, Australia.

Hendricks, M., Wilson, R., Moon, A., Stewart, I. and Flentje, P., 2005. Slope hazard assessment on a coast road in New South Wales, Australia. Joint Technical Committee on Landslides and Engineered Slopes, JTC-1, in association with Vancouver Geotechnical Society. Proceedings of the International Conference on Landslide Risk Management/18th Annual Vancouver Geotechnical Society Symposium, Vancouver. May 31 to June 4 (10 page pdf on CD).

Hendron, A.J. Jr., 1971. Analytical and graphical methods for the analysis of slopes in rock masses, NCG Tech. Rep. No-36, U.S. Army Engineers Waterways Experiment Station, 162 pp.

Hendron, A.J. Jr. and Patton, F.D., 1985. The Vaiont Slide, A geotechnical Analysis Based on New Geologic Observations on the Failure Surface, Vols. I and II, Final Report prepared for the Department of The Army, US Army Corps of Engineers, Washington, DC, Monitored by Geotechnical Laboratory, US Army Engineer Waterways Experiment Station, Vicksburg, Mississippi, USA.

Henkel, D.J., 1960. The shear strength of saturated remolded clays, Proc. ASCE, Conf. on Shear Strength of Cohesive Soils, Boulder (Colorado); 533–554.

Henkel, D.J., 1967. Local geology and the stability of natural slopes, J. Soil Mech. Found. Div., ASCE, 93, SM4; 437–446.

Henkel, D.J., 1970. Geotechnical considerations of lateral stresses, Proc. ASCE Geotech. Eng. Div. Specialty Conf. in Lateral stresses in the Ground and Design of Earth Retaining Structures, Cornell University; 1–50.

Herrman, L.R., 1965. Elasticity equations for incompressible and nearly incompressible materials by a variational theorem, AL4-A Journal, 3, 10.

Higginbottom, I.E. and Fookes, P.G., 1970. Engineering aspects of periglacial features in Britain, Quarterly Journal of Engineering Geology, 39(2); 85–119.

Hiroaki, F., Nishimura, S., Shimada, K. and Hori, T., 1999. Application of FEM on the basis of elasto-viscoplastic model to landslide problems, Proc. International Conference IS-Shikoku'99, Matsuyama, Shikoku, Japan, Slope Stability Engineering Edited by N Yagi, T Yamagami, J Jiang, Vol. 1, 219–224.

Hirschfeld, R.C. and Poulos, S.J., 1973. (Editors) Embankment Dam Engineering-Casagrande Volume, Wiley Interscience, 454 pp.

Hobbs, D.W., 1970. The behaviour of broken rock under triaxial compression, Int. J. Rock Mech. & Min. Sci., 7: 125–148.

Hoeg, K., Andersland, D.B. and Rolfsen, E.N., 1969. Undrained behaviour of quick clay under load tests at Asrum, Geotechnique, 19(1); 101–115.

Hoek, E., 1970. Estimating the stability of excavated slopes in open cast mines, Inst. Min. and Met., Transactions, 79: 109A–132A.

Hoek, E., 1976. State-of-the-art-paper on rock slopes, ASCE Geotech. Eng. Div. Specialty Conf., Boulder (Colorado), volume 2.

Hoek, E., 1987. General two-dimensional slope stability analysis, in E T Brown (Editor): Analytical and Computational Methods in Engineering Rock Mechanics, Allen and Unwin, 95–128.

Hoek, E., 1990. Estimating Mohr–Coulomb friction and cohesion values from the Hoek-Brown failure criterion, Int. J. Rock Mech. Min. Sci., 27, No. 3, 227–229.

Hoek, E. and Bray, J.W., 1974. Rock Slope Engineering, Inst. of Min. and Met., London, 310 pp.

Hoek, E. and Bray, J.W., 1977. Rock Slope Engineering, Revised Second Edition, Inst. of Min. and Met., London, 402 pp.

Hoek, E. and Londe, P., 1974. Surface workings in rock, Advances in Rock Mechanics, Proc. 3rd Congress, Int. Soc. Rock Mech., Denver (Colorado), 1, A; 613–654.

Hooker, V.E. and Johnson, C.F., 1969. Near surface horizontal stresses including the effects of rock anisotropy, U.S. Bureau Min. R.I., 7224.

Hough, B.K., 1957. Basic Soils Engineering, Ronald Press, New York.

Hovland, H.J., 1977. Three-dimensional slope stability analysis method, J. Geotech. Eng. Div., ASCE, 103, GT9; 971–987.

Hsu, K.J., 1978. Albert Heim: Observations on landslides, in Rockslides and Avalanches, Vol. 1, Ed. B. Voight, Elsevier, 833 pp.

Hult, J., Kvapil, R. and SLmdkvist, H., 1966. Function and scope of stress meters in rock mechanics, Int. J. Rock Mech. & Min. Sci., 3(1); 1–10.

Husein Malkawi, A.I., Hassan, W.F. and Sarma, S.K., 2001a. An efficient search method for finding critical circular slip surface using Monte Carlo techniques, Can., Geotech. J., Ottawa.

Husein Malkawi, A.I., Hassan, W.F. and Sarma, S.K., 2001b. Global search method for locating general slip surface using Monte Carlo techniques, Journal of Geotechnical and Geoenvironmental Engineering, Vol. 127, No. 8.

Hutchinson, J.N., 1995. Landslide hazard assessment, Proc. VI Int Symp Landslides,Christch- urch, 1: 1805–1842.

Hutchinson, J.N. and Del Prete, M., 1985. Landslides at Caltiri, Southern Appenines reactivated by the earthquake of 23rd Nov. 1980, Geologia Applicata Idrogelogia,, Vol. XX, part I, 1985, 9–38.

Hynes-Griffin, M.E. and Franklin, A.G., 1984. Rationalising the seismic coefficient method, Miscellaneous Paper No. GL-84–13, U.S. Army Engineering Waterways Experiment Station, Vicksburgh, Mississipi.

Ireland, H.O., 1954. Stability Analysis of Congress Street Open Cut in Chicago, Geotechnique Vol. 4, 163–168.

Ishizaki, H. and Hatakeyama, N., 1962. Considerations of the vibrational behaviour of earth dams; Bulletin No-52, Disaster Prevention Research Institute, Kyoto University, Kyoto, Japan.

Jaeger, J.C., 1970. The behaviour of closely jointed rock, Proc. llth Symposium on Rock Mechanics, Berkeley, 57–68.

Jaeger, J.C., 1971. Friction of rocks and stability of rock slopes, Rankine Lecture, Geotechnique, 21(2); 97–134.

Jaeger, C., 1972. Rock Mechanics and Engineering, Cambridge University Press, England, 417 pp.

Jaeger, J.C. and Cook, N.G.W., 1968. Fundamentals of Rock Mechanics, Chapman and Hall, London, 515 pp.

Jaky, J., 1944. The co-efficient of earth pressure at rest, Magyar Mernok es Epitesz Egglet Koz-lonye.

James, P.M., 1971a. The role of progressive failure in clay slopes, Proc. lst Australia-New Zealand Conf. Geomechanies, 1: 344–348.

James, P.M., 1971b. Some effects of structure on the behaviour of argillaceous sediments, Proe. lst Australia-New Zealand Conf. Geomechanics, 1: 154–159.

James, R.G. and Bransby, P.L., 1971. A velocity field for some passive earth pressure problems, Geotechnique, 21(1); 61–83.

Janbu, N., 1954a. Stability analysis of slopes with dimensionless parameters. Harvard Soil Mechanics Series No. 46, 811 pp.

Janbu, N., 1954b. Application of composite slip surfaces for stability analysis, European Conference on Stability of Earth Slopes, Stockholm, Discussion, 3.

Janbu, N., 1957. Earth pressure and bearing capacity calculations by generalised procedure of slices, Proc. 4th Int. Conf. Soil Mech. Found. Eng., 2: 207–212.

Janbu, N., 1973. Soil Stability Computations, Embankment Dam Engineering, Casagrande Volume, Ed. by R.C. Hirschfeld and S.J. Poulos, Wiley, New York, 47–87.

Janbu, N., 1977. State-of-the-art report on Slopes and Excavations in Normally and Lightly Overconsolidated Clays, 9th Int. Conf. Soil Mech. Found. Eng., Tokyo, 2, 549–566.

Janbu, N., Bjerrum, L. and Kjaernsli, B., 1956. Soil mechanics applied to some engineering problems, Norwegian Geotech. Institute, Publication No. 16.

Jenike, A.W. and Yen, B.C., 1963. Slope stability in axial symmetry, Proc. 5th Symp. Rock Mechanics, 689–711.

Jennings, J.E., 1970. A mathematical theory for the calculation of the stability of slopes in open cast mines, Proc. Symposium on Open Pit Mining, Johannesburg.

Jiang, G.L. and Magnan, J.P., 1997. Stability analysuis of embankments : comparison of limit analysis with method of slices, Geotechnique, 47, No. 4, 857–872 (See Table 2, see also discussion in Geotechnique 2002, 52, No. 4, 305–306 where more results are given by Donald and Giam which complement Table 2 of this paper).

Jibson, R.W., 2007. Regression models for estimating coseismic landslide displacement, Engineering Geology, Volume 91, 209–218.

Jibson, R.W., Harp, E.L. and Michael, J.A., 1998. A method for producing digital probabilistic seismic landslide hazard maps: an example from the Los Angeles, California area. Open-file report 98–113, 1998, 17 pp + 2 maps, USGS, Denver Federal Center, Denver, CO, USA.

Jibson, R.W., Harp, E.L. and Michael, J.A., 2000. A method for producing digital probabilistic seismic landslide hazard maps, Engineering Geology 58(3–4); 271–289 Dec 2000.

Jibson, R.W. and Jibson, M.W., 2003, Java programs for using Newmark's method and simplified decoupled analysis to model slope performance during earthquakes: U.S. Geological Survey Open-File Report 03-005, version 1.1, on CD-ROM".

Jitno, H. and Byrne, P.M., 1995. Predicted and observed liquefaction-induced deformations of La Palma dam, Third Int. Conf. Recent Advances in Geotechnical Earthquake Eng. and Soil Dynamics, St Louis, Missouri (USA), 6 pp.

John, K.W., 1968. Graphical stability analysis of slopes in jointed rock, J. Soil Mech. Found. Div. ASCE, 94, SM2; 497–526.

John, K.W., 1969. Civil Engineering approach to evaluate strength and deformability of regularly jointed rock, Proc. llth Symp. Rock Mech., Berkeley; 69–80.

Johnson, S.J., 1975. Analysis and design relating to embankments, Proc. Geotech. Eng. Div. Spec. Conf. on Analysis and Design in Geotech. Eng., University of Austin, Texas, 1974. 2: 1–48.

Johnston, M.M., 1969. Laboratory comparison tests using compacted fine-grained soils, Proc. 7th Int. Conf. Soil Mech. Found. Eng., Mexico, 1: 197.

Karal, K., 1977a. Energy method for soil stability analyses, J. Geotech. Eng. Div., ASCE, 103, GT5; 431–447.

Karal, K., 1977b. Application of energy method, J. Geotech. Eng. Div., ASCE, 103, GT5; 381–399.

Katrina, 2008. Contributions from several authors to Katrina Special Issue, Journal of Geotechnical and Geoenvironmental Engineering, ASCE, Vol. 134, No. 5, May 1, 2008, 555–717.

Kavazanjian, E., Jr., Matasovic, N., Hadj-Hamou, T., Sabatini, P.J., 1997. Design Guidance: Geotechnical Earthquake Engineering for Highways, Vol. 1, Design Principles, Geotechnical Engineering Circular 3, Publication FHWA-SA-97-06, FHA, US Dept of Transportation, Washington, DC.

Kawakami, H. Suwa, Marui, H., Sato, O. and Izumi, K., 1999. The Otari debris flow disaster occurred in December 1996, Proc. Int. Symposium on slope stability engineering, Matsuyama, Japan, November, Vol. 2, 1379–184.

Keefer, D.K., 1984. Landslides caused by earthquakes, Geol. Soc. Annual Bulletin, 95, 1984, 406–421.

Keefer, D.K., 1994. The importance of earthquake-induced landslides to long-term slope erosion and slope-failure hazards in seismically active regions, Geomorphology, 10, 1994, 265–284.

Keefer, D.K., 2007. Landslides caused by recent earthquakes: Anomalies and relations to general trends, First North American landslide Conference, Vail Colorado, USA, June 3–10, 2007, CD-ROM, 2007, pp. 876–883.

Keefer, D.K. and Wilson, R.C., 1989. Predicting earthquake-induced landslides, with emphasis on arid and semi-arid environments, in P.M. Sadler & D.M. Morton (editors) Landslides in a semi-arid environment with emphasis on the inland valleys of Southern California, 2, Inland Geographic Society of Southern California Publications, Riverside, CA Pt 1, 1989, 118–149.

Kehle, R.O., 1964. Determination of tectonic stresses through analysis of hydraulic well fracturing, J. Geophys. Res., 69, 259.

Kenney, T.C., 1967a. Field measurement of in situ stresses in quick clays, Proc. Geotech. Conf., Oslo, 1: 49–55.

Kenney, T.C., 1967b. The influence of mineral composition on the residual strength of natural soils, Proc. Geotech. Conf., Oslo, 1: 123–129.

Kenney, T.C., 1967c. Stability of the Vajont Valley Slope, Rock Mech. Eng. Geol., 5, 1.

Kenney, T.C., 1977. Residual strength of mineral mixtures, Proc. 9th Int. Conf. Soil Mechanics and Found. Eng., Tokyo, 1: 155–160.

Kjellman, W., 1936. Report on an apparatus for the consummate investigation of mechanical properties of soils, Proc. Ist Int. Conf. Soil Mech. Found. Eng., 2: 16–20.

Kjellman, W., 1955. Mechanics of large Swedish landslides, Geotechnique, 5: 74.

Knight, K. and Blight, G.E., 1965. Studies of some effects resulting from the unloading of soils, Proc. 6th Int. Conf. Soil Mech. Found. Eng., 1: 282–286.

Ko, K.C., 1972. Discrete element technique for pit slope analysis, Stability of Rock Slopes, 13th Symp. Rock Mechanics, Ed. by E.J. Cording, ASCE; 183–199.

Ko Ko, C., 2001. Landslide Hazard and Risk Assessment Along a Railway Line, Ph.D. Thesis, University of Wollongong, Wollongong, New South Wales, Australia.

Ko Ko, C., Flentje, P. and Chowdhury, R., 2003. Quantitative Landslide Hazard and Risk Assessment: a case study, Quarterly Journal of Engineering Geology and Hydrogeology, Vol. 36, 261–272.

Ko Ko, C., Flentje, P. and Chowdhury, R., 2004. Landslide qualitative hazard and risk assessment method and its reliability, Bull Eng Geol ENv (2004) 63: 149–165.

Kobayashi, Y., 1981. Causes of fatalities in recent earthquakes in Japan, Journal of Disaster Science, Vol. 3, 15–22.

Koerner. R.M., 1998. Designing with Geosynthetics, 4th edition, Prentice Hall, New Jersey, USA.

Kojan, E. and Hutchinson, J.N., 1978. Mayunmarca rockslide and debris flow, Peru, in Rockslides and Avalanches, Ed. B. Voight, Elsevier, 833 pp.

Kondner, R.L. and Zelasko, J.S., 1963. A hyperbolic stress-strain formulation for sands, Proc. 2nd Pan American Conf. Soil Mech. Found. Eng., Brazil, 1: 289–324.

Kondner, R.L., 1963. Hyperbolic stress-strain response: cohesive soils, J. Soil Mech. Found. Div., ASCE, 89, SMI; 115–143.

Koppula, S., 1970. The consolidation of soils in two dimensions and with moving boundaries, Ph.D. Thesis, University of Alberta, Edmonton, Canada.

Krahn, J., 2001. The R.M. Hardy Lecture: The limits of limit equilibrium analyses, Can. Geotech J, Vol. 40, 643–660.

Krahn, J. and Morgenstern, N.R., 1976. Mechanics of the Frank Slide, Rock Engineering for Foundations and Slopes, ASCE Geotech. Eng. Specialty Conf., Boulder (Colorado), 1: 309–331.

Kramer, S.L., 1996. Geotechnical Earthquake Engineering, Prentice Hall, New Jersey, USA.

Kramer, S.L., and Smith, M.W., 1997. Modified Newmark Model for Seismic Displacements of Compliant Slopes, Journal of Geotechnical and Geoenvironmental Engineering, ASCE, 123(7); 635–644.

Krishna, J., 1962. Earthquake resistant design of earth dams, Proc. Earthquake Symposium, Roorkee University, Roorkee (U.P.), India.

La Rochelle, P., 1960. The short term stability of slopes in London clay, Ph.D. Thesis, Univ. of London.

Ladanyi, B. and Archambault, G., 1970. Simulation of shear behaviour of a jointed rock mass, Proc. llth Symp. Rock Mech., AIME, New York, 105–125.

Ladanyi, B. and Archambault, G., 1972. Evolution de la resistance au cisaillement d'lum massif rocheux fragmente, Proc. 24th Int. Geol. Congress, Montreal, 13D; 249–260.

Ladd, C.C. and Foott, R.P., 1974. New design procedure for stability of soft clays, J. Geotech. Eng. Div., ASCE, 100, GT7; 763–786.

Lambe, T.W. and Whitman, R.V., 1969. Soil Mechanics, John Wiley, New York, 553 pp.

Langer, K., 1936. Discussion by K. Terzaghi reporting observations at Provins, France, Proc. lst Int. Conf. Soil Mech. Found. Eng., 3: 152–155.

Lee, E.M. and Jones, D.K.C., 2004. Landslide Risk Assessment, Thomas Telford Ltd., 454 pp.

Lee, K.L., 1974. Earthquake induced permanent deformations of embankments, Report No. UCIA-ENG-7498, School of Eng. and App. Sci., Univ. of California, Los Angeles.

Lee, K.L. and Roth, W., 1977. Seismic stability analysis of Hawkins hydraulic fill dam, J. Geotech. Eng. Div., ASCE, 103, GT6; 627–644.

Lee, K.L. and Seed, H.B., 1967. Dynamic strength of anisotropically consolidated sand, J. Soil Mech. Found. Div., ASCE, 93, SM5; 169–190.

Lee, K.L., Seed, H.B., Idriss, I.M. and Makdisi, F.I., 1975. Properties of soil in the San Fernando Hydraulic Fill Dams, Journal of Geotechnical Engineering Division, ASCE, 101, GT8; 801–821.

Lee, K.L. and Singh, A., 1968. Direct shear report, UCIA Publ. for ASCE, Los Angeles Chapter, Los Angeles, USA.

Lekhnitskii, S.G., 1963. Theory of Elasticity of an Anisotropic Body, Translated from the Russian by P. Fern, Holden Day, San Francisco.

Leonards, G.A., 1983. Investigation of Failures, Terzaghi Lecture, Journal of Geotechnical Engineering Division, ASCE, 108, GT2; 187–246.

Leroueil, S., 2001. 39th Rankine Lecture: Natural slopes and cuts: movement and failure mechanisms, Geotechnique, April, Vol. LI, Number 3, 195–244.

Les'niewska, D. and Mro'z, Z., 2000. Limit equilibrium approach to study the evolution of shear band systems in soils, Geotechnique, volume 50, Number 5, 521–536.

Li, K.S. 1992. "Point-estimate method for calculating statistical moments", Journal of Engineering Mechanics, ASCE, 118(7); 1506–1511.

Li, K.S. and White, W., 1987. Rapid evaluation of the critical slip surface in slope stability problems, Int. J. Numer and Analytical Methods in Geomech, 11: 449–473.

Lighthall, P., 1979. Dimensionless charts for critical acceleration and static stability of earth slopes, MSc Dissertation, Imperial College (London, UK), Civil Engineering, Soil Mechanics and Engineering Seismology Section.

Ling, I., Leshchinsky, D. and Perry, E.B., 1997. Seismic design and performance of geosynthetic–reinforced soil structures, Geotechnique, 47, No. 5, 933–952.

Lo, K.Y., 1965. Stability of slopes in anisotropic soil, J. Soil Mech. Found. Div., ASCE, 91, SM4; 85–106.

Lo, K.Y., 1970. The operational strength of fissured clays, Geotechnique, 20: 57–74.

Lo, K.Y. and Lee, C.F., 1973. Stress analysis and slope stability in strainsoftening materials, Geotechnique, 23(1); 1–11.

Lo, K.Y., Lee, C.F. and Gelinas, P., 1972. An alternative interpretation of the Vajont slide, Stability of Rock Slopes, Ed. by E.J. Cording, ASCE; 595–625.

Londe, P., 1973. The role of rock mechanics in the reconnaissance of rock foundations, Quart. J. Eng. Geol., 6(1); 57–74.

Londe, P., Vigiert, G. and Vorlbringer, R., 1969. Stability of rock slopes, a three-dimensional study, J. Soil Mech. Found. Div., ASCE, 95, SMI; 235–262.

Low, B.K., 1996. Practical Probabilistic Approach Using Spreadsheets, Geotechnical Special Publication No58,Uncertainty in the Geologic Environment: From Theory to Practice, ASCE, Proc. Vol. 2, Madison, Wis. USA, 1284–1302.

Lowe, J., 1967. Stability analysis of embankments, J. Soil Mech. Found. Div., ASCE, 93, SM4; 1–33.

Lumb, P., 1975. Slope Failures in Hong Kong, Quarterly Journal of Engineering Geology, Vol. 8, 31–65.

Lutton, R.J., 1975. Study of clay shale slopes along the Panama Canal, U.S. Army Engineers Waterways Experiment Station, S-70-9, Report 21 Vicksburgh, U.S.A.

Lutton, R.J. and Banks, D.C., 1970. Study of clay shale slopes along the Panama Canal, U.S. Army Engineers Waterways Experiment Station, S-70-9, Report 1, Vicksburgh, U.S.A.

Lysmer, J., 1970. Limit Analysis of plane problems in soil mechanics, J. Soil Mech. Found. Div., ASCE, 96, SM4; 1311–1334.

Makdisi, F.I. and Seed, H.B., 1978. Simplified procedure for estimating dam and embankment earthquake-induced deformations, Journal of the Geotechnical Engineering Division, ASCE, Vol. 104, No. GT 7, 1978, 849–867.

Marachi, N.D., Chan, C.K. and Seed, H.B., 1972. Evaluation of properties of rockfill materials, J. Soil Mech. Found. Div., ASCE, 98, SM1; 95–114.

Marcuson III, W.F., Hynes, M.E. and Franklin, A.G., 1992. Seismic stability and permanent deformation analyses: the last twenty five years, Stability and Performance of Slopes and Embankments, a 25 year perspective, Geotechnical Special Publication No. 31, ASCE, 552–59.

Marsal, R.J., 1973. Mechanical properties of rockfill, Embankment Dam Engineering Casagrande Volume, Ed. by R.C. Hirschfeld and S.J. Poulos, Wiley, New York, 109–200.

Marsland, A., 1967. Discussion on 'Shear Strength of Natural Soils and Rocks,' Proc. Geotech. Conf., Oslo, 2: 160–161.

Matheson, D.S., 1972. Geotechnical implications of Valley Rebound, Ph.D. Thesis, University of Alberta7 Edmontont Canada.

Matheson, D.S. and Thomson, S., 1973. Geological implications of valley rebound, Canadian J. of Earth Sciences, 10: 961–978.

Mathur, L.P., 1953. Assam earthquake of 15th August 1950 – A short note on factual observations. A compilation of papers on the Assam earthquake of August 15, 1950, compiled by M. Ramachandra Rao, Central Board of Geophysics, Government of India, 1953, 56–60.

Matsui, T. and San, K.C., 1992. Finite element slope stability analysis by shear strength reduction technique, Soils and Foundations, 32, No. 1, 59–70.

Matthai, A.C. and Ranganatham, B.V., 1968. Stability of free and retained slopes of anisotropic, non-homogeneous soil, Sols Soils, 20: 11–19.

Matthews, M.D., 1983. Progressive Failure by the Limit Equilibrium Approach, Final Year Undergraduate Thesis, Department of Civil, Mining and Environmental Engineering, University of Wollongong, Australia.

McInnes, R., Jakeways, J., Fairbank, H. and Mathie, E., (eds), 2007. Landslides and Climate Change, challenges and solutions, Taylor & Francis Group, 514 pp.

McSaveney, M.J., 2002. Recent rockfalls and rock avalanches in Mount Cook National Park, New Zealand, in Evans S.G. and DeGraff J.V. (2002), eds., Catastrophic Landslides: Effects, Occurrence and Mechanisms, Reviews in Engineering Geology XV, The Geological Society of America, pp. 35–71.

McClintock, F.A. and Walsh, J.B., 1962. Friction on Griffith cracks under pressure, Proc. 4th U.S. National Conf. App. Mech.; 1015–1021.

Menard, L., 1957. Measures in situ des proprieties physiques des sols, Annls Ponts Chauss.

Menzies, B.K., Sutton, H. and Davies, R.W., 1977. A new system for automatically simulating K consolidation and K_o swelling in the conventional triaxial test, Geotechique, 27(4); 593–599.

Meyerhof, G.G., 1965. Discussion of paper, 'Stability of slopes in anisotropic soil', J. Soil Mech. Found. Div., ASCE, 91, SM6; 132.

Michalowski, R.L., 1995. Slope stability analysis: a kinematical approach, Geotechnique, 45, No. 2, 283–293.

Michalowski, R.L., 2007. Displacements of multi block geotechnical structures subjected to seismic excitation, Journal of Geotechnical and Geoenvironmental Engineering, Vol. 133, No. 11, 1432–39.

Michalowski, R.L., 2009. Critical Pool level and stability of slopes in Granular Soils, Journal of Geotechnical and Geoenvironmental Engineering, ASCE, Vol. 135, No. 3, 444–448.

Miles, S.B., Keefer, D.K. and Ho, C.L., 1999. Seismic slope-performance analysis: from hazard map to decision support system, 5th US Conf. on Lifeline Earthquake Engineering, ASCE, Reston, VA, 10 pp.

Mitchell, J.K., 1976. Fundamentals of Soil Behaviour, John Wiley, New York, 422 pp.

Mitchell, J.K., Seed, R.B. and Seed, H.B., 1990. Kettleman Hills waste landfill slope failure: I. Liner system properties, ASCE, Journal of Geotechnical Engineering, 116(4); 647–668.

Moon, A.T., Wilson, R.A. and Flentje, P.N., 2005. Developing and using landslide size frequency models. Joint Technical Committee on Landslides and Engineered Slopes, JTC-1, in association with Vancouver Geotechnical Society. Proceedings of the International Conference on Landslide Risk Management/18th Annual Vancouver Geotechnical Society Symposium, Vancouver. May 31 to June 4, pp. 681–690.

Morgan, G.C., Rawlings, G.E. and Sobkowicz, J.C., 1992. Evaluating total risk to communities from large debris flows, Proc. of the 1st Canadian Symposium on Geotechnique and Natural Hazards, Vancouver, Canada, 225–236.

Morgenstern, N.R., 1963. Stability charts for earth slopes during rapid draw down, Geotechnique, 13(2); 121–132.

Morgenstern, N.R., 1968. Ultimate behaviour of rock structures, Rock Mechanics in Engineering Practice, Ed. by K.G. Stagg and O.C. Zienkiewiez, Wiley; 321–346.

Morgenstern, N.R., 1977. State-of-the-art report and preliminary general report on Slopes and Excavations, 9th Int. Conf. Soil Mech. Found. Eng., Tokyo, 2: 547–603.

Morgenstern, N.R. and Price, V.E., 1965. The analysis of the stability of general slip surfaces, Geotechnique, 15(1); 79–93.

Morgenstern, N.R. and Tahmasseb, I.A., 1965. Stability of a slurry trench in cohesionless soil, Geotechnique, 15: 387–395.

Morgenstern, N.R. and Tchalenko, J.S., 1967a. Microstructural observations on shear zones from slips in natural clays, Proc. Geotech. Conf. Oslo, 1: 147–152.

Morgenstern, N.R. and Tchalenko, J.S., 1967b, Microstructural structures in Kaolin subjected to direct shear, Geotechnique, 17: 309–328.

Muller, L., 1964. The rock slide in the Vajont Valley, Rock Mech. Eng. Geol., 2: 148–228.

Muller, L., 1968. New considerations on the Vajont slide, Rock Mech. Eng. Geol., 6: 1–91.

Muller, L., 1977. Opening address to 25th Geomechanics Colloquy, Entwicklungstendenzen in der Geomechanik, Rock Mech., Suppl. 6.

Murray, E., 2001. Rainfall Thresholds for Landslide Initiation in the Wollongong Region, Internal report to Australian Geological Survey Organisation and SPIRT Project Team at the University of Wollongong.

Murrell, S.A.F., 1965. The effect of triaxial stress system on the strength of rocks at atmospheric temperatures, Geophys. J., 10: 231–281.

Navdocks, 1962. Design Manual. Soil Mechanics, Foundations and Earth Structures, Navdocks, DM-7, Dept. of the Navy, Bureau of yards and docks, Washington, U.S.A.

Newmrk, N.M., 1965. Effect of earthquakes on dams and embankments, Rankine Lecture, Geotechnique, 15(1); 139–160.

Nguyen, V.U., 1985. Determination of critical slope failure surfaces, Geotech. Eng. Div., ASCE, 111, GT2; 238–250.

Nguyen, V.U. and Chowdhury, R., 1984. Probabilistic Study of Spoil Pile Stability in Strip Coal Mines-Two Techniques Compared, Int. J. Rock Mech. Min. Sci & Geomech Abstr, Vol. 21, No. 6, 303–312.

Nguyen, V.U. and Chowdhury, R., 1985. Simulation for Risk with Correlated Variables, Geotechnique, Vol. 35, No. 1, 47–58.

Nonveiller, E., 1965. The stability analysis of slopes with a slip surface of general shape, Proc. 6th Int. Conf. Soil Mech. Found. Eng., 2: 522–525.

Obert, L., 1967. Determination of stress in rock, A state-of-the-art report, ASTM, STP 429.

Obert, L. and Stephenson, D., 1965. Stress conditions under which core discing occurs, Trans. AIME, 232(3); 227–236.

Ozawa, Y. and Duncan, J.M., 1976. Elasto-plastic finite element idealisation of sand deformations, Numerical Methods in Geomechanies, Ed. by C.S. Desai, ASCE, 1: 243–269.

Palladino, D.J. and Peck, R.B., 1972. Slope failures in an overconsolidated clay, Seattle, Washington, Geotechnique, 22: 563–595.

Palmer, A.C., 1973a. (Editor) Proc. Symp. on Plasticity and Soil Mechanics, Cambridge University Engineering Department, England, 314 pp.

Palmer, A.C., 1973b. Discussion on paper, 'some applications of classical plasticity theory for soil stability problems', Proc. Symp. on Plasticity and Soil Mechanics, Ed. by A.C. Palmer, Cambridge Univ. Eng. Dept., England.

Palmer, A.C. and Rice, J.R., 1973. The growth of slip surfaces in the progressive failure of overconsolidated clay, Proc. Royal Soc. London, A 332: 527–548.

Patton, F.D., 1966. Multiple modes of shear failure in rock, Proc. lst Int. Cong. Rock Mechanics, Lisbon, 1: 509–514.

Paulding, B.W., 1970. Co-efficient of friction of natural rock surfaces, J. Soil Mech. Found. Div., ASCE, 96, SM2; 385–394.

Peacock, W.H. and Seed, H.B., 1968. Sand liquefaction under cyclic loading sim,)le shear conditions, J. Soil Mech. Found. Div., ASCE, 94, SM3; 689–708.

Peck, R.B., 1967. Stability of natural slopes, J. Soil Mech. Found. Div., ASCE, 93, SM4; 403–417.

Peck, R.B., 1969. Advantages and limitations of the observational method in applied soil mechanics, Rankine Lecture, Geotechniqueg 19(2); 171–187.

Peck, R.B., 1973. Presidential Address, Proc. 8th Int. Conf. Soil Mech., Moscow, 4(1); 156–159.

Peck, R.B., 1977. Keynote address to Penrose Conference (Geol. Soc. of Am. and ASCE joi.qt meeting) Vail, Coloradot Oct. 9, 1977, Unpublished (notes of talk by courtesy of Dr. James V. Hamel).

Peck, R.B., 1980. Where has all the judgment gone? Laurits Bjerrum Mineforedrag No. 5, Norges Geotekniske Institut, Oslo p. 5, also published in Canadian Geotechnical Journal,17, 1980, 585–590 and in Norwegian Geotechnical Institute Publication, 134: 1–5.

Peck, R.B., 1982. Proc. Dam Safety Research Coordination Conf., Interagency Committee on Dam Safety, Research Sub-committee, Denver, II-2-11.

Peck, R.B., Hanson, W.E. and Thornburn, T.H., 1974. Foundation Engineering, 2nd Edition, John Wiley, New York.

Peterson, R., 1954. Studies of Bearpaw shale at a damsite in Saskatchewan, Proc. ASCE, 80, Separates No. 476 and 759.

Petley, D.N., Dunning, S.A. and Rosser, N.J., 2005. The analysis of global landslide risk through the creation of a database of worldwide landslide fatalities, Landslide Risk Management-Hungr, Fell, Couture&Eberhardt (eds), Conference Proceedings of an International Conference held at Vancouver, Canad, 31 May–3 June, Taylor&Francis Group, London, 367–373.

Potts, D.M., 2003. 42nd Rankine Lecture: Numerical analysis: a virtual dream or practical reality?, Geotechnique, August, Vol. LIII, Number 6, 533–574.

Potts, D.M., Kovacevic, N. and Vaughan, P.R., 1990. Finite element analysis of progressive failure of Carsington embankment, Geotechnique, Vol. 40, No. 1, 79–101.

Potts, D.M., Kovacevic, N. and Vaughan, P.R., 1997. Delayed collapse of cut slopes in stiff clay, Geotechnique, 47, No. 5, 953–982.

Poulos, H.G., 1995. Design of reinforcing pilesto increase slope stability,Canadian Geotechnical Journal, 32(5); 808–818.

Poulos, H.G., 1999. Design of slope stabilising piles, Proceedings of the International Conference on Slope Stability Engineering, IS-Shikoku, Matsuyama, Japan, 1, 67–81.

Poulos, H.G. and Davis, E.H., 1972. Laboratory determination of in-situ horizontal stress in soil masses, Geotechnique, 22(1); 177–182.

Prater, E.G., 1979. Yield acceleration for seismic stability of slopes, Journal of Geotechnical Engineering Division, ASCE, Vol. 105, No. GT5, 682–687.

Puzrin, A.M. and Houlsby, G.T., 2001. Strain-based plasticity models for soils and the BRICK model as an example of the hyperplasticity approach, Geotechnique, 51, No. 2, 169–172.

Quinlan, R., 1993. C4.5: Programs for Machine Learning, San Mateo, CA: Morgan Kaufmann.

Ramamurthy, T., Narayan, C.G.P. and Bhetkar, V.P., 1977. Variational method for slope stability analysis, Proc. 9th Int. Conf. Soil Mechanics Found. Eng., Tokyo, 2: 139–143.

Rana, M.H. and Bullock, W.D., 1969. The design of open pit mine slopes, Canadian Mining Journal; 58–66.

Rankine, W.J.M., 1862. A Manual of Civil Engineering, Griffin and Bohn, London.

Resendiz, D., 1974. Discussion of 'Aaccuracy equilibrium slope stability analysis', J. Geotech. Eng. Div., ASCE, 100, GT8, 967–970.

Resendiz, D., 1977. Slopes in compacted soils, General Report, Proc. gth Int. Conf. Soil Mech. Found. Eng., Tokyo, 2: 591–597.

Revilla, J. and Castillo, E., 1977. The calculus of variation applied to stability problems, Geotechnique 27(1); 1–11.

Rice, J.R., 1973. The initiation and growth of shear bands, Proc. Symp. on Plasticity and Soil Mechanics, Ed. by A.C. Palmer, Cambridge Univ. Eng. Dept.; 263–274.

Rice, J.R. and Simons, D.A., 1976. The stabilisation of spreading shear faults by coupled deformation-diffusion effects in fluid-infiltrated porous materials, J. Geophy. Res., 81: 5322–5334.

Richards, B.G., 1982. The finite Element Analysis of Mine Spoil Piles Using Slip Elements to Simulate Strain-softening Yield Behaviour. Civil Engineering Transactions, Institution of Engineers, Australia, Vol. CE 24, 69–76.

Richards, B.G., Coulthard, M.A. and Toh, C.T., 1981. Analysis of Slope Stability at Goonyella Mine,Canadian Geotechnical Journal, Vol. 18, 179–194.

Richter, C.F., 1958. Elementary Seismology. W.H. Freeman and Co. San Francisco.

Robertson, A. MacG. 1971. Accounting for cracks in slope stability analysis, 5th Regional Conf. for Africa on Soil Mechanics Found. Eng., Luanda, Angola; 4.3–4.10.

Rocha, M., 1964. Mechanical behaviour of rock foundations in concrete dams, Trans. 8th Int. Cong. on Large Dams, Edinburgh, 1: 785–832.

Rocha, M., 1974. Present possibilities of studying foundations of concrete dams, Advances in Rock Mechanics, Proc. 3rd Cong. Int. Soc. Rock Mech., Denver (Colorado), 1, A; 879–897.

Rodrigquez, C.E., Bommer, J.J. and Chandler, R.J., 1999. Earthquake-induced landslides: 1980–1997, SDEE, 8, 1999, 326–346.

Romani, F., Lovell, C.W. and Harr, M.E., 1972. Influence of progressive failure on slope stability, J. Soil Mech. Found. Div. ASCE, 98, SM11; 1209–1223.

Romero, S.U. and Molina, R., 1974, Kinematic aspects of the Vaiont slide, Proc. 3rd Congress Int. Soc. Rock Mechanics, Denver, Col., Sept, Vol. II, Part B, 865–870.

Roscoe, K.H., 1970. The importance of strains in soil mechanics, Rankine Lecture, Geotechnique, 20(2); 129–170.

Roscoe, K.H., Schofield, A.N. and Wroth, C.P., 1958. On the yielding of soils, Geotechnique, 8(1); 22–53.

Rosenblueth, E., 1975. Point Estimates for Probability Moments, Proc National Academy of Sciences of the United States of America, 72: 3812–3814.

Rowe, P.W., 1972. The relevance of soil fabric to site investigation practice, Rankine Lecture, Geotechnique, 22: 195–300.

Rutledge, P.C. and Gould, J.P., 1973. Movements of articulated conduits under earth dams on compressible foundations, Embankment Dam Engineering-Casagrande Volume, Ed. by R.C. Hirschfeld and S.J. Poulos, Wiley, New York; 209–239.

Saito, M., 1965. Forecasting the time of occurrence of slope failure, Proc. 6th Int. Conf. Soil Mech. Found. Eng., Montreal 2: 537–541.

Samsioe, A.F., 1936. Report on the investigation of the compressibility of the ground of the hydroelectric power plant, Svir 3, Proc. Ist Int. Conf. Soil Mech. Found. Eng., 1; 41–47.

Sancio, R.T. and Goodman, R.E., 1979. Analysis of the Stability of Slopes in Weathered Rock, 4th Int. Congress on Rock Mechanics, Vol. 1, 723–730.

Sarma, S.K., 1973. Stability analysis of embankments and slopes, Geotechnique, 23: 423–433.

Sarma, S.K., 1975. Seismic stability of earth dams and embankments. Geotechnique, 25(4); 743–761.

Sarma, S.K., 1979. Stability analysis of embankments and slopes, Journal of Geotechnical Engineering Division, ASCE,105, GT12, 1979, 1511–1524.

Sarma, S.K., 1988. Seismic response and stability of earth dams. Seismic Risk Assessment and Design of Building Structures, Ed A. Koridze, Omega Scientific, 143–160, 1988.

Sarma, S.K., 2006. Personal communications, February 2006.

Sarma, S.K. and Jennings, D.N., 1980. A dynamic pore pressure parameter An, Proc. Int. Symp. on Soils under Cyclic and Transient Loading, Swansea, England, Vol. 1, No. 2, 295–298.

Sarma, S.K. and Kourkoulis, R., 2004. Investigation into the prediction of sliding block displacements in seismic analysis of earth dams. Proc. 13 WCEE, paper no 1957, Vancouver, Canada, 2004.

Saygili, G. and Rathje, E.M., 2008. Empirical Predictive Models for Earthquake-Induced Sliding Displacement of Slopes, Journal of Geotechnical and Geoenvironmental Engineering, ASCE, 134(6); 790–803.

Schmertmann, J.H., 2006. Estimating slope stability reduction due to rain infiltration mounding, Journal of Geotechnical and Geoenvironmental Engineering, ASCE, 132, No. 9, September, 1219–1228.

Schmertmann, J.H. and Osterbergg, J.O., 1961. An experimental study of the development of cohesion and friction with axial strain in saturated cohesive soil, Proc. ASCE Research Conf. Shear Strength of Cohesive Soils, Boulder, (Colorado); 643–694.

Schofield, A.N. and Wroth, C.P., 1968. Critical State Soil Mechanics, McGraw-Hill, England, 310 pp.

Schuster, R.L., Salcedo, D.A. and Valenzuela, L., 2002. Overview of catastrophic landslides of South America in the twentieth century, in, Evans S.G. and DeGraff J.V. (2002), eds., Catastrophic Landslides: Effects, Occurrence and Mechanisms,Reviews in Engineering Geology XV, The Geological Society of America, pp. 1–34.

Seed, H.B., 1966. A method for the earthquake resistant design of earth dams, J. Soil Mech. Found. Div., ASCE, 92, SM1; 13–41.

Seed, H.B., 1967. Slope stability during earthquakes, Soil Mech. Found. Div., ASCE, 93, SM4; 299–323.

Seed, H.B., 1968. Landslides during earthquakes due to soil liquefaction, Terzaghi Lecture, J. Soil Mech. Found. Div., ASCE, 94, SM5; 193–261.

Seed, H.B., 1970. Earth slope stability during earthquakes, Chapter 15, pp. 383–401, Earthquake Engineering, Eds. Robert L. Wiegel, Prentice-Hall, Inc., Englewood-Cliffs, N.J.

Seed, H.B., 1973. Stability of earth and rockfill dams during earthquakes, Embankment Dam Engineering Casagrande Volume, Ed. by R.C. Hirschfeld, and S.J. Poulos, Wiley, New York; 239–269.

Seed, H.B., 1979. Considerations in the earthquake-resistant design of earth and rockfill dams, Nineteenth Rankine Lecture, Geotechnique, 29(3); 13–41.

Seed, H.B., Lee, K.L. and Idriss, I.M., 1969. Sheffield Dam failure, J. Soil Mech. Found. Div., ASCE, 95, sm6; 1453–1490.

Seed, H.B. and Martin, G.R., 1966. The seismic co-efficient in earth dam design., J. Soil Mech. Found. Div., ASCE, 92, SM3; 25–28.

Seed, H.B. and Sultan, H.A., 1967, Stability Analysis for a sloping core embankment, J. Soil Mech. Found. Div., ASCE, 93, SM4; 69–84.

Seed, R.B. and Harder, L.F., 1990. SPT-based analysis of cyclic pore pressure generation and undrained residual strength, in J.M. Duncan, ed. Proceedings, H. Bolton Seed Memorial Symposium, University of California, Berkeley, Vol. 2, 351–376.

Seed, R.B., Mitchell, J.K. and Seed, H.B., 1990. Kettleman Hills waste landfill slope failure II. stability analysis, ASCE, Journal of Geotechnical Engineering, 116(4); 669–690.

Serafim, J.L., 1964. Rock Mechanics considerations in the design of concrete dams, Proc. Int. Conf. on the state of stress in the earth's crust, Santa Monica, California, Elsevier, New York; 611–645.

Sevaldson, R.A., 1956. The slide in Lodalen, Oct. 69 1954, Geoteelmique, 6: 167–182.

Shahgholi, M., Fakher, A. and Jones, C.J.F.P., 2001. Horizontal slice method of analysis, Geotechnique, 51, No. 10, 881–885.

Sharma, H.D., Nayak, G.C. and Maheshwari, J.B., 1976. Generalisation of nonlinear sequential analysis – A study of rockfill dam with joint elements, Numerical Methods in Engineering, Ed. by C.S. Desai, 2: 662–686.

Sharma, S., 2007. Slope stability assessment using limit equilibrium methods, in Turner A.K. and Schuster R.L. (Editors) Landslides and Socirty, AEG Special Publication No. 22, 1st North American Landslide Conference, Vail Colorado, June, 239–260.

Sherrard, J.L., 1967. Earthquake considerations in earth dam design, J. Soil Mech. Found. Div., ASCE, 93, SM4; 377–401.

Sherrard, J.L., Woodward, R.J., Gizienksi, S.G. and Clevenger, W.A., 1963. Earth and Earth Rock Dams, John Wiley, New York.

Shreve, R.L., 1966. Sherman landslide, Alaska, Science, 154: 1639–1643.

Shreve, R.L., 1968. The Blackhawk landslide, Geol. Soc. Am., Spec. Paper 108, 47 pp.

Silva, F., Lambe, T.W. and Marr, W.A., 2008. Probability and Risk of Slope Failure, Journal of Geotechnical and Geoenvironmental Engineering, Vol. 134, No. 12, 1691–1699.

Singh, A., 1970. Shear strength and stability of man-made slopes, J. Soil Mech. Found. Div., ASCE, 96, SM6; 1879–1892.

Singh, D.N. and Basudhar, P.K., 1993a. A note on vertical cuts in homogeneous soils, Canadian Geotechnical Journal, 30(5); 859–862.

Singh, D.N. and Basudhar, P.K., 1993b. Optimal lower bound bearing capacity of strip footing, Soils and Foundations, 33, No. 4, 18–25.

Sitar, N., Anderson, S.A. and Johnson, K.A., 1992. Conditions for rainfall-induced debris flows, Stability and Performance of Slopes and Embankments II, a 25 year perspective, Geotechnical Special Publication No. 31, Vol. 1, 834–849.

Sitar, N., MacLaughlin, M.M. and Doolin, D.M., 2005. Influence of kinematics on landslide mobility and failure mode, Journal of Geotechnical and Geoenvironmental Engineering, Vol. 131, No. 6, 716–728.

Skempton, A.W., 1948. The rate of softening of stiff-fissured clays with special reference to London clay, Proe. 2nd Int. Conf. Soil Mech. Found. Eng., 2: 50–53.

Skempton, A.W., 1954. The pore pressure co-efficients A and B, Geotechnique, 4: 143–147.

Skempton, A.W., 1957. The planning and design of the new Hong Kong Airport.-Discussion, Proc. Inst. of Civil Engineers(London), Vol. 7, 305–307.

Skempton, A.W., 1960. Effective stress in soils, concrete and rock, Conf. on Pore Pressures and Suction in Soils, Butterworths, London, 4.

Skempton, A.W., 1961. Horizontal stresses in an overconsolidated Eocene clay, Proc. 5th Int. Conf. Soil Mech. Found. Eng., Paris, 1: 351–358.

Skempton, A.W., 1964. Long-term stability of clay slopes, Rankine Lecture, Geotechnique, 14: 77–101.

Skempton, A.W., 1966a. Some observations on tectonic shear zones, Proc. lst Int. Cong. Rock Mech., Lisbon, 1: 329–335.

Skempton, A.W., 1966b. Bedding plane slip, residual shear strength and the Vajont slide, Geotechnique, 16: 82–84.

Skempton, A.W., 1970. First-time slides in overconsolidated clays, Geotechnique, 20: 320–324.

Skempton, A.W., 1977. Slope stability of cuttings in brown London clay, Special Lectures Volume, 9th Int. Conf. Soil Mech. Found. Eng., Tokyo, 25–33.

Skempton, A.W. and Brown, J.D., 1961. A landslip in boulder clay at Selset in Yorkshire, Geotechnique, 11: 280–293.

Skempton, A.W. and Hutchinson, J.N., 1969. Stability of Natural Slopes and Embankment Foundations, Proc. 7th Int. Conf. Soil Mechanics & Foundation Engineering, Mexico City, State-of-the Art Volume, 291–340.

Skempton, A.W. and La Rochelle, P., 1965. The Bradwell slip, a short-term failure in London clay, Geotechnique, 15: 221–242.

Skempton, A.W. and Petley, D.J., 1968. The strength along discontinuities in stiff clay, Proc. Geotech. Conf. on Shear Strength Properties of Natural Soils and Rocks, Oslo, 2: 29–46.

Skempton, A.W. and Vaughan, P.R., 1993. Failure of Carsington dam,Geotechnique, 43, No. 1, 151–173. Discussion in Vol. 45, No. 4, 719–739.

Smith, C.K. and Redlinger, I.F., 1953. Soil properties of Fort Union clay shale, Proc. 3rd Int. Conf. Soil Mech. Found. Eng., 1: 62–66.

Smith, I.M., 1970. Incremental numerical analysis of a simple deformation problem in soil mechanics, Geotechnique, 20(4); 357–372.

Smith, I.M., 1973. Discussion of paper 'some applications of plasticity theory to stability problems in soil mechanics', Proc. Symp. on Plasticity and Soil Mechanics, Ed. A.C. Palmer, Cambridge Univ. Eng. Dept., England.

Smith, I.M. and Kay, S., 1971. Stress analysis of contractive or dilative soil, J. Soil Mech. Found. Div., ASCE, 97, SM7; 981–997.

Sokolovski, V.V., 1960. Statics of Grannlar Media, English translation, Butterworths, London.

Sokolovski, V.V., 1965. Statics of Granular Media, Revised edition, English translation, Pergamon Press, England, 270 pp.

Sowers, G.B. and Sowers, G.F., 1970. Introductory Soil Mechanics and Foundations, 3rd Edition, Collier Macmillan, New York, 556 pp.

Spencer, E., 1967. A method of analysis for stability of embankments using parallel inter-slice forces, Geotechnique, 17: 11–26.

Spencer, E., 1968. Effect of tension on stability of embankments, J. Soil Mech. Found. Div., ASCE, 94, SM5; 1159–1173.

Spencer, E., 1973. The thrust line criterion in embankment stability analysis, Geotechnique, 23: 85–101.

Starr, M.R., 1968. Discussion on paper 'use of computers for slope stability analysis', J. Soil Mech. Found. Div., ASCE, 94, SM3; 784–789.

Stead, D. 1984. An evaluation of the factors governing the stability of surface coal mine slopes, Ph.D. Thesis, University of Nottingham, United Kingdom.

Sultan, H.A. and Seed, H.B., 1967. Stability of sloping core earth dams, J. Soil Mech. Found. Div., ASCE, 93, SM4; 45–68.

Tabesh, A. and Chowdhury, R., 1997. Seismic response of natural slopes, Proc. 8th International Conference on Soil Dynamics and Earthquake Engineering, SDEE '97, Istanbul, Turkey, 1997, 236–238.

Tang, W.H., Chowdhury, R. and Sidi, I., 1985. Progressive Failure Probability of Soil Slopes, ICOSSAR'85, 4th Int. conf on Structural Safety and Reliability, Vol. III, III 363–III 372.

Tang, W.H., Yuceman, M.S. and Ang, A.H-S., 1976. Probability Based Short-Term Design of Soil Slopes, Canadian Geotechnical Journal, Vol. 13, 201–215.

Taylor, D.W., 1937. Stability of earth slopes, J. Boston Soc. Civil Engt. 24, 197.

Taylor, D.W., 1948. Fundamentals of Soil Mechanics, Wiley, New York, 700 pp.

Terzaghi, K., 1925. Principles of soil mechanics, Eng. News Record, 95, 20, 796.

Terzaghi, K., 1936. Stability of slopes of natural clay, Proc. lst Int. Conf. Soil Mech. Found. Eng., Harvard, 1: 161–165.

Terzaghi, K., 1943. Theoretical Soil Mechanics, John Wiley, 510 pp.

Terzaghi, K., 1945. Stress conditions for the failure of concrete and rock, Proc. ASTM, 45, 777.

Terzaghi, K., 1950. "Mechanisms of landslides". Application of Geology to Engineering Practice, Berkey Volume, Geological Society of America, 83–123. Reprinted in "From Theory to Practice in Soil Mechanics", New York, John Wiley and sons, 1960, 202–245.

Terzaghi, K., 1960. From Theory to Practice in Soil Mechanics, Ed. by L. Bjerrum et al., John Wiley, New York.

Terzaghi, K., 1962. Stability of steep slopes in hard unweathered rock, Geotechnique, 12: 251–270.

Terzaghi, K. and Peck, R.B., 1967. Soil Mechanics in Engineering Practice, Wiley, New York, 729 pp.

Terzaghi, K., Peck, R.B. and Mesri, G., 1996. Soil Mechanics in Engineering Practice, Third Edition, John Wiley & Sons Inc., New York, 549 pp.

Thrush, P.W., 1969. A dictionary of mining, mineral and related terms, U.S. Bureau of mines, Spec. Publ., 1269 pp.

Tika, T.E., Vaughan, P.R. and Lemos, L.J., 1996. Fast shearing of pre-existing shear zones in soil, Geotechnique, 46, No. 2, 197–233.

Trenter, A. and Warren, C.D., 1996. Further investigations at the Folkestone Warren Landslide, Geotechnique, 46, No. 4, 589–620 (see also discussion with authors' reply, published in Geotechnique, 2001, 51, No. 2, 189–192).

Turner, A.K. and Schuster, R.L., eds, 1996. Landslides: Investigation and Mitigation, Transportation Research Board, Special Report 247, National Research Council, National Academy Press, Washington DC, 673 pp.

Turnbull, W.J. and Hvorslov, M.J., 1967. Special problems in slope stability, J. Soil Mech. Found. Eng., ASCE, 93, SM4; 499–528.

Ugai, K. and Leshchinsky, D., 1995. Three-dimensional limit equilibrium and finite element analyses: a comparison of results, Soils and Foundations, 35, No. 4, 1–7.

United States Army Corps of Engineers, 1970. Stability of Earth and Rockfill Dams, EM1110-2-1902.

United States Dept. of Interior, 1977. Failure of Teton Dam, 2 Vols; Report of Independent Panel dated Dec. 1976 and of Internal Review Group dated April, 1977. U.S. Govt. Printing Office, Washington, D.C., U.S.A.

Vanmarcke, E.H., 1977a. Probabilistic modelling of soil profiles, J. Geotech. Eng. Div., ASCE, 103, GTI1; 1227–1246.

Vanmarcke, E.H., 1977b. Reliability of earth slopes, J. Geotech. Eng. Div., 103. GTI1; 1247–1265.

Vanmarcke, E.H., 1983. Random Fields: Analysis and Synthesis, The MIT Press, Cambridge, Massachusetts.

Varnes, D.J., 1958. Landslide types and processes, Landslides and Engineering practice, Ed. by E.B. Eckel, Highway Research Board, Special Report 29, NAS-NRC Publ. 4 and 5; 232 pp.

Varnes, D.J., 1978. "Slope movement types and processes", Chapter 2 in this book, Landslides: Analysis and control (Special Report 176, TRB, National Academy of Sciences, Washington D.C., 234 pp.

Varnes, D.J., 1984. Landslide Hazard Zonation: A Review of Principles and Practice. UNESCO, Paris, 63 pp.

Vaughan, P.R. and Chandler, H.J., 1974. Notes concerning informal discussion on 'The Design of Cuttings in Overconsolidated Clay' at the Institution of Civil Engineers, London, May.

Vaughan, P.R. and Walbancke, H.J., 1973. Pore pressure changes and delayed failure of cutting slopes in overconsolidated clay, Geotechnique, 23: 531–539.

Vesic, A.S. and Clough, G.W., 1968. Behaviour of granular materials under high stresses, J. Soil Mech. Found. Div., ASCE, 94, SM3; 661–688.

Vitatjandr, C. and Michalowski, R.L., 2006. Limit analysis of slope instability caused by partial submergence and rapid drawdown. Canadian Geotechnical Journal, 43, No. 8, 802–814.

Voight, B., 1973. Correlation between Atterberg plasticity limits and residual shear strength of natural soils, Geotechnique, 23: 265–267.

Walbancke, H.J., 1975. Pore pressures in clay embankments and cuttings, Ph.D. Thesis, University of London, England.

Walker, B.F., 2007. Rainfall data analysis at Newport, Australian Geomehanics, 42(1); 1–17.

Wang, Y.J. and Voight, B., 1969. A discrete element stress analysis model for discontinuous materials, Proc. Int. Symp. on large permanent underground openings, Oslo.

Weeks, A.G., 1969. The stability of slopes in S.E. England as affected by periglacial activity, Quart. J. Eng. Geol., 2: 49–63.

Whitman, R.V., 1984. Evaluation of calculated Risk in Geotechnical Engineering, Journal of Geotechnical Engineering, ASCE, Vol. 110, 145–188.

Whitman, R.V. and Bailey, W.A., 1967. Use of computers for slope stability analysis, J. Soil Mech. Found. Div., ASCE, 93, SM4; 475–498.

WHO, 2002. WHO Collaborating Centre for Research on the Epidemiology of Disasters(CRED) 2002 EM-DAT:The OFDA/CRED International Disaster Database. Universite Catholique de Louvain, Brussels, http://www.cred.be/emdat/intro.htm.

Wilkins, J.K., 1970. A theory for the shear strength of rockfill, Rock Mechanics, 2: 205–222.

Wilson, R.C. and Keefer, D.K., 1985. Predicting areal limits of earthquake-induced landsliding, in, Ziony, J.I. (ed.) Evaluating Earthquake Hazards in the Los Angeles Region-An Earth Science Perspective, U S Geological Survey Professional Paper 1360, 316–345, C124.

Wilson, S.D., 1970. Observational data on ground movements related to slope instability, Terzaghi Lecture, J. Geotech. Eng. Div., ASCE, 969 sm6; 1519–1544.

Windle, D. and Wroth, C.P., 1977. In situ measurement of the properties of stiff clays, Proc. 9th Int. Conf. Soil Mech. Found. Eng., 1: 347–353.

Wittke, W., 1965. Verfahren Bereschnung der standsicherheit Belasteter und unberasteter Fels-boschiingen, Rock Mech. Eng. Geol., Supplement 2, 52–79.

Wolfskill, L.A. and Lambe, T.W., 1967. Slide in the Siburua dam, J. Soil Mech. Found. Div., ASCE, 93, SM4; 107–133.

Wright, S.G., 1975. Evaluation of slope stability analysis procedures, Preprint 2616, ASCE, National Convention, Denver (Colorado), 28 pp.

Wright, S.G., Kulhawy, E.D. and Duncan, J.M., 1973. Accuracy of equilibrium slope stability analysis, J. Soil Mech. Found. Div., ASCE, 99, SM10; 783–793.

Wroth, C.P., 1975. State-of-the-art Report, 'In situ measurements of initial stresses and deformation characteristics, Proc. ASCE, Geotechnical Eng. Div. Specialty Conference; 181–277.

Wu, T.H. and Kraft, L.M., 1970. Safety analysis of slopes, J. Soil Mech. Found. Div., ASCE, 96, SM2; 609–630.

Wu, F. and Wang, S., 2001. Strength theory of homogeneous jointed rock mass, Geotechnique, 51, Number 9, 815–818, C19.

Xu, B. and Low, B.K., 2006. Probabilistic Stability Analyses of Embankments Based on Finite-Element Method, Journal of Geotechnical and Geoenvironmental Engineering, ASCE, Vol. 132, No. 11, 1444–1454.

Xu, D.W., 1994. Stability and Reliability Assessments of Earth Structures Ph.D. Thesis, University of Wollongong, Wollongong, New South Wales, Australia.

Yamagami, Jiang, J., and Ueno, K., 2000. A limit equilibrium stability analysis of slopes with stabilising piles, slope stability 2000,Geotechnical Special Publication 101, ASCE, Reston VA, 343–354.

Young, A.R.M., 1976. The Distribution, Characteristics and Stability of Debris-mantled Slopes in Northern Wollongong, Master of Science Thesis, University of Wollongong, Australia.

Yuceman, M.S., Tang, W.H. and AH-S., 1973. A Probabilistic Study of Safety and Design of Earth Slopes, Structural Research Series No. 402, Dept of Civil Engineering, University of Illinois at Urbana, Illinois USA, Vol. III, 204 pp.

Zaruba, Q. and Mencl. V., 1969. Landslides and their control, Elsevier, Amsterdam, 205 pp.

Zhang, S., 1989. Evaluation and Updating of Slope Reliability, Ph.D. Thesis, University of Wollongong, Wollongong, New South Wales, Australia.

Zhang, S. and Chowdhury, R., 1989. Identification of critical slope failure surfaces with critical tension cracks,in A.W. Khair (editor0 Rock Mechanics as a guide for efficient utilisation of natural resouces, A A Balkema, 185–192.

Zhang, S. and Chowdhury, R., 1995. Inter-slice shear forces in slope stability analysis-a new approach, Soils and Foundations, 35, 1, March, 65–74.

Zienkiewicz, O.C., 1968. Continuum mechanics as an approach to rock mass problems, Rock Mechanics in Engineering Practice, Ed. by K.G. Stagg and O.C. Zienkiewicz, Wiley, New York; 237–270.

Zienkiewicz, O.C., 1971. The finite element method in engineering science, McGraw-Hill, London, 521 pp.

Zienkiewicz, O.C. and Cheung, Y.K., 1967. The finite element method in structural and continuum mechanics, McGraw-Hill, London.

Zienkiewicz, O.C., Humpheson, C. and Lewis, R.W., 1975. Associated and non-associated viscoplasticity and plasticity in soil mechanics, Geotechnique, 25: 671–691.

Zienkiewicz, O.C., Valliapan, S. and King, I.P., 1968. Stress analysis of rock as a 'no-tension' material, Geotechnique, 18(1); 56–66.

Permissions

1 Figures 1.2 & 1.3, (Skempton and Hutchinson, 1969), Mexican Society of Soil Mechanics (affiliated to ISSMGE)
2 Figure 1.4, (Cooke and Doornkamp, 1974), Oxford University Press, U.K.
3 Table 1.1, (Deere and Patton, 1971), Vice President for North America, ISSMGE
4 Tables 1.4, 5.7 & 7.1, (Lambe and Whitman, 1969), John Wiley and sons, USA
5 Table 1.5, (Deere, 1963), Springer, Germany
6 Tables 1.6 & 1.8, (Hoek and Bray, 1974), Maney Publishing, U.K.
7 Table 1.7, (Hoek, 1970), Maney Publishing, U.K.
8 Figure 2.3, (Lo, 1970), Thomas Telford, U.K.
9 Figures 2.9, 2.10 & 2.11, (Bishop and Bjerrum, 1960), American Society of Civil Engineers (ASCE)
10 Table 2.1, (Bjerrum, 1967), American Society of Civil Engineers (ASCE)
11 Table C3III.1, (Ang and Tang, 1975), John Wiley and Sons, USA
12 Tables E4.2 & E4.3, (Jaeger, 1971), Thomas Telford, U.K.
13 Figures 4.12 & 4.13, (Henkel, 1967), American Society of Civil Engineers (ASCE)
14 (Table 5.1 a & b, Table E5.1 a & b), and (Figures 5.1 a & b, E5.1, E5.2, E5.3 & E5.4), (Zhang, 1989), Dr Shu Zhang
15 Table 5.2, (Whitman and Bailey, 1967), American Society of Civil Engineers (ASCE)
16 Figure E5.4, (Richards, 1982), Institution of Engineers , Australia
17 Figure E5.7, (Chowdhury, 1980), Southeast Asian Geotechnical Society (affliated to ISSMGE)
18 Table 5.8, (Lo and Lee, 1973), Thomas Telford, U.K.
19 Figure 5.12, (Revilla and Castillo, 1977), Thomas Telford, U.K.
20 Table 6.1, (Chowdhury, 1970b), American Society of Civil Engineers (ASCE)
21 Tables 6.1 & 6.2, (Duncan and Dunlop, 1969), American Society of Civil Engineers (ASCE)
22 Table 6.3, (Brown and King, 1966), Thomas Telford, U.K.
23 Table 6.4, (Wright et al., 1973), American Society of Civil Engineers (ASCE)
24 Figure 6.11, (Lo and Lee, 1973), Thomas Telford, U.K.
25 Table 7.5, (Jaeger, 1972), Cambridge University Press, U.K.
26 Figure 7.12, (Romani et al., 1972), American Society of Civil Engineers (ASCE)
27 Figure 7.15, Tables 7.6 & 7.7, (Chowdhury, 1978), Springer, Germany

The full details of references cited in this Permissions list can be found in the full Reference list (p. 683).

28 Figure 9.2, (Seed, 1967), American Society of Civil Engineers (ASCE)

29 Table 9.3, (Seed, 1968), American Society of Civil Engineers (ASCE)

30 Figures 9.8, 9.9, 9.10, 9.13, 9.14 & 9.15 and Tables 9.1, 9.2, 9.4 & 9.8, (Seed 1979), Thomas Telford, U.K.

31 Figure 9.16, (Jibson et al., 2000), first published in Jibson et al. (1998), USGS-United States Geological Survey, Denver Federal Center

32 Figures 10.8, 10.9 & 10.10, (Chowdhury et al., 1987), Thomas Telford, U.K.

33 Figures 10.11 & 10.12, (Chowdhury, 1992), NRC Research Press (National Research Council of Canada)

34 Figures 10.13 & 10.14, (Vanmarcke, 1977b), American Society of Civil Engineers (ASCE)

35 Tables C10.1 & C10.2, (Duncan, 2000 and Duncan, 2001), American Society of Civil Engineers (ASCE)

36 Table C10.3, (Chowdhury and Flentje, 2003), Springer, Germany

Appendix I

37 Tables I.1, I.2 & I.3, (Deere and Patton, 1971), Vice President for North America, ISSMGE

Appendix II

38 Figures II.5–II.18 were reproduced in Slope Analysis (1978), These stability charts were kindly made available by Mr. B.F. Cousins (since deceased), Cousins (1977)

39 Figures II.20 & II.21, (Hoek and Bray, 1977), Maney Publishing, U.K.

40 Figures II.19, II.20 & II.21, (Hoek, 1970), Maney Publishing, U.K.

Appendix III

41 With kind permission from Dr. James V. Hamel, this Appendix, based mainly on the following Report, was first published in Slope Analysis (1978)
Hamel, J.V., 1968, Morgenstern and Price Method of Slope Stability Analysis, Report by Dept. of Civil Eng., Univ. of Pittsburgh to U.S. Bureau of Mines, 149p.

Requests pending

Permissions requested but not received by time of printing

42 Tables 8.2 & C8.1, Chen, W.F., 1975. Limit Analysis and Soil Plasticity, Elsevier, NL

43 Figure 5.13, Skempton, A.W., 1977. Slope stability of cuttings in Brown London clay, Special lectures Volume, 9th Int. Conf. Soil Mechanics and Foundation Engineering, Tokyo, published by Japanese Society of Soil Mechanics

44 Figures 1.6, 1.7, 5.7, 5.10 & AII.4, and Tables 1.2 & 1.3, (Terzaghi and Peck, 1967), John Wiley, USA

45 Figures 1.1 & 1.5, (Blyth and de Freitas, 1974), Edwin Arnold

46 Figure 9.4, (Seed and Harder, 1990), University of California at Berkeley, California, USA

Subject index

Colour plates

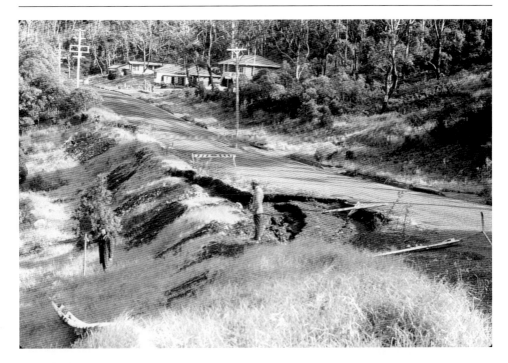

Figure C1.1 Slide in coalwash fill and colluvium along Alanson Avenue [photo by Ann Young 1974 (Young, 1976)].

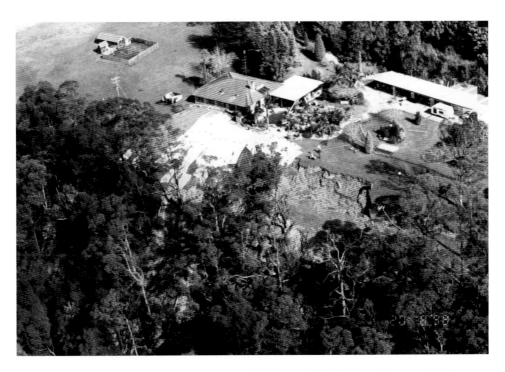

Figure C1.2 Complex slide-flow near Mount Kembla, August 1998. Coloured sheets of plastic cover parts of the slide close to the house (photo, courtesy of NSW Police and Wollongong Geotechnical Team).

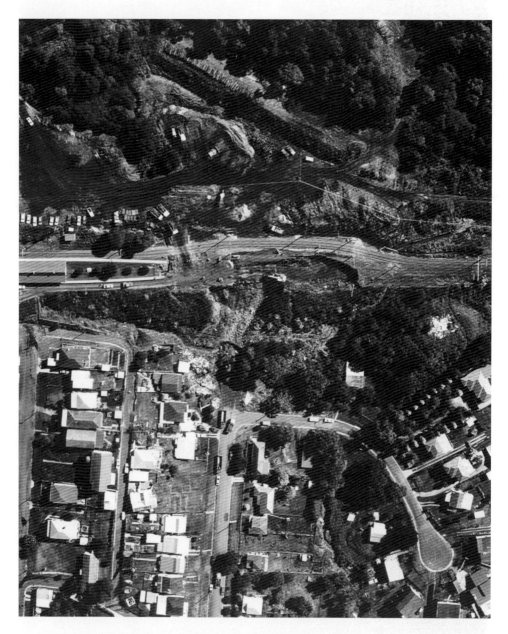

Figure C1.3 Vertical aerial photograph of the Coledale Landslide (slide-flow) which occurred on the 30th April, 1988. This landslide destroyed a house and caused two fatalities. Photo, courtesy of the New South Wales Railway Services Authority.

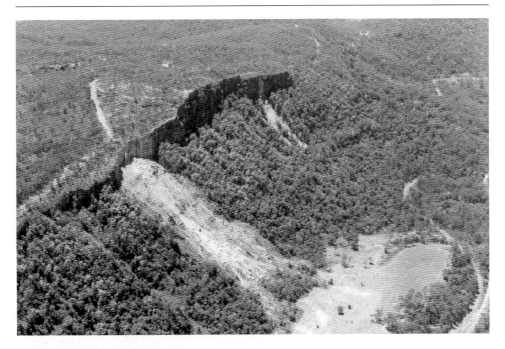

Figure C1.4 Oblique aerial photograph of a rockfall at Dombarton (Photo by Ann Young 1974).

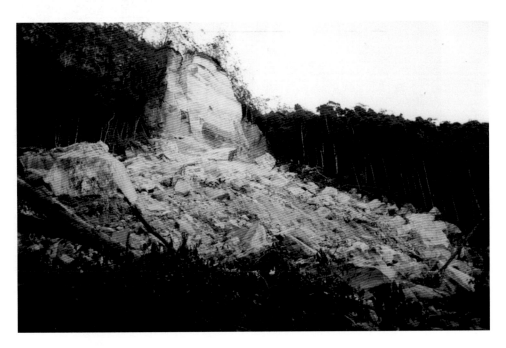

Figure C1.5 The Mount Barrengarry rockfall occurred in the early morning of the 29th of June, 1997, during heavy rainfall in the Kangaroo Valley southwest of Wollongong. The rock fall involved approximately 6000 m³ of Hawkesbury Sandstone bedrock. The ensuing debris flow also involved approximately 15000 m³ of additional colluvium on the slopes below (underlain by Kangaloon Sandstone). The debris flow completely destroyed up to 2Ha of dense forest. The toe of the flow stopped several metres upslope of the Fitzroy Falls to Kangaroo Valley Road.

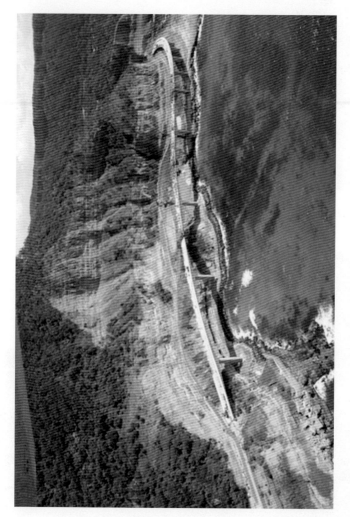

Figure C1.6 A section of the coastal road, Lawrence Hargrave Drive, between Coalcliff and Clifton affected by falls, slides and flows. Over a 1 km section the road was bypassed by a bridge (later named the Sea Cliff Bridge), shown here under construction during 2005.

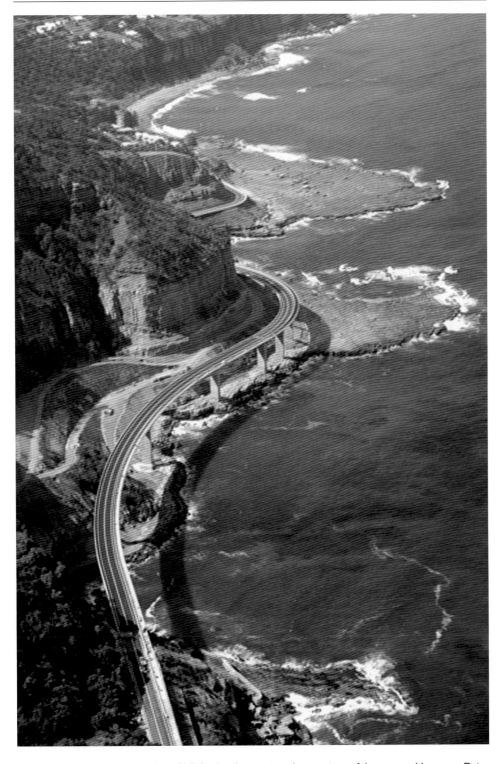

Figure C1.7 The completed Sea Cliff Bridge by-passing the section of Lawrence Hargrave Drive affected by landslides. The cover of this book shows a view of the area taken prior to the bridge construction.

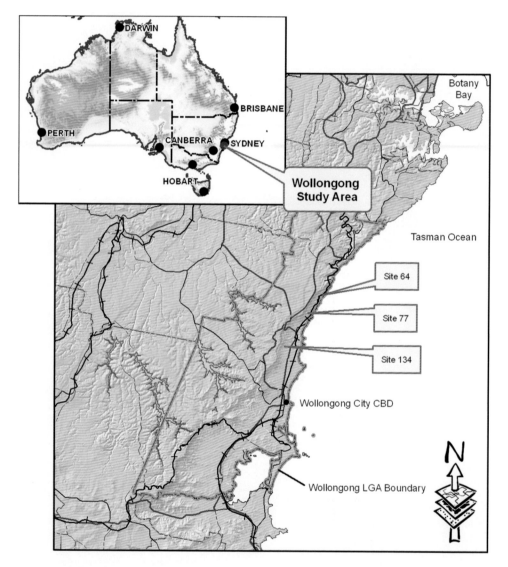

Figure 11.1 Location plan showing location of Wollongong, the Escarpment and the location of three landslides discussed herein.

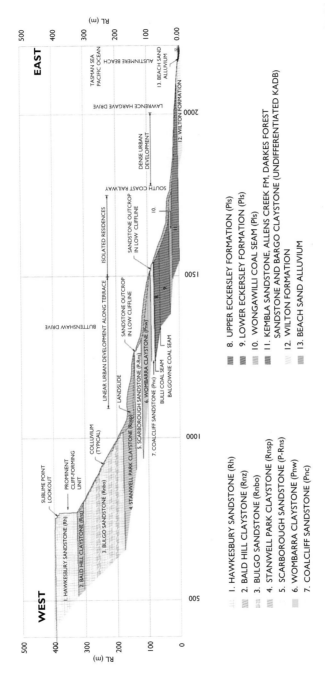

Figure 11.2 Representative Escarpment Cross-Section in the northern suburbs region of Wollongong. (P. Flentje in association with GHD)

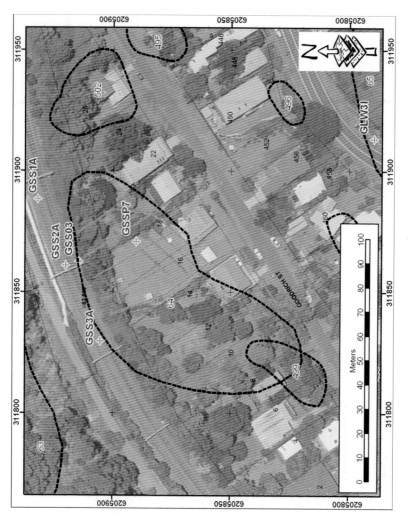

Figure 11.4 Plan highlighting the Site 64 landslide and showing extent of subsurface slot drains (marked in light blue lines).

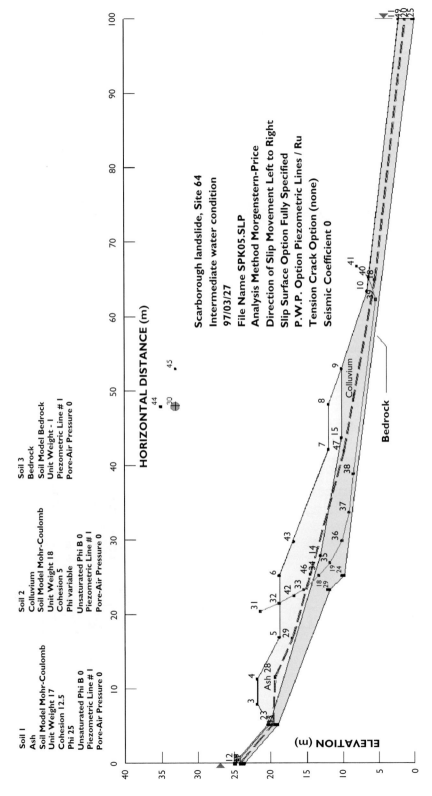

Figure 11.6 SLOPE/W model used for the stability assessment of Site 64, RSA Project 1569 at Scarborough, chainage 63.650 km.

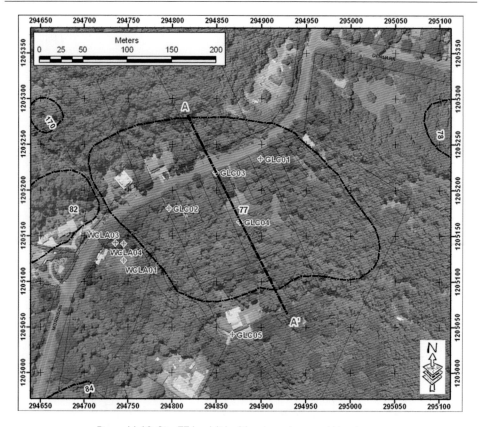

Figure 11.10 Site 77 landslide: Morrison Avenue, Wombarra.

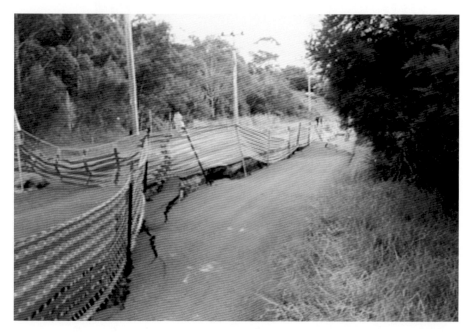

Figure 11.11 Damage to the pavement of Morrison Avenue within the Site 77. The rear main head-scarp of this landslide is approximately 40 m to the left and upslope of the road pavement.

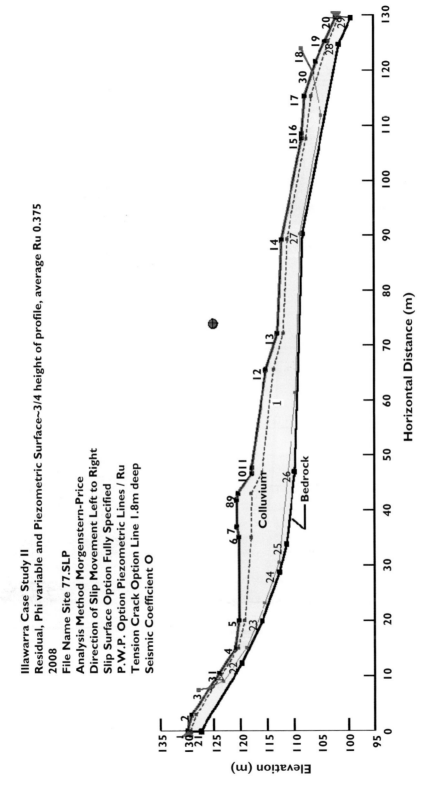

Figure 11.12 SLOPE/W model used for the stability assessment of Site 77, the Morrison Avenue landslide.

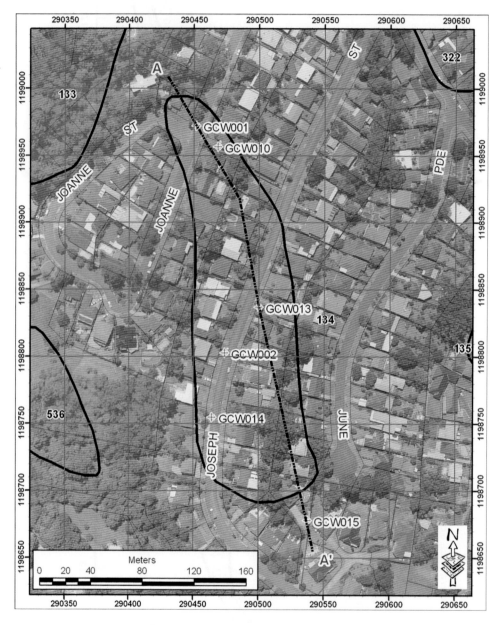

Figure 11.16 Plan of the Site 134 landslide.

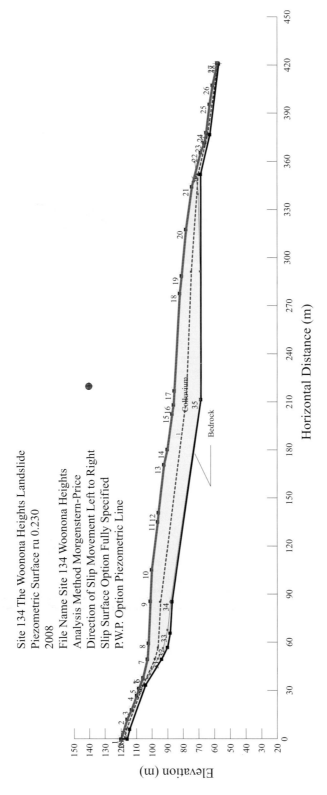

Site 134 The Woonona Heights Landslide
Piezometric Surface ru 0.230
2008
File Name Site 134 Woonona Heights
Analysis Method Morgenstern-Price
Direction of Slip Movement Left to Right
Slip Surface Option Fully Specified
P.W.P. Option Piezometric Line

Figure 11.17 SLOPE/W model used for the stability assessment of Site 134, the Woonona Heights landslide.

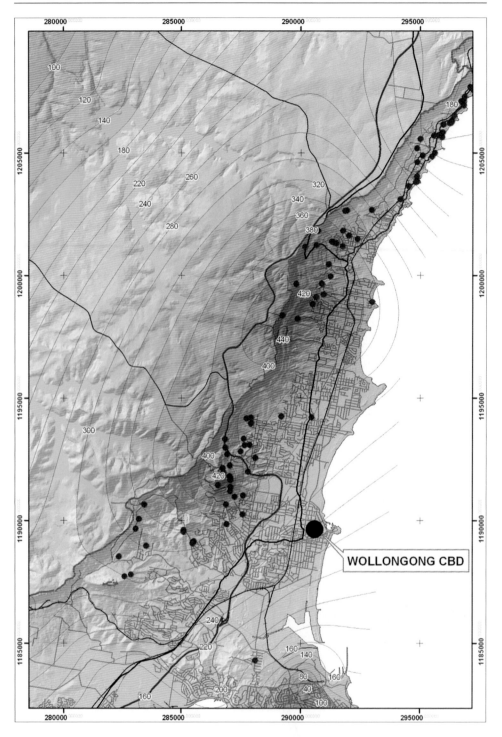

Figure 11.21 GIS based 24 hr rainfall distribution to 9am on the 18th August 1998 (contours marked in mm rain) with observed landslides shown as dots.

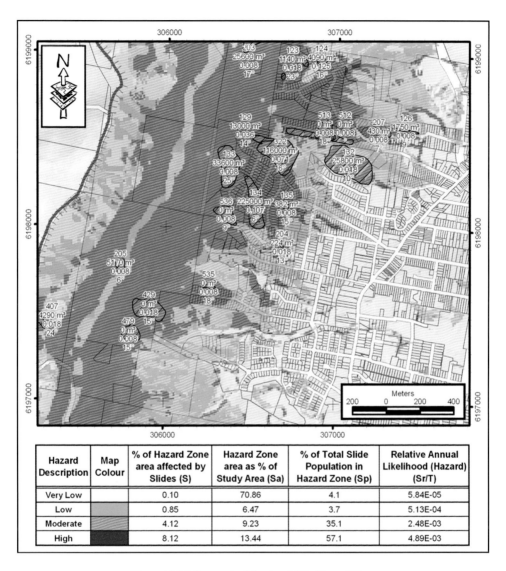

Hazard Description	Map Colour	% of Hazard Zone area affected by Slides (S)	Hazard Zone area as % of Study Area (Sa)	% of Total Slide Population in Hazard Zone (Sp)	Relative Annual Likelihood (Hazard) (Sr/T)
Very Low		0.10	70.86	4.1	5.84E-05
Low		0.85	6.47	3.7	5.13E-04
Moderate		4.12	9.23	35.1	2.48E-03
High		8.12	13.44	57.1	4.89E-03

Figure 11.24 Segment of the Landslide Hazard Map.

Date Due